Y0-CSQ-451

Controversy in Internal Medicine
II

Edited by

FRANZ J. INGELFINGER, M.D.
EDITOR, THE NEW ENGLAND JOURNAL OF MEDICINE

RICHARD V. EBERT, M.D.
PROFESSOR AND CHAIRMAN OF THE DEPARTMENT OF MEDICINE,
UNIVERSITY OF MINNESOTA MEDICAL SCHOOL

MAXWELL FINLAND, M.D.
GEORGE RICHARDS MINOT PROFESSOR OF MEDICINE, EMERITUS,
HARVARD MEDICAL SCHOOL

ARNOLD S. RELMAN, M.D.
FRANK WISTER THOMAS PROFESSOR OF MEDICINE
AND CHAIRMAN OF THE DEPARTMENT OF MEDICINE,
UNIVERSITY OF PENNSYLVANIA SCHOOL OF MEDICINE

W. B. SAUNDERS COMPANY · Philadelphia · London · Toronto   1974

W. B. Saunders Company: West Washington Square
Philadelphia, PA 19105

12 Dyott Street
London, WC1A 1DB

833 Oxford Street
Toronto 18, Ontario

Controversy in Internal Medicine—II   ISBN 0-7216-5026-0

© 1974 by W. B. Saunders Company. Copyright under the International Copyright Union. All rights reserved. This book is protected by copyright. No part of it may be reproduced, stored in a retrieval system, or transmitted in any form or by any means, electronic, mechanical, photocopying, recording, or otherwise, without written permission from the publisher. Made in the United States of America. Press of W. B. Saunders Company. Library of Congress catalog card number 73-76267.

Print No.   9   8   7   6   5   4   3   2   1

Contributors

ABRAM S. BENENSON, M.D., Professor and Chairman, Department of Community Medicine, University of Kentucky Medical Center, Lexington, Kentucky.

ROBERT L. BERGER, M.D., Professor of Surgery, Boston University, School of Medicine; Director, Cardiothoracic Surgery, University and Boston City Hospitals, Boston, Massachusetts.

JOSEPH R. BERTINO, M.D., Professor of Medicine and Pharmacology, Yale University School of Medicine, New Haven, Connecticut.

DOUGLAS A. K. BLACK, M.D., F.R.C.P., Professor of Medicine, University of Manchester; Physician, Manchester Royal Infirmary, Manchester, England.

PAUL H. BLACK, M.D., Associate Professor of Medicine, Harvard Medical School; Associate Physician, Massachusetts General Hospital, Boston, Massachusetts.

HENRY BLACKBURN, M.D., Professor of Physiological Hygiene, School of Public Health; Professor of Medicine, School of Medicine, University of Minnesota; Director, Laboratory of Physiological Hygiene, University of Minnesota, Minneapolis, Minnesota.

JEROME B. BLOCK, M.D., Clinical Associate Professor, Department of Medicine, Georgetown University Medical Center, Washington, D. C.; Associate Director, The Clinical Center, National Institutes of Health, Bethesda, Maryland.

PHILIP K. BONDY, M.D., Visiting Professor of Medicine, Institute of Cancer Research, London, England; C.N.H. Long Professor of Medicine, Yale University School of Medicine; Honorary Consultant, Royal Marsden Hospital, London; Attending Physician, Yale New Haven Hospital, New Haven, Connecticut.

ROBERT F. BRADLEY, M.D., F.A.C.P., Medical Director, Joslin Clinic, Boston; Associate Clinical Professor of Medicine, Harvard Medical School; Physician, New England Deaconess Hospital; Consultant in Medicine, Boston Hospital for Women;

CONTRIBUTORS

Senior Associate in Medicine, Peter Bent Brigham Hospital, Boston, Massachusetts.

BRYAN N. BROOKE, M.D., M. Chir., F.R.C.S., Professor of Surgery, University of London; Surgeon, St. George's Hospital Medical School, St. George's Hospital, London, England.

ROBERT A. BRUCE, M.D., Professor of Medicine, Co-Director, Division of Cardiology, University of Washington; Cardiologist, University Hospital, Seattle, Washington.

HENRY BUCHWALD, M.D., Ph.D., Associate Professor of Surgery, University of Minnesota School of Medicine; Attending Surgeon, University of Minnesota Hospitals, Minneapolis, Minnesota.

JOHN PHILIP BUNKER, M.D., Professor of Anesthesia, Stanford University School of Medicine; Department of Anesthesia, Stanford University Medical Center, Stanford, California.

THOMAS C. CHALMERS, M.D., Professor of Medicine, George Washington University School of Medicine, Washington, D.C.; Director, The Clinical Center, National Institutes of Health, Bethesda, Maryland.

REX S. CLEMENTS, Jr., M.D., Associate Professor of Medicine, University of Alabama School of Medicine; Division of Endocrinology and Metabolism, University of Alabama Hospitals, Birmingham, Alabama.

MORRIS F. COLLEN, B.E.E., M.D., Director, Medical Methods Research, Kaiser Foundation Research Institute and Permanente Medical Group, Oakland California.

JEFFREY J. COLLINS, Ph.D., Department of Microbiology and Molecular Genetics, Harvard Medical School, Boston, Massachusetts.

ROBERT WOLF COLMAN, M.D., F.A.C.P., Associate Professor of Medicine, Associate Professor of Pathology, University of Pennsylvania School of Medicine; Head, Coagulation Unit of the Division of Hematology, Hospital of the University of Pennsylvania, Philadelphia.

JAMES J. CORRIGAN, Jr., M.D., Associate Professor, Department of Pediatrics, University of Arizona Medical Center; Consultant, Tucson Medical Center and St. Joseph's Hospital, Tucson, Arizona.

WILLIAM H. CROSBY, M.D., Adjunct Professor of Medicine, University of California School of Medicine, San Diego; Director, L. C. Jacobson Blood Center, Scripps Clinic and Research Foundation, La Jolla California.

LESLIE J. DeGROOT, M.D., Professor of Medicine, University of Chicago, Pritzker School of Medicine; Endocrinologist and

CONTRIBUTORS

Thyroid Specialist, Billings Hospital, University of Chicago, Chicago, Illinois.

FRANK J. DIXON, M.D., Chairman, Department of Experimental Pathology, Scripps Clinic and Research Foundation, La Jolla, California.

WILLIAM DOCK, M.D., Emeritus Professor of Medicine, State University of New York, Downstate Medical Center, Brooklyn; Consultant, Veterans Administration Hospital, New York, New York.

RICHARD V. EBERT, M.D., Professor and Chairman, Department of Medicine, University of Minnesota Hospitals, University of Minnesota Medical School, Minneapolis, Minnesota.

PHYLLIS Q. EDWARDS, M.D., M.P.H., Chief, Tuberculosis Branch, Center for Disease Control, Atlanta, Georgia.

FRANKLIN H. EPSTEIN, M.D., Professor of Medicine, Harvard Medical School; Director, Harvard Medical Unit and Thorndike Memorial Laboratory, Boston City Hospital, Boston, Massachusetts.

MAXWELL FINLAND, M.D., George Richards Minot Professor of Medicine, Emeritus, Harvard University Medical School; Distinguished Physician, U.S. Veterans Administration.

DONALD S. FREDRICKSON, M.D., Director, Division of Intramural Research, National Heart and Lung Institute, National Institutes of Health, Bethesda, Maryland.

SAMUEL O. FREEDMAN, M.D., Professor of Medicine, McGill University, Montreal; Director, Division of Clinical Immunology and Allergy, Montreal General Hospital, Montreal, Canada.

FRANK GLENN, M.D., Professor of Surgery Emeritus, Cornell University Medical College; Consultant in Surgery, New York Hospital, New York, New York.

DONALD J. GLOTZER, M.D., Associate Professor of Surgery, Harvard Medical School; Surgeon, Beth Israel Hospital, Boston, Massachusetts.

PHIL GOLD, M.D., Ph.D., Professor of Medicine, McGill University, Montreal; Associate Physician, Montreal General Hospital, Montreal, Canada.

MONTE A. GREER, M.D., Professor of Medicine, University of Oregon Medical School, Portland, Oregon.

LAURAN D. HARRIS, M.D., Associate Professor of Medicine, Boston University School of Medicine; Attending Physician, University and Boston City Hospitals, Boston, Massachusetts.

CONTRIBUTORS

NORMAN G. G. HEPPER, M.D., M.S. (Medicine) Associate Professor of Clinical Internal Medicine, Mayo Graduate School of Medicine, University of Minnesota, Minneapolis; Consultant, Division of Thoracic Diseases and Internal Medicine, Mayo Clinic and Mayo Foundation, Rochester, Minnesota.

JAMES F. HOLLAND, M.D., Professor and Chairman, Department of Neoplastic Diseases, Mount Sinai School of Medicine of City University of New York;; Director, Cancer Center, Mount Sinai School of Medicine and Hospital, New York, New York.

JOHN HORTON, M.B., Ch.B., F.A.C.P., Associate Professor of Medicine, Albany Medical College of Union University, Albany; Head, Division of Oncology, Albany Medical Center Hospital, Albany, New York.

FRANZ J. INGELFINGER, M.D., Clinical Professor of Medicine, Boston University School of Medicine, Boston; Editor, New England Journal of Medicine.

HAROLD L. ISRAEL, M.D., Professor of Medicine, Jefferson Medical College, Thomas Jefferson University, Philadelphia, Pennsylvania.

WILLIAM McKENDREE JEFFERIES, M.D., Assistant Clinical Professor of Medicine, Case-Western Reserve University School of Medicine; Endocrinologist, Euclid Clinic Foundation; Consultant in Endocrinology, University Hospitals of Cleveland, Euclid General Hospital, Highland View Hospital, Lutheran Medical Center, and St. Vincent's Charity Hospital, Cleveland, Ohio.

JOSEPH B. KIRSNER, M.D., Ph.D., Louis Block Professor of Medicine, and Deputy Dean for Medical Affairs, University of Chicago, Pritzker School of Medicine; Attending Physician, A.M. Billings Hospital University of Chicago, Chicago, Illinois.

MICHAEL J. S. LANGMAN, M.D., F.R.C.P., Professor of Therapeutics, University of Nottingham Medical School; Honorary Consultant Physician, Nottingham City and General Hospitals, Nottingham, England.

ALEXANDER D. LANGMUIR, M.D., Visiting Professor of Epidemiology, Harvard Medical School, Boston, Massachusetts.

LOUIS LASAGNA, M.D., Professor of Pharmacology and Toxicology, University of Rochester School of Medicine and Dentistry, Rochester, New York.

PAUL D. LEBER, M.D., Assistant Professor of Pathology, Harvard Medical School; Assistant Pathologist, Children's Hospital Medical Center, Boston, Massachusetts.

HERBERT LEONARD LEY, Jr., M.D., M.P.H., Medical Consultant in Foods and Drugs, Bethesda, Maryland.

CONTRIBUTORS

DONALD B. LOURIA, M.D., Professor and Chairman of Department of Preventive Medicine and Community Health, New Jersey Medical School, Newark, New Jersey.

PETER T. MACKLEM, M.D., C.M., F.R.C.P.(C) Professor, Experimental Medicine, McGill University; Director, Meakins Christie Laboratories, McGill University Clinic, Royal Victoria Hospital, Montreal, Canada.

HAQVIN MALMROS, M.D., Professor of Internal Medicine, Emeritus, University of Lund; Research Department, University Hospital, Lund, Sweden.

NINAN G. MATHEW, M.D., Assistant Professor, Baylor College of Medicine, Houston; Staff Neurologist, Methodist and Ben Taub General Hospitals, Houston, Texas.

ROBERT L. MAYOCK, M.D., Professor of Medicine, University of Pennsylvania School of Medicine; Physician, Pulmonary Disease Section, Hospital of the University of Pennsylvania, Philadelphia, Pennsylvania.

ROBERT T. McCLUSKEY, M.D., S. Burt Wolbach Professor of Pathology, Harvard Medical School; Pathologist-in-Chief, Children's Hospital Medical Center, Boston, Massachusetts.

THOMAS McKEOWN, M.D., Ph.D., D. Phil., Professor of Social Medicine, University of Birmingham, Birmingham, Alabama.

JOHN P. MERRILL, M.D., D.Sc. (Hon.), Professor of Medicine, Harvard Medical School; Director, Cardiorenal Section, Peter Bent Brigham Hospital; Consultant, Children's Hospital Medical Center, Boston, Massachusetts.

JOHN STIRLING MEYER, M.D., Professor and Chairman, Department of Neurology, Baylor College of Medicine, Houston; Chief of Neurology, Methodist, Ben Taub General, and Houston V.A. Hospitals, Houston, Texas.

R. DREW MILLER, M.D., M.S. (Medicine), Professor of Internal Medicine and Associate Director, Mayo Graduate School of Medicine, University of Minnesota; Consultant, Division of Thoracic Diseases and Internal Medicine, Mayo Clinic and Mayo Foundation, Rochester, Minnesota.

CLARK HAROLD MILLIKAN, M.D., Professor of Neurology, Mayo School of Medicine; Senior Consultant in Neurology, Mayo Clinic; Director, Mayo Cerebrovascular Clinical Research Center, Rochester, Minnesota.

JOHN D. MINNA, M.D., Chief, Section on Somatic Cell Genetics, Laboratory of Biochemical Genetics, National Heart and Lung Institute, National Institutes of Health, Bethesda, Maryland.

CONTRIBUTORS

ROBERT S. MORISON, M.D., Richard J. Schwartz Professor of Science and Society, Cornell University, Ithaca, New York.

ANTHONY D. MORRISON, M.D., Assistant Professor of Medicine, University of Pennsylvania School of Medicine; George S. Cox Medical Research Institute, Department of Medicine, Hospital of the University of Pennsylvania, Philadelphia, Pennsylvania.

EDMUND D. PELLEGRINO, M.D., Professor of Medicine, Health Sciences Center, State University of New York, Stony Brook; Vice-President, Health Sciences, SUNY Stony Brook; Consultant in Internal Medicine, Nassau County Medical Center, East Meadows, Veterans Administration Hospital, Northport, New York.

RICHARD COLESTOCK PILLARD, M.D., Associate Professor of Psychiatry, Boston University School of Medicine; Head, Basic Studies Unit, Psychopharmacology Laboratory; Associate Director, Research Training Program, Boston, Massachusetts.

ARNOLD S. RELMAN, M.D., Frank Wister Thomas Professor of Medicine and Chairman, Department of Medicine, University of Pennsylvania School of Medicine; Chief of Medical Services, Hospital of the University of Pennsylvania, Philadelphia, Pennsylvania.

STANLEY J. ROBBOY, M.D., Assistant Professor of Pathology, Harvard Medical School; Assistant Pathologist, Massachusetts General Hospital, Boston, Massachusetts.

SOL ROY ROSENTHAL, M.D., Ph.D., Professor, Preventive Medicine, University of Illinois Abraham Lincoln School of Medicine; Medical Director, Research Foundation, Chicago, Illinois.

RICHARD S. ROSS, M.D., Professor of Medicine, The Johns Hopkins University School of Medicine; Physician, The Johns Hopkins Hospital, Baltimore, Maryland.

DAVID C. SABISTON, Jr., M.D., James B. Duke Professor and Chairman of the Department of Surgery, Duke University Medical Center, Durham, North Carolina.

RICHARD D. SAUTTER, M.D., Thoracic and Cardiovascular Surgeon, Marshfield Clinic, Marshfield Clinic Foundation for Medical Research and Education, Marshfield, Wisconsin.

FENTON SCHAFFNER, M.D., George Baehr Professor and Acting Chairman, Department of Medicine, Mount Sinai School of Medicine of City University of New York; Attending Physician and Acting Director, Department of Medicine, The Mount Sinai Hospital, New York, New York.

STANLEY SHALDON, M.D., M.R.C.P., Medical Director, National Kidney Centre, London, England.

CONTRIBUTORS

HERBERT SHUBIN, M.D., Associate Director and Associate Professor of Medicine, University of Southern California School of Medicine; Associate Director, Center for the Critically Ill, Hollywood Presbyterian Hospital, Los Angeles, California.

LOUIS E. SILTZBACH, M.D., Clinical Professor of Medicine, Mount Sinai School of Medicine, City University of New York; Head, Division of Thoracic Diseases; Chief, Sarcoidosis Clinic, Department of Medicine, Mount Sinai School of Medicine; Consultant Physician, Rockefeller University, New York, New York.

B. R. SIMPSON, D. Phil. (Oxon), F.F.A.R.C.S., Professor of Anaesthetics, London Hospital Medical College, University of London; Consultant Anaesthetist, The London Hospital, London, England.

MORLEY M. SINGER, M.D., Assistant Professor of Anesthesia and Medicine, San Francisco Medical Center, University of California; Director, Intensive Care Unit, San Francisco Medical Center, University of California, San Francisco, California.

DAVID B. SKINNER, M.D., Dallas B. Phemister Professor and Chairman, Department of Surgery, University of Chicago, Pritzker School of Medicine; Chairman, Department of Surgery, University of Chicago, Hospitals and Clinics, Chicago, Illinois.

DONALD M. SMALL, M.D., Professor and Chief, Biophysics, Boston University School of Medicine; Visiting Physician, Boston City and University Hospitals, Boston, Massachusetts.

HOWARD M. SPIRO, M.D., Professor of Medicine, Yale University School of Medicine; Staff, Yale-New Haven Hospital, New Haven, Connecticut.

NORTON SPRITZ, M.D., Professor of Medicine, New York University School of Medicine; Chief of Medical Service, Manhattan Veterans Administration Hospital, New York, New York.

EUGENE A. STEAD, Jr., M.D., Professor of Medicine, Duke University Medical School, Durham, North Carolina.

L. STRUNIN, M.B.B.S., F.F.A.R.C.S., Senior Lecturer in Anaesthetics, Kings College Hospital, London University; Consultant Anaesthetist, Kings College Hospital, London, England.

H. J. C. SWAN, M.D., Ph.D., Professor of Medicine, University of California, Los Angeles; Director, Department of Cardiology, Cedars-Sinai Medical Center, Los Angeles, California.

JESSE E. THOMPSON, M.D., Clinical Professor of Surgery, University of Texas Southwestern Medical School, Dallas; Attending Surgeon and Consultant in Vascular Surgery, Baylor University Medical Center, Dallas, Texas.

ROBERT D. UTIGER, M.D., Associate Professor of Medicine, University of Pennsylvania School of Medicine; Attending Physician, Hospital of the University of Pennsylvania, Philadelphia, Pennsylvania.

RICHARD L. VARCO, M.D., Ph.D., Professor of Surgery, University of Minnesota Medical School; Attending Surgeon, University of Minnesota Hospitals, Minneapolis, Minnesota.

ROBERT LAWRENCE VERNIER, M.D., Professor, Pediatrics and Pathology, University of Minnesota, Minneapolis, Minnesota.

B. WALTON, M.B.B.S., F.F.A.R.C.S., Lecturer, London Hospital Medical College, London, University; Senior Registrar, The London Hospital, London, England.

THOMAS A. WARTHIN, M.D., M.A.C.P., Professor of Medicine, Harvard Medical School, Boston; Chief, Medical Service, Veterans Administration Hospital, West Roxbury, Massachusetts.

ANDREW S. WECHSLER, M.D., Instructor in Surgery, Duke University Medical Center, Durham, North Carolina.

MAX HARRY WEIL, M.D., Ph.D., Director and Clinical Professor of Medicine and Biomedical Engineering, University of Southern California School of Medicine, Los Angeles; Consultant Physician, Medical Staff, Cedars-Sinai Medical Center, Temple and Midway Hospitals, Los Angeles; Senior Attending Cardiologist, Children's Division, Los Angeles County/USC Medical Center; Director, University of Southern California Shock Research Unit; Director, Center for the Critically Ill, University of Southern California School of Medicine and Hollywood Presbyterian Hospital, Los Angeles, California; Visiting Professor of Anesthesia/Critical Care Medicine, University of Pittsburgh, Pittsburgh, Pennsylvania.

CURTIS B. WILSON, M.D., Associate, Department of Experimental Pathology, Scripps Clinic and Research Foundation, La Jolla, California.

ALBERT I. WINEGRAD, M.D., Professor of Medicine, University of Pennsylvania School of Medicine; Director, George S. Cox Medical Research Institute, Department of Medicine, Hospital of the University of Pennsylvania, Philadelphia, Pennsylvania.

LAWRENCE E. YOUNG, M.D., Professor and Chairman, Department of Medicine, University of Rochester School of Medicine and Dentistry; Physician-in-Chief, Strong Memorial Hospital, Rochester, New York.

JOHN YUDKIN, M.D., Ph.D., Emeritus Professor of Nutrition, Queen Elizabeth College, University of London, London, England.

Contents

INTRODUCTION 1
   Franz J. Ingelfinger

CONTROVERSY ONE REVISITED 3

1. Why Have Boards of Internal Medicine? ... 5
2. Atherosclerosis and Diet 7
3. Who Needs Drugs for Hypertension? 9
4. The "Anticoagulant Dilemma" 10
5. Fibrinolytic Therapy 11
6. Dietary Treatment of Duodenal Ulcer 13
7. Management of Gastric Ulcer 15
8. Malignant Potential of Colonic Polyps 16
9. Classification of the Cirrhoses 17
10. Is Hemochromatosis Inherited or Acquired? 18
11. Asymptomatic Bacteriuria: Significance and Management 19
12. Pathogenesis of Chronic Glomerulonephritis 20
13. To Catheterize or Not to Catheterize 21
14. Diagnosis of Unilateral Renal Disease 22
15. Treatment of Emphysema 23
16. The Control of Obesity 24
17. Are the Complications of Diabetes Preventable? 25
18. Autoimmunity in Human Disease 26
19. Treatment of Rheumatoid Arthritis 28
20. How Useful Are 5-TU and Related Substances in the Treatment of Adenocarcinoma? 30
21. Antibiotic Preparation of the Large Bowel .. 31
22. Drugs and the Anxious Patient 33
23. "Lies, Damn Lies, and Statistics" 35

CONTENTS

1. **IS INTERNAL MEDICINE OBSOLETE?** 39

    THE IDENTITY CRISIS OF AN IDEAL 41
    Edmund D. Pellegrino

    THE BROADLY BASED INTERNIST AS THE BACKBONE OF MEDICAL PRACTICE 51
    Lawrence E. Young

    COMMENT 64
    Richard V. Ebert

2. **REGULATION OF PHARMACO-THERAPY BY GOVERNMENT** 65

    FEDERAL REGULATION IS ESSENTIAL TO PROTECT THE PATIENT 67
    Herbert L. Ley, Jr.

    BUREAUCRATIC CONTROLS WILL STIFLE BOTH INDUSTRY AND INTELLIGENT MEDICAL PRACTICE 74
    Louis Lasagna

    COMMENT 81
    Maxwell Finland

3. **MULTIPHASIC SCREENING** 83

    MULTIPHASIC TESTING AS A TRIAGE TO MEDICAL CARE 85
    Maurice F. Collen

    UNVALIDATED PROCEDURES HAVE NO PLACE IN SCREENING PROGRAMS 92
    Thomas McKeown

    COMMENT 99
    Franz J. Ingelfinger

4. **THE DYING PATIENT** 101

    THE ROLE OF THE PHYSICIAN IN THE PROLONGATION OF LIFE 103
    Franklin H. Epstein

DEATH AS YOU WISH IT 110
   Eugene A. Stead, Jr.

ALTERNATIVES TO STRIVING TOO OFFICIOUSLY 113
   Robert S. Morison

5. ARE CORONARY BYPASS GRAFTS THE ANSWER TO ANGINA PECTORIS? 123

   THE EFFECTIVENESS OF CORONARY BYPASS GRAFTS IN MANAGING MYOCARDIAL ISCHEMIA 125
     Andrew S. Wechsler and David C. Sabiston, Jr.

   THE ROLE OF CORONARY BYPASS GRAFTS IN THE TREATMENT OF ANGINA PECTORIS REMAINS TO BE ESTABLISHED 137
     Richard S. Ross

   COMMENT 142
     Richard V. Ebert

6. EXERCISE FOR THE CORONARY PATIENT 143

   THE BENEFITS OF PHYSICAL TRAINING FOR PATIENTS WITH CORONARY HEART DISEASE 145
     Robert A. Bruce

   DISADVANTAGES OF INTENSIVE EXERCISE THERAPY AFTER MYOCARDIAL INFARCTION 162
     Henry Blackburn

   COMMENT 173
     Richard V. Ebert

7. THE MEASUREMENT OF CENTRAL VENOUS PRESSURE 175

   ROUTINE CENTRAL VENOUS CATHERIZATION FOR MANAGEMENT OF CRITICALLY ILL PATIENTS 177
     Herbert Shubin and Max Harry Weil

CENTRAL VENOUS PRESSURE MONITORING IS AN
OUTMODED PROCEDURE OF LIMITED PRACTICAL
VALUE 185
    H. J. C. Swan

COMMENT 194
    Richard V. Ebert

8. **PREVENTION OF ATHEROCLEROSIS** 197

SUGAR AND CORONARY DISEASE 199
    John Yudkin

PREVENTION OF ATHEROSCLEROSIS BY DIETARY
CONTROL OF HYPERLIPIDEMIA 208
    William Dock

A FAT CONTROLLED DIET FOR ALL 217
    Haqvin Malmros

CONTROL OF HYPERLIPIDEMIA BY SURGERY 228
    Henry Buchwald and Richard L. Varco

A SKEPTICAL VIEW OF A NATIONAL DIET
PROGRAM 239
    Norton Spritz

COMMENT 245
    Donald S. Fredrickson

9. **THE PLACE OF IPPB IN THE MANAGEMENT OF CHRONIC OBSTRUCTIVE LUNG DISEASE** 247

IPPB IS A USEFUL MODALITY IN THE TREATMENT
OF CHRONIC OBSTRUCTIVE LUNG DISEASE 249
    Robert L. Mayock

THE DANGERS AND LIMITATIONS OF IPPB IN
MANAGING DISEASES AFFECTING VENTILATION 263
    R. Drew Miller and Norman G. G. Hepper

COMMENT 272
    Richard V. Ebert

10. MANAGEMENT OF ACUTE PULMONARY INSUFFICIENCY 273

THE ADVANTAGES OF AN AGGRESSIVE, PROPHYLACTIC APPROACH 275
Morley M. Singer

THE INDICATIONS FOR ARTIFICIAL VENTILATIONS ARE LIMITED 280
Peter T. Macklem

COMMENT 288
Richard V. Ebert

11. TREATMENT OF MASSIVE PULMONARY EMBOLISM 291

THE EFFECTIVENESS OF THROMBOLYTIC THERAPY 293
Richard D. Sautter

THE ADVANTAGES OF EMBOLECTOMY 303
Robert L. Berger

COMMENT 310
Richard V. Ebert

12. PROPHYLAXIS AGAINST TUBERCULOSIS 311

ROUTINE CASE FINDING AND APPROPRIATE CHEMOTHERAPY DESERVE TO BE CONTINUED 313
Phyllis Q. Edwards

ADVANTAGES OF SELECTIVE USE OF BCG 322
Sol Roy Rosenthal

COMMENT 332
Maxwell Finland

13. THE KVEIM TEST 337

THE KVEIM REACTION IS NOT A SPECIFIC TEST FOR SARCOIDOSIS 339
Harold L. Israel

THE KVEIM TEST IS A RELIABLE MEANS OF
DIAGNOSING SARCOIDOSIS 349
    Louis E. Siltzbach

COMMENT 359
    Maxwell Finland

14. THE STATUS OF SMALLPOX
    VACCINATION 361

    VACCINATION SHOULD BE ABOLISHED IN THE
    UNITED STATES EXCEPT FOR SELECTED
    POPULATIONS 363
        Alexander D. Langmuir

    ROUTINE VACCINATION FOR ALL IS STILL
    INDICATED 371
        Abram S. Benenson

    COMMENT 382
        Maxwell Finland

15. MANAGEMENT OF ADULT-ONSET
    DIABETES 387

    ORAL ANTIDIABETIC AGENTS HAVE A LIMITED
    PLACE IN MANAGEMENT AND MAY BE HARMFUL ..389
        Albert I. Winegrad, Rex S. Clements, Jr.,
        and Anthony D. Morrison

    ORAL HYPOGLYCEMIC AGENTS ARE WORTHWHILE..404
        Robert F. Bradley

    COMMENT 416
        Arnold S. Relman

16. THYROID NODULES 419

    MOST SOLITARY THYROID NODULES SHOULD BE
    REMOVED 421
        Leslie J. DeGroot

    THYROID NODULES: SURGERY IS USUALLY NOT
    NECESSARY 428
        Monte A. Greer

    COMMENT 435
        Robert D. Utiger

17. THE PROLONGED THERAPEUTIC USE OF ADRENOCORTICAL STEROIDS 437

GLUCOCORTICOID THERAPY: AN OVERMALIGNED REPUTATION WITH UNTAPPED POTENTIAL BENEFIT 439
William McK. Jefferies

HAZARDS OF PROLONGED CORTICOSTEROID THERAPY 446
Philip K. Bondy

COMMENT 450
Arnold S. Relman

18. TREATMENT OF CROHN'S DISEASE 453

THE USEFULNESS OF ADRENOCORTICAL STEROIDS ...455
Joseph B. Kirsner

THE USEFULNESS OF AZATHIOPRINE 460
Brian N. Brooke

THE CASE FOR SURGICAL TREATMENT 470
Donald J. Glotzer

A CONSERVATIVE APPROACH 482
Thomas A. Warthin

COMMENT 489
Franz J. Ingelfinger

19. ASPIRIN AND THE STOMACH 491

ASPIRIN IS NOT A MAJOR CAUSE OF ACUTE GASTROINTESTINAL BLEEDING 493
Michael J. S. Langman

ASPIRIN IS DANGEROUS FOR THE PEPTIC ULCER PATIENT 500
Howard M. Spiro

COMMENT 509
Franz J. Ingelfinger

20. MECHANISMS THAT PREVENT GASTROESOPHAGEAL REFLUX 511

THE IMPORTANCE OF THE ANATOMIC CONFIGURATION OF THE CARDIA IN PREVENTING GASTROESOPHAGEAL REFLUX 513
David B. Skinner

THE IMPORTANCE OF THE SPHINCTER AT THE GASTROESOPHAGEAL JUNCTION 524
Lauran D. Harris

COMMENT 529
Franz J. Ingelfinger

21. MANAGEMENT OF GALLSTONES, PARTICULARLY THE SILENT VARIETY 531

THE ADVANTAGES OF AN AGGRESSIVE SURGICAL APPROACH 533
Frank Glenn

ADVANTAGES OF A VARIED AND INDIVIDUALIZED APPROACH 545
Donald M. Small

COMMENT 560
Franz J. Ingelfinger

22. THE HEPATOTOXICITY OF HALOTHANE 563

HALOTHANE HEPATITIS 565
Fenton Schaffner

EVIDENCE FOR HALOTHANE HEPATOTOXICITY IS EQUIVOCAL 580
B. R. Simpson, L. Strunin, and B. Walton

COMMENT 595
John P. Bunker

23. THE TREATMENT OF ACUTE GRANULOCYTIC LEUKEMIA 599

THE NEED FOR AGGRESSIVE MANAGEMENT 601
James F. Holland

THE TEMPERED APPROACH 610
William H. Crosby

24. MANAGEMENT OF DISSEMINATED INTRAVASCULAR COAGULATION 621

HEPARIN SHOULD BE USED CAUTIOUSLY AND SELECTIVELY 623
James J. Corrigan, Jr.

HEPARIN SHOULD BE USED IN THE THERAPY OF CLINICALLY SIGNIFICANT DISSEMINATED INTRAVASCULAR COAGULATION 633
Robert W. Colman, Stanley J. Robboy, and John D. Minna

25. THE USE OF STEROIDS IN TREATING THE NEPHROTIC SYNDROME 649

LIMITED ROLE OF STEROIDS IN MANAGING THE NEPHROTIC SYNDROME 651
Douglas A. K. Black

THE ADVANTAGES OF USING STEROIDS IN SOME PATIENTS WITH THE NEPHROTIC SYNDROME 658
Robert L. Vernier

COMMENT 663
Arnold S. Relman

26. TREATMENT OF UREMIA 665

DIALYSIS AS A DEFINITIVE TREATMENT FOR END STAGE UREMIA 667
Stanley Shaldon

THE INDICATIONS FOR RENAL
TRANSPLANTATION 675
    John R. Merrill

COMMENT 681
    Arnold S. Relman

27. IMMUNOLOGIC MECHANISMS IN
THE PATHOGENESIS OF
GLOMERULAR DISEASE 683

THE IMPORTANCE OF IMMUNOLOGIC
MECHANISMS 685
    Curtis B. Wilson and Frank J. Dixon

AN EVALUATION OF IMMUNOLOGIC MECHANISMS ..694
    Robert T. McCluskey and Paul D. Leber

COMMENT 710
    Arnold S. Relman

28. EVALUATION OF CARCINO-
EMBRYONIC ANTIGEN IN
DIAGNOSIS OF CANCER OF
THE COLON 713

EVALUATION OF CARCINOEMBRYONIC ANTIGEN IN
DIAGNOSIS OF CANCER 715
    Jeffrey J. Collins and Paul H. Black

COMMENT 725
    Phil Gold and Samuel O. Freedman

29. THE TREATMENT OF
HODGKIN'S DISEASE 729

THE TREATMENT OF HODGKIN'S DISEASE—
A CONSERVATIVE VIEW 731
    John Horton

THE CASE FOR AN AGGRESSIVE THERAPEUTIC
APPROACH FOR PATIENTS WITH ADVANCED
HODGKIN'S DISEASE 739
    Joseph R. Bertino

COMMENT 748
    Jerome B. Block and Thomas C. Chalmers

30. THE MARIHUANA DEBATE 751

    THE MARIHUANA DEBATE: DOUBTS ABOUT
    LEGALIZATION 753
        Donald B. Louria

    MARIHUANA IS NOT A PUBLIC HEALTH MENACE:
    IT IS TIME TO RELAX OUR SOCIAL POLICY 762
        Richard C. Pillard

31. MANAGEMENT OF CEREBRAL
    ISCHEMIA 769

    MEDICAL MANAGEMENT IN CEREBRAL ISCHEMIA ..771
        John Stirling Meyer and Ninan G. Mathew

    ANTICOAGULANT OF SURGICAL TREATMENT OF
    CEREBRAL ISCHEMIA 787
        Clark H. Millikan

    THE ROLE OF SURGERY IN CONTROLLING
    CEREBRAL ISCHEMIA 804
        Jesse E. Thompson

INDEX 815

Introduction

"It is difficult to understand the process of thought that prompted publication of this book," wrote one reviewer after he had looked at the first volume of "Controversy in Internal Medicine," and added, "The frontispiece (sic) should contain in bold red type a warning to all residents who propose to sit for the boards that they should avoid this book. If he were not confused before reading it, he would have a written guarantee for confusion before he finished it."[1] Others, less certain of the ageless verity of their medical knowledge, and agreeing that "the first dawn of wisdom lies in recognition that we know so little,"[2] were less harsh but still had their doubts. Bing, for example, took a dim view of the editorial comments which he saw as authoritarian touches gratuitously provided by "chosen experts, mainly from the Northeast Meccas of American Medicine."[2] And Feinstein saw a basic defect in having contributors submit their views without knowledge of what the opponent might write, a practice that leads to "disagreement without dispute."[3]

Yet here we go, offering "Controversy II" in a format identical to that of the first volume. We recognize the existence of a medical pedagogy devoted to turning out practical doctors, trained to go into action rather than thought. Controversy II is not recommended for medical curricula so oriented. We also admit that editors engage in many authoritarian and unattractive practices—such as selecting, rejecting, criticizing, deleting as well as commenting—but parochialism has at least been mitigated by an editorial expansion as far south as Philadelphia and as far west as Minneapolis. And although Dr. Feinstein's analysis is most accurate, we still prefer a positive statement of an author's concepts, to a negative essay bent on destroying someone else's ideas.

Although the format is similar to that of Controversy I, the subjects and contributors are, with a few exceptions, different. As in Controversy I, the intensity of disagreement varies from total, through partial to minimal. When the contributors appear to hold similar opinions, the editors' selection of the topic may have been inappropriate, or the controversy that may have appeared to exist at the time of the selection has now evaporated in the light of further developments.

One feature has been added, namely a chapter that attempts to update the controversies aired in the first volume. The lesson it teaches appears both clear and discouraging: some controversies in Internal Medicine persist for years and years; others subside gradually as interest wanes. Very few if any appear to be resolved by some elegant study that dramatically demolishes one side or the other. The glorious promise of Truth rising from the flames of Controversy is thus probably more visionary than real, but controversy has its own lessons, whether or not it is headed anywhere. Controversy, moreover, is a fact of medical life—wholesome medical life in our opinion.

References

1. Herrell, W. E.: Controversy in Internal Medicine. (Book Review.) Int. Med. Dig., July, 1966, pp. 63–64.
2. Bing, J. R.: Controversy in Internal Medicine. (Doctor's Bookshelf.) Med. World News, September 30, 1966, p. 122.
3. Feinstein, A. R.: Controversy in Medicine. (The Book Forum.) J.A.M.A. *196*:920–921, 1966.

For the Editors
FRANZ J. INGELFINGER, M.D.

Controversy One-Revisited

Whatever has happened to the issues argued in Controversy I? Have any been settled in the eight years since that book was published? These questions are answered in part by the titles of the present volume, for, to a varying degree, "Is Internal Medicine Obsolete?", "Prevention of Atherosclerosis by Nutritional Means," "The Place of IPPB in the Management of Chronic Obstructive Lung Disease," and others continue certain aspects of several discussions in Volume I. Except for the articles on atherosclerosis and diet, however, none of the controversies of Volume I is specifically extended in Volume II. Furthermore, no reference is made in the present collection to about two thirds of the controversies aired in Volume I. The editors, aided by guest editors Neil Abramson, Robert W. Colman, and A. Theologides, have therefore undertaken to submit the following comments in response to the question, "Whatever has happened to the issues argued in Controversy I?"

1. *Why Have Boards of Internal Medicine?*

Since Dwight Wilbur and Stewart Wolf discussed this topic, the Board has made several changes in procedure.[1] The final modification introduced a longer and more searching written examination at the end of at least three years of training in internal medicine following medical school graduation and abolished the oral examination. Those who pass this new written examination are certified as Diplomates in Internal Medicine. Substantiation of clinical skills by local evaluation committees is required before candidates are admitted to the examination. Subspecialty examinations are offered to Diplomates after a minimum of two years of subspecialty training. The Board has enlisted the help of the National Board of Medical Examiners and their facilities to improve the written examination so as to test the clinical skills of the applicants. The hope was expressed that no further changes will be required until the plan has been in effect long enough to permit a reasonable evaluation of the new procedures.

Meanwhile, the Board is working with the American College of Physicians on the problem of recertification to cope with the rapid obsolescence of medical knowledge and the need for continuing medical education. This is now a major controversial issue because of the reluctance on the part of those already certified to take another examination. At present a voluntary self-assessment program is being introduced and evaluated by the American College of Physicians. A new type of examination is contemplated for recertification of Diplomates by the Board.

The new procedures for evaluating clinical competence of candidates for the Board's examinations were described in detail by Petersdorf and Beck.[2] Briefly, candidates applying for examination would be required to substantiate their competence as practicing internists through documents furnished by directors of their residency program in general internal medicine in the hospitals in which the applicants were trained. The Board suggested that the program director establish a committee to assist in this evaluation and that the department of medicine evaluate the clinical skills of the trainees repeatedly throughout the period of education as interns, residents, and fellows. The Board, in turn, would require evidence of the qualification and activities of the evaluating committee of each training program.

A major criticism of the boards is that they promote increasing specialization at the expense of primary and family care, but if the Nixon administration is successful in its plans to phase out federal support of training programs in all subspecialty areas, an effective buffer against the excessive spread of specialization may be anticipated. Furthermore, as discussed elsewhere in this volume by Pellegrino and Young, specialists in primary care, or internists capable of primary care, should be available in increasing numbers to help fulfill the need of many patients for the personal attention of a physician rather than for the technology of a hospital.

References

1. Ebert, R. V.: Further changes in the requirements and procedures of the American Board of Internal Medicine. Ann. Intern. Med. 75:121, 1971.
2. Petersdorf, R. G., and Beck, J. C.: The new procedure for evaluating the clinical competence of candidates to be certified by the American Board of Internal Medicine. Ann. Intern. Med. 76:491, 1972.

M.F., R.V.E., and F.J.I.

2. Atherosclerosis and Diet

Albrink in her discussion of dietary prophylaxis of coronary disease emphasized elevation of triglycerides as a risk factor. She states that triglyceride concentration provides a better discrimination between patients with coronary disease and the normal population than does the level of serum cholesterol, and that the value of the serum cholesterol in predicting coronary artery disease is related to its association with serum triglycerides.

Recent studies have emphasized the concentration of specific classes of lipoproteins rather than the individual concentration of cholesterol and triglycerides in the plasma. The classification of Fredrickson, Levy, and Lees[1] has been widely accepted. Based on the use of electrophoresis, the lipoproteins can be separated into four classes; namely, chylomicrons, pre-beta-lipoprotein, beta-lipoprotein, and alpha-lipoprotein.[1,2] Pre-beta- and beta-lipoproteins may also be isolated by analytic ultracentrifugation. From the point of view of coronary artery disease, the beta- and pre-beta-lipoproteins are of a major interest. The former is also classed as low density lipoprotein (LDL) and contains a large amount of cholesterol as well as other lipids. The latter, also known as very low density lipoprotein (VLDL), transports triglycerides and contains a lesser amount of cholesterol. It is generally agreed that families with a marked elevation of beta-lipoproteins (Type II hyperlipoproteinemia) exhibit a marked increase in the incidence of coronary artery disease. Elevation of pre-beta-lipoproteins without elevation of beta-lipoprotein (Type IV hyperlipoproteinemia) seems to be associated with a moderate increase in risk of coronary artery disease. Other risk factors such as obesity and diabetes are often associated with this disorder.

Attempts have been made to separate the effect of elevation of serum cholesterol and increase in serum triglycerides on the incidence of coronary artery disease. Statistical analysis of the results of the Framingham Study[3] provides little evidence that elevation of very low density lipoproteins exerts an influence independent of the elevation of serum cholesterol on the incidence of coronary disease except in older women. The results may have been influenced by the fact that specimens of plasma were not obtained during the fasting state. On the other hand, two other prospective studies[4,5] showed that elevation of triglycerides without elevation of serum cholesterol led to an increased risk of coronary disease.

Further attempts to define more exactly the importance of each risk factor would appear to have limited value. It is of more importance to determine the influence of modification of risk factors on the incidence of disease in individuals without clinical evidence of coronary atherosclerosis and on the course of the disease in patients with known coronary arteriosclerosis. A number of prospective studies are underway. We can expect important information on the effect of modification of risk factors to become available in the next decade.

References

1. Fredrickson, D. S., Levy, R. I., and Lees, R. I.: Fat transport in lipoproteins—an integrated approach to mechanisms and disorders. New Eng. J. Med. *276*:32; 94; 148; 215; 273; 1967.
2. Stone, N. J., and Levy, R. I.: Hyperlipoproteinemia and coronary artery disease. Progr. Cardiov, Dis. *14*:341, 1972.
3. Kannel, W. B., Castelli, W. P., Gordon, T., and McNamara, P. M.: Serum cholesterol, lipoproteins and the risk of coronary disease. The Framingham Study. Ann. Intern. Med. *74*:1, 1971.
4. Carlson, L. A., and Böttiger, L. E.: Ischemic heart disease in relation to fasting values of plasma triglycerides and cholesterol. Lancet *1*:865, 1972.
5. Rosenman, R. H., Friedman, M., Straus, A., Jenkins, C. D., Zyzanski, S. J., and Wurm, M.: Coronary heart disease in the Western Collaborative Group Study. J. Chron. Dis. *23*:173, 1970.

R.V.E.

3. Who Needs Drugs for Hypertension?

The value of anti-hypertensive drugs in prolonging life in malignant hypertension was generally accepted in this discussion. There was a difference of opinion, however, in regard to the treatment of benign hypertension, but both Hollander and Relman stated the need for a carefully controlled prospective study. Such a study has now been done.

The results of a clinical trial conducted in Veterans Administration Hospitals and led by Fries conclusively demonstrated the value of treating patients with benign hypertension of a moderate or severe grade.[1] The mortality rate in the treated group was lower than in the control group, and there was a marked reduction in the incidence of strokes and congestive heart failure. There was little change in the incidence of myocardial infarction.

The question still remains as to whether treatment of mild hypertension unassociated with cardiovascular complications is necessary.[2,3] It has been conclusively demonstrated that the risk of developing clinical manifestations of coronary disease is greater in individuals with slightly elevated blood pressure than in individuals with a blood pressure that is average or low for the population studied. Hence, hypertension has been classed as a risk factor for coronary disease. Further prospective clinical trials will be required to demonstrate conclusively whether lowering of the blood pressure in individuals with mild hypertension will lower the risk of developing coronary disease. Data from the Framingham study have been used to show that hypertension is a major antecedent of congestive heart failure, so that vigorous treatment of even moderate systolic hypertension is recommended by the authors.[4]

References

1. Veterans Administration Cooperative Study Group on Antihypertensive Agents: Effects of treatment on morbidity in hypertension. II. Results in patients with diastolic blood pressure averaging 90 through 114 mm. Hg. J.A.M.A. 213:1143, 1970.
2. Veterans Administration Cooperative Study Group on Antihypertensive Agents: Effects of treatment on morbidity in hypertension. III. Influence of age, diastolic pressure, and prior cardiovascular disease; Further analysis of side effects. Circulation 45:991, 1972.
3. Proger, S.: Antihypertensive drugs: Praise and restraint. New Eng. J. Med. 286:155, 1972.
4. Karrel, W. B., Castelli, W. P., McNamara, P. M., McKee, P. A., and Feileib, M.: Role of blood pressure in the development of congestive heart failure. New Eng. J. Med. 287:781, 1972.

R.V.E.

4. The "Anticoagulant Dilemma"

Opinion on the use of anticoagulants in acute myocardial infarction appears to have leveled off somewhere between the positions taken by Hilden and by Griffith. Three clinical trials involving randomization of patients[1-3] have been reported recently. There was a small difference in mortality in favor of the treated men in each study, but in no instance was the difference statistically significant. A larger difference was demonstrated by Drapkin and Merskey in a small group of women. The MRC and VA studies demonstrated a large reduction in the incidence of embolic phenomena in the treated group. This included both pulmonary and systemic emboli. Thus, the evidence is clear that administration of anticoagulants does prevent the occurrence of pulmonary and systemic emboli and can logically be employed in those patients most susceptible to these complications. It is of interest that no deaths from hemorrhage were reported in these recent studies.

The question of the long-term use of anticoagulants in patients recovered from myocardial infarction is still not settled. Patients were treated for five years in two well designed clinical trials.[4,5] There was no difference in mortality between the treated and untreated groups at five years in either study. On the other hand, there is a considerable body of evidence that during the period of one to two years after an acute myocardial infarction, there is a lower mortality in patients treated with anticoagulants. This evidence has been ably analyzed in a collaborative review.[6]

References

1. Report of the Working Party on Anticoagulant Therapy in Coronary Thrombosis to the Medical Research Council: Assessment of short-term anticoagulant administration after cardiac infarction. Brit. Med. J. *1*:335–342, 1969.
2. The Use of Anticoagulants in Acute Myocardial Infarction. The Results of a Cooperative Clinical Trial. J.A.M.A. (To be published.)
3. Drapkin, A., and Merskey, C.: Anticoagulant therapy after acute myocardial infarction. J.A.M.A. *222*:541–548, 1972.
4. Cooperative Study: Long-term anticoagulant therapy after myocardial infarction. The Final Report of the Veterans Administration Cooperative Study. J.A.M.A. *207* (12):2263, 1969.
5. Seaman, A. J., et al.: Prophylactic anticoagulant therapy for coronary artery disease: A seven-year controlled study. J.A.M.A. *189*:183, 1964.
6. Collaborative analysis of long-term anticoagulant administration after acute myocardial infarction. An International Anticoagulant Review Group. Lancet *1*:203, 1970.

R.V.E.

5. Fibrionlytic Therapy

Although thrombolytic therapy has been available for 15 years, its place in the treatment of thrombotic disorders is still not fully defined. Delay in clinical usage of fibrinolytic agents can be ascribed to the problems enumerated by Oscar Ratnoff in *Controversy I*. Fortunately, progress in the past seven years has enabled many of these difficulties to be surmounted.

Investigators now agree that plasminogen activators such as streptokinase and urokinase are preferable to plasmin or other fibrinolytic enzymes, both theoretically and practically, and that systemic intravenous administration achieves as good a result as local perfusion. Both urokinase and streptokinase have been purified, resulting, in the case of the latter, in the elimination of most of the pyogenic and many of the allergic side effects. The work of an international committee on thrombolytic agents has resulted in standardization of the methods of assay and units of the preparations employed clinically. Experience has allowed the development of effective and reasonably safe dosage schedules. A fixed amount of streptokinase has been selected that contains sufficient amounts of the protein to overcome resistance, due to antibodies, in 85 to 90 per cent of the patient population. The thrombin time provides a simple method of measuring the activity of the thrombolytic state and allows for individual adjustment of dose level. Hemorrhage is a side effect usually confined to sites of invasive procedures, although life-threatening bleeding has been known to occur. Embolization of clots has not proved to be an important hazard, but rethrombosis almost always occurs unless heparin is used immediately following the infusion. Development of lung scans to monitor the effects of thrombolytic therapy on pulmonary embolism, radioactive fibrinogen localization to evaluate peripheral venous thrombosis, and refinements of arteriography to localize arterial disease now allow critical objective evaluation of therapeutic regimens.

Experience over the past 10 years has defined the possible areas of benefit of thrombolytic therapy, but definitive recommendations are still not possible. Encouraging evidence from small scale trials using ^{125}I-labeled fibrinogen scans and phlebography suggests that streptokinase may be of benefit in the treatment of deep leg venous thrombosis. About half the treated vessels are relieved of obstructing clots, especially if less than 96 hours have passed since onset of the symptoms. Proof of clinical benefit will require large controlled trials.

The results of the first phase of the multicenter urokinase–pulmonary embolism trial, sponsored by the National Heart and Lung Institute, have recently been published. A 12-hour infusion of urokinase followed by heparin accelerates the resolution of pulmonary emboli as compared to heparin alone. This conclusion was based on improvement in the pulmonary angiogram and lung scan at 24 hours, as well as decreases in pulmonary artery pressure, right ventricular pressure, and total pulmonary resistance. However, no change was noted in the recurrence rate of pulmonary embolism and no significant difference in mortality was observed. Phase II of the study is now underway to compare streptokinase to urokinase as well as the effect of longer infusion times in an attempt to decrease recurrence rate and mortality.

A considerable amount of data is available concerning acute peripheral arterial occlusion but, unfortunately all the evidence stems from uncontrolled trials. Satisfactory dissolution of thrombi occurs in about 50 per cent of patients treated with streptokinase, but the value of thrombolytic therapy as compared to surgery is not yet clear. The most exciting area for the application of thrombolytic therapy would be the treatment of myocardial infarction. The results of trials to date have been inconclusive. Of seven trials, three show no statistical difference, and four show decreased mortality with only streptokinase therapy. Plans are now underway for a streptokinase–urokinase myocardial infarction trial along the lines of the urokinase–pulmonary embolism study. The questions asked are obviously of great importance; one can only hope that definitive answers are forthcoming.

Robert W. Colman

6. *Dietary Treatment of Duodenal Ulcer*

When the antral hormone gastrin was identified and fingerprinted as to its amino acid composition, and an effective analogue in the form of pentagastrin marketed, new ways of controlling gastric acidity, and hence of peptic ulcer management, appeared to be just around the corner. Disappointingly, however, inhibitors of gastrin release or action have not been readily produced, and, with the exception of the Zollinger-Ellison syndrome, serum levels of gastrin in fasting duodenal ulcer patients appeared little different from those obtained in control populations. The possibility that gastrin has something to do with the pathogenesis of duodenal ulcer, however, is not quite dead; recent studies have shown that when duodenal ulcer patients eat, their serum gastrin levels reach higher peaks than those achieved by normal persons after a meal.[1]

So gastrin has done little to influence the controversy between Roth and Ingelfinger as to the kind of food duodenal ulcer patients should be permitted to eat. Gastrin levels, to be sure, respond differently to different foods, and even to different amino acids. The more a dietary constituent buffers gastric acidity, the more gastrin will be released, but that the initial buffering effect of proteins is later followed by increased gastric secretion is hardly news. Thus, although new knowledge of gastrin metabolism might sooner or later affect the controversy as to which foods ulcer patients should eat, the influence of gastrin on that debate has to date been negligible. Roth still entertains the hope that he can "rest the stomach" with appropriate dietary restrictions, whereas Ingelfinger has judiciously retired from the fray. Yet his place is taken by ever-growing numbers of gastroenterologists who, perhaps in tune with the culture of the times, are permissive in their dietary advice to ulcer patients. Even dieticians have become less rigorous and have issued a manifesto deploring the rigidity of ulcer diets.[2]

Although the academic establishment by and large endorses liberal diets for ulcer patients, Roth, as far as what actually goes on in the world, is still king. The diet manual and practices of practically any hospital, or of any similar health facility, still recommend slops I, white mush II, and bland tastelessness III for ulcer patients. Such aversive regimens, moreover, surely remain the kinds of diets that the average practitioner recommends to his ulcer patient.

So the controversy about what kind of food the duodenal ulcer patient should eat is rather subdued these days. But that's not because anything has been settled; it is only because the ammunition of new ideas has run out.

References

1. McGuigan, J. E., and Trudeau, W. L.: Differences in rates of gastrin release in normal persons and patients with duodenal ulcer disease. New Eng. J. Med. 288:64, 1973.
2. American Dietetic Association: Position paper on bland diet in the treatment of chronic duodenal ulcer disease. J. Amer. Diet. Ass. 59:244, 1971.

F.J.I.

7. Management of Gastric Ulcer

Back in the "good old days," a favorite subject for medical-surgical conferences was gastric ulcer. The internist could be counted on to argue for a trial of medical management, whereas the surgeon, pointing to an irreducible minimum risk that the ulcer might be cancerous, would hold forth in favor of resection. The argument has lost much of its steam, chiefly because the internist has become both wiser and more skilled. He has recognized that the management of a recurrent gastric ulcer, even if benign, is apt to have much more favorable long-term results if the surgeon is allowed to take over. At the same time the surgeon is much more willing to permit the internist to handle a first and possibly even a second attack of gastric ulcer because of the more accurate diagnosis made possible by improved techniques of radiology, cytology, and endoscopy. Perhaps the decrease in frequency of gastric cancer in North America has also helped to defuse the traditional medical-surgical confrontation over gastric ulcer.

Early clouds of renewed debate may, however, be appearing on the horizon. Several papers have presented evidence to suggest that some gastric ulcers are not merely manifestations of an acid-peptic disorder, but that complementary noxious agents are bile salts regurgitating in excessive amounts from the duodenum.[1,2] Furthermore, Fisher and Cohen[3] report that the pylorus in patients with gastric ulcer is incapable of performing its normal gate-keeping function, i.e., if the "normal gate-keeping function" of this muscle is accepted as preventing retrograde rather than forward movement in the gastroduodenal area. If such new ideas turn out to be correct, one may anticipate a medical and perhaps even surgical attempt to correct pyloric function, and new alternatives may be available to compete with gastric resection in the management of a patient with a recurrent gastric ulcer.

References

1. Rhodes, J.: Etiology of gastric ulcer. Gastroenterology 63:171, 1972.
2. Donaldson, R.: Breakdown of barriers in gastric ulcer. New Eng. J. Med. 288:316, 1973.
3. Fisher, R. S., and Cohen, S.: Pyloric-sphincter dysfunction in patients with gastric ulcer. New Eng. J. Med. 288:273, 1973.

F.J.I.

8. *Malignant Potential of Colonic Polyps*

To the best of my knowledge, Baker and Jones on one hand, and Castleman and Krickstein on the other, still believe what they wrote seven years ago. But there is no more controversy; it has petered out. Why? Because the development of fiberoptic colonoscopes has made it possible to remove polyps safely, at reasonable expense, and with only moderate trouble from almost any part of the colon without necessitating laparotomy. This technical development has made the controversy concerning the malignant potential of colonic polyps academic, for now anyone who is discovered to have a colonic polyp can have a biopsy of this lesion, and usually can have it removed from below; even those who are sure that the malignant potential of colonic polyps is very small will probably endorse polypectomy via the colonoscope.

Reference

1. Wolff, W. I., and Shinya, H.: Polypectomy via the fiberoptic colonoscope: Removal of neoplasms beyond reach of the sigmoidoscope. New Eng. J. Med. 288:329, 1973.

F.J.I.

9. *Classification of the Cirrhoses*

Here is another controversy that has petered out, but in this instance the cause can be identified as a new medical discovery rather than the development of a new technique. Those who study liver disease have become so engrossed by Australia antigen, and the new investigative vistas that it has opened up, so as to be quite unconcerned with semispeculative arguments as to the number and characteristics of various types of hepatic cirrhosis. The presence or absence of morphologic or immunologic evidence of Australia antigen in the blood or tissues of patients with liver disease obviously offers a much sounder basis for etiologic interpretations than division of cirrhotic liver lobules into those that are tiny, medium, or large in size. Moreover, even though they used different names for the varieties of cirrhosis, Popper's and Gall's concepts, described in Controversy I, as to how chronic liver disease develops were really not too radically different.

F.J.I.

10. *Is Hemochromatosis Inherited or Acquired?*

   Crosby argued that hemochromatosis is primarily a heritable disorder; MacDonald that it is principally acquired. As corollaries to these positions, Crosby in general supported vigorous phlebotomy to drain the body of excess iron; MacDonald feared that such treatment might well be excessive and lead to iatrogenic debility. If current therapeutic practices are accepted as a criterion, the Crosby view continues to predominate, for the practice of blood-letting to remove excess iron stores from the hemochromatotic patient is widely observed. Yet the controversy has by and large subsided. One hardly hears anybody arguing anymore that hemochromatotics got that way because they drank too much iron-containing wine. Those interested in this view have seemed to stop writing about it so that the issue commands little interest. All of which shows that controversy depends not only on the existence of contradictory scientific data but also on the availability of vociferous protagonists willing to espouse a cause.

F.J.I.

11. *Asymptomatic Bacteriuria*

During the past several years evidence has accumulated to suggest that asymptomatic bacteriuria in otherwise healthy women is a relatively benign condition, only occasionally leading to progressive renal damage. Even when infection is acutely symptomatic and is known to involve the kidney, the long-term prognosis is apparently not so serious as formerly thought. Thus, for example, a recent study[1] of young women followed 10 to 20 years after hospital admission for acute pyelonephritis reported that only 15 per cent had subsequently suffered significant damage to one or both kidneys, despite the fact that more than half had recurrent or persistent bacteriuria. In infancy and childhood the risk to the kidney appears to be much more substantial, and there is a growing opinion that most of the gross pyelonephritic lesions seen in adult women are the result of infections that began in childhood. Although enthusiasm for the aggressive therapy of *all* women with asymptomatic bacteriuria seems to be waning, it seems clear that *some* will develop renal disease if untreated. The question therefore still remains as to how to decide which patients need treatment.

Reference

1. Parker, J., and Kunin, C.: Pyelonephritis in young women. A 10- to 20-year follow-up. J.A.M.A. *224*:585, 1973.

A.S.R.

12. Pathogenesis of Chronic Glomerulonephritis

Careful follow-up studies published in the past few years[1,2] have helped to clarify the natural history of sporadic acute poststreptococcal glomerulonephritis in children. The evidence indicates that complete healing occurs in the great majority of children with this disease, but there are a few who die in the acute stage or go on to chronic nephritis. No comparable studies of adult poststreptococcal glomerulonephritis have been published recently, but there has been no change in the prevailing view that a much higher proportion of adults with this condition develop chronic nephritis.

The relative importance of poststreptococcal glomerulonephritis as a cause of chronic renal disease in adults remains uncertain. New classifications of chronic nephritis, based on light and electron microscopy and immunofluorescent stains of biopsy material, have tended to stress the wide variety of etiologic factors that can produce this disease. The classification suggested by Wilson and Dixon elsewhere in this volume considers poststreptococcal glomerulonephritis to be only one of many different forms of so-called "immune complex" glomerulonephritis. Also included are many other types of chronic nephritis, some apparently caused by antiglomerular basement membrane antibodies, and others without any known relation to immunologic mechanisms.

Further developments in this rapidly moving field will undoubtedly help to put this controversy in clearer perspective.

References

1. Lewy, J. E., et al.: Clinico-pathologic correlations in acute poststreptococcal glomerulonephritis. Medicine 50:453, 1971.
2. Dodge, W. F., et al.: Poststreptococcal glomerulonephritis: A prospective study in children. New Eng. J. Med. 286:273, 1972.

A.S.R.

13. *To Catheterize or Not To Catheterize*

Most of the heat has gone out of this issue as additional data have accumulated. It is now firmly established that single urethral catheterizations of patients with normal uninfected urinary tracts carry a small risk of subsequent infection, no matter how careful the technique. The likelihood of infection is least in healthy ambulatory patients and greatest in those who are hospitalized. There is some evidence that instillation of antibacterial solutions into the bladder following catheterization will reduce the rate of infection.

As for indwelling urethral catheters, the data are crystal-clear: Catheters attached to an *open* drainage system lead to infection within a week in the great majority of cases, regardless of the catheterization technique. Continuous irrigation of the bladder with antibacterial solutions through a three-way catheter significantly reduces the incidence of infection for the first 10 days or so, but thereafter the chances of infection increase rapidly. Similar results can be achieved without irrigation by the use of a completely *closed* collection system. Whether the addition of antibacterial irrigation can improve results even further has not yet been clearly established.

In short, a consensus seems to have been reached. The catheter *is* a risk, but often a necessary one. The risks can be greatly reduced—but not totally eliminated—by the use of closed drainage or an appropriate type of bladder irrigation.

References

1. Kaye, D. (ed.): *Urinary Tract Infection and Its Management.* St. Louis, The C. V. Mosby Co., 1972.
2. Kunin, C. M.: *Detection, Prevention and Management of Urinary Tract Infections.* Philadelphia, Lea & Febiger, 1972.

A.S.R.

14. *Diagnosis of Unilateral Renal Disease*

Perhaps the most important diagnostic development in this field during the past few years has been the use of bilateral renal vein renin measurements. Many patients with curable hypertension due to renal arterial lesions have normal peripheral vein renin levels and may even have normal levels in renal venous blood, but the ratio of the concentration in the blood from the ischemic kidney to that in the blood from the normal kidney is usually greater than 1.5 and this difference is enhanced by physiological stimuli that normally increase renin secretion.[1] Although *no* single diagnostic test is foolproof, this one appears to be a reasonably reliable indicator of surgically curable renovascular hypertension. Of course, this test should be used only after a screening procedure (such as the intravenous pyelogram or the radioisotope renogram) has suggested the possibility of a vascular lesion, and after an arteriogram has demonstrated the actual existence of such a lesion.

Opinion as to the efficacy of surgery in the management of renovascular hypertension has swung back in recent years to a more conservative position. Experience has shown that only about a third of patients with arteriosclerotic lesions and only two thirds of those with fibromuscular lesions will be "cured" by surgery.[2] Furthermore, it is now clear that many such patients can be successfully managed with drugs. The opinion seems to be growing that surgery in patients with arteriosclerotic lesions should be reserved for those with very severe hypertension that fails to respond to drugs. Many patients who have medial fibroplasia of the renal artery (the "string of beads" pattern) can also be treated medically, particularly since it has been shown that this type of lesion rarely progresses or leads to loss of renal function.[3]

References

1. Strong, C. G. et al.: Renal venous renin activity: Enhancement of sensitivity of lateralization by sodium depletion. Amer. J. Cardiol. 27:602, 1971.
2. Hunt, J. C., et al.: Diagnosis and management of renovascular hypertension. Amer. J. Cardiol. 23:434, 1969.
3. Stewart, B. H., et al.: Correlation of angiography and natural history in evaluation of patients with renovascular hypertension. J. Urol. *104*:231, 1970.

A.S.R.

15. Treatment of Emphysema

Since the publication of the last Controversy, little advance has occurred in the treatment of patients with emphysema. Physiologic studies of experimental emphysema as well as of the naturally occurring disease have cast further light on the relationship between the morphologic changes in the lung and function. Exposure of the lungs of animals to papain produces destructive emphysema similar morphologically to that observed in human beings.[1,2] The major physiologic effect is a change in elastic properties of the lung, with an alteration in the pressure volume curve so that less pressure is required to inflate the lung to a given volume. Little alteration in airway resistance occurs. Recent studies have suggested that naturally occurring emphysema produces a similar effect on the pressure volume curve of the lung and has less effect on resistance to airflow.[3,4] The alteration in elastic properties of the lung permits the bronchi to collapse more readily and limits the rate of expiratory airflow. Thus, the lung is more vulnerable to bronchial obstruction from complicating bronchitis.

In view of these observations, it is difficult to understand the reason for elevating the diaphragm in patients with emphysema. The low diaphragm is the result of lack of elastic recoil of the lung. Elevating the diaphragm will lower static intrathoracic pressure at the point of maximum inspiration and will render the bronchi more vulnerable to collapse during expiration. A more logical procedure would be the surgical removal of emphysematous lung and bullae, thus restoring the pressure volume curve toward normal and increasing the elastic recoil of the lung. The diaphragm would then be elevated in a physiologic manner. Unfortunately, such a surgical procedure is valuable only when large bullae are present and is not successful when there is widespread emphysema.[5]

References

1. Johanson, W. G., Jr., et al.: Effects of elastase, collagenase, and papain on structure and function of rat lungs in vitro. J. Clin. Invest. 51:288, 1972.
2. Goldring, I. P., et al.: Histopathology and mechanical properties of the lung in experimental emphysema. Path. Microbiol. (Basel) 35:176, 1970.
3. Finucane, K. E., et al.: Elastic behavior of the lung in patients with airway obstruction. J. Appl. Physiol. 26:330, 1969.
4. Park, S. S., et al.: Postmortem evaluation of airflow limitation in obstructive lung disease. J. Appl. Physiol. 27:308, 1969.
5. A Statement by the Committee on Therapy: Current status of the surgical treatment of pulmonary emphysema and asthma. Amer. Rev. Resp. Dis. 97:486, 1968.

R.V.E.

16. The Control of Obesity

When obesity starts in youth, fat cells tend to multiply so that, to use the appropriate jargon, early onset obesity is characterized by hyperplasia of adipocytes.[1] In adult onset obesity, to the contrary, the number of fat cells may increase little if at all, but each cell just gets bigger, i.e., it hypertrophies.

As of the present, however, the distribution of the fat that engulfs and submerges the obese has no import for therapy. Adipocytes, whether more numerous or just larger, thumb their noses with equal indifference at all types of treatment. Indeed, as compared to the time when the treatment of obesity was argued in Controversy I, the art has regressed rather than advanced, with anorectic agents now not only officially questioned as to their efficacy[2] but also suspected of having aggravated the mania for "speed" and related substances.

In view of B. F. Skinner's impact on the tenets of psychology, it is not surprising that behavior therapy has been applied to the obese person (called, for some reason, a "client" rather than a patient.[3]) "In the area of obesity," the theory runs, "the target behaviors are the set of habits contributing to excessive caloric intake and decreased energy expenditure. Obesity, or overweight, is seen as the consequence of such habits rather than as a symptom of some underlying psychologic disorder."[3] According to Stunkard, "behavior modification is more effective than previous methods of treatment for obesity."[4] Self-help groups, the members of which encourage each other much in the fashion of Alcoholics Anonymous, have also had some success—at least as long as the group has had a charismatic leader. Indeed, the treatment of obesity and of alcoholism have much in common in that medical science has accomplished little, but mysticism and evangelic fervor sometimes have done the trick. After all, St. Simeon Stylites did not manage to keep down his weight because he took amphetamines or had his small bowel bypassed.

References

1. Hirsch, J., and Knittle, J. L.: Cellularity of obese and non-obese human adipose tissue. Fed. Proc. 29:1516, 1970.
2. FDA Bulletin: Anorectics Have Limited Use In Treatment of Obesity. 1972.
3. Levitz, L. S.: Behavior therapy in treating obesity. J. Amer. Diet. Ass. 62:22, 1973.
4. Stunkard, A.: New therapies for the eating disorders. Arch. Gen. Psychiat. 26:391, 1972.

F.J.I.

17. Are the Complications of Diabetes Preventable?

This controversy continues to simmer without signs of resolution. Nothing has recently appeared in print that, in my opinion, adds any decisive new clinical information on the question of whether good control of blood sugar will prevent vascular complications. Indeed, I think it unlikely at present that the kind of controlled, prospective clinical study necessary to answer this question could ever be successfully carried out. I suspect that, instead, the problem will ultimately be resolved in other ways, probably by further research information on the pathogenesis of vascular disease in diabetes.

One of the most interesting recent leads in this direction has been provided by the studies of Winegrad and his colleagues, who have shown that an elevated glucose concentration causes significant alterations in glucose metabolism, respiration, and water content of isolated strips of rabbit aorta.[1] Whether or not these in vitro observations have any relevance to the development of vascular disease in diabetic patients remains to be determined, but the possible implications of this work have aroused wide interest.

Reference

1. Morrison, A. D., Clements, R. S., Jr., and Winegrad, A. I.: Effects of elevated glucose concentrations on the metabolism of the aortic wall. J. Clin. Invest. 51:3114, 1972.

A.S.R.

18. *Autoimmunity in Human Disease*

Autoimmunity has become a vast expanse of diseases in which a serum antibody is present for no apparent reason. Basic to the controversy raised by Mackay and Waksman, in the previous edition of this textbook, is whether antibodies are present in man as a self-destructive process or in some acceptable capacity as a mechanism of host defense. The presence of unrecognized antigens in the past led to the suggestion that autoimmunity was an aberration of the immune system in which antibodies were formed against self. More recent recognition of offending drugs and bacterial and viral antigens has shifted the emphasis of the antibody to one of defense; albeit, in so defending, an antigen-antibody complex may produce "self-destruction" when deposited on vital tissues, such as the glomerular basement membrane in acute glomerulonephritis.

An unusual feature of autoimmune disease is that no single controversy exists. Mackay and Waksman specifically addressed themselves to the significance of "auto-antibodies." In addition, other as yet unresolved controversies are concerned with the etiology of antibody formation, the nature of antigenic stimulation, the aberrations of the immune system that allow for antigenic stimulation and antibody formation, and the human genetic factors associated with the "normal" or "abnormal" (depending upon one's side in the dispute) responses to foreign substances. In view of the knowledge that antibody subclass expression is under genetic influences, one wonders whether one person's response to antigens results in efficient clearance of the foreign material, whereas another's response is attended by pathologic significance.

Several diseases have caused renewed interest in the inherited or acquired immunologic abnormalities that are associated with individual susceptibility for autoimmunity. Pernicious anemia is the latest example. This hematologic disorder, which was initially considered to be a malignancy, became a nutritional disease when described by Minot and Murphy, and later a gastrointestinal disease when Castle described intrinsic factor deficiency. Soon thereafter, pernicious anemia became an autoimmune disease as evidenced by parietal cell antibodies, intrinsic factor antibodies, intrinsic factor B_{12} antibodies, and thyroid antibodies. In recent years this disease has been reported in patients with depressed immunologic defense mechanisms (pernicious anemia in young adults with hypogammaglobulinemia, or with abnormalities in cellular immunity, or in patients with multiple myeloma and relative hypogammaglobulinemia). Therefore, a possibility exists that an immune deficiency state occurs first which allows for antigenic stimulation and, as a result, parietal cell destruction. Systemic lupus erythematosus is perhaps another example of a disease with evolutionary thought processes concerning etiology. What was first a disease of unknown etiology in which antibodies were present directed against "self" has become, according to some investigators, a disease characterized by antibodies directed against circulating DNA and to other researchers a disease associated with demonstrable viral invasion. More recent studies have suggested that some patients have an abnormality in cell-mediated immunity. Thymic derived lymphocytes have been demonstrated in decreased numbers, which raises the possibility that a defect in cellular immunity allows for undue antigenic stimulation and antibody production. An obvious unanswered question, however, is whether the drugs employed for treatment of the disease result in a diminution of thymic-derived lymphocytes or the reverse. The congenital T cell, B cell, and stem cell abnormalities and the acquired lymphoproliferative diseases are yet other examples of defects in immunity associated with excessive antibody production, some antibody directed against "self." Although it is tempting to attribute antibody production to abnormal clones, one must recognize the possibility that antibody may be present for its ascribed purpose, that is, for self-protection and not for self-destruction.

Neil Abramson, M.D.

19. *Treatment of Rheumatoid Arthritis*

After reviewing some recent clinical reports on the management of patients with rheumatoid arthritis and the summaries and recommendations by some of the leading workers currently active in the field and then rereading the three contributions on this subject in the first volume of Controversies in Internal Medicine, I could not help but be struck by the healthy conservatism of our earlier essayists. All three of them stressed the value of rest and physical therapy and the predominant reliance on aspirin as the major anti-inflammatory and analgesic agent.

Alan S. Cohen quickly dismissed adrenocorticosteroids without discussion because of the limited role he felt that they play in the current management of rheumatoid arthritis. He saw no need for gold salts in this disease and, indeed, neither he nor any of his many associates in the arthritis clinics of two large hospitals where he works had used them in their patients in recent years.

Evan Calkins discussed the indications, proper usage, contraindications, untoward effects, precautions, and dangers of the adrenocortical steroids as applied to patients with rheumatoid arthritis. He ended by noting that he employs them in about only 3 per cent of his patients and urged that they be avoided if at all possible.

Theodore L. Bayles discussed conservative management, generally following the same line as Cohen. He dismissed phenylbutazone and oxyphenylbutazone as not useful and not worth the risk of the toxic effects their use entails. Antimalarials he considered only mildly suppressive in early cases. However, he felt that gold salts do have a place in severe cases refractory to other therapy, to relieve and reduce, even though only temporarily, the progressive inflammation and synovial destruction in certain patients. From the length he goes to explain to his patients the potential toxicity and actual serious dangers of the use of the gold salts, he must simultaneously convey some strong conviction of their potential value in order to gain consent from any of them to accept the course of chrysotherapy he prescribes, with all its attending problems.

Goldman and Hess (Bull. Rheum. Dis. *21*:609, 1970) came to a similar conclusion with regard to chrysotherapy and called attention to observation of the British multicenter controlled trial, that if a patient does not respond to an initial trial of gold therapy, a second course is not useful. They, like others, noted the contraindication of various immunosuppressive therapies in women of childbearing age who are not on contraceptives, and the need for close supervision of patients receiving cytotoxic drugs.

Recent reports and studies on the management of rheumatoid arthritis have been dealing increasingly with the use of immunosuppressive and cytotoxic agents, and they have become a major controversial issue. In their review of advances in rheumatic diseases for 1967 through 1969, Ferguson and Worthington (Ann. Intern. Med. 73:109, 1970) seem to agree that aspirin is still the most generally useful agent in the management of rheumatoid arthritis. In their view, most of the studies of newer anti-inflammatory and analgesic drugs, including indomethacin, and the less well known flufenamic acid, ibuprofen and mefenamic acid, have failed to establish any consistent advantage over aspirin or phenylbutazone. They note that chloroquine and related compounds are being used less frequently because of the occasional retinopathy they may produce, but many physicians continue to use antimalarial drugs in low dosage. These reviewers indicate that most American rheumatologists continue to rely on gold as the preferred supplement for those patients who are refractory to conservative therapy. Among cytotoxic and immunosuppressive drugs, in addition to cyclophosphamide and azathioprine, other agents such as nitrogen mustard, 6-mercaptopurine, methotrexate, and chlorambucil have all been subjected to clinical trials. The question of whether these agents act by exerting an anti-inflammatory effect or by an immunosuppressive action has not been settled. They conclude that the hazards of toxicity (in up to 90 per cent of those receiving large doses) and the uncertainty of benefit require that all the cytotoxic agents must still be regarded as highly experimental. A similar view on the use of cytotoxic agents in rheumatoid arthritis was expressed in an editorial in Lancet (2:1231, 1970).

As a physician interested in infectious diseases, I believe that the use of these toxic agents, especially for the long periods that would be required in longstanding and refractory cases of rheumatoid arthritis, cannot be justified unless the benefits were remarkable, consistent, and reliable, which does not seem to be the case. Although not so frequent as in recipients of organ transplants, serious "opportunistic" infections may be expected, as with long-term steroid therapy. Indeed, they have been encountered and some of those infections have been fatal. It is doubtful whether the risks are warranted in such a disease as rheumatoid arthritis, which itself is not fatal.

20. How Useful Are 5-FU and Related Substances in the Treatment of Adenocarcinoma?

The points of view expressed by Lemon, Foley, and Zubrod regarding 5-fluorouracil are still valid and acceptable. There have been some recent changes in dosage and schedules of administration of 5-FU; in general, the weekly I.V. administration is favored as less toxic but equally effective as the five-day intermittent courses. 5-FUDR did not show significant advantages over 5-FU and it is used less frequently. 6-Mercaptopurine is not used at present in therapy of carcinoma and sarcoma because it has been shown to be ineffective. Methotrexate is seldom used in the treatment of sarcomas and carcinomas except as part of combination chemotherapy. Both drugs, of course, are still used in acute leukemias as part of combination regimens. Since these papers were written, some new cytotoxic drugs have been used in various malignancies mentioned by the authors.

As far as the biochemical and biologic explanations and hypotheses given by Lemon, most of these remain controversial or are accepted as valid observations on specific animal tumors under special experimental circumstances.

References

1. Jacobs, E. M., et al.: Treatment of cancer with weekly intravenous 5-fluorouracil. Study of the Western Cooperative Cancer Chemotherapy Group. Cancer 27:1302, 1971.
2. Hall, T. C.: Biochemical factors predicting response to chemotherapeutic agents. In Brodsky, I., and Kahn, S. B. (eds.): Cancer Chemotherapy II. New York, Grune & Stratton, 1972, pp. 93–101.

A. Theologides, M.D.

21. Antibiotic Preparation of the Large Bowel

The controversy on the value of using antibiotics in addition to cathartics and cleansing enemas in the preoperative preparation of patients undergoing resections of the colon is by no means resolved, judging from the conflicting results that continue to be reported.

In the previous volume Isadore Cohn, Jr., expressed his long-held conviction, based on experience with a succession of regimens involving different antibacterial agents used preoperatively, that they were effective in reducing postoperative wound and peritoneal infections after surgery on the colon. On the other hand, Robert Tyson and his bacteriologist colleague, Earle H. Spaulding, who had likewise conducted careful clinical and bacteriologic studies in successive groups of patients receiving various active antibacterial agents orally in the same manner, had abandoned their routine use. In an addendum to their contribution, the latter called attention to the interesting experiments in rabbits reported by Vink, who demonstrated a higher incidence of tumor recurrences when antibiotics were used in the preparation of the large bowel. They also noted that Borgstrom failed to confirm Cohn's reported protection against peritoneal infection following devascularized anastomoses of the colon by preoperative administration of antibiotics.

In a later report, Bornside and Cohn (Gastroenterology 57:569, 1969) tested the effect on the fecal flora of normal volunteers of oral clindamycin given for three days along with purgatives and enemas, as employed in the preoperative preparation for large bowel surgery. This antibiotic is well absorbed and is highly active against the anaerobic flora of the bowel and against gram-positive cocci, except for most enterococci, but is inactive against the aerobic gram-negative bacilli. In a double-blind study they found that the fecal flora of those who received a placebo remained remarkably constant during the three days of therapy and the following two days. They interpreted this as indicating that the mechanical cleansing reduced the mass of feces, but what remained contained the same number of bacteria and, hence, was potentially a major hazard for infection. During the clindamycin therapy, those fecal streptococci (nonhemolytic enterococci and alpha hemolytic streptococci) that were sensitive to clindamycin were replaced by clindamycin-resistant enterococci. Staphylococci, nearly all of which were sensitive, were not prominent in these subjects, so the effect on this species could not be evaluated. However, the coliforms were unaffected by the clindamycin treatment and were found in similar numbers as in placebo-treated subjects, although high concentrations of the antibiotic were demonstrated in the feces. The authors interpreted these results as supporting their thesis that "both mechanical cleansing and antibiotics are essential for an effective three-day bowel preparatory procedure."

At Royal Melbourne Hospital, Hughes and collaborators (Med. J. Aust. 1:305, 1970) carried out a double-blind trial in 108 patients on the effect of intravenous administration of a large dose of penicillin immediately before large bowel surgery. In the patients who underwent open anastomosis without resection, the incidence of postoperative wound infections was not significantly different in the placebo group (12.5 per cent) and in those who received antibiotic treatment (8.8 per cent). However, among those who underwent colon resection without anastomosis, 58.3 per cent of patients who received a placebo and only 12.5 per cent of those who were given penicillin intravenously became infected. The reduction in infection attributed to penicillin in the patients whose colon was resected was statistically significant at the 5 per cent level. Mechanical cleansing and laxatives, but no oral antibiotics, were used in the preoperative preparation of the bowel.

In an extension of a study mentioned by Tyson and Spaulding, the group at the Wadsworth Veterans Administration Hospital in Los Angeles—H. Earl Gordon, D. W. Gaylor, and others (Calif. Med. 103:243, 1965)—reported the results of an investigation of 183 patients to whom kanamycin, neomycin, or a placebo was administered in a double-blind fashion during a 72-hour period preceding operation in an attempt to evaluate the role of antibiotics in surgery of the colon. Considering only the criteria of mortality and the incidence of postoperative wound and peritoneal infections, there apparently was no significant difference between patients receiving antibiotics and those receiving a placebo.

Another extensive experience was reported at the 1966 meeting of the Society for Surgery of the Alimentary Tract by Herter and Slanetz (Amer. J. Surg. 113:165, 1967). They reviewed the results of the 1042 colonic resections performed between 1951 and 1956 and between 1958 and 1962 at the Presbyterian and Francis Delafield Hospitals in New York City. During these periods 724 patients received various intestinal antibiotics and 318 were prepared by mechanical measures alone. General postoperative complications were equally frequent in both groups. Staphylococcal enteritis, though not common, was more frequent after antibiotic prophylaxis, and two deaths were ascribed to this complication. The rate of wound infections after colonic operations entailing only intraperitoneal anastomoses was similar in both groups. However, after anterior resections in which the bowel was anastomosed extraperitoneally, antibiotic bowel preparation appeared to afford significant protection against local complications. These authors therefore recommended antibiotics for use preoperatively when an extraperitoneal resection is anticipated.

M.F.

22. *Drugs and the Anxious Patient*

This controversy has become almost historically quaint, for it focused on the needs of the individual anxious patient, and meprobamate was the drug on nearly everyone's tongue—literally! Now, just eight short years later, an anxious society in its entirety appears at risk, and meprobamate has a hard time keeping up with the benzodiazepine agents in the mood-drug popularity race. So the controversy has broadened to include the larger question—i.e., whether doctors, by prescribing tranquilizers, exalters, and apatheticizers indiscriminantly, are responsible for a iatrogenic disease of society.

The role of the doctor in fostering drug abuse is not easily assessed. It is all a matter of opinion, and usually an emotionally conditioned opinion at that. The same basic facts, for example, are used to support contrary conclusions. In Sweden amphetamines were classified as narcotics in 1944, and phenmetrazine (Preludin) and methylphenidate (Ritalin) were withdrawn from the market in 1965 and 1968, respectively.[1] Yet abuse of these agents is continuing—obvious evidence according to one side that Swedish doctors cannot be blamed for misuse of these stimulants. Not at all, runs the counter argument, which holds that doctors were so profligate in their prescriptions of Preludin and Ritalin for fat girls and depressed boys that this, at the time licit practice, initiated the illicit use that continues. In this country, Mellinger et al.[2] surveyed a cross-section of adult San Francisco residents in 1968–1969 and found that 45 per cent of women and 30 per cent of men had used a mood-affecting agent at least once in the course of the preceding year. Balter and Levine think that practitioners, rather than overprescribing and overusing psychotherapeutic drugs, actually "err in the conservative direction."[3] In other words, Balter and Levine believe that one third of the population does suffer from bona fide stress and anxiety. Obviously the prevalence of such disorders will determine whether or not a given level of psychotropic drug use is excessive.

If doctors do withhold psychotrophic agents, they must as a group be impervious to pharmaceutical advertising. The advantages of this or that pacifying or stimulating agent have been widely touted, not only for the treatment of serious anxieties, but also to sustain nerves frayed by traffic noise, to relieve the insomnia of worry, and to subdue the fretfulness of fatigue. Even more suspect are the advertising practices used to promote OTC agents. It is not surprising that a public incessantly encouraged to gobble or to apply some special brand of medication for every conceivable ache or distress will be conditioned to seek stronger (i.e., prescription) medicine when the solace so persuasively promised along with the latest newscast fails to materialize.

The benzodiazepines may cause drowsiness, ataxia, fatigue and confusion,[4] but lethal complications, and the drugs' potentials for addictive and suicidal use, are negligible. The popularity and relative safety of anti-anxiety agents have changed the nature of the decision that the doctor must often make when consulted by an anxious patient. The consequences for both the individual and for society are more moral than medical when the purpose of a prescribed drug is to dull the patient's sensibilities to the knocks, annoyances, and frustrations of everyday life.

References

1. Perman, E. S.: Speed in Sweden. New Eng. J. Med. 283:760, 1970.
2. Mellinger, G. D., Balter, M. B., and Manheimer, D. I.: Patterns of psychotherapeutic drug use among adults in San Francisco. Arch. Psychiat. 25:385, 1971.
3. Balter, M., and Levine, J.: Character and extent of psychotherapeutic drug usage in the United States. Excerpta Medica. (To be published.)
4. Antianxiety drugs in organic and functional syndromes. The Medical Letter, Vol. 14, No. 25, December 8, 1972.

F.J.I.

23. "Lies, Damn Lies, and Statistics"

The meaningful use and interpretation of statistics from the point of view of one trying to identify causal factors in noncommunicable diseases was ably discussed by Ernest L. Wydner. J. Yerushalmy, in a parallel presentation, stressed the importance of recording and analyzing observations from which further well planned and designed studies can be carried out to determine the specificity of associations thus discovered. The relevance of the association established with respect to the original disease would depend to a great extent on such associations.

In commenting on these papers, the point was made that statistics are useful only to the extent that the one employing them is acquainted with the subject matter to which the statistics are applied. The more thoroughly acquainted an individual is with all the factors that may influence the data and the more accurately those data are obtained and recorded, the more useful, precise, and reliable are the results of the analyses and the more valid their interpretation.

Of course, the improper application of the scientific principles to the design of a study and statistical analysis of the data may raise serious doubts as to the interpretation of the results, as Feinstein has pointed out with respect to the now famous and controversial report of the University Group Diabetes Program (Clin. Pharmacol. Ther. *12*:167, 1971, and *13*:609, 1972). The defense of that expensive and laborious "prospective" study, which was so carefully designed by this sophisticated group of experienced investigators, was ably presented from the personal perspective of a participant by Theodore B. Schwartz (Ann. Intern. Med. 75:303, 1971). He pointed out another potential weakness in the study built in by chance, because the patients assigned to tolbutamide happened to have included a greater number of vascular abnormalities at the start of the study. These differences in baseline characteristics were not "statistically significant" but may well have affected the final results, although the writer did not think so. He also noted the marked differences among the principal investigators about discontinuing tolbutamide therapy on the basis of the results of this study. Dr. Schwartz, acting on the conviction that the results were meaningful, felt he could not continue to offer tolbutamide to his patients.

The reports on the use of hormones in the treatment of acute rheumatic fever and carditis offer another example of the difficulties in designing and executing long-term, controlled studies and gaining acceptance for the interpretation of the results. In 1965 a group of distinguished clinical investigators and statisticians in the United Kingdom and the United States reported the results of cooperative clinical trials of the effects of treatment with ACTH, cortisone, and aspirin on the course of acute rheumatic fever and rheumatic heart disease (Circulation 32:457, 1965). They concluded: "At the end of 10 years there is no evidence that, on the treatment schedules used in this study, the prognosis has been influenced more by one treatment than another. This confirms the findings reported at 1 year and 5 years." They found the most important features determining the prevalence at the end of 10 years to be the status of the heart at the time treatment was begun. In those without carditis, the prognosis was excellent (94 per cent had no residual heart disease). The rate of recurrences of acute rheumatic fever and the sex of the patient had to be taken into account in evaluating therapy of rheumatic fever.

After the results of the first year's follow-up were reported, Roy and Massell (Circulation *14*:44, 1956) criticized the study for the small doses of steroid used. These authors reported the disappearance of murmurs to be twice as common in 47 rheumatic children treated with large doses, as compared with 41 children treated with small doses. They concluded that the divergences of opinion regarding the efficacy of hormones in the treatment of acute rheumatic carditis may be explained on the basis of differences in doses of hormone, duration of therapy, and duration of illness before beginning therapy.

It was May G. Wilson, a highly respected and experienced student of rheumatic fever who, in an earlier study of 55 patients with rheumatic carditis of three to 21 days' duration, noted rapid termination of the disease with short-term steroid therapy. In a second study she and W. N. Lim (New Eng. J. Med. *260*:807, 1959) reported on 53 patient attacks of acute carditis that were treated and concluded: "In active carditis short-term therapy will terminate the inflammatory process irrespective of its duration. Only with early, adequate hormone therapy can residual cardiac damage be expected to be prevented or minimized."

Impressed by Wilson's early results, a Combined Rheumatic Fever Study Group, coordinated by Ann G. Kuttner, was set up in several hospitals and rheumatic fever clinics to compare the effects of short-term, "intensive" prednisone and acetylsalicylic acid in the treatment of acute rheumatic fever (New Eng. J. Med. *272*:63, 1965). In the early phase of this study (Markowitz, N., Kuttner, A. G.: Ch. 10, pp. 96–114, in *Rheumatic Fever—Diagnosis, Management and Prevention*. Philadelphia, W. B. Saunders Company, 1965) no evidence was obtained to indicate that prednisone in large doses given for 12 weeks was more effective than aspirin for the prevention of residual heart disease. This was a single-blind study, and four patients were changed during the study from aspirin to prednisone, of whom one died. In a further study employing double-blind controls, the difference in incidence of cardiac sequelae after short-term, intensive treatment was found to be small and not statistically significant. In eight patients rheumatic activity was not terminated in spite of two courses of 7 days of intensive steroid therapy. In their recommendations for therapy of acute rheumatic fever, Markowitz and Kuttner include progressively increasing doses and duration of aspirin therapy for those with arthritis alone, minimal carditis, definite carditis without cardiac enlargement, and for those with severe carditis. Prednisone is not recommended for the first two categories, but, interestingly enough, this drug in a dose of 1 mg./lb./day for 6 to 8 weeks is recommended for those in the third category, and for 3 to 6 months for those with severe carditis. The evidence for the value of such prolonged use of the hormone was not clearly presented.

The new insistence of the Food and Drug Administration on statistically significant data from well designed studies, double-blind wherever possible, in establishing efficacy for acceptance of new drugs, has led to concern that statistical significance would be equated with "clinical significance." Murray Weiner (Amer. J. Med. Sci. 262:4, 1971) discussed this aspect and the difference in attitude toward the results of controlled, double-blind, and statistically evaluated studies between the clinical investigator in an academic setting on the one hand and the practitioner directly responsible for the immediate care of an individual patient requiring treatment on the other. The latter must make his choice on the basis of the attributes of that patient and his knowledge of the action of the drug.

Weiner expressed the view, "Perhaps the revolutionary pendulum which is attempting to make drug evaluation a more exact science, is now swinging a bit too far to the other side." Uncontrolled variables still operate to frustrate the expert in experimental design and even he often desperately needs help from the clinician to point out what these are and how they could influence the interpretation of "clinical significance." Benefit-to-risk ratio is another often crucial and determining factor in the choice of a drug, and is difficult to work into the design of any controlled experiment, since that, again, may become a very personal assessment by each physician for each patient.

References

New statistical methods are: "The Monte Carlo Monitoring Procedure" (Bailey, N. T. J.: The Mathematical Approach to Biology and Medicine. New York, John Wiley & Sons, Inc., 1967, pp. 41–44); "The Derivation of Relative Betting Odds" (Cornfield, J.: The Bayesian outlook and its application. Biometrics 25:617, 1969) and "Betting on the Winner" (Zelen, M.: Play the winner rule and the controlled clinical trial. J. Amer. Stat. Ass. 64:131, 1969).

M.F.

1

Is Internal Medicine Obsolete?

THE IDENTITY CRISIS OF AN IDEAL
    by Edmund D. Pellegrino

THE BROADLY BASED INTERNIST AS THE BACKBONE OF MEDICAL PRACTICE
    by Lawrence E. Young

COMMENT
    by Richard V. Ebert

The Identity Crisis of an Ideal

EDMUND D. PELLEGRINO

State University of New York at Stony Brook

The man who is unwilling to accept the axiom that he who chooses one path is denied the others must try, I suppose, to persuade himself that the logical thing is to remain at the crossroads.

Dag Hammarskjold, *Markings*[1]

Intellectual disciplines and professions, like persons, must periodically confront the question of identity. Internal medicine, though less than a century old and at the height of its powers, is today challenged to re-examine its pristine image of itself and choose new directions more consonant with the changing medical scene. Not to choose is to remain at the crossroads, and this is tantamount to obsolescence.

The internist's self-image today is the fusion of two ideals born late in the nineteenth century: the ideal of the Oslerian scholar-consultant and the German ideal of the physician-scientist. In more recent years internists have modulated these two conceptions by seeing themselves as personal physicians, as synthesizers of the totality of the patient's problems, and even as sophisticated variants of the family physician.

This pastiche of images is undergoing fragmentation and polarization. Pediatrics and family and community medicine have asserted their independence; geriatrics and hebiatrics promise to do the same; the specialties are flourishing and organizing along interdisciplinary lines that transcend the boundaries of internal medicine. The clinical scientist is in the ascendant and the scholar-consultant is becoming a rare species: the two are much less in communication with each other than ever before.

Is the unity of internal medicine doomed to obsolescence, or can it be restructured in some new way more congruent with the forces altering the whole of medicine? What paths are open? Which are most consistent with whatever is unique to internal medicine, and which will enable it to serve most effectively the needs of patients and society?

I shall posit that today's dominant image is somewhat pretentious and unrealistic and that it does demand reassessment. Internal medicine's unique contributions to the whole body of medicine are in danger of becoming obscured by too vigorous defense of an apotheosized ideal no longer tenable. One may dare believe that Osler himself, in the spirit of detachment he recommended so highly in his essay on medical chauvinism, would applaud an honest look at his beloved vocation.[2]

Genesis of the Image

No physician so thoroughly embodied an ideal as did William Osler his own ideal of internal medicine. Yet, in his essay on *Internal Medicine as a Vocation*, he was forced to define it by exclusion as ". . . the wide field that remains after the separation of surgery, midwifery, and gynecology."[3]

Osler conceived the internist as the scholar-clinician and general medical consultant. To attain this ideal, he prescribed 20 years or so of time devoted to understanding the pathophysiology of disease and to the refinement of the aspirant's clinical craftsmanship. He was most emphatic that ". . . the student of internal medicine can never be a specialist."[4]

This was in 1897. The terms *internal diseases* and *internal medicine* had already been in common use in Germany for 15 years.[5] By the end of the nineteenth century, the German ideal of internal medicine emerged as a clinical specialty covering all adult nonsurgical disorders, excluding dermatology. The internist was distinguished from the general practitioner by his deeper understanding of the chemistry, physiology, and pathology of disease and by his investigative spirit. From this *anlage*, the present-day clinical scientist and the subspecialist have gradually developed.

It is the fusion of these two somewhat contradictory ideals that has most influenced academic departments of internal medicine in this country. The leading teachers and practitioners were bred first to the Oslerian ideal. Increasing numbers of late have, however, concentrated their efforts in scientific investigations and in the subspecialties. Nonetheless, most departments and training programs have tried to preserve the idea of the generalist. Even the subspecialists are presumed to be internists first and specialists second. The majority of residents in medicine have been nurtured on these ideals. While excused from investigative work if they enter practice, they are still expected to remain clinical scholars. There is the further presumption that the internist so educated is best equipped to be the personal or family physician and the synthesizer-manager of the patient's comprehensive care.

Departments of medicine hold tenaciously to these images of themselves and the people they train. But in actuality, the whole of internal medicine is undergoing erosion by the inherent contrarieties of the Oslerian and German ideals, which exert an increasingly centrifugal effect on each other.

Erosion of the Ideal

Osler's ideal of internal medicine was probably tenable when it was uttered in 1897. It was exemplified in the first edition of his textbook, which had appeared five years earlier.[6] A single author could then encompass all the major non-surgical disorders authoritatively. The infectious diseases were well described clinically, although etiologic agents were still unknown for many; pathology was the only significant basic science for clinicians; the blood and endocrine systems could be treated together in 30 pages; beriberi was listed as an infection, pellagra as an intoxication, and ptomaine poisoning was a legitimate heading. Specific treatments were virtually nonexistent, and nosography, as Knud Faber was to iterate in 1922, was, indeed, the major intellectual skill of the internist.[7]

One good head could hold all the information needed for prudent clinical decision making. The cost of incorrect diagnosis was small, since therapeutics was largely empiric or fanciful. The internist could function as an across-the-board consultant, bringing his ordered thinking and tempered judgment to the assistance of the general practitioner, whose practicality was innocent of the internist's scholarly nosology.

The problem with this view of internal medicine is epitomized by contrasting Osler's first edition with Harrison et al. in the latest edition—seven editors, 150 contributors, and 401 headings.[8] Concepts of chemistry, physics, genetics, immunology, and virology compete with pathology as the scientific fundament of clinical medicine. Specific chemical therapeusis and specific prevention have gradually replaced empiric remedies. Complex and effective surgical techniques have become available for a wide range of disorders. A host of laboratory procedures and technical diagnostic aids have challenged the neat nosographic entities of former years.

The enormously enhanced capabilities of medicine have sharpened the clinician's responsibilities for precision in diagnosis and therapeutics. The cost of error in increasing numbers of disorders is now measurable in avoidable death, disability, and discomfort. Ignorance of the detailed information collated by the flourishing subspecialties is culpable. The conscientious general consultant must perceive the impossibility of his position as the subspecialist becomes more widely available. One man's competence can no longer span the whole of internal medicine. Indeed, to be proficient even in a limited field, the subspecialist must exhibit the same dedication Osler called for. The consultant can be authentic now only in a subspecialty. Practitioners in other fields increasingly realize this, as do the more sophisticated patients. With disturbing frequency, they skip over the general consultant and go directly to the subspecialist for help.

The growth of the subspecialties and the expansion of knowledge pose another challenge in organization. Interest in an organ system is a more powerful organizing principle than identification with internal medicine per se. Thus, physicians, surgeons, physiologists, pathologists, and radiologists interested in the cardiovascular system, for instance, have more in common, and work more closely together, than do cardiologists and hematologists or endocrinologists and gastroenterologists. Identification with an organ system rather than with the department of medicine is a centrifugal force that will have increasing impact on the future development of departments of medicine.

Additional challenges are posed by the delineation of community medicine and family medicine as academic disciplines. Internal medicine can no longer be adequately defined in any institution without taking into account that institution's commitment to these two new areas.

Family medicine uses internal medicine extensively, but it is not, as some internists would hold, the same as general internal medicine. Family medicine is no longer being defined by default but is asserting itself as the medicine of the small human aggregate—the household and the family—emphasizing primary, preventive, and comprehensive care. It focuses on the dynamics of small group interactions and preventive psychiatry—all with an emphasis on the ambulant patient. The generally trained internist who wishes to become a bona fide family practitioner will find it necessary to acquire knowledge and skills beyond those he is apt to attain in the usual medical residency. His background in internal medicine is an excellent but far from a sufficient preparation.

Family medicine is achieving departmental or at least divisional status in many schools and undertaking major responsibility for undergraduate and graduate education in this specialty. Internal medicine supplies an essential set of clinical skills, but surely cannot substitute for the whole of family medicine in any sophisticated way.

Community medicine also puts constraints upon internal medicine. Community medicine is the medicine of the large human aggregate—the whole community. It deals with all the forces—social, political, behavioral, epidemiologic—that produce illness and that bear on health in the community. Family medicine and internal medicine are, on the one hand, two varieties of medicine *in* the community, but they are not synonymous with medicine *of* the community—the true domain of community medicine departments.

Some academic departments of medicine, sensing the erosion of the Oslerian ideal, are attempting to resuscitate general internal medicine by claiming the new specialties of family and community medicine as part of their domain. This is a vain and self-defeating maneuver that only obstructs the growth of these other fields temporarily and dilutes the major efforts of internal medicine. Family and community medicine need strong departments of internal medicine, not as competitors but as essential resources, much as engineers need physics and mathematics departments.

Perhaps the most divisive influence is within internal medicine itself, growing out of the rapid expansion of clinical investigation as a scientific discipline.

The bedside investigation of disease, using truly scientific techniques, will surely be a major intellectual advance to which our era can lay claim. The focusing of energies, enthusiasm, resources, and prestige of departments of medicine in this direction has brought incontestable benefits to the whole of medicine. It is a natural outgrowth of the German ideal of internal medicine as a scientific specialty, but it has made the concurrent development of the general internist along Oslerian lines difficult or impossible to maintain.

Finally, the body of general internal medicine is undergoing fission along lines of age groupings. The pediatricians split out many years ago and now have their own subspecialties; specialists in adolescence, middle age, and old age are ever more insistently demanding separate recognition. Without debating the validity of these claims, they are another set of forces fragmenting the whole of internal medicine, so that today its territory is lost in the overlappings of a huge Venn diagram in which the original circle has been completely encompassed by all the others.

The reality of these divisions in the concept of internal medicine has been felt by residents and practicing internists for some time. For at least a decade, residents have pressed for increased training in the subspecialties, as they learned from internists in the community that the internist was not the general consultant he had hoped to be. Indeed, most young internists, out of necessity as much as preference, have become general, personal, or primary physicians to middle-class America. Others have extended themselves beyond their training and taken on the care of families. Still retaining the image of the physician-scholar, however, they have limited the numbers of their patients and have not addressed the problem of volume care of the primary, emergency, and preventive type that is the major unmet need in this country today.

The cumulative effect of these changes is to cast serious doubt on the survival of today's dominant notion of internal medicine. Internal medicine has occupied a commanding position of influence in medical schools and in practice for many decades. To retain this influence, it must confront these fragmenting tendencies consciously and define its mission more precisely in the immediate future.

What of the Future?

In defining its future paths, the first task of internal medicine is consciously and directly to limit some of its pretensions. Family and community medicine are valid disciplines specifically directed to tasks of primary, preventive, and general care of the common ills of mankind—the 85 per cent of human disabilities that rarely enter the hospital. The motivations, capabilities, or interests of those who enter internal medicine are unsuited to these tasks. Those who do enter with these motivations and interests, as internists, are sure to be disappointed. Increasingly, they will be able to achieve their goals more easily in family and community medicine.

The same is true of the cherished Oslerian ideal of the internist across-the-board consultant. Most departments have already abandoned this idea in practice, but they have not yet done so conceptually. Residents, colleagues, and the public may be misled by our failure to make this point explicit. There is still a role for the general consultant, but it must be defined in a different way. It is patently impossible to train such general consultants in large numbers. The mere acquisition of training in general internal medicine cannot confer the capabilities of the generic diagnostician on the average resident or practicing internist.

The first major manpower contribution of departments and services of medicine must be in the field that is the most natural extension of the history, capabilities, and interests of departments of medicine: the production of organ system specialists. These will constitute the majority of authentic consultants, even as they now do. They are essential resources for their colleagues in family medicine and the surgical specialties. They are the clinician-scholars and the physician-scientists of today, whom no other department can train.

As patient care and research in the future are organized more completely on organ system lines, the medical subspecialists will function in interdisciplinary teams organized orthogonally to the usual departmental lines. But these medical specialists will be united by a common set of attitudes and skills which will continue to constitute another unique contribution that internal medicine must retain and emphasize. I refer to the cultivation of the arts, skills, and craftsmanship of clinical diagnosis—the capability for collecting clinical data, correlating these with laboratory and x-ray data, reasoning logically about them, and synthesizing them into a comprehensible whole with the aim of arriving at optimal and prudent actions. These are the same attitudes of mind that have made internal medicine the intellectual center of the medical disciplines, and they will not become obsolete. What is different about the future of internal medicine is that these intellectual attributes will be developed over limited sets of data and not over the entire spectrum of diseases, as the older conception of the physician–general consultant would require.

But what then of the generalist function? Who will serve the needs of the noncategorized patient or the one who has several disorders simultaneously? Who will see to the needs of the "whole" patient? Is his care merely the sum total of the specialties whose configuration is described by the diseases from which he suffers? Patently, this is not the case. There will always be a need for the physician who can manage the patient and the clinical situation, assess his needs, determine how each shall be met, and integrate data of varied sources and validity into a rational pattern of understanding and action.

These activities constitute the generalist function, which, in the future, as now, will continue to be best exemplified by internal medicine, though it cannot be exclusively the domain of that specialty.[9] The generalist function is essential in primary, secondary, and tertiary medical care, but its specific expression will be defined differently by the settings in which it occurs. Whatever the setting, however, this integrating function will always be more than the arithmetic sum of the subspecialties of internal medicine.

In primary care, the generalist function is best carried out not by the internist but by the family or primary care physician—the physician who encounters the patient first in the course of a medical event. Here, it consists in the entire process of making the prudent decisions that determine which problems can be handled immediately, and which must receive more extensive study or treatment at secondary or tertiary centers. Included are decisions about what may be delegated to medical assistants, what must be done by the physician himself, and what requires the participation of other team members—nurses, social workers, pharmacist, specialist. This is more than the triage function to which it is reduced only by those who do not understand its complexities. Emergency care, health maintenance, and the competent management of those common ills of mankind which constitute the major volume of health care in any community—these are the major functions of the primary care generalist and his team. They must manage the initial steps when the patient makes contact with the health care system and when anxiety may be at its highest. This is a segment of medical care for which the internist is now ill-prepared and one which does not make maximal use of his training in complex disorders.

On the other hand, the generalist function is becoming a more important task for the internist in the community hospital and in *secondary care*. The general internist, educated not as an across-the-board consultant but as the manager and synthesizer of the patient's diagnostic and therapeutic program, has his strongest contribution to make here. He should function as a full-time practitioner charged by the hospital with the major responsibility for coordinating the care of the more complex adult non-surgical disorders. In some more enlightened future day, this responsibility may well extend to the surgical patient as well.

The generalist in this setting must be capable of assessing the full template of the patient's needs and formulating a logical plan of management. This requires coordination of the activities of a team of subspecialists, of nurses, and of other health professionals. He must apprehend and correlate the data from these varied sources and make the whole comprehensible to the patient, his family, and the primary or family physician who will undertake continuing care of the patient when he leaves the hospital. The knowledge and skills demanded for this role are of an order different from those required of the primary or family physician. They are based in that group of the general features of complex disorders which has characterized the best-trained general internists, but which is available with diminishing frequency nowadays.

But additional skills are also required and these are not part of the current training of the general internist: experience in working with small groups (group dynamics), functioning as captain and as a member of a multidisciplinary team, making optimal use of the capabilities of other professionals, and knowing how to negotiate agreements instead of relying on an order to handle a complex clinical situation. The new generalist's synthesizing functions must obviously extend beyond the data and the disease to the human resources which must be integrated in hospital care today. He will, in fact, be required to add the attributes of a systems engineer to his basic clinical sciences to function optimally in this capacity.

These same coordinating functions are essential in the larger hospitals and other tertiary care institutions. The generalist is least understood and least appreciated in such a context, but all the more necessary since the degree of specialization and technical dominance in these settings is even more intense than in secondary care. Like his counterpart in the community hospital, the generalist in the university hospital should be a full-time practitioner, as well as a faculty member with the same set of coordinating and synthesizing responsibilities. He will, of course, be called upon to deal with the most complicated disorders and he must coordinate a more complex team of specialists, using the most sophisticated technical modalities. His assignment will, in consequence, be more difficult, so that his grasp of his clinical and coordinating skills must be quite firm.

The preparation of internists who can perform the generalist function in secondary and tertiary care is, along with the preparation of subspecialists, a major responsibility of departments of medicine. This is a more valid and more appropriate responsibility for tomorrow's academic departments than guarding the illusion of the across-the-board consultants or trying to transform general internal medicine into family and primary care medicine. Through these generalists, specifically trained both in the general clinical craftsmanship and in coordinating skills in newer patterns of care, internal medicine will retain and even strengthen its traditional central position among the clinical disciplines. No other discipline can better assume this function or better safeguard the integrity of the person against the fragmenting pull of the subspecialties.

Most departments are not oriented to, or organized for, the education of the generalist as we have defined him. To do so requires that the care of patients on medical services be cast in a new mold in which coordination of the total care is assigned to a specific division of general internal medicine. Dedicated to this purpose, experiments designed to explore optimal models of delivering patient care in an integrated fashion are needed within the daily operations of university medical services. Unless the generalist function can be concretely demonstrated for students and house staff, it will lack the credibility and academic respectability without which it cannot survive. While one form of the general internist is perforce becoming obsolete—i.e., the internist as polymath consultant—the more contemporary version described here should thrive and give new life to internal medicine in the immediate future.

What we must not fail to appreciate is that there are few alternatives. The generalist function as described here derives from the needs of patients who do not come prepackaged into categorical diseases and who cannot be disassembled into disease entities without violence to their humanity and the quality of care they receive. To make optimal and sane use of our specialized knowledge is to attend with equal enthusiasm and skill to the synthesizing function.

Any medical need so firmly rooted in the needs of patients will ultimately be satisfied, even if internal medicine does not undertake the responsibility. The integrating function should not be permitted to go by default to some group of systems engineers or clinical managers. Internal medicine is best suited by tradition and intellectual resources to undertake this function and, indeed, its own continued evolution is in considerable measure dependent upon it.

If internal medicine can renew itself in terms more congruent with its uniqueness and its role in emergent patterns of care, it will assure several highly important intellectual and pedagogic functions: (1) preparation of consultants in the organ system specialties; (2) continued cultivation of the discipline of clinical investigation; (3) education of the new generalist for roles in secondary and tertiary care, and (4) underlying all of these, maintenance of the traditional emphasis on mastery of the fundamentals of clinical craftsmanship, collection of data by history, physical examination, and laboratory tests, together with the intellectual process of using these data to understand disease and manage the clinical situation optimally.

The last two of these functions also represent the contribution internal medicine must make to its sister disciplines—those preparing for the subspecialties, for family medicine, primary care, the clinical nursing specialties, and physician assistants. These are more appropriate and more effective aims than providing other disciplines wtih a potpourri of the organ system specialties in the hope that thereby gross errors of omission and commission in referral will be avoided.

Internal medicine is assuredly not obsolete—only ailing and in need of the courage to examine itself critically. If it can refurbish its image in more realistic terms, it can resolve the centrifugal tendencies of the two ideals which originally gave it birth. When this is done with the intellectual honesty our discipline has always cultivated, the future can be as bright as Osler envisioned in 1897 when he said, ". . . but I maintain (and I hope to convince you) that the opportunities are still great, that the harvest truly is plenteous and the laborers scarcely sufficient to meet the demand."[10]

Even the Oslerian ideal of the master consultant can survive in the newer patterns of care, for there will always be a need for those rare physician's physicians who are distinguished less by a large fund of detailed information than by the clarity of their thought and judgmental processes. These will be the few general consultants of the future; they will emerge from the ranks of the generalists by the acknowledgment of their peers and not as the result of any training program. They will be sought by specialists in medical and surgical fields alike, precisely because they can critically and rigorously examine their colleagues' formulations in a large variety of clinical situations. They bring the tool of a highly sharpened clinical intelligence to bear on the detailed knowledge of the specialist and help him to examine his reasoning about the data in which he is so much more the expert.

Summary

Internal medicine, like general surgery and pediatrics, is today forced to confront a crisis of identity in which it may become lost as an entity or renewed as the synthesizing element in medical care. As it seeks to redefine itself in contemporary and future terms, it will find that some of its cherished attitudes and commitments are, indeed, obsolete. It will gain new strength and identity, not by holding uncritically to its outworn elements or by extending itself into fields like family and community medicine that demand a wholly different orientation. Rather, internal medicine must renew itself by cultivating those regions in which it is particularly adept and even unique. This renewal can grow easily and consciously by a redefinition of the ideals out of which internal medicine was originally generated.

> No single thing abides, but all things flow, fragment to fragment clings; the things thus grow until we know and name them. By degrees they melt and are no more the things we know.
>
> *Lucretius*: De Rerum Natura[11]

References

1. Hammarskjold, D.: *Markings.* New York, Alfred A. Knopf, 1966, p. 67.
2. Osler, Sir W.: Chauvinism in medicine. In *Aequanimitas.* 3rd ed. 1932. New York, Blakiston Division, McGraw-Hill Book Co., 1943, p. 263.
3. Osler, Sir W.: Internal medicine as a vocation. In *Aequanimitas,* p. 133.
4. Ibid.
5. Bloomfield, A. L.: The origin of the term "internal medicine." J.A.M.A. *169*(14):1628–1629, 1959.
6. Osler, Sir W.: *Principles and Practice of Medicine.* New York, D. Appleton, 1892. Sixteenth edition, Appleton-Century, 1947.
7. Faber, K. H.: *Nosography: The Evolution of Clinical Medicine in Modern Times.* 2nd ed. New York, Paul B. Hoeber, 1930.
8. Harrison, T. R.: *Principles of Internal Medicine.* Editors, M. M. Wintrobe et al. 6th ed. McGraw-Hill Book Co., 1970.
9. Pellegrino, E. D.: The generalist function in medicine. J.A.M.A. *198*:541–545, 1966.
10. Osler, Sir W.: Internal medicine as a vocation. In *Aequanimitas,* p. 133.
11. Carus Lucretius, *De Rerum Natura.* W. H. Mallock translation quoted in Charles P. Curtis Jr. and Ferris Greenslot, 3rd ed., Houghton Mifflin Co., Boston, p. 611.

The Broadly Based Internist as the Backbone of Medical Practice

LAWRENCE E. YOUNG

University of Rochester School of Medicine and Dentistry and Medical Service, Strong Memorial Hospital

The Role of Personal Physicians

In an ideal society, every person, young and old, should have a personal physician who renders comprehensive medical care with continuity and who seeks aid of professional colleagues when needed.[1-15] The personal physician, as I see him or her, will function increasingly as a member of a group of physicians and nurse practitioners, and in many instances will be aided by other team members such as physician's assistants, business managers, social workers, secretaries, and perhaps neighborhood health advisors or advocates.

To many patients, legislators, health care planners, and some medical educators, the term "personal physician" means general practitioner or his modern counterpart, the family physician. The role played by internists as personal physicians is grossly underestimated and poorly understood except by the patients who benefit from their services.[11-18] A still larger role that should be assumed by internists in the future is the basis for this essay.

Concern for the role of the personal physician was felt long before the 1970's arrived. William White wrote in 1926: "One of the outstanding features of the medicine of today is specialization. The movement in this direction has been rapid and all inclusive until not only has the whole field of medicine been split up into specialties, but no place has been left for the general practitioner of old."[19] As rapid advances in the medical sciences are incorporated into the delivery of health care, specialization is inevitable. It should be coordinated, not resisted. Services of personal physicians, especially in the delivery of primary care, are nevertheless of growing concern and are the focus of this paper.

The "general practitioner of old" is being replaced in many localities by the family physician whose work consists chiefly of pediatrics and internal medicine, except in smaller communities where he may provide a large share of the obstetrical care. He performs only relatively minor surgical and gynecological procedures.

In the study reported by Riley, Wille, and Haggerty in 1969, 94 per cent of randomly selected family physicians in Upstate New York reported that internal medicine constituted the predominant part of their practice; 84 per cent reported that pediatrics constituted a large but not predominant part of their practice.[20] Thirty-seven per cent of the urban practitioners cared for obstetrical patients and 20 per cent practiced hospital surgery, while 63 per cent of the rural physicians practiced obstetrics and 65 per cent performed surgery. A study of general practitioners in both urban and rural areas of Virginia in 1964 yielded similar figures.[21]

As a consequence of modern transportation and continuing shift of population toward larger communities, urbanization of health care and development of group practices seem both inevitable and desirable.[14,16] The family physician will no doubt be involved less and less with obstetrical and surgical care and his practice will thus consist largely of pediatrics and of general internal medicine for adults.

Should the personal physicians in both urban and rural areas be family physicians functioning by Plan I of the diagram in Figure 1, or should they be pediatricians and internists, dividing family health care by Plan II? For reasons to be explained, I favor Plan II, although it is acknowledged that no data are available upon which to compare the quality and cost of care rendered by these two basic plans. Such data should be obtained, if possible, by use of recently developed methods of evaluating health services, especially those measuring the outcome of health care,[3,22,23] but avoiding common pitfalls in these types of measurements.[24] In the meantime, medical educators should give all possible encouragement to medical students and house officers to prepare for a career as personal physicians by either Plan. Except for differences related to the age group served, the body of knowledge required of the personal physician is the same whether he functions as family physician or as pediatrician or internist. The difference between Plans I and II is one of function or organization rather than of knowledge of the family or other aspects of social medicine. The pediatrician or internist should be as fully interested in and as informed about the family and the community health care system as the family physician.[3,11]

This view with its related challenge to general pediatricians and internists was expressed well by Richardson in 1945: "To say that patients have families is like saying that the diseased organ is a part of the individual. Both facts seem too obvious to discuss, yet for a long time neither received due recognition from the medical profession."[25]

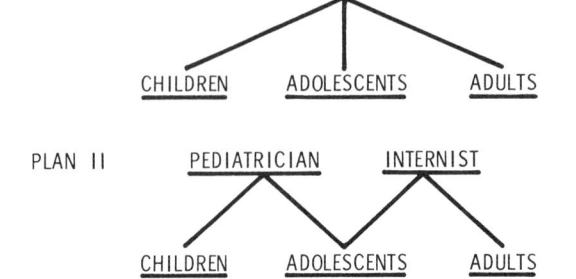

Figure 1. Plans for service of personal physicians.

Functions and Opinions of General Internists in the Rochester Region

The large role of internists as personal physicians was studied by obtaining data and opinions on the practices of internists in the Rochester region. A brief questionnaire was sent in February, 1972, to 140 internists in Monroe County, including Rochester and suburbs, and 10 additional counties extending southward to the Pennsylvania border. Previous reference has been made to the survey of Riley et al. on family physicians in this same region.[20] All internists surveyed had been certified by the American Board of Internal Medicine or had been given appointment in the Department of Medicine of the University of Rochester School of Medicine and Dentistry. Of the 94 internists based full time in the Medical School and associated hospitals, only four were included in the survey because of their known heavy engagement in rendering service as personal physicians in a pilot service and teaching unit, the Internal Medicine Group, within the University Medical Center. The other full-time internists were known to be devoting most of their private practice time to the medical subspecialties, and the remainder of their time to teaching, research, and administration. The population of the region studied is about 1,300,000, with slightly more than 700,000 in Monroe County. The number of questionnaires submitted and returned are given in Table 1.

Table 1. *Survey of Internists in Rochester Region, 1972*

	QUESTIONNAIRES		
	Submitted	Returned	% Returned
Monroe County	110	91	83
Other counties	30	24	80
All counties	140	115	82

The estimates of practice time in Table 2 are only rough approximations since they are not based on actual survey of office records. The data obtained from internists other than hospital-based subspecialists in this survey, as in my study of internists in Monroe County in 1962,[11] indicate that internists in this region devote a large share of their time to general internal medicine and to service as personal physicians. It is especially noteworthy that 51 of the 91 reporting physicians in Monroe County stated that they spent 100 per cent of their time in general internal medicine. The slightly greater engagement of internists in medical subspecialties and in consultations outside Monroe County was anticipated, since a large share of consultations within Monroe County are provided by full-time hospital-based internists.

Table 2. *Use of Practice Time by 115 Internists in Rochester Region*

	AVERAGE %		
	Monroe County	Other Counties	All Counties
General internal medicine	90	86	89
Service as personal physician	87	77	84
Consultations in subspecialty	10	16	10

Table 3. *Medical Subspecialties in Which Practicing Internists Serve as Consultants in Addition to Service as Personal Physicians*

SUBSPECIALTY	91 INTERNISTS MONROE COUNTY	24 INTERNISTS OTHER COUNTIES	TOTAL REPORTS FROM 115 INTERNISTS
Cardiology	10	7	17
10 Other subspecialties	31	6	37
Total	41	13	54

Table 3 summarizes a portion of the data on distribution of medical subspecialties in which practicing internists serve as consultants in addition to service as personal physicians. Thirty-six of the 91 practicing internists surveyed in Monroe County reported engagement in a subspecialty and five reported engagement in two subspecialties, thus giving a total of 41 subspecialty engagements. In the other counties a total of 13 subspecialty engagements were reported. Despite the fact that there are 20 senior full-time cardiologists based in five hospitals in Rochester, there are, in addition, 10 internists in Monroe County and seven in the other counties, all based in private offices in the larger communities and devoting from 5 to 50 per cent of their time to consultations in cardiology. These figures are not surprising in view of the high incidence of heart disease and the additional demands for services of cardiologists resulting from recent development of intensive care units.

Table 4 records the opinions solicited from practicing internists in our region. Ninety-three of the 115 respondents believe that their adult patients prefer to have the family health care divided between a pediatrician and an internist, while 18 believe that a family physician might be preferred by their adult patients; four express no opinion. Thirty-three believe that care of adolescents is neglected when family health care is divided between pediatricians and internists, and many of those responding in this manner suggest that training programs for internists should include more experience with adolescent medicine. All but four of the 115 internists surveyed believe that internists should serve as personal physicians for a large share of the adult population in their respective counties if sufficient numbers of internists were available. The comments of many are well summarized in the brief statement by a member of multispecialty group outside Monroe County: "We need group practice rather than family practice." Opinions of *patients* served by the 115 internists included in this study, as well as opinions of patients served

Table 4. *Opinions of 115 Internists in Rochester Region*

Do you believe your patients:		
Prefer a pediatrician for children?		93
Prefer family physician in lieu of internist and pediatrician?		18
No opinion		4
Do you believe health care of adolescents is neglected when family care is divided?	Yes	33
	No	80
	No opinion	2
Should internists serve as personal physicians for adults in your county?	Yes	111
	No	4

by family physicians in this region, would be of great interest, but thus far have not been obtained.

At the end of the questionnaire general comment was invited and the internists were asked: "What major changes do you recommend for the postdoctoral education of internists who plan to serve as personal physicians for a large share of their patients? That is, what changes do you urge in internship and residency in the institution(s) with which you are most familiar?" Since there is no significant difference in the responses from internists in Monroe County and those in other counties, the responses are presented together in Table 5, as was done in Table 4.

Table 5. *Recommendations of 115 Practicing Internists for Changes in Postdoctoral Education of Personal Physicians*

	NUMBER RECOMMENDING
No change specified	32
Total number recommending one or more changes	83
Less time in medical subspecialties	11
More time devoted to study of:	
Ambulant patient care	54
Psychiatry, sex, and marital counseling	26
Nonsurgical gynecology	19
Health services delivery	13
Otorhinolaryngology	13
Nonsurgical orthopedics	12
Dermatology	10

A total of 158 recommendations were made by the 83 internists responding to this question. Eleven believe that they were overtrained in a subspecialty and that the same is true of many house officers undergoing training in internal medicine today. On the other hand, eight of the physicians heavily engaged in the practice of general internal medicine believe that there is an advantage in practicing a subspecialty along with general medicine.

It is especially noteworthy that 54 of the 83 respondents to this question make a plea for more experience with ambulant patient care, and 26 of the 54 specify that such experience should be obtained partly in the offices of practicing internists, or with a group of physicians who could acquaint the intern or resident with a wider range of health care activities than is feasible in traditional hospital clinics. The other recommendations listed are of interest and should be taken into account in planning educational programs for internists who will serve as personal physicians in the years ahead.

Education of General Internists

The responses obtained from the internists in the Rochester region are similar in many respects to those reported by Engstrom from 107 internists in the Milwaukee area[12] and by Ebert from 140 internists in Minneapolis and St. Paul.[17]

Although there are large differences in the distribution of physicians from one part of this country to another and in relationships between generalists and specialists and between practicing physicians and teaching hospitals, these surveys have value in documenting the major role of the internist as a personal physician. These studies also point to desired changes in educational programs if personal physicians of sufficient numbers and quality are to be available in the years ahead, i.e., if the general internist is to become more available, more competent, and more appreciated, and if the diversion of young physicians into subspecialties is to be related more appropriately to the health care needs of our country. Additional surveys of these types are needed on a national basis.

I concur with other recent authors that medical students should have experience with an efficient health care team providing comprehensive care with continuity and a high degree of competence.[26-29] The experience should be predominantly with ambulant patients, since a very large share of health care is so rendered in the real world. Such experiences might be obtained within a university hospital, a community hospital, or in professional office buildings close to hospitals, in neighborhood health centers, or in other settings apart from hospitals. The student should become acquainted with the many ingredients of good health care as he works with dedicated, carefully chosen personal physicians and learns what other members of the team can contribute.

There should be a reasonable commitment of time in the undergraduate curriculum for such experience under continuing surveillance and evaluation of both students and teachers. New and rigorous types of ambulant patient clerkships as well as inpatient clerkships in the major clinical disciplines should be served before the student is required to make important career decisions and to seek postdoctoral internship or residency appointment. If such experiences are postponed to the postdoctoral years, many students will not give due consideration to the opportunities and satisfactions in careers as personal physicians and they may instead gravitate into various specialties, some of which may be overcrowded in relation to the needs of our society. Moreover, the student who chooses a career involving little or no primary care, either in practice or in an academic setting, may be handicapped by self-centered and parochial views if he has never had experience with the core of the health care system, the primary health care unit.

This movement will require increasing engagement on the part of community hospitals, which should be brought unequivocally into the mainstream of medical education.[16,29-31] We are moving in this direction in Rochester, with four private community hospitals and a county-owned chronic disease hospital closely affiliated with the Medical School and the university-owned Strong Memorial Hospital. Chief residents and other senior residents in medicine are being encouraged to acquire proficiency in primary care and to serve as program innovators and teachers of students and junior house officers in primary health care teams. This set of options is urged for an increasing proportion of senior residents in lieu of more traditional advanced training in medical subspecialties. Steel has written persuasively on these new challenges to chief residents.[32]

Table 6 lists the numbers of approved programs and residencies in the U.S.A. offered in family practice, general practice, internal medicine, and pediatrics.[33] Family practice programs are increasing in number and apparent popularity, while programs in general practice have difficulty in recruiting residents. The

Table 6. *Residencies in U.S. Hospitals 1972-73*

	NO. OF APPROVED PROGRAMS	TOTAL POSITIONS OFFERED
Family practice	87	1,024
General practice	121	734
Internal medicine	421	9,006
Pediatrics	258	3,180
Total for family and general practice, internal medicine and pediatrics	887	13,944
Total for all hospital residencies	4,576	50,948

Council on Medical Education of the American Medical Association reports 87 family practice programs, with 1,024 residencies offered.

For purposes of comparison, Table 6 lists about 9,000 residencies currently offered in internal medicine and about 3,000 in pediatrics. A high proportion of the residencies offered in these disciplines are filled as compared with nationwide data for both family practice and general practice. Accurate current data are not available to indicate the proportion of residents in internal medicine and pediatrics who will serve predominantly in academic careers and/or in subspecialties rather than as personal physicians. Data are also lacking on the national need for medical and pediatric subspecialists in the various categories now recognized. However, data to be cited illustrate the need for increased numbers of residencies in internal medicine designed to prepare more medical school graduates for careers as personal physicians with heavy involvement in primary care.

During each of the last 20 years I have interviewed at length from 25 to 35 members of the fourth year class in our Medical School to discuss career plans and choice of hospitals for internship and residency. I have interviewed still larger numbers of students from other medical schools who were applying for internship in the Strong Memorial Hospital. These students did not represent a random sample since most of them already had made a decision to prepare for a career in internal medicine. Many expressed interest in serving ultimately as a personal physician with only a minor degree of subspecialization, if any. When such students were asked about preparing for a career in family medicine, they usually replied that they could not encompass both pediatrics and adult medicine to their satisfaction because the approach to patient care might be too superficial to meet their standards. I accumulated no data for analysis of these interviews, nor did I try to obtain data from my colleagues in academic pediatrics. However, pediatricians who serve as internship advisors or interviewers of applicants for pediatric internship and residency programs inform me that students give them the same impression about difficulties anticipated in trying to care for the entire family.

Numbers of Personal Physicians Needed

Dr. Kerr White points out that at least 20 per cent of the population in this country moves annually, that the average family moves every seven years, and that physicians themselves have an appreciable degree of mobility as well as finite years of active practice.[3] These facts together with the impact of specialization must be taken into account in considering the extent to which one physician can meet the health care needs of an entire family for decades.

How can we estimate the numbers of personal physicians needed in this country or in any other country? Schonfeld and colleagues estimate that 37 pediatricians and 96 internists, or a total of 133 physicians are required for delivery of primary care per 100,000 persons.[10] The estimates include care rendered in the physician's office, the patient's home, the nursing home, the emergency room, outpatient clinic and inpatient floors of the hospital. The estimates are based not upon current demands, but upon needs for health care of high quality and upon the further assumption that each pediatrician and internist devotes about 2200 hours per year to patient service. The most reliable data on hand for the 50 states and the District of Columbia for the year 1970 reveal an average availability of 28 family physicians, eight pediatricians and 22 internists per 100,000 persons.[9] The shortage of primary care physicians is apparent from these figures.

It is widely acknowledged that the population group most in need of health care are the urban poor and the residents of rural areas.[4,9] It is also generally accepted that simply increasing the physician-population ratio by one means or another will not correct these deficiencies unless other major changes in medical education and in the health care system are effected. A study of 16 state-sponsored programs in which medical students committed themselves to practice in rural communities in exchange for loans or scholarships show that about half of the young physicians did not follow through with their agreement and preferred to return the borrowed money with interest.[34]

The trends toward urbanization of health care and development of group practice are clearly established. These trends permit well recognized division of responsibilities among physicians. The general internist who is not required to care for children can study his adult patients in greater depth, both in the office and in the hospital. He is thus less dependent upon subspecialists whose services may add to the cost and fragmentation of care for the patient with complex illness.

Primary Health Care Units

Code draws an analogy between the disappearance of the solo practitioner and the disappearance of the one-room schoolhouse, both giving way to larger units for similar reasons;[14] he states: "Doctors, like teachers, know when they cannot do the whole job alone. The public is aware of it too, though it is more reluctant to give up the solo doctor's office than the one-room schoolhouse!" My observations in Upstate New York, as well as in the rural Midwest where I grew up, have given me the same impressions. The transition from the general store to the shopping center might be added to this set of analogies.

White suggests that the basic clinical unit should consist of no less than two physicians aided by two physician-assistants or nurse practitioners caring for about 5000 persons.[3] He suggests further that two pairs of internists and one pair of pediatricians together with six nurse practitioners might care for about 18,000 persons. If two nurse-midwives and an obstetrician are added to the group, the total population served might be 20,000. In comparing the recent proposals of White,[3] Code,[14] and Anlyan[16] with the manpower estimates of Schonfeld et al.,[10] one must take into account the inclusion or exclusion of nurse practitioners and other aides and the extent of the physician's responsibility for care of patients during periods of hospitalization.

Code advocates establishment of health care units, each staffed by internists, pediatricians, an obstetrician-gynecologist, a general surgeon, and a psychiatrist.[14] Like many others, he proposes that physicians establish offices for ambulant patients near a community hospital to which their patients would be admitted and which would provide laboratory facilities for their patients.[11,35] Anlyan makes similar recommendations and urges more specifically the establishment of groups of eight to 10 physicians who are chiefly primary medical care specialists.[16] He includes family physicians as well as general internists and general pediatricians in his scheme and urges the development of more training programs for primary medical care. He further specifies that "primary medical care should have a firm base in general practice and/or internal medicine." He predicts that it will become even more difficult in the future to persuade young physicians to practice in remote rural areas.

Teamwork in Primary Health Care

Recent experience has shown convincingly that nurse specialists can assume major responsibilities for patient care in intensive care units and in other settings such as instruction of patients with diabetes or chronic renal failure. Nurse practitioners in ambulant patient care facilities can interview patients, examine them and give advice within certain limitations imposed in part by law and in part by their own training and experience. The performance of nurse practitioners working with pediatricians, internists and family physicians shows that they can handle a large share of the needs of ambulant patients in many settings.[36-43] The same might be said for physician's assistants,[44,45] although the experience of our Department of Medicine has been chiefly with nurses who are establishing increasingly effective co-professional relationships with the medical staff.

Any reasonable assessment of the needs for medical manpower must indeed take into account the enormous contributions that will be made in the future by nurses, physician's assistants, and other aides having special roles. Nonprofessional workers trained on the job for special roles, such as medical interviewing, may become highly effective and thus save the physician's time for functions that he is uniquely qualified to perform, including parts of the physical examination and interview.[46] The increasing acceptance by patients of health team members other than physicians is well documented in recent studies such as that of Beloff and Korper.[47]

Physicians no doubt will become increasingly convinced that nurses and other colleagues on the team not only can save the physician's time, but also can perform many functions more effectively than the physician himself. Increasing involvement of nurse practitioners and other aides with health care in a team effort should encourage physicians to examine more critically their own roles. Internists who develop fully their potential as team leaders by modern standards will contribute increasingly to meeting the total health care needs of the public.

Internists should use more fully their well recognized background of education and experience in pathological physiology, in differential diagnosis, in clinical judgment, and in planning complex programs of management. Too often, however, internists seem content to spend large portions of their time in performing periodic physical examinations, many of which have relatively small yield except in terms of admittedly important re-affirmed doctor-patient relationships.[48] Periodic examinations may be relatively remunerative in financial terms and less arduous than other activities in which an internist should engage. Each internist should assess critically the use of his or her precious time so that the available internist manpower can be used to serve the largest possible number of patients consistent with maintenance of high quality care.

Modernization of Community and Regional Health Care Systems

The internist, like the pediatrician and the family physician, cannot fulfill his role properly unless the health care system of his region is organized and managed far more effectively than has been achieved to date in most parts of this country.[13-15,49-52] The personal physician will have increasing need for regional planning of health care facilities and educational programs, including the continuing education of various categories of health care personnel and the education of the public in personal health care and first-aid; otherwise, his efforts may be defeated in part by intolerable cost to the public, and he will have increasing difficulty keeping pace with the complexities of patient care.

Prepayment plans that encourage economy in health care will quite likely become more prevalent in one form or another, as will group practice arrangements of various types.[15,51] Personal physicians who traditionally are rugged individualists must learn that good management practices, including record keeping, are essential not only in their offices or health care units, but also in the hospitals and nursing homes to which their patients may be admitted and throughout the health care system of the region to which they relate.[53] Let us hope that necessary changes in the system can evolve rapidly and in an orderly manner as a result of combined efforts of private enterprise and public action.

Measurement of Benefits and Costs in Health Care

The health professions and the public must be educated to measure critically the contributions, if any, of the various components of the health care system. It is painfully difficult to prove that many of our current efforts, including some of the most costly, have a significant effect on comfort, morbidity, or mortality.[54]

We shall do well to bear in mind the three general levels of medical technology long recognized but recently labeled and discussed pointedly by Thomas.[55] The first is supportive "non-technology," employed to give all possible comfort and peace of mind, often at great expense, but still deserved by all persons insofar as resources permit. The second level is that of "halfway technology," which tends to predominate on the medical floors of acute general hospitals and is also very costly, especially in intensive care units. The third is "decisive technology" such as immunization to prevent infection or the effects of bacterial toxins, the highly effective treatment of certain infections by antibiotics or chemotherapy, and the remarkably definitive treatment of pernicious anemia with vitamin B-12. Decisive technology, once developed, is relatively inexpensive and represents an enormous gain from biomedical research and enlightened use of public health measures. As we reflect critically upon relative costs and benefits and upon what really makes a difference in the health of our patients, we should also pay attention to the conclusion of Dubos, that "men as a rule find it easier to depend on healers than to attempt the more difficult task of living wisely."[56]

Conclusion

Although I acknowledge the need for more data on many points under consideration, I am convinced that this country needs more general internists to serve as personal physicians. If Americans are interested in quality as well as in access and cost of health care, many more physicians should be encouraged to prepare for a career as general internists. Their education and the systems in which they serve must be changed in accordance with rapidly changing guidelines in health care.

I agree heartily with Mrs. Anne R. Somers of Rutgers, that "yearning for a personal physician and a personal doctor-patient relationship has a firm basis in realities of good medical care. It is a legitimate demand."[15] Because of their large numbers, their interests, and their high standards for patient care and teaching, internists more than any other group of physicians should continue to respond to this demand.[57,58] If they do so with necessary adjustments to the times, the general internist will not become obsolete, but instead will become even more clearly established as the backbone of medical practice.

References

1. Report of the Ad Hoc Committee on Education for Family Practice, Council on Medical Education, American Medical Association: *Meeting the Challenge of Family Practice*, Chicago, A.M.A., 1966.
2. Report of the Citizens Commission on Graduate Medical Education: *The Graduate Education of Physicians*. Chicago, A.M.A., 1966.
3. White, K. L.: Primary medical care for families: Organization and evaluation. New Eng. J. Med. 277:847–852, 1967.
4. Fein, R.: *The Doctor Shortage: An Economic Diagnosis*. Washington, D.C., The Brookings Institution, 1967.

5. Knowles, J. H.: The quantity and quality of medical manpower: A review of medicine's current efforts. J. Med. Educ. 44:81–118, 1969.
6. A special report and recommendations by the Carnegie Commission on Higher Education: *Higher Education and the Nation's Health*. New York, McGraw-Hill Book Co., 1970.
7. Magraw, R. M.: Trends in medical education and health services: Their implications for a career in family medicine. New Eng. J. Med. 285:1407–1413, 1971.
8. Geyman, J. P.: *The Modern Family Doctor and Changing Medical Practice*. New York, Appleton-Century-Crofts, 1971.
9. Mason, H. R.: Manpower needs by specialty. J.A.M.A. 219:1621–1626, 1972.
10. Schonfeld, H. K., Heston, J. F., and Falk, I. S.: Numbers of physicians required for primary medical care. New Eng. J. Med. 286:571–576, 1972.
11. Young, L. E.: Education and roles of personal physicians in medical practice. J.A.M.A. 187:927–933, 1964.
12. Engstrom, W. W.: Are internists functioning as family physicians? Ann. Intern. Med. 66:613–616, 1967.
13. White, K. L.: Personal health services systems: Desiderata. J.A.M.A. 218:1683–1689, 1971.
14. Code, C. F.: Determinants of medical care—a plan for the future. New Eng. J. Med. 283:679–685, 1970.
15. Somers, A. R.: *Health Care in Transition: Directions for the Future*. Chicago, Hospital Research and Educational Trust, 1971, pp. 90, 91, and 95.
16. Anlyan, W. G.: 1985. J. Med. Educ. 46:917–926, 1971.
17. Ebert, R. V.: Training of the internist as a primary physician. Ann. Intern. Med. 76:653–656, 1972.
18. Petersdorf, R. G.: Some contemporary issues facing academic medicine. Pharos 35:120–123, 1972.
19. White, W. A.: *The Meaning of Disease*. Baltimore, The Williams & Wilkins Co., 1926, p. 1.
20. Riley, G. J., Wille, C. R., and Haggerty, R. J.: A study of family medicine in upstate New York. J.A.M.A. 208:2307–2314, 1969.
21. Spencer, F. J.: The changing pattern of general practice and its educational implications. Med. Coll. Va. Quart. 2(2):150–153, 1966.
22. Williamson, J. W.: Evaluating quality of patient care. A strategy relating outcome and process assessment. J.A.M.A. 218:564–569, 1971.
23. Fessel, W. J., and Van Brunt, E. E.: Assessing quality of care from the medical record. New Eng. J. Med. 286:134–138, 1972.
24. Ingelfinger, F. J.: Measuring the quality of health care. New Eng. J. Med. 285:918–919, 1971.
25. Richardson, H. B.: *Patients Have Families*. New York, Commonwealth Fund, 1945, pp. VII, 3.
26. Vayda, E.: Development of primary medical care programs by university teaching hospitals: Issues relating to student and house staff teaching programs in internal medicine. Trans. Ass. Amer. Phys. 83:69–72, 1970.
27. Dorsey, J. L.: Development of primary medical care programs by university teaching hospitals: Issues related to patient care services. Trans. Ass. Amer. Phys. 83:73–77, 1970.
28. Hansen, M. F., and Reeb, K. G.: An educational program for primary care: Definitions and hypotheses. J. Med. Educ. 45:1001–1015, 1970.
29. Young, L. E.: Convictions and predictions on the role of internists in medical education. J.A.M.A. 218:72–74, 1971.
30. Haggerty, R. J.: Community pediatrics. New Eng. J. Med. 278:15–21, 1968.
31. Young, L. E.: Community hospitals in undergraduate medical education. Proceedings of the 5th Ohio Conference for Chiefs of Staff sponsored by Ohio Hospital Association and Ohio State Medical Association, Columbus, Ohio, September 18, 1971.
32. Steel, K.: The medical chief residency in university hospitals. Ann. Intern. Med. 76:541–544, 1972.
33. Medical Education in the United States. Section III, Graduate Medical Education. J.A.M.A. 218:1229–1257, 1971.
34. Mason, H. R.: Effectiveness of student aid programs tied to a service commitment. J. Med. Educ. 44:575–583, 1971.
35. Eichna, L. W.: Verities in chaos. Trans. Ass. Amer. Phys. 84:1–9, 1971.
36. Thomas, L.: Needed: New concepts in medical manpower. Hosp. Pract. 4:37–41, 1969.
37. Bates, B.: Doctor and nurse: Changing roles and relations. New Eng. J. Med. 283:129–134, 1970.

38. Silver, H. K., and Hecker, J. A.: The pediatric nurse practitioner and the child health associate: New types of health professionals. J. Med. Educ. 45:171–176, 1970.
39. Charney, E., and Kitzman, H.: The child-health nurse (pediatric nurse practitioner) in private practice: A controlled trial. New Eng. J. Med. 285:1353–1358, 1971.
40. Extending the scope of nursing practice: A report of the Secretary's Committee to study extended roles for nurses. J.A.M.A. 220:1231–1236, 1972.
41. Riddick, F. A., Bryan, J. B., Gershenson, M. I., and Costello, A. C.: Use of allied health professionals in internists' offices. Arch. Intern. Med. 127:924–931, 1971.
42. Schulman, J., Jr., and Wood, C.: Experience of a nurse practitioner in a general medical clinic, J.A.M.A. 219:1453–1461, 1972.
43. Pesch, L. A.: Education and use of nurses: It's about time! New Eng. J. Med. 286:838, 1972.
44. Estes, E. H., Jr., and Howard, D. R.: Potential for newer classes of personnel: Experiences of the Duke physician's assistant program. J. Med. Educ. 45:149–155, 1970.
45. Smith, R. A., Bassett, G. R., Markarian, C. A., et al.: A strategy for health manpower. J.A.M.A. 217:1362–1367, 1971.
46. Andrus, L. H.: The private physician—overcoming the health manpower shortage. Bull. Amer. Coll. Phys. 10:381–384, 1969.
47. Beloff, J. S., and Korper, M.: The health team model and medical care utilization. Effect on patient behavior of providing comprehensive family health services. J.A.M.A. 219:359–366, 1972.
48. Hoekelmann, R. A.: A 1969 head start program: Implications for change, Rochester, N.Y. J.A.M.A. 219:730–733, 1972.
49. Richards, D. W.: Are our medical school faculties qualified to teach medicine? Resident and Staff Physician, Oct., 1971, pp. 76–88.
50. Rogers, D. E.: The unity of health: Reasonable quest or impossible dream. J. Med. Educ. 46:1047–1056, 1971.
51. Stevens, R.: *American Medicine and the Public Interest.* New Haven, Yale University Press, 1971, pp. 528–541.
52. DuVal, M. K.: A program for rural health development. J.A.M.A. 221:168–171, 1972.
53. Battistella, R. M., and Chester, T. E.: Role of management in health services in Britain and the United States. Lancet 1:626–630, 1972.
54. Haggerty, R. J.: The boundaries of health care. Pharos 35:106–111, 1972.
55. Thomas, L.: Notes of a biology-watcher. The technology of medicine. New Eng. J. Med. 285:1366–1368, 1971.
56. Dubos, R.: *Mirage of Health; Utopias, Progress, and Biological Change.* New York: Harper & Row, 1959.
57. Atchley, D. W.: Science and medical education. J.A.M.A. 164:541–544, 1957.
58. Hecht, H. H.: Research and patient care. J.A.M.A. 217:190–197, 1971.

Comment

Is Internal Medicine Obsolete?

No issue is more likely to be hotly debated in the next few years than the role and manpower requirements of the various medical and surgical specialties. At the very center of this controversy will be the specialty of internal medicine. Before discussing the future role of the internist, it is well to be reminded of his present function. Young has emphasized that most internists in private practice serve as personal physicians for their patients and give continuing primary care. This is combined with a hospital practice involving more complex and urgent medical problems.

Pellegrino suggests that the general internist of the future will confine his efforts largely to a hospital practice where he will coordinate the efforts of a team of highly specialized physicians. He also predicts that most internists will become subspecialists and confine their work to complex medical problems. The family practitioner, with the aid of other health professionals, will provide primary care. This proposed division of responsibility is very much like the British system, where the general practitioner provides primary care and the complex and difficult problems are referred to hospital-based specialists.

Pellegrino correctly interprets the interests of the young man who has recently completed a residency in internal medicine. He prefers a hospital-based practice and often is educated to serve as a consultant in a subspecialty. He thrives in an academic environment and often has an interest in clinical investigation. But if the internist is to cease providing primary care to his patients, a flood of new family physicians will be required. These new family practitioners will have to be convinced that the care of patients with more difficult and complex problems should be turned over to the internist. In Great Britain this is done because of the organizational pattern of the National Health Service. How would it be done in the United States?

Young emphasizes that both the internist and family physician must give primary care if the need is to be met. This is undoubtedly true in view of the present distribution of medical manpower and the current participation of the internist in primary care. The older internist will continue to provide primary care. What about the young internists leaving the training programs? Will they accept comprehensive responsibility for patients on a continuing basis? Must there be a change in emphasis in training programs if internists are to serve as primary physicians? The answers to these questions will determine the future of the specialty of internal medicine.

RICHARD V. EBERT

2

Regulation of Pharmacotherapy by Government

FEDERAL REGULATION IS ESSENTIAL TO PROTECT THE PATIENT
    by Herbert L. Ley, Jr.

BUREAUCRATIC CONTROLS WILL STIFLE BOTH INDUSTRY AND INTELLIGENT MEDICAL PRACTICE
    by Louis Lasagna

COMMENT
    by Maxwell Finland

Federal Regulation Is Essential to Protect the Patient

HERBERT L. LEY, JR.

Former Commissioner, Food and Drug Administration

In the first three years of the decade of the 1970's the medical press has been highly vocal in its criticism of the role of the Federal government in the regulation of drug products. The Food and Drug Administration (FDA) has been the most common target of such criticism, although the Federal Trade Commission has not been immune from similar attacks in its area of responsibility, the regulation of advertising to the laity of non-prescription or over-the-counter (OTC) drug products. That the preponderance of criticism has been directed at FDA's regulation of prescription drug products is understandable on two counts. First—in the opening years of the decade the majority of Federal regulatory actions against drug products have involved prescription drug products as a result of the Drug Efficacy Review of the National Academy of Sciences–National Research Council.[1] Second—it is the practicing physician or the groups representing him whose comments are accepted by the medical press for publication. The medical journals do not, as a rule, publish letters from patients!

It is not reasonable to base a judgment of the effectiveness of and the need for Federal regulation of drug products solely on the role of the Federal government in regulating prescription drug products without also considering the role of the Federal government in regulating OTC products. The critics of Federal prescription drug regulation have in most cases not looked further than their own parochial areas of interest. It is my purpose to provide a broader perspective for the reader so that he may reach his own conclusions regarding the need for Federal drug regulation to protect the patient.

First of all, it is important to recognize that until the year 1906 the Federal government played no role in the regulation of drug products in the United States. The United States Pharmacopeia,[2] beginning in 1820, did fill an important need in specifying the standards for drug items utilized by medical practitioners, but it received no Federal recognition until the Federal Food, Drug, and Cosmetic Act (FD&C Act) was passed in 1906. The stimulus for the passage of that law was the blatant, irresponsible promotion of the so-called patent medicines to the

American public as household remedies for the majority of serious illnesses affecting mankind. It is difficult at this point in history to grasp the abuses of that promotion. Some glimpse into that phase of the past may be gained from James Harvey Young's *The Toadstool Millionaires: A Social History of Patent Medicines in America Before Federal Regulation*,[3] and also from Gerald Carson's *One for a Man, Two for a Horse: A Pictorial History, Grave and Comic, of Patent Medicines*.[4] The patent medicine era of home therapeutics, with the self-treatment of tuberculosis, rheumatism, and dozens of other major illnesses, disappeared with the passage of the FD&C Act in 1906. Undoubtedly some will say that it would be impossible for such abuses to be repeated in the 1970's were the FD&C Act repealed. To the degree that effective cures for such diseases as tuberculosis are known to the public, such comments are probably valid. On the other hand, for diseases such as multiple sclerosis, cancer, and others for which no legitimate therapy is available, one does not have to look far to be convinced that similar abuses could and would occur if the FD&C Act disappeared from the Federal Statutes.

In his second major work, *The Medical Messiahs: A Social History of Health Quackery in Twentieth-Century America*,[5] Young describes the gullibility of the public regarding cancer cures which were unsupported by scientific evidence of medical benefit to the patient. Two examples are the so-called Hoxsey Cancer Cure and Krebiozen. Where there is no hope, the public is all too eager to utilize unproved cures, frequently at great expense, and sometimes erroneously in those types of cancer which are amenable to legitimate chemotherapy. It is not sufficient to say that the public of the 1970's is so well informed that it will not be misled by misleading claims or rumors of claims of benefit. The record proves otherwise.*

In the area of prescription drugs the situation is both simpler and more complex because of the role of the physician in the choice of therapy. The physician is educated to use the healing arts and sciences for the benefit of the patient. Where the healing art is practiced pharmacologically rather than surgically, it is the physician's responsibility and intent to select the medication that is most likely to produce the maximum benefit with the least adverse effects for the particular patient under his care. This task was once much easier than it is today. When the United States Pharmacopeia was created in 1820, it included 217 drugs which were then considered worthy of recognition. The present 1970 XVIII Edition of the Pharmacopeia listed 1103 articles upon publication, approximately five times more than the first edition. The National Formulary, XIII Edition,[6] listed a total of 992 articles upon publication in 1970. Both publications list principally single-ingredient drugs, except for a few restricted categories; the articles listed may fall into either the prescription or OTC categories. The First Edition of *American Medical Association Drug Evaluations, 1971*,[7] contains 44 pages in its drug index

---

*An argument can be advanced for making such unproved cancer cures available *at cost* to the public as a placebo in those instances in which the patient's condition is evaluated medically as hopeless. In the two examples of cancer cures mentioned above, evidence presented in the courts demonstrated that the originators of the cures became wealthy at the expense of the hopeless patients who received "treatment." A patient has the right to try "last resorts" where all else has failed, perhaps, but no individual has the right to wealth wrung from such desperate patients. The issue is beyond the scope of this paper.

section, each one of which lists approximately 100 drug products, both single-ingredient and combination, and also prescription and OTC products.

It is apparent that the physician of the 1970's has several thousands of drug products at his disposal to "prescribe" for his patients, either by formal written prescription or by verbal instruction to the patient. His pharmacologic resources are many-fold greater than those of his counterpart in the United States a century and a half ago. Looked at in one light, this is a highly commendable situation; in another light, one can question whether any single physician can master the use of several thousand different drug products. It is the multiplicity of products available that makes the physician's role in pharmacologic therapy complex.

Many, and probably most, physicians concentrate their efforts in drug therapy to a small proportion of the total number of drugs available and, where this is the case, they gain by direct observation an intimate and detailed knowledge of the effects of the drug in terms of both its benefits and its adverse reactions in their patients. However, each time a new drug product is introduced to the market a physician starts from zero as far as his personal experience with the drug is concerned. He must in his initial use of a new product trust the observations of other physicians in their use of the drug, and hope, if he cannot speak personally to the other physicians involved, that their experiences have been accurately communicated to him by the medium through which he first learns of the drug.

The media of communication of such information are rather limited, and are usually oriented to the medical profession, although they may occasionally involve the public media of the press, radio, and television. Use of the public media for communication of information on prescription drugs is, except for items having genuine public health or news impact, prohibited by the FD&C Act. Prescription drugs, in contrast to OTC drugs, may not be promoted to the laity. Most commonly a physician learns of a new drug product through an advertisement in a medical journal, a research report in a similar journal, or the visit of the representative of its manufacturer, the drug sales agent or detail man. If the physician is to utilize the new drug product effectively and safely in the treatment of patients, the information reaching him through these channels must be scientifically and medically accurate.

It is not the purpose of this discussion to evoke the specter of the thalidomide birth defects which led to the passage of the 1962 amendments to the FD&C Act, or even that of the sulfonamide deaths which led to the passage of the 1938 amendments to the Act. These incidents are history. They were the critical events which stimulated the Congress and the President of the United States to impose more severe drug regulation on the total drug industry in an effort to prevent similar situations from occurring in the future. It is inconceivable that any physician would have prescribed either of these products if he had been informed of the consequences of the use of the drugs in patients. The important point to be gleaned from these events is that the information available to the physicians using these products was incomplete. In an effort to protect the patient, the Federal government chose, after protracted public hearings, to impose more restrictive regulations on the drug industry that would improve the reliability of information reaching the physician regarding the drugs which he prescribed.

The role that the Federal government plays in the regulation of the drug industry is not unlike the roles it also plays in the regulation of air transport or the securities and financial market. In air transportation the passenger's safety is totally dependent upon the skill and training of the pilot and the reliability of the aircraft in which he is traveling. The Federal government, through the Federal Aviation Administration, regulates or approves both of these critical elements in air transportation. In the stock markets the individual investor is dependent upon the honesty of his broker and the accuracy of the information in the prospectus or annual report of the firm in which he wishes to invest. The Securities and Exchange Commission is responsible for the protection of the interests of the public and the investors against inaccurate or misleading information in the securities and financial markets. In both of these examples the individual's safety or well-being is dependent upon another person in much the same fashion that the patient is dependent upon the physician. The pilot or investment advisor, in providing services to the individual, utilizes an aircraft or investment documents which are regulated by the Federal government much as a physician uses drugs which are regulated by the Federal government. A significant difference is that the physician is licensed or registered by state jurisdictions, whereas the pilot or advisor is licensed or registered by the Federal government. In both of the non-medical analogies experience has shown that some form of regulation is necessary to protect the individual.

The topic of this discussion is whether the individual patient also requires a form of Federal regulation to protect him from either ineffective forms of treatment or pharmacologic hazards of drug therapy. In attempting to answer this question, we are *not* addressing the question of whether the pilot, investment advisor, or physician has met the standards of his profession. That is another question which lies far outside the scope of this discussion. It is most important to make the distinction between the personal skills and training of the pilots, advisors, and physicians and the mechanical, financial, or chemical tools with which they practice their respective professions. Unless this distinction is made sharply and cleanly, the discussion of the regulation of drug supply becomes clouded by the extraneous but related issue of the competence of the person in whom the patient places his trust.

In viewing the problems of Federal regulation of drug products the physician frequently and understandably takes the position of spokesman for his patients. This is natural, for few patients have the background and training to understand the pharmacology of drug therapy, and for that reason they are unable to speak for themselves on pharmacologic topics. On the other hand, there are topics and issues on which the patient can be expected to speak with both feeling and authority, and these are three in number.

First, the patient expects the same drug product purchased at different locations in this country and at different times to be reproducibly similar in efficacy, quality, and safety. One needs only to read the weekly FDA drug recall lists to recognize that even with the present level of drug regulation by the Federal government this objective is not always met. Some lots of drugs may be superpotent, others subpotent, and still others contaminated with inactive or even harmful substances. Is it logical to believe that the quality of the drug supply destined for patient use would improve if the Federal government ceased to regulate drug products? What purpose is served by standards of drug quality established by the United States Pharmacopeia or the National Formulary if regulatory control is not exercised to ensure that products in the marketplace meet the established standards? Unless the patient and his physician are prepared to conduct the quality control analyses on the drugs consumed, some governmental regulatory agency should perform such testing. If it is not done the patient must accept significant and sometimes dangerous variation in the potency or purity of the drugs he utilizes at the recommendation of his physician. In this area the patient feels very strongly that the drugs he purchases should meet appropriate standards for potency and purity established by a qualified body. Federal regulation of the quality of drug products is patently necessary.

Second, the patient expects, through his trust in his physician, that the drug prescribed for treatment of his disease condition will be efficacious and reasonably safe. He expects his physician to alert him or warn him of possible dangers and major side effects which he may anticipate from use of the drug prescribed. For the physician to provide this information, he himself must be well informed regarding the drug. This requires the availability of factual, concise information to the physician. If the drug in question was in use during the period the physician was in training, he was probably exposed to this information as a part of his preparation to practice medicine. If not, and this represents a large proportion of the drugs prescribed today, the physician must seek other sources of information. These may take the form of refresher courses, textbooks, journal articles, *Physicians' Desk Reference*,[8] medical journal advertisements, or information presented by the drug firm through the mails or by a drug detail man. Rarely, the physician may turn to the document prepared jointly by the manufacturer and the FDA, the package circular or insert, for the information which he seeks. Whether the physician actually utilizes the package circular directly is of little consequence because its content is reflected in the *Physicians' Desk Reference* and all other information presented to the physician by the manufacturer. The patient expects accurate information from the physician, regardless of where he obtains it. The role of Federal regulation in assuring the accuracy of that information in the package circular will be discussed after considering the patient's third expectation.

Third, the patient believes and expects that all drug products in the marketplace have received a government "Seal of Approval" in regard to efficacy and safety. Not all patients are able to identify which agency gives this seal of approval, but they believe it exists. This belief on the part of the patient is not adequate justification for Federal regulation, but if the Federal government does not regulate the drug supply the public must be informed of this fact. At present the FD&C Act has convinced both the Congress and the public that the drug supply is regulated, as indeed it is. If the regulatory statutes were to be terminated, the nation would have to be informed of the cessation of oversight of the industry, and it is highly likely that the patient and the public would object strongly and vocally to such a change. To a degree, the famous quote of Voltaire, "If God did not exist, it would be necessary to invent him," applies to government regulation of drugs, whether by the present FDA or by any other designated agency given the responsibility of administering the Federal statutes. On all three counts of patient expectations it is almost impossible to conclude that Federal regulation of drugs is unneeded and unnecessary.

The package circular or insert, mentioned earlier as the basis for all information communicated to physicians by the manufacturers of drugs, has been much maligned in recent years. Its origin predates the 1938 amendments to the FD&C Act, and, as nearly as can be determined, it began as a courtesy of the manufacturers to physicians in providing them with a concise, factual summary of the known information on the drug. The package circular came to be included in the term "labeling" in the FD&C Act, a term much more inclusive than the label on the drug bottle and the box containing the bottle. The present FD&C Act states that a drug is misbranded if its *labeling* is false or misleading in any particular (Sec. 502(a)),[9] so that the contents of the package circular must be an accurate reflection of what is known about the drug. Because the package circular is also the basis of all advertising claims that may be made for the drug, it becomes a very important document in the eyes of both the manufacturer and the FDA. It is therefore not surprising that the final text of the package circular, which is intended to summarize the contents of a voluminous New Drug Application, is the subject of extended and sometimes heated discussion between the manufacturer and the FDA. It is also not surprising that clarity of expression is sometimes lost in the argument regarding the manner in which a claim is expressed in the circular. In fact, the physician rarely sees the circular itself, although all subsequent promotion and advertising materials which he does see are held to the limits defined in the package circular. A document of this importance must be held to high standards of scientific and medical accuracy if the physician is to have the benefit of concise information on the several thousand drugs available for prescription for patients. From a purely practical viewpoint the level of power and authority to monitor the package circular can be provided only by Federal regulation of the circular. Thus, Federal regulation appears essential to achieve this end.

The physicians' views of the package circular have been colored by the role the document has played in malpractice litigation. There are signs that the courts are finally seeing the light of reason in respect to the position that the package circular occupies among the spectrum of information available on any given drug. Neil L. Chayet has summarized in two articles in the *New England Journal of Medicine* both the legal dilemma posed by the package circular and the evolving legal opinion that the information in the package circular is not legally binding but rather "no more than a recommendation" to be given a position among other valid sources of medical information.[10,11]

After reviewing these several needs for drug regulation, it is almost impossible to conclude that regulation is unnecessary to protect the patient's interests. On the other hand, it is also apparent that much of the criticism of the role of the Federal government in drug regulation is more a plea for enlightened Federal effort based on sound scientific and medical evaluation than it is for the repeal of the FD&C Act. Unfortunately the task of regulation of drugs is not considered an exciting, all-consuming career as, for example, the medical research career has been considered for the past 25 years. As a result, the Federal regulatory agencies concerned with drug regulation have suffered from the lack of personal involvement on the part of those scientists and physicians who are best qualified to assist the agencies with their task of regulation. If progress is to be made toward more enlightened Federal drug regulation in the patients' interest, more physicians and scientists must become a party to the regulatory process and participate in the process. To use the current idiom, they must "become involved" in a constructive role rather than merely criticize Federal regulation of drugs from the sidelines. Whether "involvement" means a year's post-doctoral fellowship in the FDA, membership on its advisory committees, or brief periods of one or two years' employment in Federal government must be left to the individual concerned. Regardless of the method of involvement, the end results will be better understanding of the regulatory mechanism on the part of the involved physicians and scientists and better decision making on the part of the regulatory agencies. The persons benefiting most from such an exchange of ideas will be the recipients of the drugs regulated—the patients—who are, after all, the reason that the drug regulatory mechanisms were created in the first place.

References

1. Drug efficacy study: Final report to the Commissioner of Food and Drugs. Washington, D.C., National Academy of Sciences–National Research Council, 1969.
2. *The Pharmacopeia of the United States of America.* 18th Rev. Easton, Pa., Mack Publishing Co., 1970.
3. Young, J. H.: *The Toadstool Millionaires: A Social History of Patent Medicines in America Before Federal Regulation.* Princeton University Press, 1961.
4. Carson, G.: *One for a Man, Two for a Horse; A Pictorial History, Grave and Comic, of Patent Medicines.* New York, Bramhall House, 1961.
5. Young, J. H.: *The Medical Messiahs: A Social History of Health Quackery in Twentieth-Century America.* Princeton University Press, 1967.
6. *The National Formulary.* 13th ed. Easton, Pa., Mack Publishing Co., 1970.
7. *AMA Drug Evaluations.* 1st ed. Chicago, American Medical Association, 1971.
8. *Physicians' Desk Reference*, Ed. 26. Oradell, N.J., Medical Economics, Inc., 1972.
9. Federal Food, Drug, and Cosmetic Act as amended, January 1971. Washington, D.C., U.S. Government Printing Office, 1971, p. 36.
10. Chayet, N. L.: Law-medicine notes: Power of the package insert. New Eng. J. Med. 277:1253, 1967.
11. Chayet, N. L.: Law-medicine notes: Malpractice—a break with the past. New Eng. J. Med. 278:1275, 1968.

Bureaucratic Controls Will Stifle Both Industry and Intelligent Medical Practice

LOUIS LASAGNA

University of Rochester School of Medicine and Dentistry

A decade ago many academicians were vigorously battling to strengthen the Food and Drug Administration. The Blatnik and the Kefauver committee hearings had accused the pharmaceutical industry of promotional excesses, high profits, and shoddy clinical investigation. The failure of previous legislation to spell out proof of efficacy as a prerequisite to FDA approval was considered a serious deficiency, and the inclusion of this requirement in the 1962 Kefauver-Harris Amendments was backed by a series of academic and professional witnesses at the hearings that preceded the legislation.

Now, 10 years later, a certain disenchantment has set in. It is not, to be sure, universal. There are still many who believe the drug industry to be a work of the devil, its leaders eager only to increase their share of filthy lucre, regardless of the consequences of such policy for the pocketbooks or the bodies of the American public. For these anti-industry types, the FDA is either performing its task well or not being "tough enough" on industry. It is from this direction that pressure has been exerted on the FDA, via the threat of litigation, to move more rapidly in following through on the judgments of the expert panels involved in the NAS-NRC Drug Efficacy Review.

Nevertheless, there is considerable evidence that all is *not* well in the FDA. Since the retirement of Commissioner Larrick, a small parade of physicians has passed through the FDA, holding the reins of power briefly, only to leave under more or less unpleasant circumstances. Dr. Sadusk, Dr. Goddard, Dr. Ley, and now Dr. Edwards have occupied important posts, the latter three having been Commissioners during the brief period of time since Larrick's resignation. All competent men, their difficulties cannot be glibly written off. Many reviews of the agency, including that of the recent Ritts Committee appointed by Dr. Edwards himself, have recorded at length and in detail the deficiencies in the organization and workings of the agency. Off the record, agency personnel will talk despondently of the lack of scientific talent within the FDA and of the poor morale among its personnel. In 1972 a contract was let to a Philadelphia firm to review (and presumably improve) the processing of NDA's (new drug applications). Several medical officers with a reputation for a "negative" philosophy toward approval of new drugs have been reassigned within the agency. A group of well known medical scientists (the so-called Dripps Committee) has petitioned Congressman Paul Rogers, Chairman of the Subcommittee on Public Health and Environment of the House Interstate and Foreign Commerce Committee, to institute a high level review of the current status of drug development. Respected academic and NIH researchers have publicly decried what they consider unseemly difficulties in getting permission for the use of chemicals as research tools or as potential new therapeutic agents. Editors and AMA officials have crossed swords with the FDA in regard to infringements on the right of the physician to practice medicine.

Whatever the reasons, therefore, there is almost constant critical ferment in and around the FDA. The agency is usually under attack from at least one quarter. Since the criticisms are at times opposite in thrust (urging more restrictions or less simultaneously), it is not easy to be sure where to lay the blame. This paper will attempt to convince the reader that FDA is pursuing policies that are deleterious to drug development, intelligent medical practice, and the public welfare.

To begin with, there is evidence that the United States has for some time been lagging behind other countries in the introduction of new drugs. The approval of new pharmaceuticals is, of course, not ipso facto beneficial for a society. A chemical always produces toxicity (unless it is biologically inactive), and its capacity for benefit and harm can never be assessed with assurance before many years of extensive use in different patients and situations by practitioners of various experience and competence. Hence, a policy that results purposely or accidentally in delay of approval until other countries have provided such experience is likely to provide benefit in a negative kind of way to the society thus protected from harm that is not predictable prior to marketing. The availability of each new drug, further, requires the doctor to integrate additional data into his already overcrowded store of information and is potentially a source not just of therapeutic flexibility but of confusion as well.

It is unfortunate that one cannot describe with precision this balance sheet for the United States, but measurement of the harm accruing from *not* having good new drugs available in America is matched in difficulty by the measurement of the harm that we have been spared by the FDA's failure to approve poor or excessively toxic drugs.

Let us consider the latter problem first. How many "bad" drugs have we been spared? There are countries, certainly, where trivial, worthless, or irrational products have been marketed even in recent years with relative ease. No one with any sense of responsibility can argue for such ultra-permissiveness. But even countries with reasonably effective supervision of new drugs have occasionally approved chemicals that turned out to be unpredictably toxic. Thalidomide is the most famous example. Aminorex, an appetite suppressant thought by some to have induced pulmonary hypertension in certain obese patients, may be another. Stolley[1] has suggested that the increased mortality from asthma experienced in certain countries in the 1960's was related to the marketing of aerosol nebulizers containing a higher concentration of isoproterenol than was available in countries (such as the U.S.) spared this excess mortality. While the evidence for this hypothesis is incomplete in some respects, the thesis is an attractive one. So far as I have been able to find out, the failure of American manufacturers to market the incriminated preparations was not due to denial of such a request by the FDA. Apparently U.S. manufacturers did not consider such a high concentration to be desirable and, hence, did not seek approval. Nevertheless, the failure of regulatory mechanisms abroad, formal or informal, to prevent such marketing indicates that occasionally the United States population may indeed be spared serious toxicity by differences between our country and others in regard to the ease of obtaining approval for marketing pharmaceuticals. (For the U.K., at least, the marketing of the suspect preparations was really a matter of *no* controls, since marketing began there in 1959, before the Dunlop Committee was even formed.)

In contrast to the relative paucity of examples of this first type, however, there is a lengthy list of drugs to suggest that the American patient has suffered considerably from FDA policies. The least controversial and most easily analyzable group of drugs is that which has ultimately received marketing approval in the United States and other countries. It has been pointed out that the United States was the 41st country to approve lithium for the treatment of mania[2] and the 51st country to approve rifampicin for the treatment of tuberculosis.[3] Neither of these drugs is a "me-too." Each is an important addition to the therapeutic armamentarium. So is ethambutol, considered by many now to be a first-line drug in the treatment of tuberculosis. Lidocaine was used for years all over the world as an antiarrhythmic agent before the FDA approved this indication for the drug. Propranolol, despite convincing evidence as to its efficacy as an antianginal drug, is still approved only as an anti-arrhythmic in this country.

Recently, I surveyed 82 new single entities that had been marketed in the United States during the years 1965 to 1969.[4] For 43 of these, introductory dates in at least one foreign country were available. France showed an average lead time of one year, i.e., the products were introduced one year earlier on the average than in the U.S. The average lead time for Germany was 1.6 years, and for England 2.1 years. This list included such important products as clofibrate, propranolol, cloxacillin, allopurinol, azathioprine, amantadine, furosemide, ethambutol, methotrimeprazine, amytriptyline, haloperidol, ethacrynic acid, and clomiphene. Wardell, in a more recent analysis,[5] has reviewed the data on new single chemical entities marketed during the years 1966 to 1971. As of December 31, 1971, 58 were mutually available in both the U.S. and U.K. Of these, 12 had been marketed simultaneously, 13 had been marketed first in the United States, with a mean lead time of 2.7 years, while 33 had been marketed first in the United Kingdom, with a mean lead time of 3.3 years. More recent figures collected by Paul DeHaen show that of 50 products selected as "worth watching," 31 have already been marketed abroad—four of them for 10 to 12 years. It has been alleged that the decline in new drugs is a worldwide phenomenon, but the drop in U.S. approvals has been matched by a rise in some European countries and in Japan.

Wardell has also looked at the record for drugs approved abroad but not yet approved in the United States, and vice versa. A long list of beta-blockers, antihypertensives, antianginal agents, diuretics, beta-agonist bronchodilators, antiallergic compounds, psychotropic drugs, anesthetic agents, anti-inflammatory drugs, and agents to treat gastrointestinal complaints have been introduced in the United Kingdom, but not in the United States, some of them as long as nine years ago.

Examination of a few specific therapeutic areas, such as anticancer drugs and antibiotics, by Wardell showed that the lag does not exist categorically across all therapeutic subgroupings. Bloom[6] pointed out earlier that the cardiovascular-respiratory area, in contrast to the ones just mentioned, shows a record extraordinary in the paucity of new compounds approved in this country in recent years. These facts suggest either different standards for therapeutic areas or different standards or philosophies of individual monitors in charge of the several divisions within the FDA.

My own experience suggests that the differences lie with individual monitors within the FDA, and with their personal standards and philosophy. There are some FDA physicians, for example, who believe that the public is best protected if no new drugs are approved, or if the delay until approval is made as long as possible. Others demand extraordinary amounts of clinical investigation or animal testing, or have standards of "adequacy" that are so unrealistically high that no real life research is likely to meet their standards. Still others, infatuated with the controlled clinical trial as a way of providing evidence, are unwilling to consider seriously any other forms of information. For still others, three or four well done and positive studies are "inadequate," and many hundreds or even thousands of cases are required of the sponsor, even when past experience suggests a rapidly diminishing proportion of new information from such prolonged trials.

These are not the only problems. I have presented elsewhere[4] case histories of specific drugs to show how sequential requests for clarification or for new data can prolong interminably the processing of a new drug application. In addition, the conference system for NDA's often seems to work poorly, with head-to-head confrontations between FDA and industrial personnel resulting in impasses rather than compromise and agreement. (I do not, however, imply that these impasses are always the fault of the FDA or that poor quality of submitted data may not delay the process.)

The FDA also suffers from its inept use of experts. All too often expert opinion is not effectively received to help make the fundamental judgments concerned with evaluation of evidence and the decision to grant approval for marketing. On other occasions fairly superficial opinions by experts, such as occurred during some of the NAS-NRC Drug Efficacy Review, are equated with Universal Truth, with resultant pressures upon pharmaceutical firms to generate new data, or to revise claims, or to remove drugs from the marketplace. Another example of such blind worship of experts is the case of fixed-ratio combination drugs. Since the academic mind is inclined to oppose such combinations categorically, the

FDA seems disposed to remove most such preparations from the market, despite the impressive case that can be made for some of them.

The absence of any effective appeal procedures for manufacturers who are unconvinced of the wisdom of a given FDA regulatory act makes it possible for the FDA to impose a pharmacologic Lysenkoism on the medical community. A former chief counsel for the FDA justified the arbitrary refusal of such appeals by the rule of expediency, i.e., it would take too long to do it by observing due process, an unconvincing, unattractive, and cynical justification (unless traditional American legal avenues are to be summarily closed as not worth the trouble).

Still another example of inflexibility has been the FDA position that one "modern" standard should be applied to all drugs, be they old or new, ethical or over-the-counter. While attractive in theory, and perhaps bureaucratically easier to apply than a more flexible stand, it seems hardly in the public interest to demand "modern" controlled trial data for every medication now on the market. To demand such evidence for old over-the-counter remedies, whose ingredients and dosages are chosen so as to be safe when self-prescribed, would strain the economic and personnel resources available to perform such studies, many of which would be doomed to failure because of the technical difficulties involved in their performance (such as failure of outpatients to comply with directions).

Modell[7] has eloquently attacked the FDA for trying to limit proper practice of medicine by imparting to what he contemptuously calls the "package stuffer" a legal authority which it does not possess. As Archer[8] has pointed out, "the regulation of the practice of medicine involves a large body of laws, statutory and common, federal and local. Ethics and standards of competence set by the profession itself are equally demanding, but nothing in the Federal Food, Drug, and Cosmetic Act constrains a practicing physician to have his medical decisions determined by a pharmaceutical company and the FDA through a package insert that the physician has been no party to preparing."

A considerable controversy exists in regard to the action of the Food and Drug Administration in constructing labeling for oral hypoglycemic drugs which attempts to impose on the physician a priority of approaches to the management of the diabetic patient. Thus, the physician is supposed to consider insulin before using oral hypoglycemic agents after diet and weight reduction have failed, despite the fact that insulin is notoriously unsuccessful in the management of many of the patients treated with oral agents, and despite failure to distinguish insulin from placebo in the very study used as a basis for the new labeling! A group of diabetic experts filed a brief with the Commissioner enjoining him to reconsider this decision and not to require such labeling. Their request fell on deaf ears.

Another example of this tendency is evident in the current posture of the FDA in regard to comparative efficacy. Despite the absence of legal backing for this position, the FDA seems to feel it important to take an official stand, via labeling, on comparative efficacy. While information of this sort is obviously desirable and useful to the physician, clear-cut judgments about the relative merits of drugs are often difficult to make in the generality, and impossible in the particular. In this regard, the British equivalent of the FDA, the Dunlop Committee, has assiduously avoided such postures as inappropriate and unwise.

A further blurring of the boundaries between the FDA and medical practice is evident in the plan of the FDA to construct "monographs" for both ethical and over-the-counter remedies, which may prove "convenient" for the FDA in dealings with pharmaceutical firms, but which will tend to restrict labeling and other advertising to "class" claims that will inevitably ignore differences between compounds that may (and should) tilt the balance in favor of a given member of a drug class when dealing with individual patients.

Archer[8] has also referred to the lack of legal foundation for "private IND's," i.e., the filing of investigational new drug applications by private or academic physicians who have no desire to accumulate data for the ultimate filing of an NDA, but merely want to use a drug in a way somewhat different from that which the labeling approves. Archer's stand, if legally correct, would mean that the discomfort of many academic investigators produced by their attempts to acquire IND "permission" from the FDA has been just so much wasted effort and needless frustration.

Certain other areas of difficulty exist. One concerns the increased cost and time required for development of a new pharmaceutical compound. Current estimates are that it takes from four to 15 million dollars, and five to seven years, on average, to market a new drug.[4] There is evidence that this increasing cost and difficulty is responsible for a more conservative and less adventuresome approach to drug development by the pharmaceutical industry (conservative in a pejorative sense, i.e., avoiding research programs to come up with badly needed new drugs in areas where predicting utility is difficult, or where sales would be less than in other areas). Much drug research is now being done abroad that would have been done in the United States in other times. At least part of the increased cost and time seems attributable to excessive demands in regard to animal toxicology and clinical data and inept processing of NDA's. An inevitable victim of this tendency is the "unprofitable drug," i.e., the chemical designed (or accidentally discovered) to ameliorate a rare medical condition. Such drugs have never had high priority within the pharmaceutical industry, but the facts of life dictate that the energetic pursuit of such new drugs will now make even less economic sense to most pharmaceutical firms.

A serious problem arises from the absence of adequate numbers and quality of personnel within the FDA. It is not easy to attract to a regulatory agency scientists of high caliber, at least with the FDA organized as it now is. Certain past delays in the processing of applications have been acknowledged to be attributable to the paucity of experienced statisticians within the FDA. One section head at the FDA has told me that he believes quality decision-making will not be possible until the scientific judgments are rendered by experts from outside the agency, and he has declared his preference for the summarizing of data for presentation to such experts to be prepared by extra-agency scientists as well.

It is essential that decisions be made by competent, courageous, prestigious individuals; the introduction of any new drug is a calculated risk, and we must have hard-headed weighings of the estimated costs and benefits. At times, to be sure, the FDA's hands have been tied by legislation (such as in the case of the Delaney Amendment, which makes it impossible to consider cost-benefit analyses in dealing with food additives that have been shown to be carcinogenic in any species when given by an appropriate route). On most occasions, however, the cost-benefit analyses can be made without such legal restraints, but at the present time such judgments are too often made within the FDA by people who espouse the philosophy that the public is best served if the approval of new pharmaceutical products is delayed for long periods of time. Such a philosophy makes no attempt to enter into the equation the losses that come from not having important new agents available promptly. It fails to appreciate how data on drug efficacy and safety can never be complete prior to marketing. It fails to encourage the development of effective postmarketing monitoring of a drug's performance that would allow earlier approval with a minimum of risk. Too rarely now—such as when L-dopa came along, and fierce pressures for its approval were omnipresent—does the FDA show its ability to make prompt, wise, and courageous judgments. Medical progress and intelligent medical practice are bound to suffer if inept bureaucratic controls are allowed to strangle scientific judgment and medical wisdom. As Pelletier[9] has written: "Dogmatism . . . is . . . an artificial reinforcement of our sense of security. . . . The definition of relativistic knowledge, on the other hand, carries no implication of absolute truth. An idea is held to be accurate until it has been proved inaccurate. The mark of relativistic knowledge is in its permanent acceptance of challenge. The scientific spirit is the very essence of relativism, because it not only accepts challenge but systematically encourages it."

References

1. Stolley, P.: Asthma mortality. Why the United States was spared an epidemic of deaths due to asthma. Ann. Rev. Resp. Dis. *105*:883–890, 1972.
2. Editorial: America first—or 41st? Lithium and manic-depressive reactions. Med. Tribune, Oct. 27, 1971.
3. Editorial: America first—or 51st? New treatment for tuberculosis. Med. Tribune, Nov. 3, 1971.
4. Lasagna, L.: Research, regulation, and the development of new pharmaceuticals: Past, present, and future. Amer. J. Med. Sci. *263*:8–18; 67–78, 1972.
5. Wardell, W.: Introduction of new therapeutic drugs in the United States and Great Britain: An international comparison. Clin. Pharmacol. Ther. In press.
6. Bloom, B. B.: The Rate of Contemporary Drug Discovery. Presented before Division of Medicinal Chemistry, A.C.S., Chicago, Sept. 15, 1970.
7. Modell, W.: FDA censorship. Clin. Pharmacol. Ther. *8*:359–361, 1967.
8. Archer, J.: Instrument or impediment? The regulatory monograph in medical communications. J.A.M.A. *220*:1474–1477, 1972.
9. Pelletier, G.: Science, Technology, and the Political Response. In *Civilization and Science in Conflict or Collaboration?* Elsevier. Excerpta Medica, North-Holland, 1972.

Comment

Regulation of Pharmacotherapy by Government

Most laws and governmental regulations which restrict our actions are really reactions of the people, through their elected representatives, either to an accumulation of flagrant excesses that have been committed and which they consider unacceptable, or to serious and sometimes catastrophic events, the recurrence of which the laws are intended to prevent. Regulations are made by the bureaucrats within the staff of the agency charged with administering the law; they are intended to codify what the agency sees as the requirements for implementing the laws.

In the United States the earliest attempts to regulate drugs were voluntary and privately inspired; they were intended to set uniform standards of purity and efficacy as well as safety for the therapeutic agents available at the time. Thus, the Pharmacopeial Convention was first called by a group of physicians and pharmacists in 1820, nearly three quarters of a century before the first of the major federal laws was passed to control biological and medicinal agents. There followed the successive editions of the U.S. Pharmacopeia, the National Formulary, and various activities and publications of the AMA's Council on Pharmacy and Chemistry. All these were reactions to the multitude of nostrums and quackeries rampant among the patent medicines that were sold in quantities to a gullible public.

Our Federal laws were essentially the direct consequence of a series of catastrophic events: a number of deaths from tetanus among children being immunized against diphtheria; the total impact of the nostrums, and the revelation of the deplorable and unhealthy state of the meat packing plants in Chicago; more than a hundred deaths from diethylene glycol used as a solvent in Massengill's Elixir of Sulfanilamide; and, finally, the several thousand hideously deformed infants born with phocomelia whose mothers had taken thalidomide during pregnancy. These events led successively to Biologics Control Act of 1902; the Pure Food and Drug Laws of 1906; the Food, Drugs and Cosmetics Act of 1938, and the Drug Amendments (Kefauver-Harris Amendments) of 1962. The early laws were designed to prevent adulteration of biologics, food, and drugs, and to insure that their labeling was not false and misleading; the 1938 laws were meant to insure the safety of new drugs, and the 1962 amendments to guarantee their effectiveness for the purposes for which they are recommended.

The essays by Doctors Ley and Lasagna must be considered against this background. Dr. Ley is a former Commissioner of the Food and Drug Administration; in fact, one of those mentioned by Lasagna who left that office under more or less unpleasant circumstances. Nevertheless, he defends the need for and the general quality of the performance of that agency within the limitations of its budget and staff. He tends to justify their actions as necessary if we are to insure the safety and effectiveness of the new drugs as the Congress has legislated.

On the other hand, Lasagna, as an investigator who may feel hampered by needless constraints resulting from the regulations made and administered by the FDA, has much to complain about. In a sense his complaints are essentially those of the drug industry which has been greatly, and perhaps excessively, restricted by new regulations and by requirements that may be sound in theory, but excessively demanding, almost prohibitively expensive, sometimes even impossible to comply with, and, for the ethical and experienced clinical investigators, sometimes totally impractical and generally repulsive. He, like others, complains about the failure of the agency to attract and to retain people of high caliber and ability, and also the manner in which they select advisors and utilize or fail to heed their advice.

At the time of these writings the FDA was burdened with the implementation of the decisions of the Drug Efficacy Study conducted for the agency under the auspices of the National Academy of Sciences–National Research Council and intended to evaluate all new drugs approved between 1938 and 1962 with respect to the new requirement of efficacy written into the Drug Amendments of 1962. Unfortunately the recommendations of the Drug Efficacy Study also reflect the excessive zeal of the academic clinicians and investigators aiming at perfection in performance of their tasks in the face of defective guidelines of their own making, which were not consonant with the letter of the laws that the FDA has to administer.

However, with respect to Lasagna's stand on fixed-ratio combination, which he has reiterated on several occasions, my own competence and experience is limited to those with antibiotics for use systemically. He can rest assured that the available evidence for each and every such combination and indication was carefully scrutinized and found to be unacceptable as fixed combinations. There were some for topical use which were considered as lacking in acceptable evidence of effectiveness and left for further study. A few for topical use have indeed been declared effective. In his own field, he may disagree with the majority of his colleagues who made the decisions, but some combinations, very few to be sure, were indeed declared to be effective.

Lasagna may be somewhat overly concerned about the recently declining number of new drug entities and the increasing costs of drug innovation, but he is properly distressed about the potential deterioration of the research activities within our drug industry, the shrinking of our scientific and clinical investigative talents within the academic community. There is little doubt that the recent actions will restrict our potential and we cannot afford to abdicate our position of leadership in this, as in many other fields of intellectual, scientific, and economic endeavor.

MAXWELL FINLAND

The individual components previously described have all been demonstrated in a variety of environments. Wherever multiphasic testing has been isolated from a medical care delivery system it has usually failed. For this systems concept to succeed, it will require all of these components to be integrated into an overall medical care delivery system. It will need to be supported by a suitable administrative and fiscal organization (such as a foundation, medical center, cooperative, governmental or similar agency) with adequate numbers of physicians and allied health personnel to provide these services to a sufficiently large defined population.

References

1. *Provisional Guidelines for Automated Multiphasic Health Testing & Services. Vol. 1 & 2.* Washington, D.C., U.S. Government Printing Office, 1970.
2. Collen, M. F.: Guidelines for multiphasic health checkup. Arch. Intern. Med. *127:* 99–100, 1971.
3. Garfield, S. R.: The delivery of medical care. Sci. Amer. *222:* 15–23, 1970.
4. Garfield, S. R.: Multiphasic health testing and medical care as a right. New Eng. J. Med. *283:*1087–1089, 1970.
5. Collen, M. F.: Periodic health examinations using an automated multitest laboratory. J.A.M.A. *195:*830–833, 1966; also Editorial in Arch. Environ. Health *12:*275, 1966.
6. Collen, M. F.: The multitest laboratory in health care of the future. Hospitals *41:*119, 1967.
7. Soghikian, K., and Collen, F. B.: Acceptance of multiphasic screening examinations by patients. Bull. N.Y. Acad. Med. (2nd Series) *45:*1366–1375, 1969.
8. Collen, M. F.: Automated multiphasic screening. Sharp, C. and H. Keen (eds.), *In Presymptomatic Detection and Early Diagnosis.* London,: Pitman Med. Pub. Co., Ltd., 1968, Chapter 2, pp. 25–66.
9. Collen, M. F.: Statement in *Detection and Prevention of Chronic Disease Utilizing Multiphasic Health Screening Technique.* Hearings before the Sub-committee on Health of the Elderly of the Special Committee on Aging of the United States Senate, Sept. 20–22, 1966. Washington, D.C., U.S. Government Printing Office, pp. 214–223.
10. Collen, M. F., Kidd, P. H., Feldman, R., and Cutler, J. L.: Cost analysis of a multiphasic screening program. New Eng. J. Med. *280:*1043–1045, 1969.
11. Collen, M. F., Feldman, R., Siegelaub, A., and Crawford, D.: Dollar cost per positive test for automated multiphasic screening. New Eng. J. Med. *283:*459–463, 1970.
12. Friedman, G., Goldberg, M., Ahuja, J., Siegelaub, A., Bassis, M., and Collen, M.: Biochemical screening tests, effect of panel size on medical care. Arch. Intern. Med. *129:*91–97, 1972.
13. Collen, M. F., Siegelaub, A., Cutler, J. L., and Goldberg, R.: Aspects of normal values in medicine. Ann. N.Y. Acad. Sci. *161/2:*572, 1969.
14. Cutler, J. L., Collen, M. F., Siegelaub, A. B., and Feldman, R.: Determination of normal values for blood chemistry tests. Pathologist, Oct. 1969, p. 319–326.
15. Ramcharan, S., Cutler, J., Feldman, R., Siegelaub, A., Campbell, B., Friedman, G., Dales, L., and Collen, M.: Disability and Chronic Disease After Seven Years of Multiphasic Health Checkups. A.P.H.A. Meeting, Minneapolis, Oct. 11, 1971.

Unvalidated Procedures Have No Place in Screening Programs

THOMAS McKEOWN

University of Birmingham, England

At first sight the case for screening as a major development in medical care seems irrefutable. Interpretation of past improvements in health shows that they have been due mainly to preventive measures. Such measures have proved less effective or ineffective in preventing the main residual health problems, particularly the chronic noninfectious diseases—congenital, psychiatric, and geriatric—which are now predominant in technologically advanced countries. In some of these diseases treatment has something to offer; but they are usually recognized too late for treatment to be really effective. In these circumstances is it not reasonable to hope that early identification of disease by screening will make an important contribution to the solution of some of the most intractable contemporary medical problems? That this hope is well grounded is suggested by the undoubted success of procedures such as mass radiography in the control of tuberculosis and inspection of teeth in the treatment of dental caries.

The case for screening is widely believed to be strengthened by recent advances in medical technology, particularly automation of laboratory procedures and computing. Although screening can be applied to individuals, it is essentially a method for application to populations, preferably large populations. There are several reasons for this view. In the first place the detection of pre-symptomatic disease involves investigation of groups in which a majority, usually a large majority, of those examined are not affected. Secondly, the grounds for screening are in part that it is economical, and the economies depend to a considerable extent on large-scale methods of collecting, analyzing and interpreting data. And thirdly, when a screening procedure has been proved to be effective, its benefits should be shared as widely as possible. Hence, it is concluded, the requirements of screening are precisely those which modern technology is equipped to meet. It is a natural extension of this viewpoint to suggest that the most effective type of screening is likely to be multiphasic, in which several tests and examinations are combined in a convenient and efficient procedure.

I have put the general case for screening in terms which I believe would be acceptable to its advocates, not only on the principle that "You should bury your adversary in the avalanche of your moderation," but also because no one who has thought seriously about the subject is likely to reject the concept of screening or to deny its value in a handful of well tried procedures. What is in question is the wisdom of a rapid proliferation of screening programs and the acceptance of multiphasic screening as an established feature of good medical practice.

Before considering these questions we should note that those who favor the widespread application of screening are not necessarily unaware of the associated problems. They recognize that diagnostic methods may be unreliable, that treatment may be ineffective or dangerous, that costs may be high and the administrative and managerial problems of large programs quite formidable. However, such difficulties are thought to be inseparable from the practice of medicine and are not seen to arise uniquely in the case of screening.

But screening is distinguished fundamentally from conventional medical practice, and the requirements that should be met before a procedure is accepted as suitable for general application arise from this distinction. It is due essentially to the difference in the position of the doctor in relation to the patient in the two cases: in the one when the patient seeks the assistance of the doctor; in the other when the doctor undertakes to identify the patient who needs his assistance.

When the patient seeks medical advice, the doctor's ethical position is relatively simple: he attempts to do his best with the knowledge and resources available to him. He cannot fairly be criticized when the state of medical knowledge does not enable him to treat effectively or even to diagnose accurately the condition about which his advice is sought; nor can he undertake in all cases to assemble the full range of facilities for investigation and treatment from which his patient might conceivably benefit.

The position is quite different in screening, when a doctor or public authority takes the initiative in investigating the possibility of illness or disability in people who have not reported signs or symptoms. There is then a presumptive undertaking, not merely that abnormality will be identified if it is present, but that those affected will derive benefit from subsequent treatment or care. This commitment is at least implicit, and except for research or the protection of public health, no one should be expected to submit to the inconvenience of investigation or the anxieties of case finding without the prospect of medical benefit. This obligation exists even when the patient asks to be screened or to have a health examination, for his request is based on the belief that the procedure is valuable, and if it is not, it is for medical people to make this known.

The ethical considerations are so fundamental to the concept of screening that it seems desirable to reflect them in its definition. Most definitions put the emphasis on the pre-symptomatic character of the investigations; that is to say, they focus on their timing in relation to the stage of disease rather than on the circumstances in which they are initiated. A review of screening* sponsored by the Nuffield Provincial Hospitals Trust led to the following definition: *medical investigation which does not arise from a patient's request for advice for specific*

---

* Screening in Medical Care. Nuffield Provincial Hospitals Trust. London, Oxford University Press, 1968.

complaints. This was considered to comprise "investigation of patients (a) who have not sought medical assistance (as with mass radiography), (b) who have sought medical assistance only for a screening test or health examination which they believe will be of value to them, and (c) who have sought assistance for a condition unrelated to a screening procedure." This interpretation regards as the unique feature of screening the fact that investigation is initiated by the doctor rather than by the patient. It is "the medical initiative which creates the obligation which . . . makes a strict validation procedure essential."

There is another consideration which makes it imperative to adopt for screening a more rigorous approach than that which is followed in ordinary clinical practice: this is the scale on which a program may be and, if it is properly validated, should be applied. The application of a new therapeutic measure is developed gradually because its use is determined by the practicing physician who assesses its merits in relation to the alternative treatments available to him. But a screening program believed to be of value invites large scale application which may involve deployment of extensive resources at regional and national levels. Inevitably it is developed at the expense of other possible uses of health manpower and equipment. For example, a decision to introduce national screening for breast cancer would make heavy demands which could be met only by substantial new expenditure or by diverting staff and facilities from other work. This diversion may be justified, but it is clearly essential to show that it is before accepting breast cancer screening as suitable for widespread application. The main tasks confronting those concerned with the practice of screening are therefore to decide on an appropriate validation procedure, and to apply it to existing programs and to new programs before they are brought into general use.

The review of screening referred to above outlined an evaluation scheme with the following requirements:

Definition of the problem. Screening programs are sometimes difficult to evaluate because they have no clearly defined aims. It therefore seems essential to remove ambiguity by clarifying at the outset the abnormality to be detected, the treatment to be offered, the groups to be screened, the tests to be used, and the stage of the disease at which they are aimed.

Review of the position before screening. To evaluate the contribution of screening it is necessary to assess the position before it is introduced, particularly knowledge of the disease (its prevalence, natural history, etc.) and the effectiveness of existing preventive and therapeutic measures.

Review of the screening procedure. This is an appraisal of the diagnostic methods to be used in screening (their error rates, applicability to the population under investigation, cost, etc.) and of the treatment or care it is proposed to offer to those identified as abnormal.

Summary of conclusions concerning the screening procedure. Here it is intended to prepare a balance sheet, assessing the contribution of screening in relation to its costs, risks, and displacement of other medical measures.

Proposals for organization of further evidence and initial applications. The preceding review will summarize the current position and will reveal the areas in which knowledge is seriously deficient. With this information it should be possible to make proposals for additional investigations and to recommend the policy to be adopted in relation to the screening procedure. Broadly this might be (1) that the procedure is ready for general application, (2) that limited application is needed for further study of medical and/or managerial problems, or (3) that present evidence does not justify the introduction of the screening program.

In the Nuffield Provincial Hospitals Trust exercise an evaluation of this type was applied to a number of screening procedures in current use, and it has since been employed in Britain in planning national policies with respect to screening. Used in this way the method is an effective instrument which quickly exposes deficiencies of knowledge. It focuses attention on the major requirements which should be considered before a screening program is regarded as acceptable for general use.

However, while this approach is effective in revealing deficiencies of evidence, it is arguable that it is too exacting to be applied in all cases. In the history of medicine there are numerous examples of measures which were effective before they were understood: for example, improvements in hygiene were advocated and partially implemented without knowledge of the nature of infectious disease, and mortality is declining in British doctors who have stopped smoking in advance of full understanding of the etiology of lung cancer. Not unreasonably, therefore, it may be said that if early detection of breast cancer were shown to reduce mortality, the introduction of screening would be justified without requiring a full picture of the natural history of the disease, or even a critical appraisal of the results of treatment. This point is important because extensive and prolonged investigation is usually needed to unravel the natural history of disease, and there may be ethical and other objections to an objective assessment of treatment.

However, while we may accept that we do not always need to know *how* measures work, in view of the unique ethical obligations in screening we do need to know *that* they work. We must also be sure that they do not expose patients to excessive risks and that a new service will not be introduced at the expense of other more effective uses of the same resources. These requirements suggest five points which it seems essential to consider carefully in relation to screening: reliability of diagnosis; effectiveness and availability of treatment; assessment of risks; operational problems; and cost and benefit. These points will be illustrated by reference to screening for breast cancer.

RELIABILITY OF DIAGNOSIS

Since diagnostic methods in screening are intended for use in large populations, they are likely to be less reliable than the methods employed in ordinary clinical practice. Moreover, failure to recognize abnormalities when they are present may lead to unjustified reassurance which delays diagnosis and treatment, and erroneous identification of disease may result in unnecessary treatment which may be costly, unpleasant, or even harmful. The latter risk is far from negligible, for most screening tests have low yields and with even a small error rate the number of normals incorrectly treated may exceed the number of abnormals correctly treated.

The aim of most screening tests is, of course, identification of those needing further investigation, rather than precise diagnosis. But the further investigation required may expose patients to anxiety and risk. For example, in screening for breast cancer, among women considered suspect after clinical examination, nearly nine tenths were found at biopsy not to have the disease. With clinical examination and mammography, the proportion who were negative was four fifths.

In response to such figures it may be said that patients gladly accept the anxieties associated with biopsy for the reassurance it usually gives. But it is one thing to reassure a woman already concerned about signs or symptoms for which she seeks medical attention, and quite another to reassure one who has no reason for alarm until it is created by gratuitous examination which she has not sought. It seems inexcusable to screen in such circumstances unless patients confirmed as abnormal will receive certain and substantial benefit. Furthermore, in assessing benefit it is essential to identify accurately the real objective of the procedure. If we fall into the trap of accepting the aim of implementing the surgical aphorism that "no lady should have a lump," then all removals of lumps count as credit. If we require the saving of life, then lump removals which do not prolong life count as a cost to be set against such benefits as can be demonstrated; this notwithstanding that the aphorism reflects good clinical practice.

Effectiveness and Availability of Treatment

In ordinary clinical practice it is often necessary to use treatments whose effectiveness has not been determined fully or, sometimes, at all. In screening, however, the ethical obligations and potential costs make it essential to know that treatment is effective before a test is accepted for general application. Ideally this requires a fairly complete picture of the natural history of the disease and a critical appraisal of treatment (the evidence available as a basis of screening for tuberculosis, for example); in practice it may be necessary to accept an evaluation of the effects of early detection and treatment on survival (the type of evidence becoming available in respect of screening for breast cancer).

Since it is obligatory to provide the appropriate care for those discovered to require it, the operational relationship between screening and subsequent treatment services is important. It is irresponsible to leave patients to make their own arrangements, and less than satisfactory merely to inform the patient's physician about the results of a screening exercise in which he had no part and in whose results he may have little confidence.

Assessment of Risks

The obligations of screening in relation to diagnosis and treatment apply particularly to exposure to risk. Regrettably it must be accepted that the ordinary practice of medicine involves risks which may arise from ignorance—as in the case of exposure to excessive radiation in the earlier treatment of tuberculosis— or because the risks, like the effectiveness of treatment, cannot be fully assessed. But when the initiative in investigation of an ostensibly healthy person is taken by the physician, any risks must be quantified and weighed carefully in relation to the benefit from treatment. In breast cancer screening, for example, it is not enough to believe that the risks of mammography are acceptably low; these risks must be measured accurately in relation to the frequency and type of examination, and when, as with such indices, the risks fall within a range, it is the upper limit which should be used in coming to a decision about the advisability of screening. It is also necessary to take account of the stress and risk associated with biopsy, particularly since the majority of those investigated will be found not to have the disease.

Operational Problems

In addition to the problems associated with the provision of all medical services, screening presents others which are unique to itself. One of these problems is that of public response to a service which is offered rather than requested; experience of cervical cytology suggests that the response may be least from those who have most to gain from being screened. Another problem arises from the use of staff. Screening for breast cancer, for example, makes heavy demands on the time of surgeons, radiologists, and radiographers, and unless it can be shown that less expensively trained staff can be substituted, it seems unlikely that a national service could be offered. But perhaps the largest operational issue is the relation between screening and other health services. It is not difficult to imagine the unsatisfactory position which in time would result if screening programs were developed independently, each with its own finance, administration, staff, and facilities, and all separate from the main body of medical practice. In some respects the situation would be analogous to that created by malaria eradication campaigns, before it was realized that it was essential to link them with the public health services as a whole. Hence, screening should not be developed in isolation but should be linked closely in its execution and follow-up with the rest of medical, diagnostic, and treatment services.

Cost and Benefit

Slowly, and rather reluctantly, it is becoming recognized that in time all health services will have to submit to appraisal of their cost and benefit; but in screening, for reasons discussed previously, this appraisal should precede its introduction. Clearly it is not enough to know that a program provides some benefit; before accepting it as suitable for general use we need to know how much benefit and at what risk and cost. The final decision whether to screen turns on a value judgment, but the data on which this judgment is based should be as precise as we can make them.

Again this point may be illustrated by reference to breast cancer screening. It would not be sufficient to show that after a number of years there are fewer deaths from breast cancer among women screened than among those not screened. Ideally we need to know the increase in expectation of life which results from screening in a population of women, and this benefit should be weighed in relation to the costs of screening in manpower and resources, to the anxieties associated with biopsy, and to the risks from mammography.

No such rigorous validation procedure has been applied to most of the screening procedures in current use. In the Nuffield exercise it was concluded that the evidence was seriously deficient in respect of six of the 10 procedures evaluated. The requirements were met in screening for rhesus hemolytic disease, deafness in children, phenylketonuria, and pulmonary tuberculosis, and to this list could be added a few other conditions not examined in the Nuffield investigation.

There remains for consideration multiphasic screening, which raises issues additional to those which arise in relation to individual procedures. Needless to say, it is not a screening procedure in the usual sense, but a mechanism for executing a number of procedures at the same time. It must therefore be judged as an operational mechanism.

There is clearly no objection in principle to the coordination of a number of screening tests in time and place; indeed, it was suggested before that the procedures should be linked operationally not only with one another but with medical practice as a whole. What is unfortunate, however, in multiphasic screening as currently practiced, is that most of the tests it comprises have not been validated; indeed, the approach seems to invite inclusion of procedures in the hope, rather than in the knowledge, that they will be useful. Inevitably this results in two major problems. First, it is difficult, if not impossible, to assess the credentials of individual tests when they are incorporated in a multiphasic program. And secondly, if multiphasic screening in its present form comes to be regarded as an established feature of good medical practice, it may well displace alternative and more rewarding uses of the same resources. This problem is in some respects analogous to that associated with school health work, where the long established but unvalidated practice of routine examinations has diverted attention and effort from other and probably more effective methods of identifying the child who needs medical assistance.

To sum up: In principle we should prefer in medicine never to use diagnostic or therapeutic measures whose value has not been established, but in clinical practice, where the patient seeks medical assistance, it is often necessary to do so. In screening, however, where investigation is initiated by the physician, unvalidated procedures should have no place; for the inconvenience, anxieties, risks and costs of screening are justified only if it is known to result in substantial benefit. Before a screening program is regarded as suitable for general use it is therefore necessary to establish that diagnostic methods are sufficiently reliable, that treatment is effective and will be provided, that any risks are known and can be accepted, and that the benefits justify the inevitable displacement of resources from other forms of care. These requirements are not met by some of the screening procedures in current use, or by multiphasic screening which packages together a number of tests, most of which are still unvalidated.

Comment

Multiphasic Screening

Since it appears likely that medical care in the U.S.A. will become increasingly organized so that groups of providers will take care under contractual arrangements of groups of consumers, and since increasing emphasis will be placed on keeping consumers from becoming patients, screening programs will surely be used more and more. In other words, as Garfield (cited by Collen) points out, screening programs will be used whether or not any evidence is available that they improve the health of the people. The essays of Collen and McKeown, seen in this context, should therefore serve as guidelines promoting what should be done, and cautioning what should not be done, if the unavoidable proliferation of screening programs is to be helpful rather than harmful.

The technical aspects of screening programs have been extensively debated. All agree that they have to have well defined aims, that tests must be validated, that costs must be calculated, that the impact of false negatives and positives must be assessed, and that the programs must be well integrated in the total health care system. Dr. McKeown, however, raises an ethical issue. He argues that medical procedures, when initiated by doctors or society, must be much more stringently examined than when the same procedures are used in response to a patient's request. A year ago I would have thought this proposition philosophically interesting but of little practical consequence. But the varied and often remarkable reactions to sickle cell screening programs[1-3] illustrate the real-life practicality of Dr. McKeown's concerns. There are few technical problems with sickle cell screening programs. Precise goals can be set, tests are accurate and simple, and the population at risk can be either reassured or advised as to various potential health risks. But since the population at risk is a sensitive minority group, questions are being raised. How can society presume, for example, to lay down eugenic rules for one segment of the population—"as if they were cattle"? What justification is there for testing when inadequate facilities are available to instruct those tested in what it means to have the disease or the trait? Why should the health status of an ethnic group be stigmatized? Reactions such as these show there is more to a screening program than biochemical accuracy.

One can think of other groups that for genetic or environmental reasons are more susceptible to certain diseases than the population at large. Theoretically such groups should benefit from appropriate screening programs: gallbladder x-rays for the American Indian, glucose tolerance tests for families of diabetics, lipoprotein studies for those of certain body build, pulmonary studies for those exposed to dust and smoke. Though society may initiate with the best of intention special screening programs for such groups, the sickle cell experience shows that the potential examinees want a strong voice in deciding whether or not they want the programs and, if so, what kind of programs they will be. As McKeown indicates, whatever deficiencies a medical procedure may have, it is more readily accepted if it is patient-initiated.

Inevitably the consumer will be given an increasing voice in the design and implementation of screening programs. Furthermore, screening programs, as Collen points out, will to a large part be carried out by ancillary personnel. Doctors should thus be prepared for yet another important social consequence of more and bigger screening programs: the gradual emergence of a new health care system that will emphasize prevention and triage, that will be as important as the traditional sick care system, but that will be quite independent of the medical profession.

References

1. Culliton, B. J.: Sickle cell anemia: The route from obscurity to prominence. Science 178:138–142, 1972.
2. Culliton, B. J.: Sickle cell anemia: National program raises problems as well as hopes. Science 178:283–286, 1972.
3. Whitten, C. F.: Sickle-cell programming—an imperiled promise. New Eng. J. Med. 288:318–319, 1972.

FRANZ J. INGELFINGER

4

The Dying Patient

The Role of the Physician in the Prolongation of Life
    by Franklin H. Epstein

Death as You Wish It
    by Eugene A. Stead, Jr.

Alternatives to Striving Too Officiously
    by Robert S. Morison

The Role of the Physician in the Prolongation of Life

FRANKLIN H. EPSTEIN

Harvard Medical School

> "He would have it that to *cure* a patient was simply to *care* for him . . . to stand guard at every avenue that disease might enter, to leave nothing to chance; not merely to throw a few pills and powders into one pan of the scales of Fate, while Death the skeleton was seated in the other, but to lean with his whole weight on the side of life, and shift the balance in its favor if it lay in human power to do it."
>
> *Oliver Wendell Holmes,* referring to Dr. James Jackson, in *Medical Essays 1842–1882.* Boston, Houghton-Mifflin, 1891, p. 308.

In an era of concern over the social cost of medicine, it has become fashionable to question the doctor's traditional duty to preserve life. Liberal churchmen indicate their up-to-date orientation by proposing "a category of allowing to die." Grieving relatives, racked by the strain of a terminal illness in the family, write powerfully about the callousness of doctors who tried to keep the patient alive. Honestly distressed physicians, recalling the simpler days when there was no anxiety-provoking alternative to therapeutic nihilism, talk of "the patient's right to die" with all the fervor of a Rousseau declaiming the natural rights of man. There is often in all this well-meaning and genuine concern an undertone of distrust or resentment of the science that makes it possible to stave off death. There is also an underlying assumption that the patient's physician has a duty to the patient's family, to society, or to the state that is separate from his duty to his patient. When doctors could do little to alter the natural course of disease, such questions might serve chiefly to amuse armchair philosophers. But now that medicine is more and more effective and expensive, the questions and our answers are increasingly important.

My point of view is that of a doctor who has been daily concerned with the immediate details of caring for desperately ill patients and for their families. I believe that there are very practical as well as philosophical reasons to hew to the ancient Hippocratic dictum. The doctor's duty is to his patient, to preserve his life and relieve his suffering. The rule should be: preserve life as long as you can.

Life after death. I will take as axiomatic for the purpose of this discussion that there is no life after death—that after a person dies he ceases to exist. If some kind of life continued after death, it would be easier to think of death as a favor to the deceased. If death is really the end, then we must look very carefully at any argument that suggests death for the patient as a gift on his own behalf.

Relief of pain. My second assumption is that with proper care and modern techniques, physical pain can be relieved in almost every instance. If necessary, a patient can be put to sleep or made drowsy for most of the day; there is a clear distinction between putting a person to sleep and taking his life. Most terminal patients, contrary to lay belief, do not suffer pain. Excruciating pain is almost never present in dying patients and when it is, it can be controlled.

Euthanasia vs. suicide. Whether a patient has a right to take his own life is a separate question that will not be discussed here. The issue is rather whether the physician should cooperate with death. It is not hard to commit suicide if one really wants to. A sick patient who wants to die and who thinks his doctor is keeping him alive against his will can always discharge the doctor. But though in the course of a lifetime almost everyone has a suicidal thought, a good measure of the general will to live is that so few suicides are actually attempted. A firmly expressed and genuine wish to die is usually encountered in depressed people with few physical problems rather than in terminally ill patients.

Acts of omission vs. commission. A distinction is sometimes made between the positive act of killing a patient, and the negative act of omitting therapy that would save his life. To the thoughtful practicing physician this will appear a distinction without much of a difference. It may be true that the man who pushes his victim overboard into an icy sea is culpable in a different legal sense than is he who, standing on the stern of the boat, sees the drowning man float by and gives him a smile and a wave instead of a life preserver. But every doctor knows that when an 83 year old patient develops pneumonia, the physician must make a decision about antibiotics, and that the decision-making process is the same whether or not the drug is given. It may be comforting to take shelter in the thought that to others sins of omission can be represented as venal rather than cardinal, but the great issues of life and death should not be dodged in that way. *If a therapeutic option is really available, the doctor's responsibility is to offer or withhold it; he cannot pretend it does not exist.* The important question is not: "Is therapy an act of commission or omission?" but "What is the chance that therapy will help?"

Useless treatments. It should be clear that when life is irretrievable, useless treatments should not be employed—and in fact by common consent they are not. No doctor transplants a heart when the patient is dying of gangrene; no one amputates a limb when the problem is pneumococcal pneumonia. Drastic surgery, unusual medical treatments, or simple maintenance therapy with oxygen and intravenous fluids are usually undertaken because there is some hope of either cure, prolongation of life, or relief of pain. The difficult problem is that in practically all cases it is impossible to know whether life is really irretrievable, whether all hope is really lost. The difficulty is compounded by the nature of statistical prediction. It may be possible, for example, for the doctor to say that the chances are only one out of ten that treatment will help. For the tenth man, however, this is not a 90 per cent chance of failure—it is a 100 per cent chance of success. It is never possible to know except in retrospect whether one is dealing with the nine men who will die or with the tenth man who will respond to treatment. If the doctor is convinced that treatment will neither prolong life nor relieve suffering, he should of course withhold it. But he bears the heavy burden of being quite certain of his ground.

The doctor is not omniscient. Doctors are fallible. Their omniscience tends to be greatly exaggerated by the popular press and too often by doctors themselves. There is also a powerful psychological need for patients to believe that their doctors know everything and can prognosticate with great accuracy. But the fact is that the most accurate prognosis is only reliable in a statistical, not an individual, sense. The kindest, best intentioned doctor can be wrong. We are surprisingly ignorant of the natural history of the most commonplace diseases. A doctor's prognosis tends to be weighted toward pessimism because patients who do badly claim most of his time and attention and remain in his memory longer than those with the same disease who do well. And for all too human reasons, doctors tend to forget the times when their predictions were wrong.

The pathology service of any general hospital will supply arguments against letting the doctor decide to give up:

A 38 year old housewife had had a carcinoma of the cervix treated by hysterectomy and irradiation two years previously. She entered the hospital in a uremic and anuric state. Her physician, an experienced and eminent gynecologist, made the obvious diagnosis: carcinomatous invasion of the ureters with obstruction. He decided that she had suffered enough and that further investigation was unwarranted. She died quietly under heavy sedation with morphine. At autopsy there was no trace of cancer; the ureters were occluded by postradiation fibrosis, causing obstruction that could easily have been relieved.

A 58 year old businessman entered the neurosurgical service with signs of a cord tumor that had invaded the spine. The attending neurosurgeon, able and well trained, kindly and sympathetic, thought to spare the patient and his family pain and expense, and forbade invasive diagnostic procedures while treating the paralyzed patient with narcotics and judicious neglect. Under great pressure from the house staff he consented to undertake a biopsy, which showed lymphoma. Local irradiation resulted in complete regression of all symptoms for three years.

The assumption that an incurable illness is causing symptoms when in fact a coincidental curable disease is at fault is a common mistake in medicine. An argument often used against euthanasia is that science may at any moment develop a cure for a previously fatal condition—a new insulin, another penicillin. Much more likely is that if euthanasia is permitted, a curable disease will be overlooked. *The best way to insure that a cure is not overlooked is to make it very hard for the doctor to give up.* If the doctor has the option of agreeing with the family that (their) suffering should cease by curtailment of the patients' life, mistakes will inevitably multiply. And some patients will die unnecessarily.

One error doesn't balance another. Of course, mistakes happen on the other side. Time and money are invested vainly: the patient dies. An error made in the mistaken hope that a patient's life will be prolonged by treatment is not a catastrophe. A trial that fails may be expensive, but it is usually a small cost looked at overall. But if the mistake is in the other direction and one does not try where he could have succeeded, that is a big mistake. That is a human life, and if one believes that once that life is lost it will never come again, it is an irretrievable loss. One mistake does not balance another in such an equation.

Practical consequences of interrupting therapy in dying patients. More than pain, loneliness and depersonalization are the most common causes of suffering in the dying. Studies of dying patients have shown that there is no more effective way to increase the inevitable barrier between the patient and his visitors and nurses than to suspend therapy on the grounds that the patient is incurable. Doctors hurry past the foot of the bed, nurses find more urgent tasks at their desks; it takes longer to answer a summons from the bedside, for no one likes to look at the face of death. It is impossible to keep the decision secret. The patient down the hall discovers what is going on and begins to wonder about his own treatment. Intense anxiety is generated in doctors and nurses that mounts the longer the patient lives. The relatives bear a special burden of guilt that is intensified cruelly if the patient doesn't die on time. If the patient is conscious, he soon senses that he is regarded by family and staff as already dead—at a time when he is most lonely and most needs human contact.

Prolongation of life vs. prolongation of dying. Proponents of euthanasia refer to therapeutic efforts to prolong life in desperately ill patients as "prolongation of dying," but in one sense, we are all dying from the moment we are born. Most of us carry within us the biochemical seeds of our decay. From the standpoint of the Creator, or of geological time, or of the life of the species, we live for an infinitesimal moment. Without some simple and unmistakable rule, it would be impossible for the doctor to decide, on an *ad hoc* basis, how long his patient should live. What length of life is worth fighting for? I suppose that nearly everyone would agree that a 20-year prolongation of life would be desirable. Five years seem worth fighting for, at least according to the cancer statisticians. One year? There might be some dissent. But some men would give a million dollars for a month more. Is another week worth it? A day? An hour? Who is to decide?

It is sometimes suggested that the "quality of life" should be entered into an equation in which length of life multiplied by "quality" would equal a number that would guide the doctor's conduct. The only judge of the quality of his life, however, is the living patient. If his alternative is death, it would be arrogant indeed for an outsider, a physician, employed by the patient to fight for his life, to judge its quality so poor as not to merit the effort. If we say that for the physician-as-judge, life itself is less important than its quality, that it must be life where a man can appreciate a poem, or read the Sunday *Times*, or love his wife, or recognize her, or perceive the difference between light and dark, or heat and cold, then we put ourselves in the position of saying that there is a human life that is not worth living. That is not the doctor's prerogative.

Under special circumstances—for example, on the battlefield, or whenever resources are artificially limited—the doctor must of course devote his energies to those who can best benefit from them and he must establish some sort of triage.

Patients with mortal wounds should not get all the plasma that would save others who might recover. But these are exceptional situations and do not apply to most hospitals in civilized countries at peace.

The doctor's contract. The doctor's obligation to ameliorate his patient's pain is sometimes distorted into an obligation to prevent suffering of relatives, friends, and other onlookers. In fact, much of the "suffering" of terminally ill patients from nasal oxygen tubes and intravenous drips is entirely imaginary and projected by shocked relatives who are sickened and frightened by unfamiliar procedures and apparatus. Such suffering by the spectator is often compounded by guilt. The loudest pleas to "end her suffering, Doctor," come from the neglectful children of a comatose mother who is not suffering at all. In this situation the doctor must remember that he has only one client—the patient. His contractual and moral obligation is to the patient, not to the family, not to the welfare agency, certainly not to the kindly clergymen, squeamish at the sight of tracheostomy.

Anything else, any conflict of loyalties, would place the relationship between doctor and patient in jeopardy. In the words of the British Medical Association Panel on Euthanasia, "to be a trusted physician is one thing; to appear as a potential executioner quite another."

Death and dignity. The term "dignity in death" is sometimes used as a euphemism for a terminal illness in which little is done to help the patient, aside from minimal nursing care. Talk about a "dignified death" comes from onlookers, not usually from the patient. Most patients want to live, need to have some hope of staying the inevitable end, and like to feel that the doctor is helping to keep hope alive. Much dignity lies in their fight for life and in their struggle to maintain contact with humanity. It is unfortunate that the climate of opinion has brought some elderly people to believe that they are a burden to others and to fear that their lives may be unduly prolonged in an "undignified" way by modern medical developments. But the elderly are generally kept alive not by drugs but by kindness, good nutrition, and good nursing. Euthanasia for old people whose bodily functions and control are failing would relieve primarily the distress of the relatives and not that of the patient. For such a reason it can never be justified.

The doctor as an interested party. An elementary principle of justice is that interested parties should be excluded from impartial decisions affecting the rights of others. Physicians must be forbidden to cut their patients' lives short—whether by injecting air into their veins or by "judicious neglect"—because the psychological pressures on the doctor caring for terminally ill patients conspire against his impartiality. *The doctor suffers when the patient doesn't get well, and his suffering ends when the patient dies.* Only the practicing physician can appreciate how difficult it is to visit a dying patient day after day, with support, condolence, and hope; how frustrating it is to contemplate months of decline, of weary, anxious relatives, of *nothing working*, of vague complaints poorly understood—or all too well understood. Only he knows the overwhelming sense of relief that floods over him when, on hurrying to the patient's room in the morning, nerving himself to face the ordeal of a man not getting better, he learns that death has come, unexpectedly, an hour earlier. How wise (and dignified) not to have attempted resuscitation! The sense of relief that envelops doctor and relatives can be so intense that it is hard to remember that the patient cannot share it. The doctor is an interested party, and the decision to stop trying should not be left to him. The line should be drawn so clearly that he does not have to make that decision.

Definition of human life. A corollary of this is that there must be a simple definition of a single human life, both at the beginning and the end of its span Since in the sense of modern biology life is continuous from generation to generation, any such definition must be arbitrary. The important thing is that it be generally and impartially applied and easy to recognize. It should be framed in such a way that as few conflicts as possible arise in efforts by the medical profession to save "human lives," as defined. A convenient definition of the starting point of human life is, therefore, that stage at which the fetus can sever its connection with the mother and live independently. The recently proposed definition of "brain death" would appear to be a reasonable endpoint.

The cost of trying. It is clearly wrong that a family's lifetime savings should be eaten away while an unconscious man is kept alive with a respirator in a hospital. But this is not a difficult problem to solve by society as a whole. With proper general national health insurance, catastrophic illness would not be an individual burden. It would be the kind of financial burden society thinks nothing of carrying for a lifetime when a mentally defective child is born, or when a patient with paralytic poliomyelitis or shrapnel wounds in his spine is kept alive for years by mechanical respiration. We take care of thousands of such patients from birth to grave. Why do we do it? The reason is that it is a small price to pay to preserve our sense of the uniqueness of human life.

The uniqueness of human life. This is, in the last analysis, the most powerful philosophical argument for resisting euthanasia. It has to do with the integrity of the medical profession and the quality of a civilized society. There is an analogy with the constitutional safeguards in criminal prosecution. Under constitutional law a convicted murderer may be set free if the evidence used to convict him was unlawfully obtained so as to encroach on his civil rights. The idea, of course, is that it is not only the individual criminal's rights that are encroached on—it is the rights of all. It is bad that a murderer should go free, but it is worse that the civil rights of all should be threatened. Imagine the unlikely circumstance of a man unconscious for years, without hope of recovery, kept alive by medical attention, unable to feel or think. It might be considered unfortunate that he should be kept alive (though this would largely be a function of the cost), but it is worse that his right to live should be threatened. The rights of all of us are bound up with his. It is important for the profession and for society that doctors should not be asked to determine who is worth saving. If a doctor can decide arbitrarily that one human being's life should be shortened (or not prolonged if prolongation is feasible), then the way is open to arbitrary decisions about everyone.

Nowhere is the evidence for this thesis more brutally convincing than in the detailed history of the "Doctors of Infamy," studied by the Allied War Crimes Commission and summarized by Dr. Leo Alexander in his classic article, "Medical Science under Dictatorship."

Whatever proportions these crimes finally assumed, it became evident to all who investigated them that they had started from small beginnings. The beginnings at first were merely a subtle shift in emphasis in the basic attitude of the physicians. It started with the acceptance of the attitude, basic to the euthanasia movement, that there is such a thing as a life not worthy to be lived. This attitude in its early stages concerned itself merely with the severely and chronically sick. Gradually the sphere of those to be included in this category was enlarged to encompass the socially unproductive, the ideologically unwanted, the racially unwanted, and finally all non-Germans. But it is important to realize that the infinitely small wedged-in lever from which this entire trend received its stimulus was the attitude toward the non-rehabilitable sick.

Physicians belong to an ancient profession, standing apart from all others in its primary concern and respect for human life and its enmity to death. In the long run, that attitude of the profession may be as important for society as any miracle that modern technical medicine can perform.

Attitudes toward the prolongation of life are invested with a peculiar emotional ambivalence that springs from the horror most people have of contact with the ill, or with any reminder of their own vulnerability. The nightmare that men might live forever as vegetables springs from this irrational horror. It should be relegated to science fiction. The world will never be peopled with cripples and corpses. The fact is that for all our miracles, life cannot be prolonged indefinitely. For all our talk and our science, we do only a little. Death comes at last. The comatose patient treated with antibiotics falls victim a few weeks later to a resistant organism, or to a heart attack. Patients die, and always will, despite the best efforts of doctors. But the little we can do has an importance that transcends the patient, for it carries a message to all our patients and to the world: Human beings are important. Humanity is to be preserved.

Death as You Wish It

EUGENE A. STEAD, JR.

Duke University Medical Center

The patient does the dying, but the doctor determines the speed of the dying, the place of the dying, the emotional cost to the family of the dying, and the dollar cost of the dying. Since the presence of the patient is essential but the services of the doctor are optional, it is reasonable to give the patient a larger role in the decision-making.

The patient, when he is of age, and the family of the minor need to have in sharp focus what medicine really has to offer. This information is surprisingly hard to come by. Medical records are not kept in a way that allows the doctor to write out an accurate description of his patient and match him with like patients whose courses are known. Only with this type of record can the doctor know whether modern therapy has been useful or meddlesome. Statistics on young patients with acute myelogenous leukemia treated at the National Institutes of Health do not help one in determining the best way to care for a 60 year old man with acute leukemia in a community hospital in North Carolina. Too often the doctor attempts curative therapy when he really has nothing to offer.

The patient with a sound mind can at least ask the questions and have a hand in the decision-making. But what about the patient who is confused or comatose? What can he do to have a hand in determining the place and the manner of the dying? Any input he wishes to have must be planned before he loses control of the situation. We need some mechanism which will help patients in good health to determine how their bodies are to be handled when their brains are no longer functioning. What can be done when the rewards of living are gone but heart beat and respiration persist?

People for years have been urged to face up to the fact that they are not immortal and to have prepared a will which will allow the creator of an estate to determine its uses after his death. The legal profession is willing to face the inevitability of death. The person drawing the will rarely remembers that the majority and, not infrequently, the totality of the estate may be consumed by medical expenses between the time the patient became incompetent and the time that respiration and heart beat cease. The medical profession, having no guidance, assumes that its mandate is to keep the heart beating and the lungs working.

In our mobile society, with small living quarters and no domestic service, families become unglued. People end up in nursing homes unattended by family doctor or by family. There are commonly no instructions about how the dying patient is to be handled and no mechanism to determine how much of medical science and technology should be applied to prolong life. When acute illness occurs, the patient is sent to the emergency room. The doctor there knows only that he has an acutely ill person; he has no knowledge of the previous condition of the patient or the desires and wishes of the patient when he was capable of controlling his destiny. Before this information is obtained—if it ever is—many useless procedures may have been performed and many thousands of dollars wasted.

I believe the time has come to offer to our people consultative services to help them plan for dying. The expense of this program should be borne by third-party carriers who will profit from the saving in hospital charges resulting from a successful program. I would offer the opportunity for planning for death to the segment of our society who are accustomed to paying their own bills. This will assure that those entering the program have done so with no coercion. If the least constrained portion of our society profits by planning for death, the time will naturally come when such planning might be done with those supported by public funds. If the idea should prove unsuccessful with the most flexible portion of our society, its time has not come and no further action is indicated.

I am not worried about the fact that documents thoughtfully drawn by persons in their right mind may not have legal validity if challenged in the courts. In the majority of instances, the information about the wishes of the patient would be appreciated by the doctor and by other health professionals. Ninety per cent compliance within the medical profession would seem likely, and that would determine the amount of "gold" in the concept.

The first step is to make available to people the services of doctors who have thought about planning for death and are not frightened by it. The second step is to draw up a document which defines the situations which commonly cause the patient to be confused, demented, stuporous, and comatose and to determine where and how he wishes to be treated when he becomes mentally incompetent. Many years ago, I wrote the following letter to my doctor to guide him in my dying:

> If I become ill and unable to manage my own affairs, I want you to be responsible for my care. To make matters as simple as possible, I will leave certain specific instructions with you.
>
> In event of unconsciousness from an automobile accident, I do not wish to remain in a hospital for longer than two weeks without full recovery of my mental faculties. While I realize that recovery might still be possible, the risk of living without recovery is still greater. At home, I want only one practical nurse. I do not wish to be tube-fed or given intravenous fluids at home.
>
> In the event of a cerebral accident, other than a subarachnoid hemorrhage, I want no treatment of any kind until it is clear that I will be able to think effectively. This means no stomach tube and no intravenous fluids.
>
> If, in spite of the above care, I become mentally incapacitated and have remained in good physical condition, I do not want money spent on private care. I prefer to be institutionalized, preferably in a state hospital.
>
> If any other things happen, this will serve as a guide to my own thinking.
>
> Go ahead with an autopsy with as little worry to my wife as possible. The Anatomy crematory seems a good final solution.

The third step is to have a mechanism whereby the family, the director of the nursing home, or the doctor knows when the terms of the bond are to become operative. The fourth step is to have the health professionals accept the fact that a hospital may be used as a place for dying. One should be able to die in a hospital without tubes in each orifice. One should have the services one could obtain from a good wife and so die in peace. Infections need not be treated by antibiotics, dehydration does not have to be combated, nutrition does not have to be forced on the patient, tracheotomy and ventilation machines do not have to be used, diagnostic procedures are not in order. Morphine can be used freely to control pain and ease suffering.

The hardest step is the third. How does one determine whether the patient is living or merely existing? When do the terms of the bond become operative? The family doctor and the family can usually make the decisions by themselves when the patient is part of a closely knit family. What of the person living in a nursing home separated by distance and age from any family? Frequently such persons do not have a doctor who knows about the family or the resources and ambitions of the patient. Here we need a new approach. The director of the nursing home needs a committee composed of a doctor, minister, and lawyer who periodically review the documents signed by the patient when he was in full possession of his mental faculties and then determine whether the time has come to follow the instructions given then by the patient.

Many persons prefer to die at home when the family is not afraid and when they can obtain the necessary help to keep the patient comfortable. In our society the home frequently is not structured for dying, and the family would prefer that the patient die in an institution cared for by professionals who are accustomed to tending the dying. The hospital can serve this purpose if the professional staff know that their role does not involve diagnostic testing or curative medicine. Ideally one should be able to use any reasonably private area in the hospital in this way and avoid the multiple problems which arise among personnel when persons in a given area are responsible for the care of all terminal patients. Members of the professional staff enjoy the day more when they have a variety of roles. With patience, they can be trained in the art of allowing persons whose time has come to die in quietness and dignity.

I believe that our society has reached the point where many people would like to enroll in the program described above. The bather can never be sure of the temperature of the water until he tests it with his toe. We will never be sure what society will allow and support until several programs become operational. Then we can collect data to determine whether planning for death gives us happier lives and families than our present catch-as-catch-can methods.

Alternatives to Striving Too Officiously

ROBERT S. MORISON

Cornell University Medical College

The composers of fairy tales have long warned against wishes too completely granted, but it is only in the 20th century that science has conclusively demonstrated that all roses have thorns. Thus, we now know that the manufacture of the power that relieves man of manual labor also darkens his skies, overheats his trout streams, and hastens the deterioration of his own cardiovascular system. But even against this background, and prepared though we may have been made by a William Osler to welcome the old man's friend, it is a shock to realize that success, even in the struggle against death, has its peculiar penalties and terrors.

In a statistical sense the general triumph over early death has brought us the population problem. In the dimension of the individual, abnormal prolongation of life extends suffering and imposes spiritual and material stress on family and friends. From the public health point of view, it is obvious that personnel and facilities are not infinite. It would seem to be simple common sense to employ them in maintaining the health of young people in a position to enjoy life and to contribute something in return rather than to tie them up in rear-guard actions against deaths which by any reasonable definition must be regarded as postmature.

It is to the more personal aspects of the survival problem that this article is principally directed. The basic change in our position as physicians is profound. Death can no longer be regarded as simply an opponent whose comings and goings remain strictly in the hands of other powers. The doctor must somehow learn to mix his responsibility for the life of his patient with an intelligent and sympathetic concern for his death. The recognition is, of course, not wholly novel. Doctors have always been acquainted with death; in the care of most patients, there has probably come a moment when the physician has accepted the inevitability of death and ceased to busy himself with new remedies. The two important novelties are the elaborateness and effectiveness of the means for prolonging life and the fact that the majority of lingering deaths occur not in the privacy of the home but in the pitiless exposure of the hospital ward. The doctor is thus confronted with a large number of things he must decide either to do or not to do.

Worst of all, he is required to make these decisions in front of a vast array of interested onlookers, from student nurses to the august experts on the tissue committee. No longer can decisions to allow to die be taken more or less automatically or implicitly, perhaps even unconsciously. They must be faced up to, discussed with colleagues, and often given explicit visibility in a written order.

It is this growing explicitness that has led to a sudden increase in public discussion of death and dying and a flood of lectures and papers.[1] If anyone doubts the public concern on this issue and the bitterness with which many laymen view the fanatical determination of conscientious physicians to postpone death until the last possible moment, let him write an article on the subject, even for a relatively obscure scientific journal, and then read his mail.

So far the discussion has centered on the following topics: the definition of death, improving the care of the dying patient, and the ethical and legal implications of allowing a patient to die. The business of devising a more practical "definition of death" has received the attention of some of the most conscientious and clear-headed members of the profession and much sensitive commentary from theologians and legal experts. The recommendations of a group of Harvard physicians[2] have gained rapid acceptance by individual scholars, hospital staffs, and interdisciplinary groups interested in the ethical and legal implications of biomedical advance.[3] With the passage by all the states of the uniform Anatomical Gift Act, which defines procedures for determining the appropriate time for removing organs for transplantation,[4] and more recent recommendations for further legislation,[5] the move to update the definition of death has achieved somewhat of a plateau of acceptance. During the debate the title evolved from "redefining death" to "updating the criteria for declaring that an individual has died." This change from an apparently simple to a more cumbersome phraseology avoids some important metaphysical difficulties and focuses attention where it should be, on an operational consideration of what doctors should or should not do in certain definable circumstances.

Another aspect of the debate, which many observers found uncomfortable, was the fact that it arose in part because of the growing importance of ensuring a supply of organs in the best possible condition for transplantation. Much though the philosopher, theologian, or lawyer[6] may deplore the introduction of a third party interest into the new definition itself, it remains undeniably true that some of the incentive to reconsider was derived from this source.[7]

As is now well known, the current consensus centers on the Boston recommendation to use neurological rather than cardiologic criteria as the basis for pronouncing a person dead. As presently stated, these criteria include a complete absence of reflexes, spinal as well as cerebral, and, if convenient to obtain, a flat EEG. Already a move to liberalize the criteria by limiting the required areflexia to the upper levels of the nervous system is under way. This is based on an increasing accumulation of cases which appear to have lost all possibility of human interaction or consciousness, even though spinal, medullary, and pontine reflexes are retained for many months.[8]

Discussions of definition often become confused with the question of allowing to die and the not very well concealed hope that embarrassing decisions may be avoided by declaring the patient in question already dead. This attitude is clearly reflected, for example, by the recommendation of the Boston committee that a patient exhibiting the central nervous signs referred to above be declared dead *before* someone finally turns off the respirator. The concern about allowing to die, however, includes many patients who, by no stretch of the Harvard criteria, could be considered dead. The problem is that the quality of their continuing existence does not appear (at least to some people) to justify a vigorous therapeutic regimen. In such cases, no refinements of definition would appear to get the profession off the hook of weighing the tangible and the intangible qualitative factors before arriving at a decision to act or not to act.

Before entering this tangled and rather frightening frontier, some words should be said about the kind of care now given to the terminal or dying patient. There is a good deal of evidence to back up one's clinical intuition that many, perhaps most, doctors do not do a particularly good job of conducting their patients through their last days. There may have been a time when the doctor did more for the spirits of his patients, though somewhat less for their bodies. In those days, however, death was a much more familiar visitor in everyone's home, and the doctor had the help of other experienced professionals from the church. Our civilization has not only made death a rare event; it also rivals the ancient Egyptians in devising ceremonials, monuments, and embalming procedures with the primary purpose of denying that death is real.

Doctors participate in the general neglect, if not the actual denial of death, and turn away from it with a sense of failure. Indeed, the few quantitative studies available tend to show that in spite of their familiarity with dissecting rooms and morgues, doctors are even more frightened and repelled by death than is the average man.[9] The result is a vacant chair at the bedside of the dying and a growing tendency to fill it with a new specialty. Dr. Elizabeth Kübler Ross[10] is perhaps the most active charter member of a growing group of physicians, pastors, and nurses dedicated to investigating the special problems of the dying and providing instruction for young professionals. She and her associates have already done a great deal to remind us of the loneliness that has always attended the dying and that has inevitably been intensified by the current cultural denial of death. A movement to instruct individuals who attend the dying in how to listen to them and share their thoughts and feelings is now well under way in many hospitals and medical schools. First year students are reading *The Death of Ivan Ilyich* along with Gray's *Anatomy*, and there seems some hope, for a time at least, that there will be more sympathy and understanding at the bedside.

There is still room for disagreement, of course, and eminent physicians will no doubt go on arguing about the ethics and the practicalities of revealing or suppressing the truth about fatal illness. The pendulum now seems to be swinging in the direction of more openness between doctor and patient. Though all experienced physicians can cite anecdotes to prove that at least some patients don't really want to hear the truth they ask for, the preponderant evidence is on the side of those who feel that the professional relationship is soundest when there is a sharing of the truth rather than a conspiracy to perpetuate a falsehood. In the latter case there is always a danger that sooner or later the falseness will be revealed, either by physical event or an inadvertent word, and the patient will be left literally with no one he can trust.

The damaging effects of such revelations may be devastating, especially on children, with whom, unhappily, the temptations toward a conspiracy of optimism are often most intense. The published literature is still rather confused and uncertain on what to tell the patient,[11] so one inevitably falls back on personal experience and prejudice. Recently, for example, I had an opportunity to conduct a seminar for some 20 doctors, nurses, psychologists, and ministers, most of whom had professional experiences with dying patients. When this subject came up, almost all of them could cite experiences in which much damage had been done by efforts to prevent the patient from knowing his real condition. Particularly poignant were stories about children dying of leukemia. Not one of the participants attempted to defend a policy of suppression.

Clearly this is an area for individualized treatment. If any general guidelines can be laid down, they may properly take the form of recommendations for open discussion of the probabilities and a warning against the dangers of suppressing the truth in an increasingly sophisticated age. At the very least the physician should be constantly conscious that his attribution to his patients of an unwillingness to discuss the possibility of death may be most simply explained as a projection of his own fears.

In the care of the terminal patient there often comes a time when one is forced to ask what is to be gained and what may be lost by continuing vigorous measures to prolong life. Almost everyone, from the firmest believer in a God-given code of objective ethics to the most relativistic utilitarian, recognizes that there is a problem here. Indeed, it is probable that today there are very few patients for whom "everything possible" is actually done until the very last moment. A half dozen years ago even the Pope, the most outspoken and revered defender of an ethical code which carries the explicit sanction both of the will of God and the reason of man, spoke forcefully to the effect that a physician is not required in all cases to exhibit "extraordinary means" to prolong life.

It is generally agreed that the doctor's obligation to preserve life is mixed in some fashion with a responsibility for its quality. The disagreement arises over quantitative matters. How much interaction with other human beings does one need to lead a life of dignity? How much need one remember? What are the degrees of consciousness that qualify one as a human being? On the other side of this equation are other quantitative questions. How many attempts at resuscitation are compatible with death with dignity? How many tubes lying in what orifices and for how long?

What indeed are "extraordinary means"? Some of us remember when blood transfusions and even venoclyses had something extraordinary about them. More of us recall the altogether extraordinary changes in the wards of our city hospitals brought about by the introduction of penicillin. Then as now, however, it would have been entirely unacceptable to deny penicillin to a vigorous middle-aged man with lobar pneumonia on the grounds that an antibiotic constituted "extraordinary means" (which it certainly was). On the other hand, now that antibiotics are commonplace, there are many who doubt the wisdom of initiating antibiotic therapy in, for example, an 80 year old man whose bones are riddled with metastatic malignancy and who develops bronchial pneumonia as his natural resistance weakens.

The point is that we perforce appraise the extraordinariness of the means not on some absolute scale, or even by criteria inherent in the means themselves, but rather in relation to the quality of the current life and the probable future of the patient in question. Thus, it turns out that just as in the case of updating the definition of death, efforts to hide behind the complexities of "extraordinary means" cannot for long protect us against harsh reality. Inevitably we are being pushed into doing what no inheritor of the Judeo-Christian tradition can feel comfortable about doing[12]—assigning degrees of value to an individual life and weighing that value against the welfare of other individuals and of the society as a whole.

The precedents are not entirely reassuring. Many of us were brought up to abhor the "exposing" of unwanted infants by the Lacedemonians or the tacit understanding in certain societies that old and worn-out members should voluntarily leave the community and go off by themselves to die. Particularly revolting, of course, were announced attempts of Nazi Germany to eliminate "defectives" of all ages and to include in the definition those who did not conform to an almost wholly mythical standard of Aryanism. This terrible example, besides demonstrating the depths of depravity into which presumably civilized people may rather easily fall, carries the additional burden of having made it almost impossible to think in an unprejudiced way about any deliberate termination of life, however much that life may have deteriorated below any practical definition of humanity. It may be well to recall here that there is a school of moralists who subscribe to what is known as the slippery slope or camel's head argument. This holds that any departure from the strictest and most absolute standard of conduct leads inevitably to the uttermost ends of depravity. My grandmother, an admirable woman of the old school, would not put a teaspoonful of brandy in the sauce for a Christmas pudding on the grounds that it might start some unsuspecting visitor or even one of her grandchildren on the way to skid row. Similarly, I have several friends today who believe that to allow abortion for Tay-Sachs disease will lead our society inevitably to the massacres of St. Bartholomew and Belsen. I regard such absolutist thinking as an archaic intellectual and moral luxury which can have no place in a complex modern society where everything one does may benefit some people and harm some others. To put it another way, there are now few if any overarching generalizations which can save us from the arduous business of making our ethical decisions one by one.

What society and especially the medical, legal, and theological professions are confronting is an increasingly obvious need and, in fact, an increasing public demand for some way to allow people to die without weakening our hard-won sense of the inviolability of the individual human life. It would be a mistake, of course, to expect anything like a quick or comprehensive resolution of a cultural dilemma of this kind. Fear of death and horror of murder lie very deep in the human psyche, and our present respect for the sanctity of human life is one of the most cherished achievements in man's long and twisted march toward a civil existence. No one really wants to tamper with the rules, and there are many people who quite understandably feel that the whole matter would better be left to the quiet good judgment of the individual physician. Premature attempts to crystallize procedures in the form of ethical codes or legal definitions, they fear, may only confuse matters or tempt the unscrupulous to seek financial gain by suing physicians for under- or overtreating the dying.

It is the opinion of the present writer that increased public discussion of death with dignity will in the long run do more good than harm, and that indeed the time has come to proceed with all deliberate speed to clarify and make somewhat more explicit the guidelines for managing terminal illness.

Let us first consider certain informal modifications of the doctor-patient relationship. These measures hold considerable promise for ameliorating some of the greatest discomforts in the present situation without presenting more than minimum risks of abuse. In the first place doctors must realize that they are at least as responsible for the *quality* of a patient's life as for its duration. The pendulum is already swinging in this direction, and more and more articles are being written which weigh a possibly slight improvement in life expectancy against a certain decrease in normal function. Note, for example, the increasing doubt about radical as opposed to conservative surgery for malignancy. Similarly, in the past couple of years we have seen a general, though probably temporary, abandonment of cardiac transplantation on the grounds that the advantages of a few months' extension of life are outweighed by the pain, distress, anxiety, and simple economic costs attendant on the procedure as currently practiced.

What remains obscure is the number of doctors prepared to discuss probable costs and benefits and to leave it to the patient to make the final choice. The tradition that the doctor knows everything best is hard to dislodge. Frank discussion of the contingencies likely to arise in terminal care is beset by more than normal embarrassment. The doctor is embarrassed to admit that his role as lifesaver is faltering, and the patient hesitates to open a subject likely to be painful to both parties. Some may be inhibited by a fear that preference for rapid termination of pain and suffering may be interpreted as a lack of courage or a pathological impulse toward suicide. Clearly there are problems here. Nevertheless, there may be many advantages in centering as much of the decision-making as possible on the patient himself, aided and supported, of course, by his physician. There may be no better way to protect the patient's individual freedom and his sovereignty over his own body, for example.

Unfortunately there are also severe practical difficulties in the way of solving the problem through a series of frank discussions between patient and doctor. Many, perhaps most, people nowadays do not have family physicians who know them well. The illnesses from which they suffer do not always offer clear-cut alternatives that can be discussed effectively before the actual event. The influence of family and friends can complicate matters, and so on.

The lack of a regular family physician and the inadequacy of the modern apartment house as a place to be sick combine to place most patients with terminal illness in large general hospitals attended by a specialist in a subsection of surgery or the medical aspects of the cardiovascular system. We have already noted that most of the influences in large general hospitals press toward a simple prolongation of life regardless of its quality. The magnitude of this institutional aspect of the problem may be estimated if we remember that in 1958, the year for which the most recent national data are available, approximately 61 per cent of the recorded deaths in the United States occurred in institutions, 47.6 per cent of them in general hospitals.[11] The general hospital is the scene of a much higher proportion of the lingering or difficult deaths, since most of those which occur in public places and many of those in other institutions and the home are of the sudden uncomplicated variety.

Although it is, of course, theoretically and legally possible for a patient simply to refuse treatment and, so to speak, take command of his own terminal illness, this is relatively rarely done in practice. Among the several obstacles is the simple fact that the more one approaches the situation in which being allowed to die is the wisest, most dignified course, the less likely one is to be in a condition to arrive at a decision, much less to enforce it on a set of technicians with quite different objectives and habits. In order to circumvent this problem, a variety of suggestions has been made for ensuring a certain course of action in advance. These take the form of letters to one's physician or more formal documents instructing "whom it may concern" how one is to be treated.[13] In addition to letting one's desires be known, such procedures are proposed in the hope of relieving the attending physician from a presumptive obligation to do everything possible to prolong life. Some lawyers are sufficiently concerned about this possibility that they have drawn up legislation specifically legalizing benign neglect.[14]

The legal aspects of the situation are far from clear. Although there have been a small number of criminal proceedings against physicians who have actively hastened the death of a suffering patient, few convictions have been obtained. There is no record of a criminal action against a physician for neglecting to engage in active treatment of a dying patient. More surprisingly, in these days when so many people regard lawsuits as a normal source of income, there seems to have been no successful civil action against a physician for deliberately withholding treatment from a dying patient. This means that we may still have a few years to experiment with informal arrangements before becoming entangled with the law. In the long run, however, the interest of the tidy-minded and the fears of those who distrust the increasing sophistication and avarice of the public will combine to produce regulatory legislation. It is not too early, then, to be thinking about what ought to be in it. My own taste runs in the direction of the simple, permissive statute which recognizes that judgments regarding the intensity of treatment for presumably terminal patients may legitimately take into account such factors as the quality of the life of the patient, the pain and suffering to be endured by him and his relatives, the unlikelihood of substantial recovery of function, and so on.

The previously expressed wishes of the patient to be let alone in certain circumstances should ordinarily be respected and regarded as relieving the physician of legal responsibility to continue active therapy. Others with less confidence in the medical profession and more faith in formal arrangements would try to define situations and criteria more explicitly and even set up court-appointed agents or committees to share the decision to treat or not to treat. That such machinery can even be suggested at this time testifies to the growing public awareness that there is a problem. At the very least it should serve as a warning to doctors to show more concern for the dignity of dying if they don't want to be reduced to mere technical advisors at the deathbed.

For some time to come it is unlikely that substantial numbers of people will have the foresight to arrange in advance their thoughts on dying. The great majority of the decisions will continue to be made as they are now—without benefit of a recorded opinion of the patient himself. The physician will presumably have to rely on his professional conscience and what he can divine of the real wishes of the relatives, aided perhaps by a gradually changing climate of opinion. Just this change in climate may be most important in helping the more active type of physician to lose some of his self-assurance and gain some respect for differences of opinion.* At the very least, one hopes that eminent professors will cease from holding parents up to public obloquy for refusing intercurrent therapy in a grossly defective child or from seeking court orders to overrule a spouse who decides against a new battery to keep the heart beating in her dehumanized husband.

Still another approach to ensuring death with dignity is through modification of institutions. We have already noted that in many advanced countries, and especially in the United States, death commonly occurs in big general hospitals where the very idea of death with dignity becomes swallowed up in professionalized opposition to death of any kind. Although other types of institutions are available, the most explicit and thoughtful effort to change the atmosphere is represented by the invention of the "hospice" in England. The most notable of these appears to be St. Christopher's outside of London, presided over by Dr. Cecily Saunders. Here the emphasis is on accepting the probability of death and on making the last days not only as comfortable but as intellectually and emotionally satisfying as possible to both patient and relatives. Among other things, the development of an institutionalized solution allows a patient, his family, and his doctor to make a decision without coming quite face-to-face with its final meaning. The problem of dying is handled simply by choosing an appropriate place in which to be terminally ill.

Finally, there is the possibility of dying quietly at home. Because of the peculiarities of many medical insurance plans and the aversion of most Americans to providing personal services outside of institutions, the potential of this solution seems limited to the very rich or the abysmally poor. Since death is basically a personal or family matter, however, the possibility is worth further exploration by those who have responsibilities for devising better ways of distributing medical care.

The observant will have noticed that the word "euthanasia" has not been used in this article and no suggestion has been made of positive measures to hasten the approach of death to the hopelessly ill. "Euthanasia" has been avoided since the word has accumulated too many confusing overtones. Nor is positive intervention included under any other name since, as a practical matter, it seems very unlikely that many doctors will want to undertake what they think of as positive measures. In any case lawyers are sure to raise strong objections on the grounds that sanctioning positive steps would run counter to the distinction the law has always made between deliberately hostile acts and criminal negligence. From the point of view of scientific rather than legal rationalities, there seems to be very little difference between doing something that will speed the process of dying and not doing something else that might slow it down. In either case the intent may be the same—to shorten the period of distress. Admittedly one may feel differently when he turns off a respirator than when he simply fails to turn one on, but it is hard to see how this feeling has any rational basis.

---

* For a thoughtful review of the many subtleties facing the physician, as seen by the experienced theologian, see Ramsey, P.: *op. cit.,* Chap. 3.

Usually the dichotomy is not so clear as this, and those disposed to have their cake and eat it, too, can comfort themselves with the thought that what they are "really doing" when they discontinue cumbersome treatments is making the patient more comfortable. Death may then occur as a surprising, though welcome, side effect.

Probably the most common positive way of hastening the time of death is to give the patient morphine or other sedatives. This is not looked upon by the virtuous as positive euthanasia, however, since the stated objective is to keep the patient quiet and comfortable. Secondarily, of course, the respiration and cough reflex may be depressed with who knows what effect on the condition of the lungs, but even the strictest moralists find no fault with this procedure since it falls under what is known as the law of double effect. The same doctrine protects those who abort a fetus as the inevitable side effect of a hysterectomy for a diseased uterus. Given existing cultural norms, it thus appears that very few people will engage in positive euthanasia, and that those who do will find ways of persuading themselves that this is not what they are really doing. Given the strong reasons for maintaining an inviolable reverence for human life, this seems a trifling homage for vice to pay to virtue.[15]

References

1. Vernick, J. J.: *Selected Bibliography on Death and Dying.* Washington, D. C., U.S. Department of Health, Education, and Welfare.
2. Beecher, H. K., Adams, R. D., Burger, A. D., et al.: A definition of irreversible coma: Report of the Ad Hoc Committee of the Harvard Medical School to Examine the Definition of Brain Death. J.A.M.A. *205*:337–340, 1968.
3. Cassell, E., Bass, L. R., Lappe, M., et al.: Refinements in criteria for the determination of death: An appraisal. A Report by the Task Force on Death and Dying of the Institute of Society, Ethics and the Life Sciences. J.A.M.A. *221*:48–53, 1972.
4. Sadler, S. M., Jr., Sadler, B. L., and Stason, E. B.: Transplantation and the law: Progress toward uniformity. New Eng. J. Med. *282*:717, 1972.
5. Capron, A. M., et al.: A statutory definition of the standards for determining human death, an appraisal and proposal. University of Pennsylvania Law Review, November, 1972.
6. Ramsey, P.: *The Patient as a Person.* New Haven, Yale University Press, 1970, pp. 101–112.
7. Biörck, G.: On the definitions of death. World Med. J. *14*:137–139, 1967.
8. Brierly, J. B., Adams, J. H., Graham, D. I., and Simpson, J. A.: Neocortical death after cardiac arrest. Lancet *2*:560–565, 1971.
9. Feifel, H., Honson, S., Jones, R., and Edwards, L.: Proceedings of the 75th Annual Convention of the American Psychological Association *2*:201–202, 1967.
10. Ross, E. K.: *On Death and Dying.* New York, the Macmillan Company, 1969.
11. Brim, O. G., Jr., Freeman, H. E., Levine, S., and Scotch, N. A. (eds.): *The Dying Patient.* New York, Russell Sage Foundation, 1970.
12. Kass, L.: Death as an event: A commentary on Robert Morison. Science *173*:699–702, 1971.
13. Downing, A. G. (ed.): *Euthanasia and the Right to Death.* Los Angeles, Nash, 1969, pp. 205–206.
14. Brill, H. W.: Death with dignity, a recommendation for statutory change. University of Florida Law Review. *XXII*:368–383, 1970.
15. Rochefoucauld, F., Duc de La: *Maxim 218,* 1665.

5

Are Coronary Bypass Grafts the Answer to Angina Pectoris?

The Effectiveness of Coronary Bypass Grafts in Managing Myocardial Ischemia
    by Andrew S. Wechsler and David C. Sabiston, Jr.

The Role of Coronary Bypass Grafts in the Treatment of Angina Pectoris Remains To Be Established
    by Richard S. Ross

Comment
    by Richard V. Ebert

The Effectiveness of Coronary Bypass Grafts in Managing Myocardial Ischemia*

ANDREW S. WECHSLER and
DAVID C. SABISTON, JR.

Duke University Medical Center

An estimated 50,000 aorto-coronary bypass procedures have been performed since the introduction of this technique six years ago in the management of myocardial ischemia. The majority of physicians knowledgeable in this field favor the operation when the appropriate indications are present. Nevertheless, others seriously question the use of this procedure. The objective data currently available which support this procedure will be reviewed and a reply given to its critics concerning the controversial issues.[1-3]

Historical Aspects

Previous attempts to improve coronary flow in ischemic states have been characterized by many original ideas and numerous disappointments. Although little was gained directly in the treatment of atherosclerosis by sympathectomy, epicardectomy, epicardial abrasion, and internal mammary ligation, the involvement of the surgeon stimulated interest and provided an additional approach in management. Many studies were initiated to gain an improved understanding of the coronary circulation. An obvious need was to document the natural history of coronary atherosclerosis and especially in those patients with angina pectoris.

---

* This work was supported by National Institutes of Health Training Grant No. GM 01709-07 and National Institutes of Health Research Grant No. HL 09315-10.

The Natural History of Patients with Angina Pectoris

Since the original and classic description of angina pectoris by Heberden in 1759, the clinical manifestations of this serious disorder have been clearly appreciated. That the underlying basis for these symptoms is most often the presence of severe coronary atherosclerosis, however, has been much more recently recognized. Is it possible that after 30 years of intensive study we do not know the natural history of angina pectoris? The issue speaks for itself. In fact, a more pertinent point may be a redefinition in terms of the natural history of coronary atherosclerosis rather than of angina alone. The need for redefinition is emphasized by data from the Framingham study in which 77 per cent of patients presenting with myocardial infarction had *no* preceding angina pectoris.[4] For 119 men and 110 women who were admitted to the study with the diagnosis of angina uncomplicated by myocardial infarction, the overall yearly mortality rate was 4 per cent. Since angina in the Framingham study was diagnosed by clinical manifestations and not necessarily by electrocardiographic confirmation, the mortality figures for angina were derived from a population at risk that may have included up to 20 per cent of false positives, approximately the percentage of patients with anginal symptoms who are referred for coronary arteriography but who do not have obstructive coronary disease. By adjusting the figures for this probable error, the yearly mortality for all patients with angina becomes 5 per cent or a mortality of about 25 per cent at five years.

Quite pertinent to a comparison of the effects of coronary artery surgery with the natural history of angina pectoris is the prospective study of Friesinger, Page, and Ross based on a system in which the severity of coronary obstruction was graded.[5] With this grading, it became apparent that patients with minor single vessel involvement had a five-year survival of 95 per cent compared with 47 per cent for patients with scores of 10 or more, indicating severe involvement with two and three vessel disease. This latter group had a yearly attrition rate slightly above 10 per cent. However, since the overall age in the population with single vessel disease was 39 years, these patients will perhaps advance to a more serious form of atherosclerosis with increasing age.[5] Such data offer better prognoses for single vessel disease than data presented by Sones, which indicate a 4 per cent yearly death rate from isolated left anterior descending lesions and a 1.8 per cent death rate with isolated right or circumflex lesions. The seven-year mortality for two and three vessel involvement was 44 per cent and 70 per cent, respectively, in this series.[6]

Establishment of Surgical Technique

The fate of saphenous vein autografts in vascular reconstructive surgery has been demonstrated in the peripheral arterial system. Long-term follow-up studies have demonstrated the durability of these bypass grafts in femoropopliteal reconstruction, with 79 per cent of the grafts open one month postoperatively remaining patent at death or after five years.[7] In another study of 295 consecutive saphenous vein grafts in the leg, the yearly interval failure rate ranged from 1.2 to 5.1 per cent over a seven-year period, averaging 3.2 per cent per year. Eighty per cent of the grafts which were patent at one month were also patent at the time of death or after seven years. In this series no correlation was found between long-term patency and anatomic run-off.[8] "Run-off" refers to the ability of the distal vascular bed to accept and transmit blood from a more proximal source. In the series quoted, this was assessed by the extent to which patent distal vessels were visualized by contrast medium. Thus, the "run-off" was anatomically defined but not quantitated as flow per unit time.

The advent of microsurgical vascular techniques and the application of these to the coronary arteries by Johnson and Favaloro firmly established the ability to perform the coronary anastomoses.[9-11] Two-year patency rates of 86 per cent have been demonstrated by Favaloro and 30-month patencies of 87 per cent by Morris, and most recently long-term patency as high as 90 per cent has been demonstrated when initial flow exceeds 41 cc./min.[12-14] In fact, it might be held that the coronary graft has a more favorable outlook for long-term patency than peripheral grafts since graft distance is less, there are no fascial tunnels to traverse, and occlusion is not promoted by change in position, such as leg crossing. Moreover, the vast majority of coronary obstructions are proximal and the estimate is that suitable vessels exist for anastomosis in over 90 per cent of patients with coronary artery disease.[15]

The ultimate fate of venous grafts in the aorto-coronary position remains to be determined. Despite initial optimism, it is well documented that pathologic changes occurs in these aorto-coronary saphenous vein grafts.[16-18] Eight grafts obtained at necropsy three and a half to nine months after operation had two distinctive lesions. Firstly, thrombosis was present in two of the eight grafts and was associated with severe distal coronary artery obstruction. Secondly, six of eight grafts had "intimal fibrous proliferation" with varying degrees of luminal narrowing. This lesion was accentuated in the patients with the poorest distal coronary run-off.[16] Further anatomic studies on these vein grafts are needed. It should be emphasized that the pathology described above was highly selected in that it occurred in patients who had expired and, hence, may not represent the situation in the numerous living patients with patent grafts.

Retrospective Analysis of Performance

Four major areas will be discussed that are responsible for the belief that aorto-coronary bypass grafts are more likely to be beneficial than harmful to the patient with obstructive coronary artery disease. These include: (1) evidence for increased myocardial oxygen delivery, (2) augmentation of ventricular function, (3) improvement in exercise tolerance correlated with augmented hemodynamic function and graft patency, and (4) the influences of surgical therapy on the natural history of coronary obstructive disease.

Objective Data for Augmented Myocardial Oxygen Delivery

Since the symptom of angina pectoris results from an inadequacy of myocardial oxygen delivery relative to demand, any procedure designed to reduce angina and protect against infarction must increase myocardial tissue O_2 delivery. Initial mean vein bypass graft flows for patients in several studies have varied from 35 to 68 ml./min.[19-21] The capacity for increasing flow in our series was demonstrated by administration of isoproterenol and by reactive hyperemia in the coronary bed supplied by the graft that was present in 17 of 32 patients studied. On the basis of experimental studies by Khouri and Gregg, flows in the graft would be expected to increase with time as collaterals regress.[22] Further documentation of augmented myocardial flow was documented by Gorlin's group, who showed increased rates of myocardial ^{133}xenon washout when bypass grafts were opened.[23] Gardner and Gott et al. measured significant increases in myocardial oxygenation associated with bypass grafting by mass spectrophotometric monitoring of intramyocardial oxygen levels, and Kaiser and his associates showed regional improvement in surface electrograms.[24, 25] The relationship between these observations and the syndrome of clinical angina is purely inferential, but flow measurements, surface electrograms, and intramyocardial O_2 tensions all document improved oxygenation at the tissue level in response to bypass grafting.

Further evidence for augmented myocardial aerobic energy metabolism after vein grafting emerges from studies utilizing the fact that the myocardium responds to diminished O_2 delivery by decreased lactate utilization and increased lactate/pyruvate ratios. Beer and Kremkau and their associates independently have evaluated the effects of bypass grafting on myocardial lactate production. Both studies demonstrated increased aerobic metabolism after grafting in response to pacing-induced stress.[26, 27] Finally, using the ^{84}rubidium bolus technique, Knoebel and co-workers determined that preoperative abnormal myocardial blood flow responses to isoproterenol converted to normal following bypass grafting for patients with patent grafts.[28]

Augmentation of Ventricular Performance Following Grafting

If myocardial function is limited by ischemia, and if bypass grafting diminishes ischemia, then improved left ventricular performance should be one benefit of the procedure. Contractile element velocity during isovolumetric systole extrapolated to zero end-diastolic pressure (V_{max}) was evaluated and found significantly increased in 50 per cent of the patients undergoing surgery.[29] In our own studies at Duke on 13 patients, both mechanical contractile indices and hydraulic performance indices demonstrated that opening the vein graft(s) resulted in improvement in left ventricular function in 46 per cent of the patients. If the effect of the graft during the stress of isoproterenol infusion is studied, then opening the graft improved cardiac function in 89 per cent of the patients ($P<.01$) as measured by increased stroke work, stroke index, and contractility.[30]

These observations are summarized in Figure 1. In one group of patients

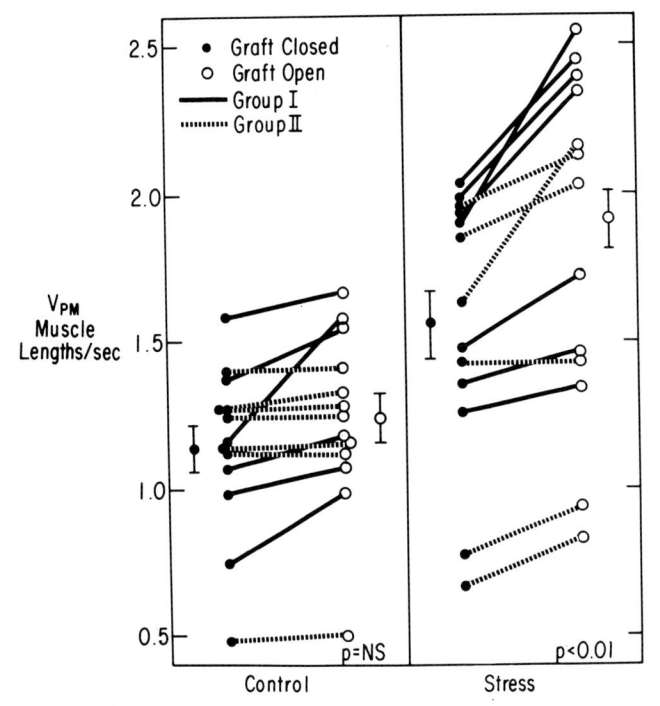

Figure 1. Contractile response to opening aorto-coronary vein grafts at rest and during isoproterenol infusion (stress). All but one patient augmented V_{pm} when the grafts were opened during isoproterenol infusion. Six patients (solid lines) significantly increased V_{pm} when the grafts were opened in the resting state. (Reproduced from Wechsler, A. S., et al.: Norepinephrine induced augmentation of myocardial contractility as a means for assessing the immediate efficacy of aorta to coronary artery bypass grafts. J. Thorac. Cardiov. Surg. 64:861, 1972.)

(solid lines) peak measured contractile element velocity (V_{pm}) increased when the grafts were opened in the resting state and this increase was accentuated when the grafts were opened during isoproterenol infusion. The second group of patients (broken lines) had no increase in V_{pm} in the resting state, but when the grafts were opened during isoproterenol infusion there was significant ($P<.01$) augmentation of contractility.

Of great importance is the study of Rees and Bristow et al. correlating decrease in end-diastolic volume, increase in ejection fraction, and increase in velocity of circumferential fiber shortening with graft patency; patients with occluded grafts had deterioration of ventricular performance as measured by those parameters. Their investigations were in patients with moderate impairment of left ventricular function. The pre- and postoperative left ventricular contour from one of the patients who experienced augmentation of function when studied three months after operation is reproduced in Figure 2. This study emphasizes the high correlation between an anatomically successful operation, a physiologically improved heart, and subjective relief of symptoms. Such correlations were distinctly lacking in earlier procedures. In a similar manner, Grondin

PREOPERATIVE

E.D.V. = 88 ml/m²
E.S.V. = 41 ml/m²
E.F. = 0.53

POSTOPERATIVE

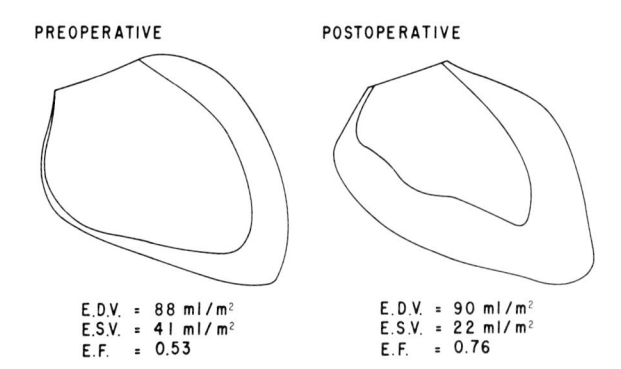

E.D.V. = 90 ml/m²
E.S.V. = 22 ml/m²
E.F. = 0.76

Figure 2. Outline of left ventricle before and three months after aorto-coronary bypass grafting. The mildly diminished ejection fraction is restored to normal. This patient was selected from the group demonstrating improved function associated with a patent graft. (Reproduced from Rees, G., et al.: New Eng. J. Med. 284:1116, 1971.)

and co-workers determined reversal of left ventricular akinesis or hypokinesis in 66 per cent of patients with patent vein grafts, and Chatterjee et al. observed similar improvement in segmental contraction patterns in the majority of patients with patent grafts but no improvement, or worsening, in patients with obstructed grafts.[31-33]

Subjective and Objective Influence on Exercise Tolerance

Early surgical therapy for angina pectoris suffered many hardships. Some of these related to inadequacies in the understanding of the abnormal cardiovascular physiology of myocardial ischemia and its attendant anatomic aberrations, while others were the result of an inability to diagnose adequately and to follow the disease in a scientific manner. Relief from angina, independent from mortality, is an acceptable end itself, but subjective improvement without accompanying hemodynamic alterations is an unacceptable criterion for successful surgery. A surgical procedure is best evaluated by tests obtained in an exercise laboratory equipped for simultaneous hemodynamic determinations. With coronary arteriography it is possible to correlate augmented exercise capacity with graft patency, and, unlike the paradoxical data obtained for myocardial implant procedures, the correlation between increased exercise or functional capacity and graft patency is high. Uniformly, poor exercise responses are found in patients with obstructed grafts. Functional capacity of the vast majority of patients improves and subjective relief of angina is reported as high as 95 per cent.[13] In our own series at Duke, 28 of 57 patients converted from electrocardiographically positive to negative exercise tests, but of nine patients with occluded grafts, six had less satisfactory postoperative tests. Particularly important is the study of Mason and associates in which pre- and postoperative bicycle ergometry, along with estimates of myocardial oxygen demand as determined from pressure-rate product indices, were used to assess changes in exercise tolerance. In the group of patients studied, fatigue at a higher pressure-rate product limited postoperative exercise but not angina.[34] The exercise studies for that group of patients are summarized in Figure 3. Following aorto-coronary bypass, a greater pressure-rate product was achieved without pain than preoperatively, when pain occurred at a low pressure-rate product even after propranolol administration.

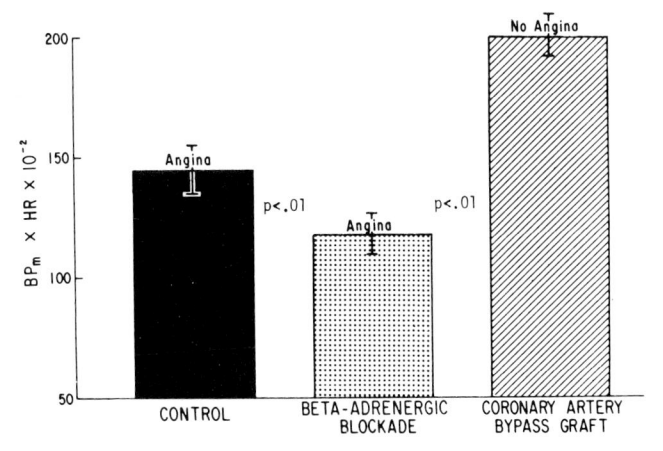

Figure 3. Pressure-rate product during exercise testing. After aorto-coronary bypass grafting these patients were able to exercise at a higher pressure-rate product, without pain, than in the preoperative period. Propranolol did not significantly increase the maximum pressure-rate product tolerated without angina before operation. (Reproduced from Mason, D. T., et al.: Amer. J. Cardiol. 28:608, 1971.)

OPERATIVE HISTORY VERSUS NATURAL HISTORY

Operative mortality for bypass grafts should be subdivided very finely for ultimate statistical analysis, and this division should be made on both the basis of arterial involvement and functional impairment. Although large compilations of such data are not yet available, at present immediate operative mortality ranges from 2 to 10 per cent, but most encouraging are the low attrition rates, even for patients with two and three vessel disease, in the months after surgery. These rates are reported in the range of 2 to 4 per cent for all patients grafted, with some 85 per cent of patients returning to full activity.[13]

Prospective Randomization

"Randomization is most ethical when there is no knowledge about relative efficacy and toxicity, and this state exists in its purest form at the time the first patient is to be treated."[35] Demands for complete prospective randomization of patients for coronary bypass grafts have reached a zenith, but the acquisition of experience and data confirming the efficacy of the operative procedure renders ethical randomization of patients difficult.[1-3]

The random allocation of patients to operative or nonoperative treatment of coronary artery disease justifiably supersedes the classic subjective physician-determined therapy only when the relative merits and risks of the procedure are completely unknown; that is, when there is a "50-50 chance" that a given mode of therapy might prove beneficial or injurious.[36] The entire ethic of randomization, however, becomes altered when a legitimate retrospective analysis of performance indicates that objective benefit has been acquired by one portion of the sample population. At this point the basic probability ratio is no longer 50-50 (pure chance), and the physician is obliged to apply a therapeutic program that he believes has the greatest potential for success. No matter how great the desire for trial by randomization may be at present, the reality is that the 50,000 procedures already performed cannot be relegated to nonexistence in order to set the record straight. Ethical practice dictates that as much information as possible be obtained from these experiences. When this is done, the result is apt to shift the 50-50 probability ratio such that a demand for complete randomization is no longer justifiable. Retrospective analysis of aorto-coronary bypass procedures to date has emphasized several areas where randomization is clearly needed and justified and should be applied. These are discussed later in the text.

The second major factor precluding complete randomization is more complex. It involves the superimposition of a "psychic reality" onto "objective reality" such that randomization of the population at risk becomes pragmatically impossible because of patient and physician conditioning. This is an illegitimate factor and introduces bias into any future study by allowing preselection. *Bias* is the result of premature reporting by participants seeking individual acclaim and conducting studies in inadequately controlled circumstances. Bias results from confusing idle speculation with accomplishment of defined scientific objectives, and from channeling scientific data through lay media to audiences inadequately trained to assess critically the information obtained. Bias results from improper initial control over any new procedure, and the guilt for this dwells within the scientific community. In the use of aorto-coronary bypass grafts, both major factors are operative and preclude a completely randomized study. Scientific evidence supports the contention that bypass grafting is an effective way to treat proximal obstructive coronary artery disease and the population of physicians and patients at large is a highly biased group.

The failures of the past should not serve to influence the present controversy. The same statistically oriented proponents of random patient selection paradoxically point to the demonstrated efficacy of sham internal mammary artery ligation in curing angina as another of the shortcomings of the past. Closer examination of these studies, however, demonstrates that the experiments prove only that subjective relief of angina (in some cases) is not a valid indicator of the physiologic effectiveness of the treatment. The total number of patients, combining both studies, was 35 (14 sham, 21 ligated), and we do not know how many of the patients with angina actually had coronary arterial obstruction since coronary arteriography had not evolved to its current sophisticated state. The most important fact evolving from the studies was that the electrocardiograms (the best objective evidence for ischemia then available) were reliable.[37, 38] If something is to be learned from this period of "trial and error," it is that objective data must be used in assessing efficacy of procedures for angina. Let the critics of contemporary surgical data and procedures forego the absurdity of using the past to condemn the future. Rather, they should stress the acquisition of objective data as a primary goal of any study.

The Future

The 50,000 aorto-coronary bypass grafts performed to date suggest the following conclusions:

1. A patient and physician bias has been established that probably precludes *effective* randomization. Physicians refer their patients to selected centers for specific treatment. Failure of a referral center to perform bypass surgery in the presence of appropriate indications will unquestionably divert "ideal" operative candidates away from the randomizing institution to other centers and result in randomization of an already preselected population.

2. Retrospective analysis and careful characterization of subjects may well be inferior to randomization at day one, but the knowledge gained from study of the procedures performed to date no longer allows the assumption of a 50-50 chance that the procedure will be harmful (or no good). Thus, for the individual physician, convinced by favorable reports, it becomes impossible in good conscience to allow randomization of his patient.

3. Randomized studies recently initiated are apt to be questioned because of biased selection. The Veterans Administration program probably suffers from some degree of preselection since the population is a relatively restricted one. Moreover, the administrative "escape" clause, allowing veterans in the study to have surgery if they so desire as well as the option to seek treatment of their choice outside the confines of the study, compromises the meaning of the results.

4. Coronary arteriography is attended by a risk of 2 per cent in ischemic heart disease and as high as 5 per cent for left main coronary lesions.[39] If no surgery is to be performed, is the risk of repetitive arteriography ethically justifiable?

5. Studies of the natural history to date indicate that the mortality rate from coronary obstructive disease is unacceptably high for patients with two and three vessel disease, and early retrospective analyses favor a surgical approach to these patients. Many hold that bypass procedures should be recommended strongly to patients with two and three vessel disease in view of the high mortality associated with such lesions if no correction measures are used.

6. Patients with single vessel involvement comprise a special group because of their better long-term prognosis, and surgical intervention should probably be limited to patients incapacitated from their angina and acquiring little medical relief.

7. Unlike procedures of the past, a high degree of correlation exists between subjective relief of angina, augmented exercise tolerance, improved ventricular function, and graft patency. Although relief of angina is a subjective result of aorto-coronary bypass grafting, the association of subjective relief, a good anatomic result, and restored physiology justify surgical intervention for relief of angina and its attendant improvement in the "quality" of life. This argument is not thwarted by the observation that angina is capricious and may spontaneously regress. The association of surgical intervention and relief of angina (with adequate hemodynamic improvement) is too high to be coincidental.

8. Certain *special* groups of patients exist who comprise disease categories

with *inadequately* described natural histories. These patients can be subdivided and randomized for therapy in good conscience. These groups are:

    a. Patients with "pre-infarction angina" or the acute progressive coronary insufficiency syndrome. The problem with this group is very much the problem of definition of the syndrome, but working criteria must be established for standardization of patient selection.

    b. Patients studied after full recovery from acute myocardial infarction and found to have significant proximal disease without angina. From the Framingham study, many of these subjects are statistically apt to suffer subsequent infarction *without interim angina*. No studies on this group have yet been undertaken, and there is no existing bias and no a priori reason to assume anything other than a 50-50 probability situation. This group is ideal for randomization for long-term analysis.

    c. Patients with acute myocardial infarction responding poorly to management or with extensive infarction as determined by enzyme analysis in whom the prognosis is now known to be unfavorable.

    d. Patients experiencing myocardial infarction as a direct result of coronary arteriography.

    e. Patients with severe left ventricular failure and accompanying angina. This group may have an operative mortality high enough to warrant separate treatment.

These groups readily fulfill all the criteria for ethical randomization. Other patients undergoing operation should be subjected to intensive pre- and postoperative investigation so that the best retrospective analysis of data will be possible in a situation where the need for randomization was initially great but where the opportunity has since passed. The conscience of the present can best be satisfied by diligent analysis of the past rather than by denial of its existence. The lessons learned will set the trends for the future with avoidance of past mistakes.

References

1. Zimmerman, H. A.: And now—vein grafts. Amer. Heart J. 80:585, 1970.
2. Spodick, D. H.: Coronary revascularization. Circulation 44:302, 1971.
3. Spodick, D. H.: Revascularization of the heart—numerators in search of denominatiors. Amer. Heart J. 81:149, 1971.
4. Kannel, W. B., and Feinleib, M.: Natural history of angina pectoris in the Framingham Study. Amer. J. Cardiol. 29:154, 1972.
5. Friesinger, G. C., Page, E. E., and Ross, R. S.: Prognostic significance of coronary arteriography. Trans. Ass. Amer. Phys. 83:78, 1970.
6. Moberg, C. H., Webster, J. S., and Sones, M. F.: Natural history of severe proximal coronary disease as defined by cineangiography (200 patients, 7 year followup). Amer. J. Cardiol. 29:282, 1972.
7. DeWeese, J. A., and Rob, C. G.: Autogenous venous bypass grafts five years later. Ann. Surg. 174:346, 1971.
8. Darling, R. C., Linton, R. A., and Razzuk, M. A.: Saphenous vein bypass grafts for femoropopliteal occlusive disease: A reappraisal. Surgery 61:31, 1967.
9. Favaloro, R. G., Effler, D. B., Groves, L. K., Sheldon, W. C., and Sones, M. F.: Direct myocardial revascularization by saphenous vein graft. Ann. Thorac. Surg. 10:97, 1970.
10. Johnson, D. W., Flemma, R. J., Lepley, D., and Ellison, E. H.: Extended treatment of severe coronary artery disease. Ann. Surg. 170:460, 1969.

11. Green, G. E., Spencer, F. C., Tice, D. A., and Stertzer, S. H.: Arterial and venous microsurgical bypass grafts for coronary artery disease. J. Thorac. Cardiov. Surg. 60:491, 1970.
12. Favaloro, R. G.: Surgical treatment of coronary arteriosclerosis by the saphenous vein graft technique. Amer. J. Cardiol. 28:493, 1971.
13. Morris, G. C., Reul, G. J., Howell, J. F., Crawford, E. S., Chapman, D. W., Beazley, H. L., Winters, W. L., Peterson, P. K., and Lewis, J. M.: Follow-up results of distal coronary artery bypass for ischemic heart disease. Amer. J. Cardiol. 29:180, 1972.
14. Walker, J. A., Friedberg, H. D., Flemma, R. J., and Johnson, W. D.: Determinants of angiographic patency of aortocoronary vein bypass grafts. Circulation 43 and 44 (Suppl. 2):108, 1971.
15. Glassman, E., Spencer, F. C., Tice, D. A., Weisinger, B., and Green, G. E.: What percentage of patients with angina pectoris are candidates for bypass grafts. Circulation 43 and 44(Suppl.1):101, 1971.
16. Vlodaver, Z., and Edwards, J. E.: Pathologic changes in aortic-coronary arterial saphenous vein grafts. Circulation 44:719, 1971.
17. Johnson, W. D., Auer, J. E., and Tector, A. J.: Late changes in coronary vein grafts. (Abstract.) Amer. J. Cardiol. 26:640, 1970.
18. Grondin, C. M., Meere, C., Castonguay, Y., Lepage, G., and Grondin, P.: Progressive and late obstruction of an aorto-coronary venous bypass graft: A case report. Circulation 43:698, 1971.
19. Johnson, D. W., Flemma, R. J., Manley, J. C., and Lepley, D.: The physiologic parameters of ventricular function as affected by direct coronary surgery. J. Thorac. Cardiov. Surg. 60:483, 1970.
20. Grondin, C. M., Lepage, G., Castonguay, Y. R., Meere, C., and Grondin, P.: Aortocoronary bypass graft. Circulation 44:815, 1971.
21. Greenfield, J. C., Rembert, J. C., Young, G. W., Oldham, H. N., Alexander, J. A., and Sabiston, D. C.: Studies of blood flow in aorta-to-coronary venous bypass grafts in man. J. Clin. Invest. 51:2724–2735, 1972.
22. Khouri, E. M., Gregg, D. E., and McGranahan, G. M.: Regression and reappearance of coronary collaterals. Amer. J. Physiol. 220:655, 1971.
23. Smith, S. C., Gorlin, R., Herman, M. V., Taylor, W. J., and Collins, J. J.: Effects of coronary artery bypass and coronary collaterals on myocardial bloodflow. Circulation 43 and 44(Suppl.2):60, 1971.
24. Gardner, T. J., Brantigan, J. W., Perna, A. M., Bender, H. W., Brawley, R. K., and Gott, V. L.: Intramyocardial gas tensions in the human heart during coronary arterysaphenous vein bypass. J. Thorac. Cardiov. Surg. 844:62, 1971.
25. Kaiser, G. A., Waldo, A. L., Bowman, F. O., Hoffman, B. F., and Malm, J. R.: The use of ventricular electrograms in operation for coronary artery disease and its complications. Ann. Thorac. Surg. 10:153, 1970.
26. Beer, N., Keller, N., Apstein, C., Kline, S., Tarjan, E., Carlson, R. G., and Brachfeld, N.: The cardiac hemodynamic and metabolic responses to coronary arteriovenous bypass surgery. Amer. J. Cardiol. 20:252, 1972.
27. Kremkau, E. L., Kloster, F. E., and Neill, W. A.: Influence of aorto-coronary bypass on myocardial hypoxia. Circulation 43 and 44(Suppl.2):103, 1971.
28. Knoebel, S. B., McHenry, P. L., Phillips, J. F., and Jacobs, J. J.: Objective assessment of saphenous vein bypass grafts. Circulation 43 and 44(Suppl.2):187, 1971.
29. Bolooki, H., Rubinson, R. M., Michie, D. D., and Jude, J. R.: Assessment of myocardial contractility after coronary bypass grafts. J. Thorac. Cardiov. Surg. 62:543, 1971.
30. Wechsler, A. S., Gill, C., Rosenfeldt, F., Oldham, N., and Sabiston, D. C.: Norepinephrine induced augmentation of myocardial contractility as a means for assessing the immediate efficacy of aorta to coronary artery bypass grafts. J. Thorac. Cardiov. Surg. 64:861–868, 1972.
31. Rees, G., Bristow, J. D., Kremkau, E. L., Green, G. S., Herr, R. H., Griswold, H. E., and Starr, A.: Influence of aortocoronary bypass surgery on left ventricular performance. New Eng. J. Med. 284:1116, 1971.
32. Saltiel, J., Lesperance, J., Bourassa, M. G., Castonguay, Y., Campeau, L., and Grondin, P.: Reversibility of left ventricular dysfunction following aorto-coronary bypass grafts. Amer. J. Roentgenol. 110:739, 1970.
33. Chatterjee, K., Parmley, W. W., Sustaita, H., Matloff, J. M., and Swan, J. C.: Influence of aortocoronary artery bypass on left ventricular asynergy. Amer. J. Cardiol. 29:256, 1972.
34. Mason, D. T., Amsterdam, E. A., Miller, R. R., Hughes, J. L., Bonanno, J. A., Iben, A. B., Hurley, E. J., Massumi, R. A., and Zelis, R.: Consideration of the therapeutic roles

of pharmacologic agents, collateral circulation and saphenous vein bypass in coronary artery disease. Amer. J. Cardiol. 28:608, 1971.
35. Chalmers, T. C.: When should randomisation begin? Lancet 1:858, 1968.
36. Chalmers, T. C.: Mortality rate versus funeral rate in clinical medicine. Gastroenterology 46:788, 1964.
37. Cobb, L. A., Thomas, G. I., Dillard, D. H., Merendino, K. A., and Bruce, R. A.: An evaluation of internal-mammary-artery ligation by a double-blind technic. New Eng. J. Med. 260:1115, 1959.
38. Dimond, E. G., Kittle, C. F., and Crockett, J. E.: Comparison of internal mammary artery ligation and sham operation for angina pectoris. Amer. J. Cardiol. 5:483, 1960.
39. Cohen, M. V., Cohn, P. F., Herman, M. V., and Gorlin, R.: Diagnosis and prognosis of main left coronary artery (LCA) obstruction. Circulation 43 and 44(Suppl.2):102, 1971.

The Role of Coronary Bypass Grafts in the Treatment of Angina Pectoris Remains To Be Established

RICHARD S. ROSS

The Johns Hopkins University and Hospital

It has been estimated that 20,000 coronary artery bypass procedures were done in the United States during the calendar year of 1971, and it seems likely that an even greater number of procedures will be done in the future. Each procedure costs about $10,000, and if this unit cost is multiplied by the number of procedures a figure of $200,000,000 is obtained. This new operation is, therefore, not only a major medical problem but also a major national economic problem to patients and insurance companies.[1,2]

Despite this widespread use and tremendous cost, the role of this procedure in the treatment of ischemic heart disease has yet to be clearly defined. There are, however, certain facts upon which there is general agreement by all physicians and surgeons concerned with the problem. First and foremost is the effect of the procedure on the patients' symptomatology. It seems clear that symptomatic relief from angina pectoris can be expected in 85 to 100 per cent of patients. This is a worthwhile objective because angina is a disabling disease and limits the effectiveness of patients as contributors to society and interferes with the enjoyment of their personal life. It is also possible to demonstrate that exercise tolerance is improved in a similar fraction of patients who have successful bypass surgery. The improvement in exercise tolerance is, however, not clearly dissociated from the relief of symptoms because it is often the chest pain that limits exercise tolerance; and, if this is removed, exercise tolerance will be improved.

Improvement in symptoms and exercise tolerance is far easier to demonstrate than improvement in ventricular function. It is possible to find a few patients who have dramatic improvement of ventricular function as evidenced by improved hemodynamics, an increase in ejection fraction, and improved contractility as viewed cineangiographically,[3,4] but this is by no means universal, and certainly does not approach the 80 per cent frequency of symptomatic improvement. Most investigators find that in no more than 20 to 25 per cent of patients is it possible to demonstrate improved wall motion on cineangiography. There is little or no change in conventional hemodynamic measurements such as cardiac output, left ventricular filling pressure, or ejection fraction.[5] Improvement has, however, been reported in several of the noninvasive methods of evaluating cardiac performance such as the systolic time intervals and the ballistocardiogram.[6, 7]

Probably the most important unanswerable question concerning the efficacy of aorto-coronary vein bypass surgery is that concerning its effect on natural history of the disease. It has not been demonstrated that the construction of a successful bypass to the distal coronary vessel will significantly reduce the probability of that patient's having a myocardial infarction or dying suddenly as a consequence of his ischemic heart disease. It is tempting to reason that the disease shortens life because the obstructing lesion interferes with blood supply; therefore, the lesion can be bypassed by this simple straightforward operative procedure, the distal blood supply will be improved and life prolonged. The assumption that prognosis will be improved is often made in advising surgery, although it is not recognized to be just an assumption by either the physician or the patient.

The duration of the favorable effect on the quality of life also remains unknown. The symptoms are relieved initially, but we do not know yet how long this will last. The duration of the effect on symptoms depends to a certain extent on another unknown and that is the long-term fate of the veins used to construct the bypass between the aorta and the coronary arteries. Veins become occluded by a progressive intimal fibrous proliferative process.[8] It is difficult to compare figures from one center to another, but in general it would appear that when the veins are examined angiographically in the first month after operation approximately 85 per cent will be patent, indicating that 15 per cent become occluded very soon after surgery. With longer intervals after operation, as for example six months to one year, patency rates of between 65 and 70 per cent seem to be common. This probably indicates that the fibrous proliferative process is slowly progressive during the first year and only produces a total occlusion after the passage of time. The figure of 65 per cent is not unexpected as it is similar to the long-term patency observed with veins put into the arterial system in the lower extremities to bypass arteriosclerotic lesions in that segment of the circulation. It has been suggested that there is a greater likelihood of occlusion when the veins are used in the chest because they are not supported externally by the tissue as they are in the leg.

The relatively high incidence of obstruction of the veins at six months to a year has stimulated some surgeons to use internal mammary arteries to bypass the obstructing lesion. The early results with the arterial grafts are very encouraging, with reports of close to 100 per cent patency at one year. The operation, using an arterial rather than a venous graft, is technically more difficult but may well turn out to be the procedure of choice.[9]

The postoperative evaluation must not be limited to determination of the patency of the bypass. The intrinsic or native circulation of the heart must also be re-examined at the time of the postoperative study. The operative procedure does nothing to change the basic atherosclerotic process which afflicts the patient's intrinsic coronary circulation. Several groups who have studied patients after the construction of the vein bypass have been able to demonstrate new obstructive lesions in previously patent segments of the intrinsic or native coronary circulation.[10, 11] These occlusions in the native coronary circulation are associated with changes in the electrocardiogram and in segmental contractility and therefore have resulted in loss of myocardial tissue. At the time of restudy six to nine months after operation the likelihood of a new occlusion in the intrinsic circulation is approximately 25 per cent if the graft to the vessel is open and 60 per cent if the graft has become occluded. New lesions or occlusions have also been observed in vessels to which no graft was connected. These changes in "nongrafted" vessels appear to be more common when the intrinsic vessel was exposed by the surgeon in contemplation of bypass which was not completed because the vessel appeared to be unsuitable. In other cases in which the vessel was not touched by the surgeon, the new lesions can be attributed either to the natural progression of the disease or to effects of pump oxygenator perfusion and periods of anoxic arrest.[12]

These observations of new occlusive lesions in the native circulation are supported by the 15 to 25 per cent reported incidence of clinically identifiable myocardial infarction in the postoperative period.[13] The new occlusive lesions in the native coronary vessels into which the bypass has been placed can be divided into two groups on the basis of the location of the occluded segment. If there is failure to visualize a previously patent segment distal to the graft there can be no question about the significance of the finding. The area which was underperfused by the native circulation before operation is now totally without perfusion from either the native vessel or the graft. The second type of segmental lesion of native circulation is that which involves the segment proximal to the graft and distal to the bypassed lesion. It is sometimes argued that the occlusions in this proximal portion of the native vessel are of no importance because the large caliber bypass is open and carrying the blood to the distal vessel. The weakness of this argument is easily appreciated when we realize that there is at least a 30 per cent chance that the vein will become occluded in approximately six months; therefore, we are making the patient dependent upon a blood-carrying system with a known probability of occlusion of 30 per cent.

In view of these disturbing unknowns about the procedure it would seem appropriate to consider possible reasons for the extremely high incidence of symptomatic relief which has been universally reported.[14] The first possible explanation of symptomatic relief is that the intended objective has been achieved and that the vein has provided an increased supply of blood to a segment of the intrinsic native coronary circulation which was previously undersupplied with blood. Myocardial ischemia has been relieved in the distribution of the bypassed vessel and therefore the patient's pain has been relieved. In 40 to 50 per cent of patients this is the true sequence of events. The evidence for this depends on the identification of an ischemic segment of the myocardium prior to operation by the demonstration of a localized electrocardiographic abnormality with stress testing which corresponds to a specific anatomic lesion. Postoperative angiography demonstrates that the blood flow to this portion of the intrinsic circulation is improved, and the electrocardiographic abnormality and the pain disappear. Unfortunately, however, this neat sequence of events cannot be demonstrated in the majority of patients who report symptomatic improvement. Furthermore, in every series there are a number of patients who report symptomatic improvement in the presence of total occlusion of the vein bypasses. Obviously, in those with totally obstructed grafts, it is impossible to say that the improvement is related to increased blood flow through the bypass. In between these two extremes there are many other patients in whom there is the possibility that a direct effect of increased blood flow may be responsible for improvement, but this cannot be proved. The challenge for the future is to develop techniques whereby the patients who will be benefited by increased blood flow can be identified in advance.

Other possible explanations for the improvement do, however, exist. For example, if a myocardial infarction occurs at the site of previous myocardial ischemia one might expect that the symptoms would be relieved, because it is generally agreed that infarcted muscle is not a source of pain. Another possibility is that improvement may be related to some nonspecific effect of surgery. This might have an anatomic or physiological basis in the form of enhanced flow from the pericardium into the myocardium, diminution of the ischemic area, or an enhancement of collateral development secondary to the surgical manipulation at or about the coronary vessel. We must always keep in mind that there is a tremendous placebo effect of surgery and that this is a confusing factor in the interpretation of any or all changes in symptomatic status.

The placebo effect of surgery has been demonstrated in the past by the elegant clinical investigations of Cobb[15] and Diamond[16] and their associates, who showed that many patients with angina pectoris experienced significant relief of symptoms following a sham operation consisting of merely a skin incision on the chest. The experience with internal mammary implant surgery also provides some data about the placebo effect of surgery. The studies of Björck and associates[17] in Sweden have shown that 50 per cent of implanted mammary arteries are occluded at the time of restudy. The frequency of improvement in symptoms and improvement in exercise tolerance is approximately the same in the group with occluded vessels as it is in the group with patent vessels. Beecher[18] pointed out that the placebo effect of surgery is related to the emotional status of the patient. The more the patient wants to get well the more likely he is to experience a favorable placebo effect. He also stressed the fact that the placebo effect is a function of the enthusiasm of the surgeon. When the surgeon is confident and enthusiastic, improvement is more likely than when the surgeon approaches the patient and the operation with a questioning attitude of an investigator.

This is not to say that the aorto-coronary vein bypass operation benefits patients only because of the placebo effect. It has already been stated that there are clearly some patients in whom increased blood flow to a previously ischemic segment seems to be evident; and, therefore, it is reasonable to believe that improvement is a function of better blood flow and less ischemia. The placebo effect, however, is present to a greater or lesser degree in all patients with angina undergoing surgery. When there is no other good explanation for improvement, as for example in a case with all grafts occluded, the placebo effect may be responsible.

In summary, it is clear that the vein bypass operation will relieve the symptoms of angina pectoris in the vast majority of patients. The mechanism whereby symptoms are relieved is not always that of improving blood flow to an ischemic segment. Other possibilities include the nonspecific effects of surgery which might include a placebo effect and infarction of previously ischemic portions of the myocardium.

The intense enthusiasm for this operation is based upon the assumption that creating a surgical bypass around an obstructing lesion will impove the natural history of the patient and decrease the likelihood of myocardial infarction and sudden death. This remains an assumption at the present time.

References

1. Friedberg, C. K.: Caution and coronary artery surgery: Timeo chirurgos et dona ferentes. (Editorial.) Circulation 45:727, 1972.
2. Glenn, W. W. L.: Some reflections on the coronary bypass operation. Circulation 45:869, 1972.
3. Rees, G., Bristow, J. D., Kremkau, E. L., Green, G. S., Herr, R. H., Griswold, H. E., and Starr, A.: Influence of aortocoronary bypass surgery on left ventricular performance. New Eng. J. Med. 284:1116, 1971.
4. Chatterjee, K., Swan, H. J. C., Parmley, W. W., Sustaita, H., Marcus, H., and Matloff, J.: Depression of left ventricular function due to acute myocardial ischemia and its reversal after aortocoronary saphenous vein bypass. New Eng. J. Med. 286:1117, 1972.
5. Conti, C. R., Page, E. E., Humphries, J. O., Pitt, B., and Ross, R. S.: Objective evaluation of aortico-coronary vein bypass surgery. Trans. Ass. Amer. Phys. 84:272, 1971.
6. Johnson, A., and O'Rourke, R.: Effect of myocardial revascularization on systolic time intervals in patients with left ventricular dysfunction. Circulation 43(Suppl.2):103, 1971.
7. Starr, I., and MacVaugh, H., III: Objective tests of cardiac contractility before and after 3 operative procedures designed to improve the coronary circulation. Clin. Res. 20:621, 1972.
8. Vlodaver, Z., and Edwards, J. E.: Pathologic changes in aortic-coronary arterial saphenous vein grafts. Circulation 44:719, 1971.
9. Green, G. E., Stertzer, S. H., Gordon, R. B., and Tia, D. A.: Anastomosis of the internal mammary artery to the distal left anterior descending coronary artery. Circulation 42(Suppl.2):79, 1970.
10. Griffith, L., Achuff, S., Conti, C. R., Humphries, J. O., Brawley, R. K., Gott, V., and Ross, R. S.: Changes in intrinsic coronary circulation and segmental ventricular motion after saphenous vein coronary bypass graft surgery. New Eng. J. Med. 288:589, 1973.
11. Aldridge, H. E., and Trimble, A. S.: Progression of proximal coronary artery lesions to total occlusion after aorta-coronary saphenous vein bypass grafting. J. Thorac. Cardiov. Surg. 62:7, 1971.
12. Gensini, G. G., and Kelly, A. E.: Incidence and progression of coronary artery disease. Arch. Intern. Med. 129:814, 1972.
13. Hultgren, H. N., Miyagawa, M., Buck, W., and Angell, W. W.: Ischemic injury during coronary artery surgery. Amer. Heart J. 82:624, 1971.
14. Griffith, L., Achuff, S., Humphries, J. O., Conti, C. R., Brawley, R., Gott, V., and Ross, R. S.: Mechanisms of symptomatic improvement after coronary bypass graft surgery. Amer. J. Cardiol. 31:137, 1973.
15. Cobb, L. A., Thomas, G. I., Dillard, D. H., Merendino, K. A., and Bruce, R. A.: An evaluation of internal-mammary-artery ligation by a double-blind technique. New Eng. J. Med. 260:1115, 1959.
16. Dimond, E. G., Kittle, C. F., and Crockett, J. E.: Comparison of internal mammery artery ligation and sham operation for angina pectoris. Amer. J. Cardiol. 5:483, 1960.
17. Björck, L., Culhead, I., Hallen, A., and Strom, G.: Result of internal mammary artery implantation in patients with angina pectoris. Scand. J. Thorac. Surg. 2:1, 1968.
18. Beecher, H. K.: Surgery as a placebo: A quantitative study. J.A.M.A. 176:1102, 1961.

Comment

Are Coronary Bypass Grafts the Answer to Angina Pectoris?

No one can question that the development of the coronary bypass graft for the relief of myocardial ischemia represents a triumph of surgical skill. Within a brief period of time it has almost completely superseded previous techniques of myocardial revascularization. The flow through these grafts is often large, and symptoms of angina pectoris are relieved in a high proportion of cases. In many but not all patients there is improvement in left ventricular function and disappearance of electrocardiographic evidence of ischemia with exercise.

In view of these demonstrable desirable effects, how can anyone question the widespread use of the operation for the relief of angina pectoris? The uncertainty is related to two unanswered questions. The first relates to changes occurring in the wall of the graft resulting in narrowing or occlusion of its lumen over a period of years. This question will be answered with time. The second question is whether the operation prolongs life. The answer to this question is of great importance. If the answer is no, the operation will represent merely a palliative procedure with relief of pain as a goal. If the answer is yes, it represents a major advance in the treatment of coronary disease and will be recommended for the majority of patients. Most patients with angina pectoris fear death and will clutch at a procedure which promises a prolongation of life span.

Wechsler and Sabiston feel that the time has passed for a carefully designed clinical trial utilizing the procedure of random allocation of patients. They have faith that knowledge of the natural history of coronary artery disease will permit evaluation of the effect of the operation on longevity without use of the technique of randomization. This hope may be unfounded. The lesson learned in the evaluation of the long-term use of anticoagulants in the treatment of coronary disease should not be forgotten. The critique of early studies of the use of anticoagulants by McMichael and Parry[1] should be read by those contemplating studies on the effect of coronary bypass surgery on duration of life. It would be tragic to repeat the errors of the past.

Reference

1. McMichael, J., and Parry, E. H. O.: Prognosis and anticoagulant prophylaxis after coronary occlusion. Lancet 2:991–998, 1960.

RICHARD V. EBERT

6

Exercise for the Coronary Patient

The Benefits of Physical Training for Patients with Coronary Heart Disease
    by Robert A. Bruce

Disadvantages of Intensive Exercise Therapy After Myocardial Infarction
    by Henry Blackburn

Comment
    by Richard V. Ebert

The Benefits of Physical Training for Patients with Coronary Heart Disease

ROBERT A. BRUCE

University of Washington School of Medicine

Socrates: "And is not bodily habit spoiled by rest and illness, but preserved for a long time by motion and exercise?"
Theaetetus: "True."
This quotation from Plato dates back to around 400 B.C.[1]

In relation to angina pectoris an anonymous physician* reported to Heberden in 1772: "I have frequently, when in company, borne the pain, and continued the pace without indulging in it; at which times it has lasted from five to perhaps ten minutes, and then gone off."[2]

Osler described, in 1897, a patient who walked through his angina.[3] Recently other instances were documented by MacAlpin and Kattus.[4]

The Pathophysiological Problem

Physical training or exercise conditioning increases aerobic metabolism and heat production of working skeletal muscles. The heart is burdened to beat faster with greater contractile force and systolic pressure to circulate more blood to satisfy metabolic and thermal demands. Under these circumstances it seems paradoxical, if not indeed illogical, to suggest that repeated physical training should be either tolerated or beneficial to the ambulatory patient symptomatically

---

* The same physician also experienced recurrent exertional symptoms consistent with paroxysms of cardiac arrhythmia and correctly predicted sudden cardiac death; the latter occurred within three weeks of his letter to Heberden. (Bruce, R. A.: Amer. Heart J. 84:422, 1972.)

limited by ischemic heart disease secondary to coronary atherosclerosis. How then can this be defended and justified to the concerned physician and the uncomfortably restricted patient? What is the evidence that habitual physical activity may be protective before or beneficial after occurrence of angina pectoris or myocardial infarction? What are the risks, and are they balanced by clinical benefits and physiological evidence? Can physical training be advocated when witnessed physical exertion occasionally provokes sudden, unexpected cardiac death[5] and when surgical progress may not lower mortality and morbidity yet give greater promise of correcting the deficit in coronary flow of oxygenated blood? Questions such as these warrant careful consideration if physical training is to be recommended, either as an aid to primary intervention against clinical events of ischemic heart disease, or to facilitate cardiac rehabilitation after such events occur.

Experimental Studies of Exercise Training

Whereas myocardial ischemia impairs left ventricular function, the effects of physical training on the relationship of myocardial fiber to capillary perfusion remain unknown. In normal animals exercise training initiates cardiomegaly[6] and increases the number of capillaries of several[7] but not all mammalian species[8] and also the size of coronary arterial vasculature;[9] yet capillary/fiber ratio diminishes with aging of rats.[10] Tomanek trained young, adult and old male albino rats on a treadmill for 10 to 50 minutes, six days a week, for eight to 12 weeks.[11] Myocardial capillary/muscle-fiber ratio increased significantly (6.5 to 9.5 per cent for all three trained groups) even though it fell off with increasing age (to 22 months), as did capillary density, in confirmation of earlier observations by Rakusan and Poupa.[10] Eckstein in 1957 demonstrated intra-arterial collateral circulation following experimental ligation of the circumflex artery of dogs who were subsequently exercised for six to eight weeks.[12] This last study did not evaluate capillary/fiber ratios or ECG evidence of myocardial ischemia with exercise. Thus, the critical experiment requires (1) an appropriate animal model with significant coronary atherosclerosis, (2) ECG monitoring and evaluation of left ventricular function during exercise, together with (3) arteriographic studies during life and (4) adequate postmortem study of myocardial fiber structure and capillary/fiber relationship.

Role of Physical Activity on Heart Disease

In 1953 Morris and associates examined the effect of occupational physical activity on coronary heart disease; London bus drivers, who were initially more corpulent,[13] had less angina but more myocardial infarction than did the conductors.[14] Several studies reviewed by Fox and Haskell in 1968 are summarized graphically in Figure 1.[15] Angina was 36 per cent more frequent in physically

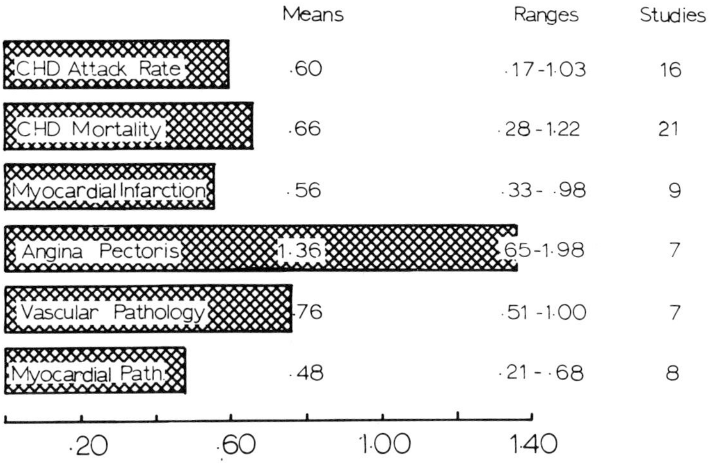

	Means	Ranges	Studies
CHD Attack Rate	.60	.17-1.03	16
CHD Mortality	.66	.28-1.22	21
Myocardial Infarction	.56	.33-.98	9
Angina Pectoris	1.36	.65-1.98	7
Vascular Pathology	.76	.51-1.00	7
Myocardial Path	.48	.21-.68	8

Figure 1. Data on the influence of physical activity on coronary heart disease summarized from several studies. Relationship of rates observed in physically active persons to those in inactive persons is given for each category. (Adapted from Fox, S. M., III, and Haskell, N. L.: Bull. N.Y. Acad. Med. 44:950, 1968.)

active than inactive persons, while myocardial infarction was less frequent and fatalities fewer. At autopsy, coronary vascular disease and myocardial pathology were less severe in patients who had been physically active. Among persons enrolled in the Health Insurance Plan of New York City, age-adjusted attack rate of myocardial infarction was twice as high in inactive as in active persons, and the effect of smoking by inactive persons was additive.[16]

Does strenuous physical activity continued over several years exert any protective effect? Although Finnish athletes were slightly shorter, weighed less, had lower blood pressures, and less frequent ST abnormalities in either resting or postexercise ECG than did sedentary shopkeepers of comparable age, Pyörälä and colleagues found larger heart volumes, higher R voltage, greater maximal oxygen intake, and less frequent clinical manifestations of coronary heart disease.[17] Studies of Chinese ricksha pullers[18] and Chinese pedicabmen occupationally involved in distance exercise also exhibited lower blood pressure, taller R waves, and larger heart size.[19]

Terminology, Significance, and Variations

Exercise "performance" refers to ordinary or submaximal energy expenditures. Exercise or work "capacity" represents the highest possible energy expenditure of which the individual is capable; it is manifested by marked fatigue, muscle weakness, and dyspnea, which quickly limit continuation of effort. Sometimes exertion is limited primarily by angina pectoris; occasionally it is stopped by intermittent claudication. Such manifestations represent pathologic restrictions of coronary or peripheral circulations, respectively. Physiologically, aerobic exercise capacity is manifested by a failure to increase oxygen intake proportional to an increased physical workload. In other words, the nearly linear relationship between oxygen intake and workload, at various levels of submaximal exertion, becomes asymptotic as maximum is approached; a deficit in oxidative metabolism for additional energy expenditure is compensated by anaerobic glycolysis until the glycogen reserves are quickly depleted. In a minority of individuals (15 per cent) who can sustain supramaximal exertion for several seconds, oxygen intake falls because of a decrement in stroke volume, presumably as limits of ventricular compliance and contractile force are exceeded.[20] Attainment of exercise capacity requires preliminary submaximal "warm-up" exertion to allow physiological adjustments in ventilation, circulation, and oxygen dissociation. Maximal oxygen intake ($\dot{V}_{O_2max}$) reflects measurements based upon methods which satisfy these requirements.

Exercise capacity of cardiovascular patients may be designated *"symptom-limited" oxygen intake*. This becomes apparent when retesting with nitroglycerin reveals significant increases in intensity and duration of exertion, faster heart rate, and higher peak levels of oxygen intake which more closely approximate the aerobic capacity of the working skeletal muscles.[21] These changes reveal differences in circulatory components, namely cardiac output and arterial-mixed venous oxygen difference, the product of which equals oxygen intake. Pathologic restrictions of left ventricular power in coronary patients limit both cardiac output and oxygen delivery despite minor compensatory increments in AV-oxygen difference. Pharmacologic vasodilation of peripheral circulation alters regional distribution of blood volume and flow, and secondarily improves exercise capacity by reducing preload and afterload of an ischemic left ventricle.

Accordingly, cardiovascular aspects of exercise *performance of submaximal exertion* need to be differentiated from *capacity for maximal work*; the latter can be altered in coronary patients by nitroglycerin, which primarily affects peripheral circulation and secondarily and transiently enhances left ventricular function in the presence of the myocardial ischemia imposed by restricted coronary circulation.

$\dot{V}_{O_2max}$ reproducibly defines the limits of aerobic metabolism; it is proportional to body weight, especially lean body mass.[22] Even when corrected for body weight, it is generally greater in males than in females, and in physically active than in sedentary persons.[23, 24] It diminishes slowly, with aging, from the first decade of life.[25] Although $\dot{V}_{O_2max}$ cannot be reliably predicted from exercise performance at submaximal workloads,[26] expected averages can be predicted from regression equations using age, sex, and habitual physical activity as independent variables.[27] $\dot{V}_{O_2max}$ decreases with enforced bed rest for a few days, and it increases slowly with physical training over several weeks.[28-30]

Physiological Effects of Physical Training

In young adults physical training increases $\dot{V}_{O_2max}$ about 15 per cent, with both an 11 per cent increase in stroke volume and an 8 per cent increase in AV-oxygen difference (Fig. 2).[28-31] Unexpectedly in middle-age a 14 per cent incre-

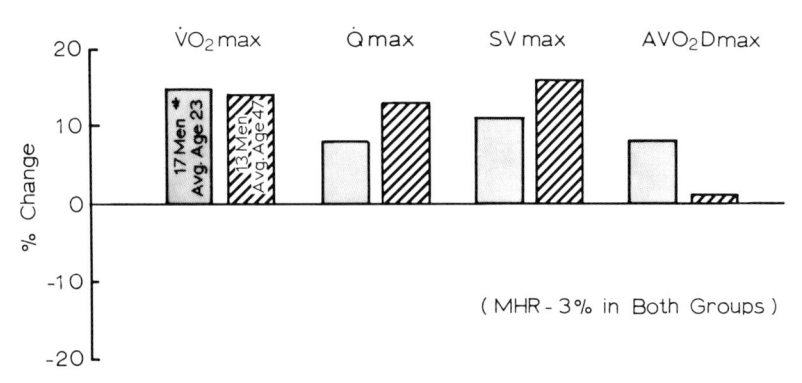

Figure 2. Cardiovascular mechanisms for increased maximal oxygen intake as a result of physical training of healthy men.[31] Note similar per cent change in $\dot{V}_{O_2max}$ in middle-aged men averaging 47 years and young adults averaging 23 years. There was a greater increase in cardiac output and stroke volume in the older men; in both groups maximal heart rate diminished 3 per cent. Conversely, AV-oxygen difference did not contribute to the increased $\dot{V}_{O_2max}$ in the older men. (Adapted from Hartley, L. H., et al.: Scand. J. Clin. Lab. Invest. 24:326, 1969. From data of Rowell, Saltin, and Ekblom.)

ment in $\dot{V}_{O_2max}$ with physical training is accomplished by a 16 per cent increase in the stroke volume, with only a 1 per cent greater peripheral oxygen extraction or widened AV-oxygen difference.[32] Another study showed 0 to 25 per cent increase in stroke volume at graded workloads and variable changes in AV-oxygen difference.[33]

Oxidative metabolism increases only in muscle groups which are trained, i.e., arm muscles conditioned by exercise do not increase capacity of leg muscles, and vice versa. With unilateral training of leg muscles, serial biopsies of trained and untrained muscle taken in each subject show ultrastructural differences between the two samples. Mitochondrial volume (Fig. 3), and oxidative energy stores of glycogen and triglycerides all increase in the trained muscle.[34] Whether parallel changes occur in the human myocardium is unknown. Usually cardiac patients have normal skeletal muscles, albeit deconditioned because of restricted activity, particularly with bed rest imposed by myocardial infarction. Such patients who participate in a program of graded exercises have the skeletal muscle potential to increase $\dot{V}_{O_2max}$ to the limits of circulatory conductance of oxygen.

Although $\dot{V}_{O_2max}$ is lower in ambulatory patients with coronary heart disease than in healthy persons of comparable age, even greater percentage increments in $\dot{V}_{O_2max}$ can be obtained with physical training (Fig. 4). Angina patients exhibit proportionally greater improvement in $\dot{V}_{O_2max}$ than do those with prior myocardial infarction but no angina; they often experience a disappearance of angina with continued exercise conditioning.

Although investigators report minor increments[35, 36] or no change in stroke volumes[37, 38] of coronary patients after physical training, other cardiovascular effects of training common to most studies of exercise performance at submaximal workloads include:

1. Minimal, but highly significant decrease in heart rate.[38]

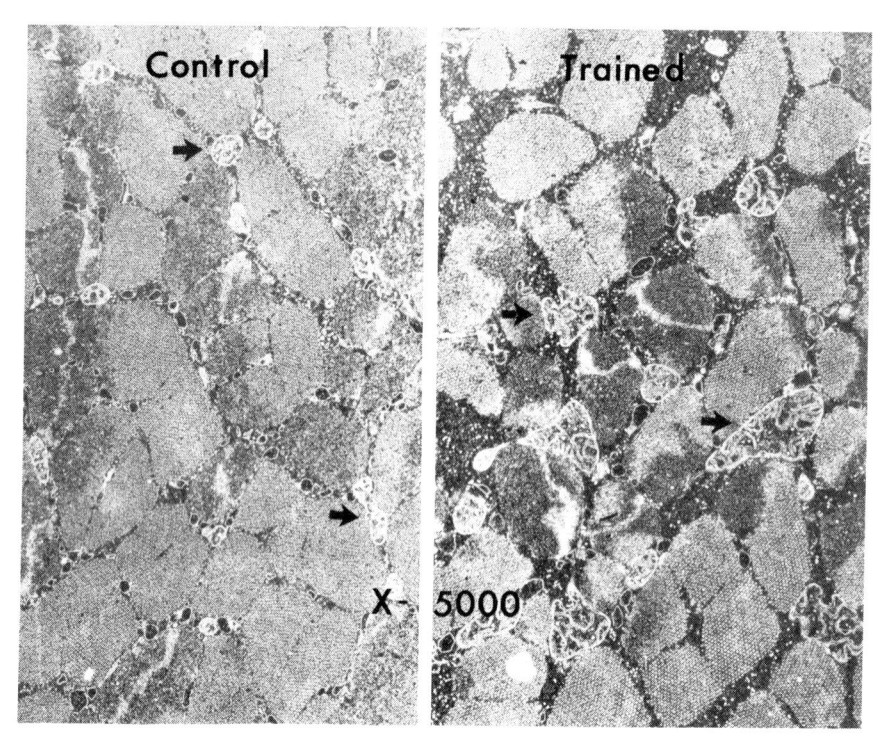

Figure 3. Electron micrographs of biopsies from control and trained skeletal muscle. The mitochondria (arrows) are considerably larger in the trained muscle (R) than in the control (L). (Morgan, T. E., et al.: In Pernow, B., and Saltin, B. (eds.): Muscle Metabolism During Exercise. New York, Plenum Press, 1971.)

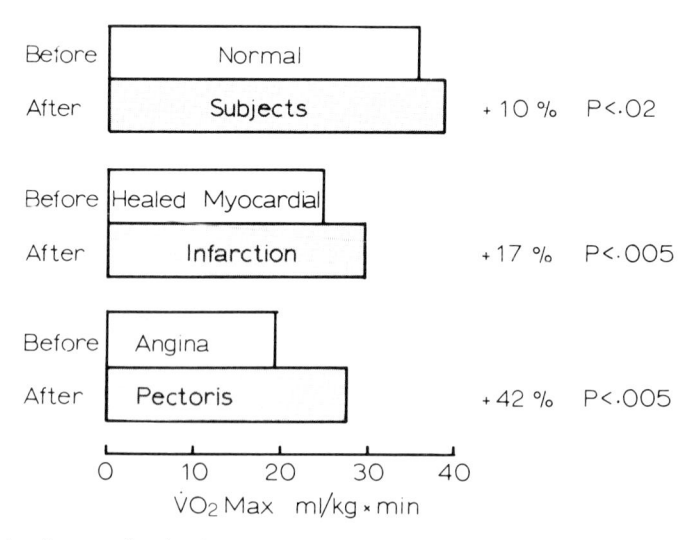

Figure 4. Average levels of maximal oxygen intake in middle-aged normal men and men with healed myocardial infarction and with angina pectoris. Note greater impairment initially of angina patients, and proportionally greater response to physical training.

2. Minimal lowering of systolic blood pressure.[38]

3. Moderate decrease in pressure-rate product/100 and, therefore, in hemodynamic stress on ischemic myocardium (Fig. 5).[38]

4. Less ST-segment depression in postexercise ECG (Fig. 6).[39]

Figure 5. Changes resulting from physical training of patients with ischemic heart disease due to coronary atherosclerosis. Product/100 of mean systemic arterial pressure and heart rate at rest and at two levels of submaximal exercise, in upright posture.[38] Patients without angina, but only history of healed myocardial infarction attain higher workloads and heart rates. However, change with physical training is equally significant in the two groups. (From Detry, J.-M. R., et al.: Circulation 44:109, 1971.)

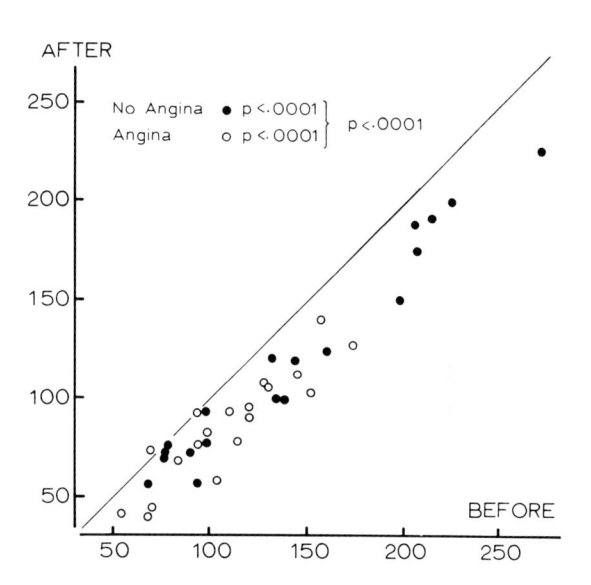

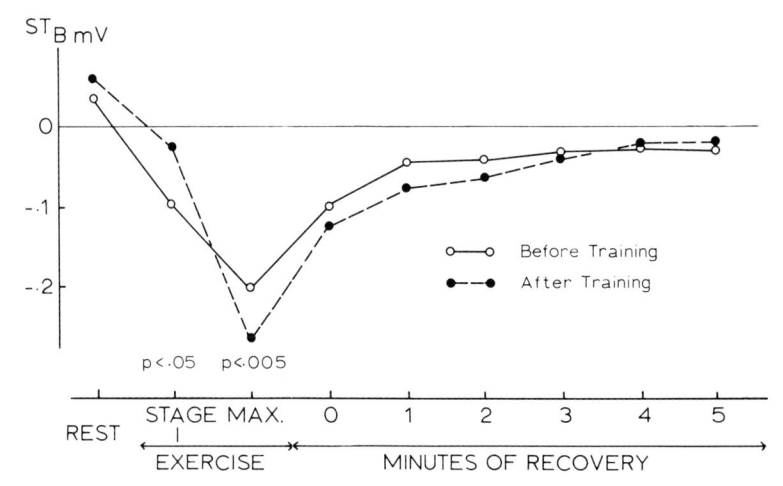

Figure 6. Mean voltages of ST_B (50 to 69 msec. after nadir of S wave, in averages of 100 consecutive heart cycles by computer analysis) at rest, submaximal (stage I) exercise, maximal exercise, and first five minutes of recovery in patients with ischemic heart disease.[39] Note higher values, equivalent to less ST segment depression, at rest and at stage I after physical training, which parallel the reductions in pressure-rate product at these workloads. At maximal exercise, however, ST_B values are more negative, consistent with greater ST depression, after training, because capacity to attain higher workloads and heart rate has increased. As a consequence, evidence of myocardial ischemia during recovery is accentuated, making the inference apparent that collateral myocardial circulation has not increased. (From Detry, J.-M. R., and Bruce, R. A.: Circulation 44:390, 1971.)

Usually AV-oxygen difference is widened,[37,38] and in some instances premature beats are less frequent.

Occasionally the oxygen requirement for a given submaximal workload is reduced if neuromuscular coordination and mechanical efficiency of a deconditioned patient are improved by physical training. Oxygen intake at rest and at submaximal loads diminishes when an apprehensive patient gains confidence with relief of disabling symptoms as a result of exercise conditioning.

Since $\dot{V}_{O_2max}$ and exercise capacity are increased in most coronary patients who participate in physical training, there is an important decrease in *relative* aerobic requirements, or per cent $\dot{V}_{O_2max}$ for any given level of submaximal exercise performance. The magnitude of such changes observed in a cooperative international study using a common protocol is shown in Figure 7.[39]

There were no changes in absolute oxygen requirements at two levels of submaximal exercise in the upright posture on a bicycle ergometer, but because of the 22 per cent increase in $\dot{V}_{O_2max}$ the relative aerobic requirement for these two workloads fell (Fig. 8).*

Is regulation of myocardial metabolism altered or collateral circulation improved by physical training? The relationship of the pressure-heart rate product/100 is altered only with respect to absolute levels of oxygen intake per unit of body weight, for there is virtually no change with respect to per cent $\dot{V}_{O_2max}$ (Fig. 9); hence, the myocardial benefit of training is merely secondary to the peripheral circulatory effects. The latter are not entirely peripheral, for much of

---

* This raises the interesting question whether reported declines[58] in catecholamine concentrations with exercise after physical training merely reflect the parallel reduction in relative aerobic demand placed upon the circulation.

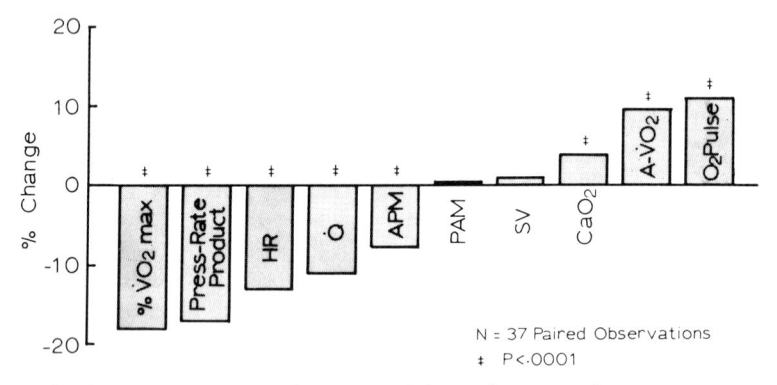

Figure 7. Average percentage decrements (L) in relative aerobic requirement (% $\dot{V}_{O_2max}$), pressure-rate product, heart rate (HR), cardiac output (Q), and systemic arterial mean pressure (AP$_M$) at rest and at the same two levels of submaximal exercise, in the upright posture, as a result of physical training of patients with ischemic heart disease.[38] The greatest fall was in metabolic demand, and the greatest decline in circulatory response was in the volume (near center). Conversely, note significant increase in AV-oxygen difference, oxygen pulse, and, to a lesser degree, in arterial oxygen content (R) as a result of physical training. Since mixed venous oxygen contents were not changed, the greater extraction was due to a higher arterial content. Consequently the latter adaptive change also provided secondary benefits to the ischemic myocardium.

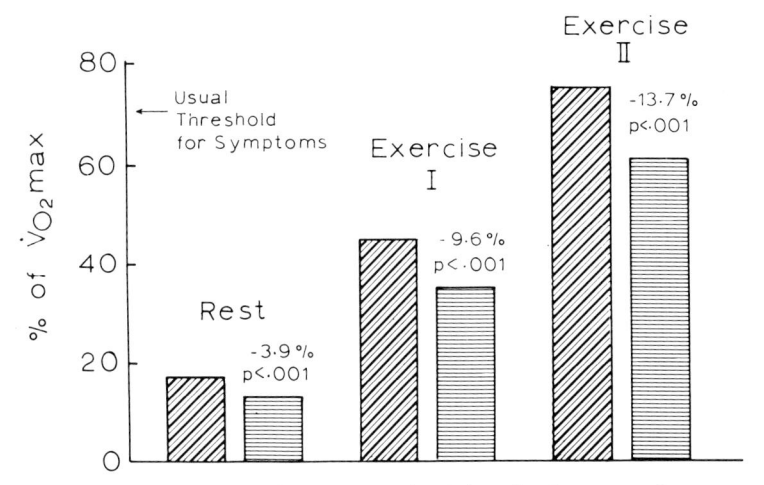

Figure 8. Changes in maximal oxygen intake (L) and relative aerobic requirements at rest and at the same two levels of submaximal exercise, in the upright posture, as a result of physical training of patients with ischemic heart disease.[38] There was no significant change in the absolute levels of $\dot{V}_{O_2}$ in ml./kg.; accordingly, the fall in relative demand was secondary to a rise in functional aerobic capacity. Unless $\dot{V}_{O_2max}$ is actually measured before and after training, the major adaptive mechanism of physical training is not apparent.

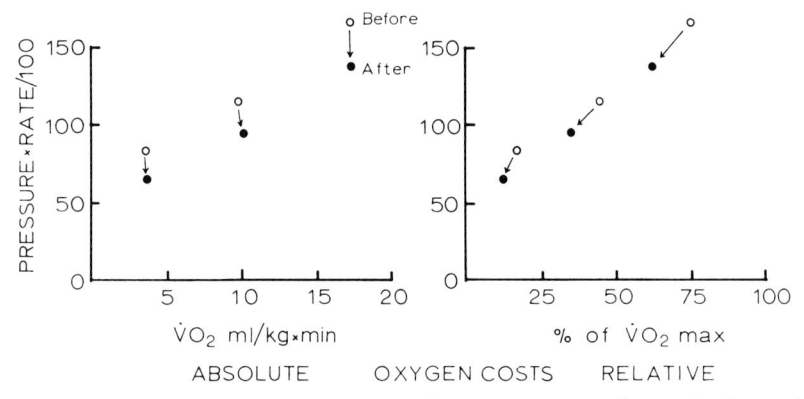

Figure 9. Relationship of pressure-rate product to oxygen intake as absolute values (L) versus relative values (% $\dot{V}_{O_2max}$-R). The former suggests a change in regulation of circulation vis-à-vis constant levels of metabolic demand, whereas the latter (R) indicates mean values are virtually on the same slope before and after physical training of patients with ischemic heart disease. Since circulation is scaled to relative aerobic requirement, reduction of this demand, as a consequence of a greater capacity ($\dot{V}_{O_2max}$), accounts for the observed changes in circulatory responses.

the significant widening of the AV-oxygen difference results from an increase in arterial oxygen contents, possibly secondary to improved pulmonary function. Similar changes in AV-oxygen difference have been reported after physical training of patients with chronic pulmonary disease.[40, 41]

"Medical revascularization" of the ischemic myocardium by exercise conditioning has been postulated,[42] but indirect assessment by computer analysis of the ST segment shows no change in relationship to heart rate (Fig. 10).[39] Lower heart

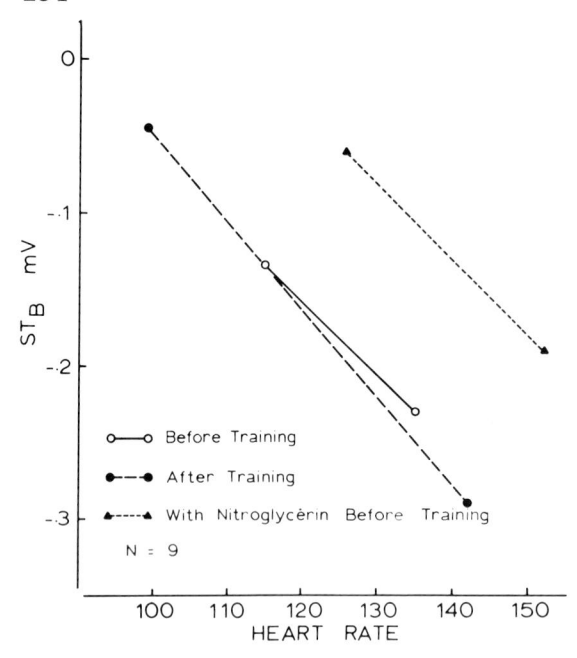

Figure 10. Comparison of relation of computer analysis of ST_B to heart rate in the same nine patients before and after nitroglycerin and after physical training. Note shift to the right with nitroglycerin treatment, which reduces blood pressure and accelerates heart rate, but no change in slope with physical training. Since after training maximal heart rate is higher and amount of ST segment depression is greater, myocardial ischemia is accentuated rather than diminished.[39]

rates and less ST depression are observed both at rest and during submaximal exercise performance, but higher rates and more ST depression occur at exercise capacity.

Personality and Psychological Effects of Training

Shephard found greater variation in ventilation than in heart rate in relation to differences in personality.[43] Hysterical subjects showed a greater ventilatory response than normals and habituated more rapidly with repetition of the same workloads. Conversely, anxious persons showed a smaller initial response and habituated more slowly. An excessive ventilatory response to unaccustomed exercise occurred equally in fit and unfit individuals.

Optimum intensity and duration of training vary with the initial state of individual and cardiorespiratory load imposed. In general this ranges between two thirds and three fourths of subject's initial $\dot{V}_{O_2max}$, further documenting the need to measure aerobic capacity before training. When this is not possible, onset of symptoms may be a guide, but variations with personality type should be considered also.

McPherson and associates recognized psychological barriers to exercise, particularly in postmyocardial infarction patients, and evaluated a hypothesis that graduated physical exercise reduced emotional tension.[44] Patients were scored by personality and anxiety scales and proved to be more tense, aloof, taciturn, fickle, emotional, hurried, and aggressive than normal subjects. The investigators related these attributes to a collapse of self-image of a strong and successful person who suffered severe and prolonged anxiety, depression, and neurotic symptoms. After about six months of physical training the patients experienced favorable changes in personality, an improved sense of well-being, and a gain in self-confidence and optimism as physical discomfort diminished and the level of physical fitness increased. Conversely, normal subjects after an equivalent period of inactivity became more anxious, inhibited, awkward, and less carefree as lack of exercise and diversionary activities caused psychophysiological regression. Finally, even a single exercise session produced favorable mood changes in all groups.

Clinical Experience with Physical Training as an Aid to Cardiac Rehabilitation

The need to rehabilitate cardiac patients has been recognized for some time, and in 1957 Hellerstein and Ford stated that "rehabilitation begins the moment the patient is first stricken with the disease, or at least when he is over the acute illness, and extends to the time when he is free of pain and out of the life-endangering stage."[45]

Whereas most physicians disregard this therapeutic modality, some have encouraged individual patients to increase physical activities of everyday living gradually and progressively. This may begin in the hospital, during convalescence from myocardial infarction,[46] and progress through a variety of steps as outlined by an expert committee of the World Health Organization.[47, 48] Some physicians refer patients to an organized community program to provide professional supervision and better adherence by reinforcement of group interaction. Hellerstein and Ford[45] found that 46 per cent of cardiac patients referred for work evaluation had important emotional limitations. Often physicians were fearful of returning patients to work, yet energy requirements of most occupations are relatively small, and most patients return to work successfully. With constructive communication and a positive approach to disabling disease, patients encouraged to participate in graded exercises subsequently showed physical and psychological improvement. With more enthusiastic and vigorous physical training, progressing to the point of participation in competitive sports, Gottheiner documented from subsequent coronary events in over 1000 patients a remarkable feasibility, adherence, and apparently lowered mortality.[49] Hellerstein reported favorable adherence to and clinical benefits from exercise and other therapy in 254 sedentary men with coronary heart disease (Fig. 2).[50] Effects of sexual activity in such patients are reported separately.[51] Kattus and associates considered exercise training "medical revascularization" of the ischemic myocardium as need for nitroglycerin therapy disappears with diminished angina.[42]

Despite these promising reports, unresolved problems persist. Which patients, how soon, what kind, and how much exercise? Uncertainties about testing, monitoring, and precautions emphasize need for practical clinical guidelines.

Local experience in Seattle developing from a pilot study initiated in 1969 by Pyfer and Doane[52] permits some clinical assessment of a medically supervised program.[39] Of 327 patients admitted up to March, 1972, 277 men and 14 women had coronary heart disease; 195 men, or 70 per cent, successfully completed an initial training course. The initial program involved walking, jogging, and over a dozen calisthenics, individual-adjusted after exercise testing to 10 levels of work intensity, for nearly an hour, three times weekly for 12 weeks.[53] During this phase five persons developed myocardial infarction, but only one case was attributable to the training activities (Table 1). After the first 12 weeks, only 159 continued training, lowering the adherence rate to 54 per cent. During this phase, four additional cases of myocardial infarction occurred outside the training regimen.* Five instances of witnessed exertional cardiac arrest occurred after the first 12 weeks, but promptly responded to ventricular defibrillation, without evolving myocardial infarction: four men voluntarily continued the training program.[54, 55] The first patient has continued training for three years, with clinical and physiological improvement after cardiac arrest. Only one cardiac arrest occurred in the past year. The attack rate now approximates one in 4700 coronary patient-hours of physical activities. Because this risk was anticipated, a policy of medically supervised group training was implemented and perpetuated from the start, and a defibrillator and one or more physicians are always present.

With a cumulative experience of over 23,500 coronary patient-exercise hours, the clinical feasibility, safety, and patient acceptability are now well established. This does not mean that coronary disease is fully controlled, for there have been six late cardiac deaths outside the training program for an observed mortality rate of 3.1 per cent. Based on concurrent experience in this community, the expected number of deaths would be 21.9 for the first six months' follow-up of 195 patients,

---

* Pyfer, H. R., Doane, B. L., and Frederick, R.: Personal communication, February 29, 1972.

Table 1. *Clinical Experience in Men with Coronary Heart Disease (Angina and/or Prior Myocardial Infarction) Who Participated in Physical Training Program Sponsored by CAPRI, Seattle, May, 1968, through February, 1972**

		MORBIDITY		CV MORTALITY		
AGE GROUP YEARS	MEN TRAINED	*Cardiac Arrest*†	*Myocardial Infarction*‡	*Observed*	*Expected*	*Ratio*§
30-39	13	1	0	1‖	0	
40-49	62	0	2	1	7.75	0.129
50-59	84	3	4	2	5.51	0.362
60-69	36	1	3	2	8.65	0.226
Altogether	195	5	9	6	21.91	0.274
Rates		2.6%	4.6%	3.1%	11.2%	

* Data, courtesy of Dr. Howard Pyfer, Executive Director, Cardiopulmonary Research Institute, Seattle.

† All occurred after initial 12-week training program; no evolving myocardial infarction, detectable residual anoxic encephalopathy and no fatalities as a result of immediate defibrillation of ventricles with a single shock.

‡ Only one occurred during training sessions, three others in everyday life during first 12 weeks, and five after first 12 weeks; only two were initial infarctions; seven were recurrent attacks.

§ Data, courtesy of Dr. Donald Peterson, based on follow-up experience of 180 patients admitted to four hospitals in this community and discharged alive; average survival of fatal cases was 6.5 months.[57]

‖ Sudden cardiac death several months after training program during whole body isometric exertion of water skiing while on vacation.

or 11 per cent. Ratio of observed to expected deaths of 0.274 clearly indicates no increased mortality risk as a result of physical training; indeed, it suggests a protective effect.* Twenty-one patients (7.5 per cent) have had coronary arteriography because of progressive exertional symptoms; 12 have had saphenous-vein-to-coronary-artery grafts, and eight have returned for further physical training. Within this limited experience, objective evidence of physiological improvement from surgical revascularization has been meager until physical training was resumed.

Clinical Guidelines for Training of Cardiac Patients†

Only ambulatory patients can participate in activities requiring between 50 and 75 per cent $\dot{V}_{O_2max}$ for short periods, at least three times weekly, for several weeks. "Interval training" with transient, peak loads of from 75 to 95 per cent $\dot{V}_{O_2max}$, repeated a few times, may facilitate adaptive changes in skeletal muscle and secondary benefits to an ischemic myocardium at submaximal levels of performance. Severity of exertion should be graded according to capacity, which requires appropriate exercise testing. Intensity of exercise is quite low initially, and increases gradually and progressively to the awareness of exertional fatigue, dyspnea, muscle weakness, or angina, which occurs about 70 per cent of $\dot{V}_{O_2max}$. Reducing intensity momentarily to relieve symptoms, then increasing it again repetitively for 20 to 40 minutes about three times weekly is desirable. Week by week the amount of exertion required to produce symptoms gradually increases. Over a period of weeks to months some patients become asymptomatic and no longer need medication for angina at activity levels which formerly provoked symptoms. Occasionally a striking recovery from a previously depressed and anxious state leads to euphoria and loss of restraint. At that time the overzealous patient may endanger himself with excessive self-imposed physical activity. Since isometric exertion rapidly increases blood pressure excessively, it is particularly hazardous, especially when it is not medically supervised. For example, I know of two coronary patients who were victims of sudden cardiac death while water skiing, when immediate defibrillatory treatment was not available.

Clinical exclusions from physical training include patients in the acute phase of myocardial infarction, severe and untreated congestive heart failure, or hypokalemia and intoxication with digitalis, as well as those undergoing intensive treatment for arrhythmias. After two months from onset of uncomplicated myocardial infarction, or two weeks after effective treatment of heart failure or relief from overdosage with cardiac drugs, training may be considered. Each patient initially should be exercise-tested, preferably with a standardized procedure to observe circulatory and ECG responses at submaximal performance and to maxi-

---

* Mortality rate in 82 drop-outs is 7.3 per cent.
† Personal opinions about how and when to initiate minimal activities in hospital and increase them progressively during convalescence from acute myocardial infarction have been summarized elsewhere.[54]

mal effort to define capacity. This can be done within a few minutes, obtaining insight into circulatory adjustments and immediate assessment of functional aerobic impairment or per cent difference in capacity from expected average normal $\dot{V}_{O_2max}$.[27]

Ideally physicians should arrange for a professionally supervised training program that provides testing, evaluation, monitoring, and most importantly, staff and facilities to defibrillate the occasional, and individually unpredictable, victim of sudden exertional cardiac arrest.[55] Until this can be achieved, most physicians and their patients have to rely upon simple, unsupervised training regimens. Fortunately for patients in class II or III functional capacity by criteria of the New York Heart Association, this rarely presents a significant problem. But it should not be forgotten that the first instance of acute myocardial infarction followed within minutes by ventricular fibrillation (which responded to defibrillatory treatment) encountered in several thousand tests under my supervision occurred in an apparently normal middle-aged individual when he was exposed to the thermal stress of a hot shower several minutes after maximal exercise testing.[56]

Class IV patients restricted to bed and chair existence should be excluded. Class I or II patients, after adequate recovery from myocardial infarction, or with clinically stable angina pectoris, can be accepted with minimal supervision to *accelerate* rehabilitation. Class III patients should be referred to medically supervised regimens to achieve rehabilitation. Regardless of classification, adherence to training is facilitated by participation in a supervised group program.

For the majority of cardiac patients, physical training is successful. *Benefits* include improvement in work performance, stamina, and capacity; lessening of symptoms at ordinary levels of activity; improved psychological outlook; reduction in need for drug therapy; and addition of "life" to years, whether or not years are added to life. Many patients and their spouses have experienced the improvement in performance, stamina, and capacity, but more experience is needed to establish the other benefits with certainty.

Risks of training are failure to attain benefits, increasing symptoms usually attributable to progressing cardiovascular disease, and the rare instance of exertional cardiac arrest. When appropriate techniques are employed, musculoskeletal complaints are minimal. Informed consent of the patient, and possibly of his spouse, is reasonable. Physician and patient should recognize that the need for other therapy may occur and that the benefits from surgical treatment may be enhanced by subsequent return to physical training.

Perhaps the greatest risk to patients is the increasing availability of premature and uncritical news releases of medical advances and the failure of physicians to provide adequate orientation about the balance of benefits established versus risk recognized. Both must face the reality that reliable evaluations emerge only from well-designed studies, carefully quantified measurements of both trained and untrained patients, in adequate numbers, who have been randomly assigned to either group. These groups must have been observed by the same protocol concomitantly, and for a long enough time to ascertain whether or not this and any other interventions actually lower frequency and severity of recurrent events of coronary atherosclerotic heart disease and prolong productive and enjoyable living. This is an educational responsibility, which the medical profession has not faced realistically. The physician who asks, "How can I deny my patient the benefits of any new treatment?" should recognize that random allocation, from the start can be done ethically by each practitioner, in good conscience, for it will protect one half of his patients from the hazards, yet to be defined, until the value of the treatment is unequivocably established. On the other hand, if it be favorable, one half of the patients will have benefited from the start. Only by this approach can the reported differences allegedly resulting from physical training be differentiated from unrecognized bias or error in sampling, which may result in invalidation of remarkably similar results reported from uncontrolled studies.

Conclusions

Physical training of coronary patients is a plausible, alternative and palliative approach to ischemic heart disease with appreciable clinical, physiological, psychological, and pathological justification. Lacking appropriately controlled studies, long-term effects on life expectancy are not well established. Like any other effective therapy, it is neither without hazard nor always beneficial, but with appropriate guidelines it may be beneficial with minimal risk. Its ultimate role in clinical management will require properly designed and controlled studies, with full understanding and cooperation of both patient and physician to achieve random allocation of the individuals evaluated. Meanwhile, uncontrolled studies of surgical treatment are more dramatic, and expensive, yet acceptable to many physicians and patients, despite greater morbidity and mortality risks. It is likely that physical training will become an important adjunct to other forms of therapeutic intervention, rather than an exclusive approach to multifactorial cardiovascular disease characterized by a variety of manifestations and complications.

References

1. Plato: *Theaetetus*. Great Books, Vol. 7, 1952 edition, p. 518.
2. Segall, H. N.: The first clinico-pathological case history of angina pectoris: Self-diagnosis by an anonymous physician: Autopsy by John Hunter: Reported by William Heberden in 1772. Bull. Hist. Med. *18*:102, 1945.
3. Osler, W.: *Lectures on Angina Pectoris and Allied States*. New York, Appleton, 1897, p. 52.
4. MacAlpin, R. N., and Kattus, A. A.: Adaptation to exercise in angina pectoris. Circulation *33*:183, 1966.
5. Yater, W. M., et al.: Comparisons of clinical and pathologic aspects of coronary artery disease in men of various age groups: A study of 950 autopsied cases from the Armed Forces Institute of Pathology. Ann. Intern. Med. *34*:352, 1951.
6. Thorner, W.: Cited by 11.
7. Petren, T. T., and Sylven, B.: Cited by 11.
8. Hakilea, J.: Cited by 11.
9. Leon, A. S., and Bloor, C. M.: Cited by 11.
10. Rakusan, K., and Poupa, O.: Capillaries and muscle fibers in the heart of old rats. Gerontologia *9*:107, 1964.
11. Tomanek, R. J.: Effects of age and exercise on the extent of the myocardial capillary bed. Anat. Rec. *167*:55, 1970.

12. Eckstein, R. W.: Effect on exercise and coronary artery narrowing on coronary collateral circulation. Circ. Res. 5:230, 1957.
13. Morris, J. N., and Crawford, M. D.: Coronary heart disease and physical activity of work. Lancet 2:1053; 1111, 1953.
14. Morris, J. N., Heady, J. A., and Raffle, P. A. B.: Physique of London busmen. Lancet 2:569, 1956.
15. Fox, S. M., III, and Haskell, W. L.: Physical activity and the prevention of coronary heart disease. Bull. N.Y. Acad. Med. 44:950, 1968.
16. Frank, C. W.: The course of coronary heart disease: Factors relating to prognosis. Bull. N.Y. Acad. Med. 44:900, 1968.
17. Pyörälä, K., et al.: Cardiovascular studies of former endurance athletes. Amer. J. Cardiol. 20:191, 1967.
18. Tung, C. L., et al.: The hearts of ricksha pullers: Study of effect of chronic exertion on cardiovascular system. Amer. Heart J. 10:79, 1934.
19. Chiang, B. N., et al.: Physical characteristics and exercise performance of pedicab and upper socioeconomic classes of middle-aged Chinese men. Amer. Heart J. 76:760, 1968.
20. Bruce, R.A.: Unpublished observations, 1972.
21. Detry, J-M. R., and Bruce, R. A.: Effects of nitroglycerin on "maximal" oxygen intake and exercise electrocardiogram in coronary heart disease. Circulation 43:155, 1971.
22. Buskirk, E., and Taylor, H. L.: Maximal oxygen intake and its relation to body composition, with special reference to chronic physical activity and obesity. J. Appl. Physiol. 11:72, 1957.
23. Åstrand, P. O.: Physical performance as a function of age. J.A.M.A. 205:105, 1968.
24. Åstrand, I.: Aerobic work capacity in men and women with special reference to age. Acta Physiol. Scand. 49(Suppl.169):1, 1960.
25. Dehn, M., and Bruce, R. A.: Longitudinal variations in maximal oxygen intake with age and activity. J. Appl. Physiol. 33:805, 1972.
26. Rowell, L. B., Taylor, H. L., and Wang, Y.: Limitations to prediction of maximal oxygen intake. J. Appl. Physiol. 19:919, 1964.
27. Bruce, R. A.: Exercise testing of patients with coronary heart disease. Ann. Clin. Res. 3:323, 1971.
28. Rowell, L. B.: Factors affecting the prediction of the maximal oxygen intake from measurements made during submaximal work. Doctoral dissertation, University of Minnesota, 1962.
29. Ekblom, B., et al.: Effect of training on circulatory response to exercise. J. Appl. Physiol. 24:518, 1968.
30. Saltin, B., et al.: Response to exercise after bedrest and after training. Circulation, Suppl. 7, 1968. (A.M.A. Monograph No. 23.)
31. Saltin, B.: Physiological effects of physical conditioning. Med. Sci. Sports 1:50, 1969.
32. Hartley, L. H., et al.: Physical training in sedentary middle-aged and older men. III. Cardiac output and gas exchange at submaximal and maximal exercise. Scand. J. Clin. Lab. Invest. 24:335, 1969.
33. Hanson, J. S., et al.: Long-term physical training and cardiovascular dynamics in middle-aged men. Circulation 38:783, 1968.
34. Morgan, T. E., et al.: Effects of long-term exercise on human muscle mitochondria. Pernow, B., and Saltin, B. (eds.): *Muscle Metabolism During Exercise*. Vol. 2. New York, Plenum Press, 1971.
35. Frick, M. H., and Katila, M.: Hemodynamic consequences of physical training after myocardial infarction. Circulation 37:192, 1968.
36. Clausen, J. P., Larsen, O. A., and Trap-Jensen, J.: Physical training in the management of coronary artery disease. Circulation 40:143, 1969.
37. Vaurnauskas, E. et al.: Haemodynamic effects of physical training in coronary patients. Lancet 2:8, 1966.
38. Detry, J-M. R., et al.: Increased arteriovenous oxygen difference after physical training in coronary heart disease. Circulation 44:109, 1971.
39. Detry, J-M. R., and Bruce, R. A.: Effects of physical training on exertional ST-Segment depression in coronary heart disease. Circulation 44:390, 1971.
40. Paez, P. N., et al.: The physiologic basis of training patients with emphysema. Amer. Rev. Resp. Dis. 95:944, 1967.
41. Bass, H., Whitcomb, J. F., and Forman, R.: Exercise training: Therapy for patients with chronic observed pulmonary disease. Chest 57:116, 1970.

42. Kattus, A. A., et al.: Diagnosis, medical and surgical management of coronary insufficiency. Ann Intern. Med. 69:115, 1968.
43. Shephard, R. J.: Initial "fitness" and personality as determinants of the response to a training regime. Ergonomics 9:3, 1966.
44. McPherson, B. D., et al.: Psychological effects of an exercise program for the post-infarct and normal adult men. J. Sports Med. 7:95, 1967.
45. Hellerstein, H. K., and Ford, A. B.: Rehabilitation of the cardiac patient. J.A.M.A. 164:225, 1957.
46. Cain, H. D., Frasher, W. G., and Stilvelman, R.: Graded activity program for safe return to self care after myocardial infarction. J.A.M.A. 177:111, 1961.
47. Rehabilitation of patients with cardiovascular diseases. Wld. Hlth. Org. Techn. Rep. Ser. No. 270, 1964.
48. "A Programme for the physical rehabilitation of patients with acute myocardial infarction." Prepared by a working group, Freiburg-im-Breisgau, March 4–6, 1968. Regional Office for Europe, World Health Organization, Copenhagen. EURO 5030 (1).
49. Gottheiner, V.: Long-range strenuous sports training for cardiac reconditioning and rehabilitation. Amer. J. Cardiol. 22:426, 1968.
50. Hellerstein, H. K.: The effects of physical activity: Patients and normal coronary prone subjects. Minn. Med. 52:1335, 1969.
51. Hellerstein, H. K., and Friedman, E. H.: Sexual activity and postcoronary patient. Ann. Intern. Med. 125:987, 1970.
52. Pyfer, H. R., and Doane, B. L.: Exercise for the cardio-pulmonary patient. Northwest Med. 68:103, 1969.
53. Pyfer, H. R., and Doane, B. L.: Cardiac arrest during exercise training. J.A.M.A. 210:101, 1969.
54. Bruce, R. A.: Exercise and the postinfarct patient. Med. World News, May, 1971, p. 82.
55. Bruce, R. A., and Kluge, W.: Defibrillatory treatment of exertional cardiac arrest in coronary disease. J.A.M.A. 216:653, 1971.
56. Bruce, R. A., Hornsten, T. R., and Blackmon, J. R.: Myocardial infarction after normal responses to maximal exercise. Circulation 38:552, 1968.
57. Peterson, D. R., and Chinn, N.: Survival after intensive coronary care: A method for evaluating therapeutic intervention. Northwest Med. 70:34, 1971.
58. Kotchen, T. A., et al.: Renin, norepinephrine, and epinephrine responses to graded exercise. J. Appl. Physiol. 31:178, 1971.

Disadvantages of Intensive Exercise Therapy After Myocardial Infarction[*]

HENRY BLACKBURN

Laboratory of Physiological Hygiene, School of Public Health and Department of Medicine, School of Medicine, University of Minnesota

Numerous arguments, theories, and claims are advanced to support the use of intensive exercise therapy for sedentary middle-aged survivors of myocardial infarction. They focus on these purported influences of such therapy:

Exercise conditioning enhances cardiovascular function and rehabilitation in all spheres of activity.

Exercise reduces known coronary risk factors.

Exercise prevents reinfarction and sudden death.

Many hypothetical mechanisms are cited to explain these presumed effects. But what is the evidence and wherein lies the controversy?

At the outset I would like to emphasize my longstanding interest, and the interest in and work of our laboratory on the role of physical activity in vascular diseases. I by no means take a negative position on exercise generally. Rather I favor more physical activity by everyone, including cardiac patients, as a part of balanced and effective living. However, I do feel that it is useful to air the issues in debate and to pose scientific criticism of the widespread use of high-level intensive exercise therapy to peak levels of physical conditioning in coronary patients. Such therapy is not yet based on evidence of long-term benefit, it is potentially dangerous and costly, and it is unnecessary for good therapeutic results. The best cure for controversy about such therapy is better data.

---

[*] Some of the work cited herein was supported by grants to this institution from the United States Public Health Service: HE 03088; CD 00333 and CD 00118; H 06314; RR 267; and from the Ober Charitable Trust Fund.

The Evidence

Does exercise enhance cardiovascular function? At the in-hospital stage of treatment of myocardial infarction it has been demonstrated that carefully supervised activity programs result in patients going home sooner, with greater physical capabilities and with no greater immediate risk than from traditionally strict bed rest treatment.[1-5] This generally favorable experience in short-term programs has been confirmed by two recent controlled studies in which patients with acute infarction were randomly assigned to bed rest care versus progressive ambulation and exercise.[4, 5]

Concerning long-term effects of therapy during the convalescent stage, numerous studies, both controlled and uncontrolled, have measured changes in cardiovascular function before and after conditioning exercise.[6-22] Circulatory changes in patients were similar to those long found among untrained healthy subjects who undertook progressive exercise, i.e., improved cardiovascular performance and efficiency. Infarction survivors admitted to such programs were a highly select group at the outset, and the majority of them showed measurable improvement in function. A minority, not identifiable beforehand, responded poorly or could not tolerate graduated exercise treatment. Some investigators have found that part of the hemodynamic changes may be due to placebo effect.[20, 23] Others, in matched-control studies of exercise conditioning after infarction, interpreted the findings of higher work heart rate and ventilation and lower stroke index and cardiac output as evidence of early left heart failure, possibly related to the exercise therapy itself.[22]

The nature of the functional changes associated with exercise therapy includes consistent and clear findings of an increased work capacity and a lower heart rate, that is, decreased oxygen requirement of the heart, for a given submaximal task. Changes in the distribution of blood flow and a higher oxidative capacity in conditioned skeletal muscle appear to contribute more to the increased cardiovascular efficiency than do changes in myocardial function. The reduction in cardiac output is largely accounted for by the lower heart rate. Contractility, contraction synergy, and sympathetic drive of the heart require more study. Changes in cardiac volume, coronary blood flow, and myocardial oxygen extraction have been minor, equivocal, or absent after exercise conditioning in coronary patients.[9, 12, 17, 19, 24]

With respect to changes in the coronary arteries, one now classic study found increased coronary collaterals in chronically exercised dogs, whereas a generally similar experiment refuted this finding.[25, 26] An occasional coronary angiogram in man has shown less obstruction, or more collaterals, associated with participation in an exercise program. Usually, however, angiographic changes have been equivocal or negative.[8, 9] There is one well-known case report of huge main coronary arteries found on autopsy in the famous marathon runner Clarence DeMar, and one systematic autopsy study suggested that the intrinsic diameter of coronary arteries was greater according to the habitual activity of occupation during life.[27, 28] However, these findings might have been expected from the greater ventricular size among the active men.[28, 29]

Changes in myocardial perfusion associated with physical conditioning have not been directly measured. Nevertheless, a couple of reports suggest that an occasional coronary patient may have an ischemic ST segment electrocardiographic response to stress, after conditioning, which is less marked than could be accounted for by simple improvement in circulatory efficiency. For example, sagging ST segments have disappeared entirely in a few patients after conditioning, irrespective of the workload imposed during a follow-up stress test. However, the majority of cases continued to show the same ST depression (or anginal pain) at a given heart rate, despite the improved work capacity after an exercise program.[30, 31]

Changes in ventricular excitability and fibrillation threshold are actively under investigation. There is a suggestive report that prolonged conditioning exercise in sedentary middle-aged, coronary-prone men might affect myocardial excitability. An exercise program was associated with reduced frequency of stress-induced ventricular ectopic beats and an elevated work threshold at which they appeared.[32] A coronary artery preparation and procedure in dogs is being used to study the influence of intensive running exercise on the threshold for ectopic and fibrillatory rhythms, and on their lethality, but the results are not yet in.[33] Damage to myocardial cell structure is apparently related to exhausting exercise in animal experiments.[34] This suggests that neither in animal experiments nor in the therapy of coronary patients is it desirable, or necessary, to push exercise repeatedly to levels of exhaustion.

Does exercise reduce risk factors? Little difference in the distributions of major "primary" coronary risk factors (blood pressure, serum cholesterol, obesity) was demonstrated in a population study that compared habitually active and sedentary working men.[35] Moreover, at the close of an 18-month program of physical conditioning no significant difference was found in blood pressure, weight, serum cholesterol, or smoking habits between exercised and sedentary control groups of middle-aged, coronary-prone men.[36] However, some reduction in risk factors occurred in both groups, and it is possible that any activity program renders it easier to influence multiple risk factors in a general hygienic approach to risk reduction.[37]

Does exercise reduce reinfarction and mortality rates? It may be that the only randomized controlled trial of survival among infarct patients is that of the Sahlgren's Hospital in Goteborg, Sweden.[38] None of the other reported conditioning programs has been a controlled study. The many existing reports of return to work after infarction are not relevant to the question of conditioning effect and have failed to analyze results in terms of clinical severity of the infarct or of other confounding variables.[39]

In the Goteborg study patients were randomly assigned at admission to the hospital into exercise or control groups and each received the same inpatient care for acute infarction. Twenty-six weeks after onset of the disease, survivors among the group originally assigned to the exercise therapy were re-examined and those considered eligible for exercise therapy were enlisted in a long-term program of dynamic activity. This was carried out in 30-minute sessions at the hospital three times a week, up to heart rate levels 10 beats below that reached during their maximal work capacity as demonstrated by a progressive ergometer test. The control group was given only general advice on home activity. At 26 weeks 75 per cent of the initial randomly assigned "exercise" group was considered eligible for the exercise program. All the original controls were left in the control group. A report at two years' follow-up revealed that 25 per cent of the exercise group still adhered to the hospital program, while 25 per cent continued an "effective" exercise program at home. Meanwhile, 10 per cent of the control group had begun personal exercise programs on their own.

Mortality for the first 26 weeks was the same in treatment and control groups. Group comparisons from 26 weeks onward during the remainder of the two-year follow-up period revealed eight total deaths in the exercise group versus 19 in the controls ($p = .05$). There were six coronary deaths versus 18 ($p = .025$), and nine nonfatal myocardial infarctions in the exercise group versus eight in the controls. Exclusion from the eventual convalescent exercise program of 25 per cent of the subjects initially randomized to exercise treatment would probably tend to minimize group differences because those excluded had relatively poor cardiac function. Longer follow-up and confirmation elsewhere of this important study is required.

The Controversy

Let us accept that early ambulation of infarct patients in the hospital is no longer controversial. This is because in any closely followed condition having a high mortality rate (15 to 30 per cent the first four weeks in hospital), treatment-related deaths would likely and soon be apparent. The uncontrolled experience of in-hospital activity programs has been generally favorable in terms of the greater capacity of patients to care for themselves, shortened hospital stay, and the patient's mood of optimism and participation in recovery. Confirmation of this uncontrolled experience by two recent well designed control studies of early ambulation for uncomplicated infarction indicates the desirability, feasibility, safety, and cost-effectiveness of this practice. The experience is adequate.

Wherein lies the controversy about exercise programs during convalescence from infarction? After all, the demonstrated improvement in work capacity and cardiovascular efficiency from such programs must be accepted as desirable. Controversy exists for many reasons. Indications, contraindications, and eligibility criteria for intensive exercise are not firm. Individual exercise prescription is difficult to ascertain, administer, or control. Danger from intensive exercise is very real in coronary patients deconditioned by years of sedentary living, climaxed by an episode of cardiac damage and further restricted activity. Moreover, there is a major deficiency in the professional interest and experience, and in medical facilities, to carry out and to evaluate exercise therapy. Surely the unknown cost of a new major mass therapy for coronary disease would be large. Most important of all, there is inadequate evidence of the beneficial influence of high level exercise on other risk factors or on the rate of recurrent infarction and death. These questions should be considered individually.

Who should have exercise therapy? Criteria are not available for the selection, even within the "eligible" functional classes 1 or 2 (New York Heart Association[40]) of those patients likely to experience improved performance—in contrast to those likely to obtain no benefit or to be in great hazard from exercise. All the exercise protagonists concur that patients must be selected and evaluated by physicians with use of a progressive exercise test to near capacity levels, before and during an exercise program. This test is limited by availability and cost, and even the stress test is not highly discriminating of those who will subsequently benefit or suffer from exercise.

How much exercise is good? This depends on what is considered "good." The question points up the essence of the problem: Is intensive exercise necessary to obtain improved performance or to delay reinfarction? Is survival related to activity at all, or, if so, to the degree of activity? Are adequate conditioning and/or health effects attainable more safely and economically from unsupervised low or moderate level exercise of longer duration than from short periods of intensive exercise which must be supervised? None of these questions can be answered adequately now.

How safe is exercise and where is skilled therapy available? In one excellent exercise program among coronary patients, seven cases of cardiac arrest occurred over a period of one and a half years. The incidence of cardiac arrest was estimated at two cases per thousand per patient-period of exercise. All seven cases in that program were successfully defibrillated, and the authors concluded that:

". . . it is prudent for physicians to (1) inform coronary patients of the risk of exertional cardiac arrest, (2) provide appropriate emergency facilities for immediate treatment of cardiac arrest, particularly in programs which involve strenuous exercise testing or training of coronary patients or both, and (3) restrict participation in vigorous physical training to group programs which are professionally supervised and provided with appropriate emergency facilities."[41]

In fact, however, there are no accurate data on the frequency of serious events, even for the best programs, not to speak of unsupervised or individual efforts. There is no voluntary or governmental agency for the collection of safety data or one even concerned with therapeutic safety, as in the case of new drug therapy. Even in the best circumstances safety is shown to be a serious problem, and ideally supervised programs and facilities are not widely available.

Are coronary risk factors influenced by exercise? The evidence for this is weak. On the one hand, exercise treatment alone is likely to be less effective and less efficient than treating the whole patient, that is, treating all known risk influences, because the relationship between other risk factors and exercise is not very strong. On the other hand, *any* demonstrated positive effect of exercise would likely be additive to other benefits—for the same reason.

Does exercise actually reduce future risk? Are the powerful arguments of the protagonists sufficient? Is the experience about the restoration of self-confidence and the performance capacity of infarct patients reason enough for intensive exercise programs on a national scale of therapy? I think not.

None of the reported uncontrolled studies answers the crucial question about the long-term preventive effects of exercise on patient and public health. Even the low death rates reported in pioneer exercise programs allow no conclusions about a real benefit.[8, 13, 14] Why? Because there was no control group and selection for exercise programs usually excludes those at high risk because they are less likely to tolerate the exercise. Moreover, some postinfarction patients may have a mortality risk approaching that of the noncoronary population and they can be identified.[42] Therefore, any comparisons made in which the treatment group is subject to bias (that is, they are selected on some basis other than random assignments) cannot provide acceptable evidence that the only difference between groups is due to the treatment itself (exercise). Moreover, because an exercise program is not blinded and involves giving health advice, the treatment is usually not confined to exercise but affects other habits and characteristics as well.[37]

Why is the existing evidence on this important question so inadequate? There are profound conceptual and practical reasons for the deficiency. With unhappy consistency in therapeutic medicine, ideas about disease mechanisms are transposed into therapeutic action—without adequate testing in man of the mechanism or empirical testing of the hypothesis. This approach can be a productive and fairly efficient way to establish the appropriate therapy for short-term, frequent diseases having largely predictable outcomes. History tells us that it has not been an efficient way to establish the effective therapy and prophylaxis of advanced chronic diseases having a variable course.

In the first place, the theory about the disease mechanism is often wrong. Potent therapy directed only at that mechanism and tested too little or too briefly by scientific empiricism very often turns out to do more harm than good. Such may be the case, for example, for treatment by insulin and insulin stimulation of the "blood glucose mechanism" in adult-onset diabetes which has apparently not favorably affected the course of the disease.[43] Conceivably the same may be found one day for cholesterol-reducing drugs in the treatment of middle-aged survivors of infarction.[44] It may also very well happen that the multimillion dollar therapeutic industry of coronary angiography–coronary surgery will go the same way. All the evidence indicates that despite this mass therapy (20,000 bypass operations last year), the death and disability rate for coronary artery disease goes unabated. In each of these instances a costly mass therapeutic system has mushroomed from a clever idea about a disease mechanism without sound empirical evidence that the natural history of the disease is favorably modified by the treatment. It is even the opinion of some that the present large-scale patchwork surgical therapy of coronary artery disease is on a course toward intellectual, ethical, and economic bankruptcy. The addition, now, of special intensive exercise programs for coronary patients would add another costly and potentially toxic mass therapy, similarly unaccompanied by demonstrated benefit in terms of the reduction or delay of morbidity and mortality. This can only further an illogical tradition and accelerate the declaration of its bankruptcy. On the other hand, the great strength in this tradition is in the incessant flow of ideas, the exploration of disease mechanisms and the proposals of therapeutic innovations. But these require, with top priority, the adjunct of good empiricism in the form of randomized controlled studies to avoid more tragically costly therapeutic fads as well as to resolve the existing controversy.[45, 46]

As to the practical impediments to obtaining good evidence about the effect of habitual high level exercise on rates of reinfarction and death, it is simply not feasible for a few investigators and centers, working separately, to answer this critical question. Simple consideration of the nature of coronary disease and the necessary sample size to study its therapy illustrates the problem and the need for scientific collaboration. Let us consider aspects of the design of an appropriate clinical trial of exercise in coronary patients which might take place over a practicable time period of five years:

The expected frequency of deaths is about 5 per cent per year among functional class 1 and 2 infarct patients who would be appropriate candidates for a controlled exercise program;[42] therefore, we can postulate something approaching 25 per cent deaths in five years for the control group which receives usual medical care and no intensive exercise.

Another guestimate necessary is the therapeutic effect to be expected from an exercise program; that is, what improvement is within reason, how much is sought, how much difference would be considered sufficient to establish the case for exercise and what the trial design would be adequate to detect. A realistic assumption and aim might be to demonstrate a 25 per cent lower mortality among the experimental group during the five-year trial.

Another estimate needed is the time lag before maximal effect of exercise therapy might be expected. If one assumes that this effect will be reached promptly, within the first year of the treatment, the lag time may be estimated as zero.

An estimate of the dropout or nonadherence rate to any formal intensive exercise program might be on the order of 50 per cent over the course of a five-year study, according to the experience in some trials.[36]

Finally, the confidence limits desired should be preset. It might be agreed that the probability of embracing a false positive conclusion should be set low for an expensive clinical trial with such important implications; for example, a 1 per cent chance or less of rejecting the null hypothesis when it is true. It would be important, of course, to avoid a false negative conclusion, that is, to fail to find a 25 per cent group difference when it actually occurred; for example, a 5 per cent chance, or less, of accepting the null hypothesis when it is false.

With these estimates, and under all these assumptions and conditions, 2665 eligible survivors of myocardial infarction would be required to answer the overriding question about the effect of exercise therapy on the five-year death rate! Clearly such a study is beyond the means of any investigator, medical center, or community. However, it is readily within the potential of collaborating investigators in this affluent nation.

What other aspects of design are desirable for an adequate demonstration of the influence of exercise on survival after myocardial infarction? The recent WHO Working Group in Prague attempted to formulate an approach.[47] Convalescent volunteers to a prevention trial would be randomly allocated to three treatment groups, one to obtain the best regular care available in the community. Another group would enter a special care program of multiple factor risk reduction to include unsupervised walking as the basic physical activity—along with modification of blood pressure and dietary and smoking habits as required. A third special care group would be offered the same hygienic regimen *plus* a supervised program of intensive exercise aimed at securing high levels of cardiovascular conditioning.

What represents a positive approach for the practitioner, and one which would do no harm, while waiting for the definitive evidence? Are there valid ethical alternatives to intensive exercise therapy? I think so. A balanced hygienic program based on current knowledge would encourage the coronary patient to seek a new way of life—to include gradually greater physical activity in the form of walking to tolerance, with advice and motivation to change eating, smoking, and alcohol habits as needed, and to remain under follow-up care where indicated for elevated blood pressure, frequent ectopic cardiac activity, and other observable and modifiable elements of risk. A rational program would include higher level exercise when the optimal conditions described here can be met, and for the individual patient who has a history of vigorous exercise habits and greatly desires to resume them.

Conclusion

Widespread, large-scale treatment of sedentary middle-aged coronary patients with intensive exercise is now beyond the skills, facilities, and means of the medical care system, while its risks are quite obvious and its preventive health benefit is undemonstrated. The possibility of benefit from intensive supervised activity in certain eligible patients, as well as that from moderate-level, unsupervised activity, urgently needs to be empirically tested in a scientific study involving ethical alternatives. Meanwhile, multiple risk factor modification to include graduated activity in the form of walking and active hobbies is a safe but reasonable and positive approach to the long-term therapy of coronary heart disease.

In closing, consider, if you will, for the sake of debate, this slightly exaggerated depiction of the ecology of coronary artery disease in man. Take it as an antagonistic view toward any widespread extension of therapy, prior to the results of adequate controlled studies, which employs high intensity physical exercise in sedentary middle-aged survivors of myocardial infarction:

Modern man in industrial society is an animal which, shortly after maturation, is confined to a system of special cages, in one of which, a mobile steel and plastic cage, he is exposed for one or two hours daily to complex decisions, frustration and danger, in an atmosphere high in carbon monoxide, while transported to and from other cages. In other cages, under constant temperature environments, the animal's physical activity is strictly constrained to many hours of sitting and a few moments daily of standing, with short, level walks, all of very low energy expenditure. The industrialized species of man is habitually overfed with animal and grain chow which usually includes 20 per cent of all calories from saturated fats, 20 per cent from refined carbohydrates, and 10 per cent from fermented spirits, plus varying concentrations of herbicides, pesticides, hormones, antibiotics, oxidizing agents, and radioactive isotopes. Man is systematically conditioned to self-administer 20 potent doses of nicotine, and five of caffeine alkaloids daily. He is also trained to lie motionless in a darkened cage for three hours and watch a cathode ray tube which continuously presents ambiguous information and repeated suggestions for unhygienic, purposeless activity. He is rewarded to the degree that he pursues this goal-less activity during the day.

Exposed to such an environment for half his life span, nearly all the animals develop largely irreparable lesions in the vascular system, and about half of the male animals experience severe damage to cardiac muscle. If the animal survives the dramatic onset of acute arterial insufficiency to the heart, it is returned as soon as possible to the same cages and systems. Recently, in a few habitats, it is placed in a special therapy cage, a humid and smelly one along with other sick animals, and there is stressed repetitively to maximal capacity for 30 to 60 minutes daily. This stress uniformly produces ischemic and arrhythmic cardiac episodes and, on occasion, sudden death. This new system to condition sick animals with high level intense exercise is associated, among surviving animals, with well documented improvement of capacity to perform physical work over a short term. It is untested with respect to the survival of animals so handled, or to their future disease and disability. However, it has been observed and reported anecdotally that following the physical conditioning process the animals appear to be more tranquil and to engage in somewhat more humping activity.

References

1. WHO Working Group on Rehabilitation: A program for the physical rehabilitation of patients with acute myocardial infarction. W.H.O. Regional Office for Europe, Copenhagen, 1968.
2. Wenger, N. K., Gilbert, C. A., and Siegel, W.: The use of physical activity in the rehabilitation of patients after myocardial infarction. Southern Med. J. 63:891–897, 1970.
3. Zohman, L. R., and Tobis, J. S.: *Cardiac Rehabilitation*. New York, Grune and Stratton, 1970.
4. Groden, B. M.: The management of myocardial infarction. A controlled study of the effects of early mobilization. Cardiac Rehab. 1:13–16, 1971.
5. Felix, J., Bloch, A., and Duchosal, P. W.: Infarctus du myocarde: readaptation à la phase aiguë. Méd. Hyg. 30:889–891, 1972.
6. Varnauskas, E., Bergman, H., Houk, P., and Bjorntorp, P.: Hemodynamic effects of physical training in coronary patients. Lancet 2:8–12, 1966.
7. Naughton, J., Bruhn, J., and Lategola, M.: Effects of physical training on physiologic and behavioral characteristics of cardiac patients. Arch. Phys. Med. 49:131–137, 1968.
8. Hellerstein, H. K.: Exercise therapy in coronary disease. Bull. N. Y. Acad. Med. 44:1028–1047, 1968.
9. Frick, M. H., and Katila, M.: Hemodynamic consequences of physical training after myocardial infarction. Circulation 37:192–202, 1968.
10. Barry, A. J., Daly, I. W., Pruett, E. D. R., Steinmetz, J. R., Birkhead, N. C., and Rodahl, K.: Effects of physical training on patients who have had myocardial infarction. Amer. J. Cardiol. 17:1–8, 1966.
11. Clausen, J. P., and Trap-Jensen, J.: Effects of training on the distribution of cardiac output in patients with coronary artery disease. Circulation 42:611–624, 1970.
12. Redwood, D. R., Rosing, D. R., and Epstein, S. E.: Circulatory and symptomatic effects of physical training in patients with coronary artery disease and angina pectoris. New Eng. J. Med. 286:959–965, 1972.
13. Brunner, D., and Meshulam, N.: Prevention of recurrent myocardial infarction by physical exercise. Isr. J. Med. Sci. 5:783–785, 1969.
14. Gottheiner, V.: Long-range strenuous sports training for cardiac conditioning and rehabilitation. Amer. J. Cardiol. 22:426–435, 1968.
15. Rechnitzer, P., Yuhasz, M., Pickard, H., and Lefcoe, N.: The effects of a graduated exercise program on patients with previous myocardial infarction. Canad. Med. Ass. J. 92:858–860, 1965.
16. Cain, H. D., Fraser, W. G., and Stivelman, R.: Graded activity program for safe return to self-care after myocardial infarction. J.A.M.A. 177:111–115, 1961.

17. Frick, M. H.: The effect of physical training in manifest ischemic heart disease. Circulation 40:433–435, 1969.
18. Hellerstein, H. K.: Effects of physical activity; patients and normal coronary prone subjects. Minn. Med. 52:1335–1341, 1969.
19. Detry, J-M. R., Rousseau, M., Vandenbroucke, G., Kusumi, F., Brasseur, L. A., and Bruce, R. A.: Increased arteriovenous oxygen difference after physical training in coronary heart disease. Circulation 44:109–118, 1971.
20. Bergman, H., and Varnauskas, E.: Placebo effect in physical training of coronary heart disease patients. In Coronary Heart Disease and Physical Fitness. Baltimore, University Park Press, 1971, pp. 48–51.
21. Siegel, W., Blomqvist, G., and Mitchell, J. H.: Effects of a quantitated physical training program on middle-aged sedentary men. Circulation 41:19–29, 1970.
22. Klassen, G. A., Woodhouse, S. P., and Johnson, A. L.: Haemodynamic responses to training. Post-infarction compared to normal controls. Clin. Res. 20:381, 1972.
23. Kavanaugh, T., Shephard, R. J., Pandit, V., and Doney, H.: Exercise hypnotherapy in the rehabilitation of the coronary patient. Arch. Phys. Med. & Rehab. 51:578–587, 1970.
24. Frick, M. H.: Coronary implications of haemodynamic changes by physical training. Amer. J. Cardiol. 22:417–425, 1968.
25. Eckstein, R.: Effect of exercise and coronary artery narrowing on coronary collateral circulation. Circ. Res. 5:230–235, 1957.
26. Cobb, F. R., Rudy, R. L., and Fariss, B. H.: Effect of exercise on acute coronary occlusion in dogs with prior partial occlusion. Clin. Res. 19:11, 1971.
27. Currens, J. H., and White, P. D.: Half a century of running. New Eng. J. Med. 265:988–993, 1961.
28. Rose, G., Prineas, R. J., and Mitchell, J. R. A.: Myocardial infarction and the intrinsic caliber of coronary arteries. Brit. Heart J. 29:548–552, 1967.
29. Morris, J. N., and Crawford, M. D.: Coronary heart disease and physical activity of work: Evidence of a national necropsy survey. Brit. Med. J. 2:1485–1496, 1958.
30. Salzman, S. H., Hellerstein, H. K., Radke, J. D., Maistelman, H. W., and Ricklin, R.: Quantitative effects of physical conditioning on the exercise electrocardiogram of middle-aged subjects with arteriosclerotic heart disease. In Blackburn, H. (ed.): Measurement in Exercise Electrocardiography. Springfield, Ill., Charles C Thomas, 1969.
31. Kattus, A., Jorgenson, C., and Alvaro, A.: ST segment depression with near maximal exercise in detection of coronary heart disease—its modification by physical conditioning. Chest, 62:678–683, 1972.
32. Blackburn, H., Taylor, H. L., Buskirk, E., Hamrell, B., Nicholas, W. C., and Thorsen, R. D.: The frequency of exercise-induced ventricular premature beats and the effect on them of physical conditioning. Amer. J. Cardiol. 31:441–449, 1973.
33. Dawson, A., and Taylor, H. L.: A controlled study of the effect of chronic exercise on ventricular fibrillation threshold. Laboratory of Physiological Hygiene, unpublished data.
34. Froelicher, V. F.: Animal studies of the effect of chronic exercise on the heart and atherosclerosis. A review. Amer. Heart J. 84:496–506, 1972.
35. Taylor, H. L., Blackburn, H., Brozek, J., Parlin, R. W., and Puchner, T.: Railroad employees in the United States. In Keyes, A. (ed.), Epidemiological studies related to coronary heart disease. Acta Med. Scand. Supplement No. 460, 1967.
36. Taylor, H. L., Buskirk, E. R., and Remington, R. D.: Exercise in controlled trials of the prevention of coronary heart disease. Fed. Proc., in press, 1972.
37. Blackburn, H.: Multifactor preventive trials in coronary heart disease. In Stewart, G. T. (ed.): Trends in Epidemiology. Springfield, Ill., Charles C Thomas, 1972.
38. Sanne, H., Elmfeldt, D., and Wilhelmsen, L.: The preventive effect of physical training after a myocardial infarction. In Tibblin, G., Keys, A., and Werko, L. (eds.): Preventive Cardiology. Stockholm, Almqvist and Wiksell, 1972.
39. Shapiro, S., Weinblatt, E., and Frank, C.: Return to work after first myocardial infarction. Arch. Environ. Health 24:17–26, 1972.
40. Criteria Committee of the New York Heart Association: Diseases of the Heart and Blood Vessels. Nomenclature and Criteria for Diagnosis. Boston, Little, Brown and Company, 1964.
41. Bruce, R. A., and Kluge, W.: Defibrillatory treatment of exertional cardiac arrest in coronary disease, J.A.M.A. 216:653–658, 1971.

42. Coronary Drug Project Research Group: The prognostic importance of the electrocardiogram after myocardial infarction. Ann. Intern. Med. 77:677–689, 1972.
43. Goldner, M. G., Knatterud, G. L., and Prout, T. E.: Effects of hypoglycemic agents on vascular complications in patients with adult-onset diabetes. J.A.M.A. 218:1400–1410, 1971.
44. Coronary Drug Project Research Group: The Coronary Drug Project. Findings leading to further modifications of its protocol with respect to dextrothyroxine. J.A.M.A. 220: 996–1008, 1972.
45. Kannel, W. B.: Physical exercise and lethal atherosclerotic disease. (Editorial.) New Eng. J. Med.: 282:1153–1154, 1970.
46. Spodick, D. H.: Uncontrolled exercise programs. (Letter to the editor.) New Eng. J. Med. 282:1435, 1970.
47. WHO Working Group on Rehabilitation Programs for Patients with Myocardial Infarction: Prague, October 4–7, 1971. EURO 8206 (6), WHO Regional Office for Europe, Copenhagen.

Comment

Exercise for the Coronary Patient

No one questions the beneficial effects of a program of rehabilitation in the management of the patient recovering from an acute myocardial infarct. Early ambulation followed by an exercise program aimed at return to normal activity has greatly decreased invalidism. The majority of patients return to an active, productive life.

The controversy is not concerned with return to normal activity but with a program of intensive exercise similar to that used by individuals preparing for athletic events. Certain changes in the circulation occur with such training. These include a reduction in heart rate, a reduction in the product of heart rate and arterial pressure, and a reduction in myocardial oxygen consumption at any given exercise level. Associated with this may be the ability to tolerate a higher level of exercise. In addition, the patient may experience a sense of well-being.

The critical issue is not whether the individual with coronary artery disease can be trained to tolerate a higher level of exercise, but rather whether intensive exercise therapy reduces the incidence of recurrent myocardial infarction and prolongs life. Few persons would engage in such a program knowing that it might produce a sense of increased fitness but that it would have no benefit in increasing longevity. Even fewer would participate if the dangers of unsupervised intensive exercise became widely known.

Blackburn and Bruce agree on the need for a large well designed clinical trial to test the hypothesis that intensive exercise improves the outlook of patients who have suffered a myocardial infarction. Such trials are difficult to organize and costly. Unfortunately there is no cheap and easy way to answer the question.

RICHARD V. EBERT

7

The Measurement of Central Venous Pressure

Routine Central Venous Catheterization for Management of Critically Ill Patients
  by Herbert Shubin and Max Harry Weil

Central Venous Pressure Monitoring Is an Outmoded Procedure of Limited Practical Value
  by H. J. C. Swan

Comment
  by Richard V. Ebert

Routine Central Venous Catheterization for Management of Critically Ill Patients*

HERBERT SHUBIN and
MAX HARRY WEIL

University of Southern California School of Medicine, the Los Angeles County/USC Medical Center, and the Center for the Critically Ill

Since the mid-1960's, central venous catheterization has been used extensively in the assessment and management of the critically ill patient.[1-4] Central venous catheterization has provided a means for obtaining: (1) measurements of central venous pressure; (2) blood samples for laboratory analyses; (3) blood phlebotomy; (4) recordings of atrial electrograms; and for administering: (5) drugs for cardiac resuscitation; and (6) hyperosmolar fluids for parenteral alimentation.

Central Venous Pressure (CVP)

Volume deficit may be an obvious cause of hypotension in patients who present with gross evidence of blood or fluid losses or with documented fluid deprivation. Less apparent are losses after trauma from a blunt object, massive infection, or protracted use of alpha or alpha beta adrenergic drugs. An increase of only 3 cm. in the circumference of one thigh may represent extravasation of 50 per cent of the total blood volume. Following blood loss, measurement of

---

* This study was supported by United States Public Health Service Research Grants HL-05570 from the National Heart and Lung Institute, GM-16462 from the National Institute of General Medical Sciences, and HS-00238 from the National Center for Health Services Research and Development, HSMHA.

hemoglobin and hematocrit values may be misleading, particularly when there has been insufficient time for volume compensation by hemodilution. Measurements of red cell and plasma volume by radioisotopic methods may be helpful under these circumstances, provided rigorous techniques are used, including multiple sampling over a period of 35 to 45 minutes to allow for complete mixing of the indicator.[5] However, the demands on technical staff and the time required for these measurements preclude their routine use in most hospitals.

The measurement of CVP provides a practical bedside guide for fluid repletion.[6] The CVP, of itself, does not indicate hypovolemia. Indeed, it may be increased to levels exceeding 10 cm. H_2O after marked blood or fluid loss, particularly in elderly patients with limited cardiac reserve. This paradoxical elevation in CVP with reduction in blood volume may be attributable to a concomitant decline in venous return to the heart. This accounts not only for a decrease in cardiac output and arterial pressure but also for a critical reduction in the blood flow to the coronary arteries. If coronary blood flow is compromised, myocardial contractility is likely to be reduced and ventricular end-diastolic volume and CVP increased. During volume repletion, cardiac output, arterial pressure, and coronary blood flow may be restored to more normal values and CVP returned to normal levels. The level of the CVP thus does not reflect the vascular volume per se; rather, it indicates the relationship between the volume of blood which enters the heart and the effectiveness with which the heart ejects that volume. As such, the CVP is primarily a reflection of ventricular filling pressure and ventricular competence. Increases in CVP reflect increases in right ventricular diastolic pressure, an early sign of heart failure.

Although individual measurements of CVP are not reliable indicators of blood volume, serial measurements of CVP nevertheless may be very useful in the management of patients with blood volume deficits. When such patients are challenged with fluid, serial measurements of CVP serve as a dynamic indicator of the competence of the right ventricle to accept and expel the blood returned to it. A question arises as to whether changes in CVP during volume loading reflect pressure changes in the left atrium (LA). Such a relationship was demonstrated in studies by Hanashiro and Weil[7] in dogs challenged with intravenous fluid. Although changes in CVP were of smaller magnitude than those in the LA, they were parallel in direction and could be expressed by the relationship

$$2 \Delta \overline{CVP} \text{ mm. Hg} + 2 = \Delta \overline{LAP} \text{ mm. Hg}$$

Fluid Challenge

CVP measurements are obtained during a 10-minute observation period. Fluid is then administered intravenously. If the CVP is less than 12 cm. H_2O, the fluid is infused at a rate of 20 ml./min. for a period of 10 minutes. If the CVP increases by more than 5 cm. H_2O above the initial pressure, the infusion is discontinued. If the CVP does not exceed the control pressure by more than 2 cm. H_2O at the end of 10 minutes, or if it decreases to within that range over a second 10-minute observation period, an additional aliquot of 200 ml. of fluid is administered over 10 minutes. If the CVP increases by 2 to 5 cm. H_2O above the initial pressure and continues to exceed the control pressure by more than 2 cm. H_2O after the second 10-minute observation period, the subsequent aliquot of fluid is reduced to 100 ml. over the next 10 minutes. The process is then repeated. Several liters of fluid may be required to restore effective circulation.

The volume of fluid contained in the venous circuit may be increased as much as threefold with relatively little pressure change, particularly in comparison to the arterial vessels. Veins are highly distensible vessels, acting as reservoirs, and the venous system functions as a capacitance bed. Its behavior is to be contrasted with that of the arterial system, which acts as a resistance bed in which pressure increases in direct relationship to the volume ejected into it.

A progressive increase in CVP indicates overloading and the need for a reduction in the rate of fluid infusion. If the initial pressure ranges from 12 to 20 cm. H_2O, the rate of fluid delivery is modified to administer only 10 ml./min. during each of the 10-minute challenge periods. Should the CVP increase by more than 5 cm. during a challenge period, an immediate phlebotomy may be performed to counter life-threatening pulmonary edema. If the initial CVP exceeds 20 cm. H_2O, no fluid challenge is undertaken, provided care has been taken to confirm the patency and proper location of the catheter tip.

A useful guide to the adequacy of venous return is the response of the CVP to abdominal pressure (hepatojugular reflux). A sustained substantial increase in CVP while pressure is applied over the right upper quadrant suggests that further augmentation of venous return may not significantly increase cardiac output. An increase in CVP also may be noted in some instances when the pressure of the examiner's hand on the abdomen triggers a Valsalva response, with a transient increase in both CVP and arterial pressure.

Pitfalls in Measurement and Interpretation of CVP

There are several potential errors to be avoided in monitoring CVP.

1. The tip of the catheter should lie inside the thorax. Measurements of venous pressure in a peripheral vein may be misleading and should not be used in patients in shock. Venoconstriction due to neurogenic or humoral stimuli may cause a rise in the peripheral venous pressure which often does not parallel CVP. The positioning of the catheter tip within the chest cavity is reflected by respiratory fluctuations in pressure. Documentation of the site of the catheter tip should be obtained on x-ray. If blood cannot be withdrawn readily from the catheter, the pressure measurements should be suspect. The catheter should then be flushed, repositioned, or replaced.

The venous pressure is related to a position on the patient's chest. In our Unit it is the mid-chest, which is presumed to reflect the location of the right atrium. However, such an estimate in a patient with chest width of 22 cm. may be inaccurate by more than 6 cm. For this reason the "absolute" value of CVP has little significance.

2. Relative changes in the CVP may also reflect changes in the zero reference level of the manometer, because of repositioning of the patient or the manometer.

This may also give rise to erroneous measurements. The zero level must be appropriately checked whenever CVP is measured to protect against such error.

3. A sudden increase in pressure may indicate that the catheter has advanced into the right ventricle. This may be confirmed by attaching the catheter to a transducer and recording the pressure wave or by demonstrating a distinct decrease in pressure on withdrawal of the catheter to the right atrium. On occasion a high pressure may be noted when the catheter is advanced into the coronary sinus, or in the presence of tricuspid insufficiency, or electrical atrioventricular heart block when cannon waves are generated.

4. Positive pressure ventilation may spuriously augment the CVP. Brief disconnection of the ventilator attachment provides an opportunity for more valid and comparable measurements.

5. In patients with extensive pneumonia, chronic lung disease, or pulmonary embolism, the CVP may exceed left ventricular end-diastolic pressure. In such patients left ventricular catheterization may be necessary to establish the level of left ventricular end-diastolic pressure.

Blood Sampling and Phlebotomy

Insertion of a central venous catheter provides a number of advantages in addition to those related to pressure measurements during fluid challenge. One of these is the facilitation of repetitive blood sampling in order to monitor acute biochemical changes in critically ill patients. Another advantage accrues to patients with acute life-threatening pulmonary edema, in whom the central venous catheter provides a ready route for phlebotomy. With a catheter lumen equivalent to No. 7 French (ID 0.046 inches), 18-gauge thin-walled Longdwel (ID 0.042 inches), pediatric feeding tube No. 8 French (ID 0.056 inches), or Intramedic PE 205 (ID 0.062 inches), blood may be rapidly withdrawn and venous return promptly reduced. Should cardiac arrest occur in a patient in whom a central venous catheter is already in place, delays in delivering emergency medications to the coronary circulation may be minimized. Injection of epinephrine, sodium bicarbonate, and calcium gluconate through the catheter, in conjunction with closed chest cardiac massage, facilitates prompt delivery while avoiding the hazards of percutaneous cardiac puncture. When a pulmonary embolus is suspected, the central venous catheter may be used for injection of contrast material, thereby facilitating the performance of pulmonary angiography on an emergency basis.

Atrial Electrogram

When the tip lies in the right atrium, the central venous catheter may be used for the purpose of differentiating between supraventricular and ventricular arrhythmias. To obtain an atrial electrogram, the catheter is filled with highly conductive 3 to 5 per cent saline or molar sodium bicarbonate solution. Alternatively, a stylet electrode may be passed through the lumen of the catheter. The atrial electrogram is particularly helpful in the recognition of atrial arrhythmias, for it magnifies P waves and allows their differentiation from ventricular complexes.

Parenteral Alimentation

The central venous catheter provides a route for sustained parenteral alimentation.[8] Solutions containing 20 to 25 per cent glucose and approximately 5 per cent protein hydrolysate, together with multivitamins and minerals, are administered to maintain nutritional and metabolic balance. This highly hypertonic solution may increase the osmolality of the plasma, from a normal range of 280-310 mM/L. to potentially lethal levels of 350 mM/L. or higher.[9] For this reason, the hyperosmolar alimentation mixture is infused at a constant rate with the aid of an infusion pump. This avoids unscheduled acceleration in the volume delivered by a gravity drip method of fluid administration.[10] Even with this precaution, plasma osmolality is repetitively measured and the rate of fluid delivery is regulated accordingly.

Pulmonary Artery Catheterization

The many other advantages of the central venous catheter notwithstanding, there now seems little doubt that measurements of pulmonary artery, and particularly pulmonary artery wedge pressure, provide a more precise indication of left ventricular function than measurements of CVP.[11-13] The development of a flow-directed, balloon-tipped catheter[14] has greatly facilitated the introduction of the catheter into the pulmonary artery. The catheter is inserted into a peripheral vein and advanced into the superior vena cava. The balloon at the tip is then inflated with air and the catheter is advanced through the right atrium and ventricle into the pulmonary artery. Arrhythmias are surprisingly infrequent and most often are limited to the brief interval when the catheter is advancing through the right ventricle. In approximately 70 per cent of patients the catheter tip can be floated into a peripheral pulmonary vessel and pulmonary capillary pressure obtained. Since this measurement closely approximates the left ventricular end-diastolic pressure (LVEDP), it serves as a measure of the preload and thus helps to delineate the relative position of the left ventricle with respect to its Starling curve. If there is evidence of perfusion failure (i.e., elevated lactate values, low cardiac output), and the pulmonary artery wedge pressure is not elevated, or is in a borderline range (12 to 20 mm. Hg), patients may be challenged with fluid. Conversely, when the pulmonary artery wedge pressure or LVEDP is greater than 20 mm. Hg, myocardial failure should be suspected and treatment with diuretic drugs may be warranted.[13] Recently, however, it has been demonstrated by Stein and associates[15] that in some patients the pulmonary artery wedge pressure may be normal in the presence of clinical and radiographic signs of pulmonary edema. This may be related in part to changes in the colloid osmotic pressure (COP). In the patients observed by Stein et al.[15] the COP had been reduced from a normal value of 26 mm. Hg to less than 17 mm. Hg.[16] Consequently the hydrostatic pressure in the pulmonary capillaries, even though in a normal range, may exceed the COP, with consequent extravasation of fluid into the pulmonary interstitium or alveoli. Other factors may be operative, for in some instances the LVEDP is not elevated and the COP is not reduced. In the clinical assessment of such patients, a reduction in PaO_2 and evidence of pulmonary congestion on the chest x-ray may serve as more reliable indicators of pulmonary edema than either measurements of pulmonary artery wedge pressure or LVEDP.

For the approximately 30 per cent of patients in whom the catheter cannot be floated into the wedge position, it has been suggested that the pulmonary artery end-diastolic pressure (PAEDP) may be used instead as an indicator of mean left atrial and LVEDP. Although a number of investigators[12, 17-19] have reported a close correlation between PAEDP and LVEDP, others have questioned the reliability of this relationship.[20] In a study of patients with left ventricular myocardial disease, Bouchard and associates[21] noted that LVEDP was consistently higher than PAEDP, with the difference ranging from 2 to 21 mm. Hg. When acute increases in LVEDP were induced by administration of methoxamine or acute decreases by atrial pacing, these changes were not reflected by comparable changes in PAEDP. In studies in patients who were given acute volume loads, or isoproterenol or epinephrine, Jenkins and associates[22] demonstrated significant correlation between PAEDP and left atrial mean pressure only when the pulmonary vascular resistance was normal. Closer correlation between pulmonary artery and left ventricular pressures has been noted when measurements at both sites are made at a time in the cardiac cycle immediately prior to atrial contraction.[21, 23]

In the assessment and management of the patient with suspected hypovolemia, monitoring of pulmonary artery and wedge pressure, with infrequent exceptions, provides a reliable indicator of the safety of fluid repletion. Serial measurements of CVP provide comparable information but are less sensitive in reflecting changes in LVEDP. Insertion of a pulmonary artery catheter thus would appear to be preferable, providing it can be accomplished with reasonable facility and without disproportionate complications. Insertion of a balloon-tip catheter into the pulmonary artery requires a cutdown over the basilic vein, whereas in most instances a central venous catheter may be inserted percutaneously. Some additional dexterity and experience may be required to position the pulmonary artery catheter in a wedged position in comparison to that required to insert a central venous catheter. These considerations notwithstanding, passage of a pulmonary artery catheter is warranted in those patients in whom left ventricular competence is most likely to be an issue, particularly those with known heart disease. If passage of the pulmonary artery catheter should prove difficult, or if percutaneous insertion of the catheter is preferred, central venous catheterization may be used alternatively.

Complications

The insertion of a central venous or pulmonary artery catheter by way of a basilic vein may be attended by some complications. In 240 patients with acute myocardial infarction who had percutaneous central venous catheterization, Walters and associates[24] noted complications in 18 per cent of patients. Among 142 patients with massive gastrointestinal hemorrhage in whom the central venous catheter was inserted by a venous cutdown, Andersen and Klebe[25] noted complications in 9 per cent. Local phlebitis was by far the commonest complication, with the highest incidence occurring in patients in whom the catheter had been in place for several days. Local infection and septicemia have been noted, with an incidence ranging from less than 1 per cent[24, 26] to as high as 5 per cent.[27] In our own experience, meticulous attention to aseptic care of the site of entry of the catheter has been associated with an incidence of infection of less than 1 per cent. Fracture of the catheter, with embolization to the heart, may occur if the catheter is advanced through a needle and then withdrawn, thereby severing the catheter on the sharp needle tip. This complication may be avoided by not withdrawing the catheter while the needle is still in the vein. Percutaneous subclavian vein catheterization may be complicated by puncture of the lung and the development of pneumothorax.[28] This may impose a substantial hazard, particularly in the critically ill patient, and for this reason percutaneous subclavian vein catheterization is best reserved for those physicians well versed in its performance. Although all these complications may be encountered with central venous or pulmonary artery catheterization, we are not aware of a single fatal outcome directly attributable to these procedures in the 10 years that they have been used routinely by us.

Considering the advantages enumerated and the relatively minor morbidity when these procedures are performed competently, the lifesaving potential of central venous and pulmonary artery measurements far outweighs their hazards.

References

1. Weil, M. H., and Shubin, H.: *Diagnosis and Treatment of Shock*. Baltimore, The Williams & Wilkins Co., 1967.
2. MacLean, L. D., and Duff, J. H.: The use of central venous pressure as a guide to volume replacement in shock. Dis. Chest 48:199–205, 1965.
3. Bradley, R. D. Diagnostic right-heart catheterization with miniature catheters in severely ill patients. Lancet 2:941–942, 1964.
4. Gunnar, R. M., Cruz, A., Boswell, J., Co, B. S., Pietras, R. J., and Tobin, J. R., Jr.: Myocardial infarction with shock: Hemodynamic studies and results of therapy. Circulation 33:746–754, 1966.
5. Ryström, L., Weil, M. H., Shubin, H., and Palley, N.: Technique of measurement of the plasma volume and red cell mass during acute circulatory failure. Surg. Gynec. Obstet. *133*:621–626, 1971.
6. Weil, M. H., Shubin, H., and Rosoff, L.: Fluid repletion in circulatory shock: Central venous pressure and other practical guides. J.A.M.A. *192*:668–674, 1965.
7. Hanashiro, P. K., and Weil, M. H.: Relationships between right- and left-sided cardiac pressures after volume overload in the intact dog. Fed. Proc. 27:445, 1968.
8. Dudrick, S. J., Wilmore, D. W., Vars, H. M., and Rhoads, J. E.: Longterm total parenteral

nutrition with growth, development and positive nitrogen balance. Surgery 64:134–142, 1968.
9. Mattar, J. A., Weil, M. H., Shubin, S. H., and Stein, L.: Hyperosmolal state following cardiac arrest. (Abstract.) Amer. J. Cardiol. 29:279, 1972.
10. Bisera, J., Peterson, E., Carrington, J. H., Palley, N., and Weil, M. H.: Computer controllable pump. (Abstract.) Association for the Advancement of Medical Instrumentation, April, 1972.
11. Bell, H., Stubbs, D., and Pugh, D.: Reliability of central venous pressure as an indicator of left atrial pressure. A study in patients with mitral valve disease. Chest 59:169–173, 1971.
12. Rackley, C. E., and Russell, R. O., Jr.: Left ventricular function in acute myocardial infarction and its clinical significance. Circulation 45:231–244, 1972.
13. Parmley, W. W., Diamond, G., Tomoda, H., Forrester, J. S., and Swan, H. J. C.: Clinical evaluation of left ventricular pressures in myocardial infarction. Circulation 45:358–366, 1972.
14. Ganz, W. W., Forrester, J. S., Chonette, D., Donoso, R., and Swan, H. J. C.: A new flow-directed catheter technique for measurement of pulmonary artery and capillary wedge pressure without fluoroscopy (Abstract.) Amer. J. Cardiol. 25:96, 1970.
15. Stein, L., Cavanilles, J. M., Weil, M. H., and Shubin, H.: Pulmonary congestion of non-cardiac causes following volume loading. Presented at the meeting of the American College of Physicians, Atlantic City, N. J., April, 1972.
16. Jacobson, E. J., Weil, M. H., Ritz, R., and Michaels, S.: Clinical measurement of plasma colloid osmotic pressure. Physiologist 14:167, 1971.
17. Rutherford, B. D., McCann, W. D., and O'Donovan, T. P. B.: The value of monitoring pulmonary artery pressure for early detection of left ventricular failure following myocardial infarction. Circulation 43:655–666, 1971.
18. Forrester, J., Diamond, G., Ganz, W., Danzig, R., and Swan, H. J. C.: Right and left heart pressures in the acutely ill patient. (Abstract.) Clin. Res. 18:306, 1970.
19. Forsberg, S. A.: Relations between pressure in pulmonary artery, left atrium, and left ventricle with special reference to events at end diastole. Brit. Heart J. 33:494–499, 1971.
20. Falicov, R. E., and Resnekov, L.: Relationship of the pulmonary end-diastolic pressure to the left ventricular end-diastolic and mean filling pressures in patients with and without left ventricular dysfunction. Circulation 42:65–73, 1970.
21. Bouchard, R. J., Gault, J. H., and Ross, J., Jr.: Evaluation of pulmonary arterial end-diastolic pressure as an estimate of left ventricular end-diastolic pressure in patients with normal and abnormal left ventricular performance. Circulation 44:1072–1079, 1971.
22. Jenkins, B. S., Bradley, R. D., and Branthwaite, M. A.: Evaluation of pulmonary arterial end-diastolic pressure as an indirect estimate of left atrial mean pressure. Circulation 42:75–78, 1970.
23. Balcon, R., Bennett, E. D., and Sowton, G. E.: Comparison of pulmonary artery diastolic and left ventricular end-diastolic pressures in patients with ischaemic heart disease. Cardiov. Res. 6:172–175, 1972.
24. Walters, M. B., Stanger, H. A. D., and Rotem, C. E.: Complications with percutaneous central venous catheters. J.A.M.A. 220:1455–1457, 1972.
25. Andersen, D., and Klebe, J. G.: Measurement of central venous pressure: Complications and possible failures of the method. Scand. J. Gastroent. 3:267–272, 1968.
26. Corso, J. A., Agostinelli, R., and Brandriss, M. W.: Maintenance of venous polyethylene catheters to reduce risk of infection. J.A.M.A. 210:2075–2077, 1969.
27. Moran, J. M., Atwood, R. P., and Rowe, M. I.: A clinical and bacteriologic study of infections associated with venous cutdowns. New Eng. J. Med. 272:554–560, 1965.
28. Schapira, M., and Stern, W. Z.: Hazards of subclavian vein cannulation for central venous pressure monitoring. J.A.M.A. 201:327–329, 1967.

Central Venous Pressure Monitoring Is an Outmoded Procedure of Limited Practical Value*

H. J. C. SWAN

University of California at Los Angeles

Central Venous Pressure

"When you can measure what you are speaking about, and express it in numbers, you know something about it. . . ." The logic of this statement, attributed to Lord Kelvin, is dependent upon the assumption that the numerical values obtained are a valid and first-order correlate of those processes of which description is desired. Otherwise, invalid concepts and conclusions are fortified by the gilt of numerical expression and error is compounded. Following reports in 1965 by Weil, Shubin, and Rosoff[1] and Wilson,[2] and by Cohn (1967),[3] central venous pressure is a numerical value which is now routinely used in the clinical evaluation of cardiac performance in seriously ill patients with and without cardiac disease. This usage is largely based on the fact that the technical procedure to obtain central venous pressure is simple and relatively safe, the data are easy to record, and the data are clearly useful in specific situations which usually are highlighted in published reports. Some experienced investigators[4] have questioned critically the justification of this stand, and indeed the majority of publications on the topic are replete with disclaimers, codicils, warnings of exceptions, and so on. Nevertheless, the procedure has been justified on the basis of simplicity, low cost, and so forth, without a clear scientific evaluation of the use which is made of such information. It is my purpose to re-evaluate the status of measurement of central venous pressure in clinical practice in the light of current knowledge. While my primary task is not to compare the value of central venous pressure measurements with the value of measurements of pulmonary artery

---

* Supported by MIRU Contract No. PH–43–NHLI–68–1333–M.

systolic and diastolic pressures and pulmonary "capillary wedge" pressures utilizing flotation catheters at the bedside,[5] some commentary on the latter is germane and will be relevant to my conclusions.

Venous pressure and central venous pressure

Blood flows from the periphery to the right atrium propelled by energy essentially derived from contraction of the left ventricle and transmitted through the arterial and capillary bed to the peripheral venous system. Hindrance to the return of blood to the right atrium by extracardiac factors or increases in the obligatory filling pressure of the right ventricle cause a substantial rise in venous pressure. In fact, a combination of the measurement of venous pressure and circulation time was classically used to define in numerical terms the presence of cardiac failure. However, when venous pressure is significantly elevated as a result of cardiac tamponade, mediastinal fibrosis, or severe right ventricular failure, other physical signs are sufficiently evident and impressive, and a numerical knowledge of venous pressure is seldom helpful. Further, in many circumstances venous tone may be altered and the venous pressure at, for example, the antecubital vein, does not necessarily reflect the venous pressure within the thorax or within the right atrium. For this reason it is current practice to advance a small catheter from a peripheral vein and locate its tip within the thorax in the superior vena cava or in the upper portion of the right atrium.[1,6] When the catheter enters this location, typical alterations in pressure, phasic with respiration, can be observed on a saline manometer, and if a sensitive strain gauge manometer is used, phasic alterations with the cardiac cycle can also be recognized and recorded. In the absence of extracardiac obstruction, the pressure in the cava is a slightly damped version of the right atrial pressure, but for our purpose it is appropriate to regard central venous pressure as essentially synonymous with right atrial pressure.

Physiological considerations

The central venous pressure is a complex phenomenon, which is a determinant as well as a consequence of venous return, venous volume, and venous tone and also the performance characteristics of the right ventricle. Nor is venous pressure related to the functional state of only the right ventricle. In a detailed consideration of circulatory pressures, Guyton[7] has pointed out that, for the right ventricle, an equilibrium in filling pressure is reached when left atrial pressure results in a level of left ventricular function to maintain inflow of blood from the systemic arterial bed into the venous vascular bed at a constant level. Similar considerations identify the partial dependency of left ventricular performance on the function of the right ventricle and the state of tone of the pulmonary vascular bed. Any factor which alters any of these functions will result in a new equilibrium between venous volume, cardiac performance, venous tone, and venous pressure. It is well recognized that these coupled interrelationships may be greatly distorted in the presence of significant cardiac disease in which cardiac performance, systemic vascular reactivity, pulmonary pressures, venous tone, and intravascular volumes and distribution are usually abnormal. Hence, pragmatic reliance on central venous pressure as an important indicator of cardiac performance would appear to be unjustified on purely physiological reasoning and, as stated by Jacobson,[8] the ready acceptance of such data as diagnostically reliable is surprising.

Central Venous Pressure and Right Ventricular Performance

In the absence of tricuspid stenosis or insufficiency, the mean central venous pressure closely approximates diastolic right ventricular pressure. As such, the central venous pressure must be a fundamental index of performance of the right ventricle. Under normal circumstances the right ventricle discharges its contents through the low resistance pulmonary arterial bed into the left atrium. The pulmonary artery diastolic pressure is usually only slightly higher than mean left atrial pressure. In fact, at low heart rates the pulmonary artery diastolic pressure also approximates right ventricular end-diastolic pressure just prior to the beginning of right ventricular systole.

The interpretation of central venous pressure necessitates an understanding of ventricular compliance. This term refers to the relation of ventricular volume to intraventricular pressure during the passive filling (diastolic) phase of the cardiac cycle. Thus, as ventricular filling proceeds the cavity pressure rises from a low point at end systole to a maximum at end diastole (disregarding the "a" wave of atrial contraction). The magnitude and rate of rise of pressure during diastole is dependent upon, among other factors, the stiffness of the ventricular wall. The normal right ventricle is a highly compliant chamber—its wall has a low stiffness factor—and, hence, the pressure volume relation is extremely flat to the pressure axis within the physiological range. In fact, it is difficult to demonstrate a clear relation between stroke volume and filling pressure in the normal right ventricle with normal pulmonary outflow impedance. However, the performance of the right ventricle is markedly affected by changes in right ventricular afterload, that is, the pulmonary artery pressure. This may be due to an acute increase in total pulmonary resistance, caused either by precapillary obstruction, as for example in pulmonary embolus, or by postcapillary pulmonary venous hypertension, as for example that resulting from left heart failure. Under these circumstances the ability of the normal right ventricle to discharge its contents completely is highly compromised, the end-systolic or residual volume is greatly increased, and the chamber is forced to operate on a stiffer segment of its passive pressure volume filling curve which has a steeper relation than normal to the pressure axis.

If changes in the pulmonary vascular bed have been present from birth or have developed gradually, then hypertrophy of the right ventricle occurs, so that right ventricular performance is maintained. However, in this instance, ventricular hypertrophy is present and the passive pressure-volume relation (compliance curve) is quite unlike the normal and resembles more that of the left ventricle. Hence, considering the central venous pressure alone as a measure of the performance of only the right ventricle, one recognizes that it is a complex function of the passive pressure-volume characteristics of that chamber, of acute or longstanding changes in impedance to outflow, as well as the contractile state of the right ventricle. Since both pulmonary venous congestion and circulatory failure result predominantly from diseases affecting the left ventricle, a description of performance of that chamber by a monitoring of central venous pressure alone is certainly unlikely to be precise. Nevertheless, it is common practice for the physician to consider that measures of central venous pressure are useful determinants of the overall state of cardiac function.

Relation Between Right and Left Atrial Pressures

In the normal human subject a relationship exists between the central venous or right atrial pressure, right ventricular filling pressure, pulmonary artery wedge pressure, and pulmonary artery diastolic pressure. The near identity of pulmonary artery diastolic and pulmonary wedge pressure is a consequence of the negligible resistance in the pulmonary circuit which allows for the passage of blood out of the pulmonary arterial bed and into the pulmonary capillaries and veins during the time course of systole and early diastole, with the attainment of near zero flow at end diastole. The data of Barratt-Boyes and Wood[9] are germane in this respect. Meticulous care and precision have characterized the work of Dr. Earl Wood's laboratory and a suitable number, 21 out of 26 subjects (Table 2, ref. 9), had near simultaneous measurements of right atrial pulmonary artery diastolic and mean pulmonary artery wedge pressures recorded. Recalculation of these data define the following regression equations: $P_{PAD} = 5.8 + 1.03 \overline{P}_{RA}$, SEE 1.27 ($r = 0.80$) and $\overline{P}_{CW} = 7.1 + 0.74 \overline{P}_{RA}$, SEE 1.27 ($r = 0.80$), where P_{PAD} and $\overline{P}_{RA}$ and $\overline{P}_{CW}$ are the pulmonary artery diastolic, mean right atrial, and mean pulmonary capillary wedge pressures, respectively. However, the error in predication of P_{PAD} or $\overline{P}_{CW}$ from these regression equations exceeds 15 per cent in a significant number of instances. Data obtained after four minutes of supine exercise showed an increase in pulmonary artery diastolic pressure of 4 mm. Hg, while the average increase in right atrial pressure was similar in magnitude.[10] Few systematic comparisons of right atrial and left atrial pressures have been made in disease states. In the presence of chronic pulmonary disease with increased pulmonary vascular resistance, the pulmonary artery diastolic pressure does not ordinarily equilibrate during one cardiac cycle with pulmonary capillary or pulmonary venous pressure levels. In mitral stenosis, increases in resistance exist at both the pulmonary arteriolar, and the mitral valvar level, rendering right or left atrial pressure remotely related to the performance of the left ventricle. As indicated above, chronic elevations of pulmonary artery pressure will change totally the compliance characteristics of the right ventricle and therefore its pressure-volume and pressure-performance relationships. Sarin and co-authors[11] reported no consistent relation between right and left atrial pressures in patients studied following cardiac valve replacement; only 28 per cent of their patients had the normal expected relationship. These authors imply that reliance on right atrial pressures alone for therapeutic decision-making results in an unnecessary incidence of "pump lung," pulmonary edema, or low cardiac output, which are avoidable if left atrial pressures are measured.

Clinical application

Although general examples and suggestions as to clinical application have been provided,[2] it is difficult to make a precise evaluation from the literature since specific goals and end-points of therapy are poorly defined—if defined at all—errors in therapy are seldom reported, and no author has attempted a critical evaluation of his own experience. The surgeon often uses central venous pressure as an index of venous volume depletion or adequacy, whereas the cardiologist frequently considers central venous pressure in a dual role, either as an index of cardiac performance and/or an index of venous volume. In the absence of a clear conceptual separation of these two quite different aspects of circulatory function, the lack of critical appraisal of the value of this technique is not surprising.

Three separate performance characteristics of circulatory insufficiency may be related to central venous pressure measurement. The first is hypovolemia with deficient venous volume manifest by a reduction in central venous pressure; a second is as an index of right ventricular performance; and the third is the relationship of central venous pressure to left atrial pressure and to the presence of pulmonary venous hypertension and left ventricular failure.

Each of these characteristics must be considered separately and appropriate end-points defined. Two approaches may be taken to the numerical values reported. Regarding the significance of the *absolute value* of central venous pressure, the normal range is said to be 2 to 8 mm. Hg. If the pressure is very high ($>$ 10 mm. Hg) or very low ($<$ 2 mm. Hg) it frequently has important prognostic and therapeutic implications. Central venous pressure values between these extremes do not usually appear to be of great significance. However, the zero reference point is not always defined, and without this reference level, data obtained by different authors cannot be compared. Hence, Wilson[2] defines central venous pressure values of 0 to 5 mm. Hg as "unelevated," and Weil et al.[1] regard the range 9 to 15 mm. Hg as "borderline," while four of the 26 normal subjects of Barratt-Boyes and Wood[9] had mean right atrial pressures of 9 or 10 mm. Hg. In spite of this, other investigators[12] have reported central venous pressure to the nearest 0.1 mm. Hg without a definition of zero reference. Others find that a single number increasing in unitary fashion is appropriate. There are no established standards or error definition for physicians, nurses, and other paramedical personnel to obtain valid and true measurements of central venous pressure in absolute terms.

The *relative changes* in central venous pressure may be more useful indicators of important alterations in cardiovascular function and in the adequacy of venous and blood volumes. The absolute magnitude of changes to be regarded as having therapeutic significance have not been agreed upon. Shubin and Weil[13] recommend a fluid challenge technique in which 200 ml. of fluid are infused over 10 minutes and observation made on the changes or absence of changes of central venous pressure. If the pressure does not rise by more than 2 cm. H_2O, a beneficial response is deduced and fluid repletion continued. But in one of the earliest reports, Nixon et al.[14] demonstrated recovery from systemic hypotension associated with a rise in central venous pressure from 9 cm. H_2O (above the sternal angle) to 18 cm. H_2O! Other investigators varied the rate and duration of fluid loading. Colton and Hamer[15] infused 500 ml. of fluid in 13 minutes for a mean rate of infusion 40 ml./min. and Loeb et al.[16] infused at a mean rate of 7.6 ml./min. for durations of up to three hours. In spite of the impossibility of extracting comparative data, it is reasonable to conclude that in patients found to have extremely low central venous pressures, there will be a significant incidence of hypovolemia, with benefit to be expected from fluid therapy. It is of interest that Colton and Hamer[15] did not find material changes in right atrial pressure measurements following fluid loading in patients with or without heart failure. In fact, in their patients with heart failure, a lowering of right atrial pressure was related to a rise in right atrial oxygen saturation, assumed by the authors to indicate improvement in cardiac performance.

Central Venous Pressure and Acute Failure of the Left Ventricle

In acute myocardial infarction, elevations of left ventricular end-diastolic pressure appear to be the rule rather than the exception. This may be due in part to a marked alteration in left ventricular compliance consequent upon the acute injury process. The relatively close relationship between left atrial mean pressure and left ventricular end-diastolic pressure which ordinarily pertains is frequently distorted in that end-diastolic left ventricular pressure can be elevated above the left atrial mean pressure. Usually with a significant rise in phasic and mean left atrial pressures, pulmonary venous congestion and the accompanying symptoms of dyspnea, orthopnea, or even pulmonary edema are consequences. It is now quite evident that central venous pressure measurements have no predictable or useful relationship to the state of filling of the left ventricle. Collins[17] and McHugh[18] and their associates have demonstrated the total absence of relation between the level of central venous pressure and the radiographic appearance of the lungs in acute myocardial infarction. Patients with severe pulmonary congestion and pulmonary edema can have normal or near normal levels of central venous pressure. On the other hand, central venous pressure may be considerably increased in patients with near normal left atrial pressures. Collins et al.[17] suggested that a raised central venous pressure was more frequently associated with dysrhythmias and posterior infarction, whereas patients with anterior infarction—and presumably more severe left ventricular dysfunction—have, as a group, a more normal level of central venous pressure. Forrester et al.[19] demonstrated the expected general biological relationship ($r=0.45$) between central venous pressure and pulmonary capillary wedge pressure in 50 patients with early myocardial infarction, but pointed out the impossibility of prediction of the mean left atrial pressure from the central venous pressure. The standard error of estimate (SEE) was 4.23 in comparison to 1.26 for normal subjects.[9] Likewise a prediction of the change in left atrial pressure from the change in central venous pressure[18] was impossible. If it were assumed that the pressure change in the left atrium was the same as in the central venous pressure then the mean error was 7.2 (S.D. 4.5) with a range of 1 to 18 mm. Hg, preliminary data of Loeb et al.[20] notwithstanding.

In acute and critical illnesses, particularly in the elderly, the incidence of chronic obstructive lung disease is significant. The occurrence of pulmonary embolus, whether small and recurrent or single and large, is not infrequent in the presence of heart disease. Elevated central venous pressure in such patients probably reflects the partially hypertrophied and compensated state of the right ventricle, as well as the impedance to right ventricular outflow.

Conclusions

The use of central venous pressure to characterize or identify changes in right ventricular function is hazardous. Right ventricular compliance and the state of impedance to right ventricular outflow are prime determinants of central venous pressure, and the value of central venous pressure alone as an index of the function of the right ventricle disease is unwarranted. The application of central venous pressure as a guide to the state of left ventricular function is totally without justification and likely to cause greater error than benefit. On the other hand, central venous pressure values approaching zero, or even in the low normal range, may suggest the presence of hypovolemia, which can be a most important yet unsuspected complication of acute illnesses. Recognition and treatment of hypovolemia may be a lifesaving intervention. For other than this specific purpose the value of central venous pressure monitoring cannot be justified on physiological grounds or from a critical view of the literature.

Alternatives

These deficiencies in the monitoring of important variables in critically ill patients have led to the development of flotation catheters.[21, 22] The provision of a balloon flotation mechanism[5] to allow the rapid placement of catheters in the pulmonary circulation at the bedside without the use of fluoroscopy has proved feasible and remarkably free of significant complications. The use of the balloon flotation catheter further permits the convenient measurement of what we, following tradition, have called the pulmonary artery "wedge" pressure.[5] Fitzpatrick et al.[23] suggest that the term pulmonary artery "occluded' pressure (P_{PAoccl}) is more appropriate. Importantly also such pressures are almost identical in phase and magnitude to left atrial pressures and are less susceptible to damping and phase delay than the conventional wedge pressure, since a larger segment of the pulmonary vascular bed is available for retrograde transmission of left atrial pressure.[24] Pulmonary artery "occluded" pressure is a direct measure of pulmonary venous and left atrial pressures and therefore a primary correlate of pulmonary venous congestion. However, it is possible that the pulmonary artery "occluded" pressure cannot be utilized as a precise indicator of the left ventricular end-diastolic pressure under all circumstances. This topic is currently under critical study. The absolute discrepancy in a group of patients with acute myocardial infarction studied by Cohn et al.[25] indicates that the end-diastolic left ventricular pressure exceeds mean left atrial pressure by approximately 7 mm. Hg in the presence of acute myocardial infarction. Our own data in this regard using conventional catheterization techniques in patients with ischemic heart disease expressed by linear regression equations is: $P_{LVED} = 8.0 + 0.75\ \overline{P}_{CW}$ and $\overline{P}_{LVD} = 0.23 + 0.87\ \overline{P}_{CW}$ where P_{LVED}, $\overline{P}_{CW}$, and $\overline{P}_{LVD}$ are left ventricular end-diastolic, pulmonary capillary "wedge," and left ventricular mean diastolic pressures, respectively. Hence, there is a limitation on the direct application of the measurement of mean pulmonary artery occluded pressures to the construction of function curves for the left ventricle.

The comparison of pulmonary artery diastolic pressure in combination with pulmonary artery "occluded" pressure is of considerable value in that a significant difference between the mean pulmonary artery "occluded" pressures and the pulmonary artery diastolic pressure suggests the presence of obstructive pulmonary vascular disease and/or pulmonary embolus.

It is now practical, utilizing the balloon flotation catheter in its double or triple lumen versions, to obtain measurements of pulmonary artery "occluded" pressure, pulmonary artery systolic pressure, and pulmonary artery diastolic pressure, as well as central venous or right ventricular end-diastolic pressure so as to define, with a high degree of precision, the state of pulmonary venous congestion, the peak pressure generated by the right ventricle, the difference between the pulmonary diastolic pressure and the pulmonary artery occluded pressure as an indicator of pulmonary arterial obstructive changes, and the mean central venous pressure as an index of right ventricular filling and the state of venous volume relative to venous vascular tone. Additionally, recent developments have allowed for the measurement of cardiac output in the acutely ill patient at the bedside.[26] With these data a reasonable, although not complete, description of the state of the circulation in disease can be obtained which is useful yet should seldom be misleading in terms of diagnosis and therapy.

Balloon flotation catheterization probably necessitates the acceptance of a slightly greater hazard to a given patient than the use of central venous pressure alone, although the latter is not without complications. However, balloon flotation catheterization can be carried out by paramedical personnel and by individuals with no specific training for this task and accomplished as readily as the placement of a central venous pressure line. The provision of simple electronic manometric systems is now within the capability of virtually all community hospitals. The coronary care concept necessitates the application of medical electronics at the bedside, and the provision of a simple control and amplifier with display in either digital or analogue form is a relatively inexpensive matter. The additional information readily obtainable more than justifies the application of flotation catheters to measure central circulatory pressure and other variables in any patient in whom, on clinical grounds, there is thought to be a need to measure the central venous pressure.

References

1. Weil, M. H., Shubin, H., and Rosoff, L.: Fluid repletion in circulatory shock. J.A.M.A. *192*:84–90, 1965.

2. Wilson, J. N.: Rational approach to management of clinical shock. Arch. Surg. 91:92–120, 1965.
3. Cohn, J. N.: Central venous pressure as a guide in volume expansion. Ann. Intern. Med. 66:1283–1287, 1967.
4. Shillingford, J., and Julian, D.: In Research on Myocardial Infarction. American Heart Association Monograph #27, page 190, Supplement IV. Circulation Vols. 39, 40, November, 1969.
5. Swan, H. J. C., Ganz, W., Forrester, J., Marcus, H., Diamond, G., and Chonette, D.: Catheterization of the heart in man with use of a flow-directed balloon-tipped catheter. New Eng. J. Med. 283:447–451, 1970.
6. Hurst, J. W., and Logue, R. B.: *The Heart.* New York, McGraw-Hill Book Co., Inc., 1970, addition to page 386.
7. Guyton, A.: *Cardiac Output and Its Regulation.* Philadelphia, W. B. Saunders Company, 1963.
8. Jacobson, E. D.: A physiologic approach to shock. New Eng. J. Med. 278:834–838, 1968.
9. Barratt-Boyes, B. G., and Wood, E. H.: Cardiac output and related measurements and pressure values in the right heart and associated vessels, together with an analysis of the hemodynamic response to the inhalation of high oxygen mixtures in healthy subjects. J. Lab. Clin. Med. 51:72–90, 1958.
10. Barratt-Boyes, B. G., and Wood, E. H.: Hemodynamic response of healthy subjects to exercise in the supine position while breathing oxygen. J. App. Physiol. 8:129–135, 1957.
11. Sarin, C. L., Yalav, E., Clement, A. J., and Braimbridge, M. V.: The necessity of measurement of left atrial pressure after cardiac valve surgery. Thorax 25:185–189, 1970.
12. Loeb, H. S., Cruz, A., Teng, C. Y., Boswell, J., Pietras, R. J., Tobin, J. R., and Gunnar, R. M.: Haemodynamic studies in shock associated with infection. Brit. Heart J. 29:883–894, 1967.
13. Shubin, H., and Weil, M. H.: Practical considerations in the management of shock complicating acute myocardial infarction. Amer. J. Cardiol. 26:603–608, 1970.
14. Nixon, P. G. F., Ikran, H., and Morton, S.: Infusion of dextrose solution in cardiogenic shock. Lancet 1:1077–1079, 1966.
15. Colton, D. J., and Hamer, J.: Response to rapid infusion of diuresis in acute cardiac infarction. Brit. Med. J. 33:72–77, 1971.
16. Loeb, H. S., Pietras, R. J., Tobin, J. F., and Gunnar, R. M.: Hypovolemia in shock due to acute myocardial infarction. Circulation 40:653–659, 1969.
17. Collins, J. V., Clark, T. J. H., Evans, T. R., and Riaz, M. A.: Central venous pressure in acute myocardial infarction. Lancet 1:373–375, 1971.
18. McHugh, T. J., Forrester, J. S., Adler, L., Zion, D., and Swan, H. J. C.: Pulmonary vascular congestion in acute myocardial infarction: Hemodynamic and radiologic correlations. Ann. Intern. Med. 76:29–33, 1972.
19. Forrester, J. S., Diamond, G., McHugh, T. J., and Swan, H. J. C.: Filling pressures in the right and left sides of the heart in acute myocardial infarction. New Eng. J. Med. 285:190–193, 1971.
20. Loeb, H. S., Gunnar, R. M., Pietras, R. J., and Tobin, J. R.: Relationships between central venous and left ventricular filling pressures prior to and during treatment of shock. Amer. J. Cardiol. 23:125, 1969.
21. Bradley, R. D.: Diagnostic right heart catheterization with miniature catheters in severely ill patients. Lancet 2:941–942, 1964.
22. Scheinman, M. M., Abbott, J. A., and Rapaport, E.: Clinical uses of a flow-directed right catheter. Arch. Intern. Med. 124:19–24, 1969.
23. Fitzpatrick, G. F., Hampson, L. F., and Burgess, J. H.: Bedside determination of left atrial pressure. Canad. Med. Ass. 106:1293–1298, 1972.
24. Mueller, H., Gensini, G., and Prevedel, A. E.: Retrograde transmission of left atrial pressure pulses across the pulmonary capillary bed in dogs. Circulation Res. 2:426–431, 1954.
25. Hamosh, P., and Cohn, J. N.: Left ventricular function in acute myocardial infarction. J. Clin. Invest. 50:523–533, 1971.
26. Forrester, J. S., Ganz, W., Diamond, G., McHugh, T., Chonette, D. W., and Swan, H. J. C.: Thermodilution cardiac output determination with a single flow-directed catheter. Amer. H. J. 83:306–311, 1972.

Comment

The Measurement of Central Venous Pressure

The use of a central venous catheter for estimation of blood volume deficits and to monitor intravenous fluid administration has become commonplace in teaching hospitals. The question at issue is whether the procedure is unnecessary in some cases and whether improper conclusions are being drawn from the measurements.

Surprisingly, the two antagonists agree on the important points. The absolute central venous pressure is commonly used as a criterion for the presence of a blood volume deficit or of an excessive volume of fluid in the circulation. It is true that if the circulation was a simple elastic system, a constant relationship between pressure and volume would exist, and knowing one, it would be possible to predict the other. Unfortunately such is not the case. Right ventricular failure, pulmonary hypertension, and alteration in venous tone may modify the pressure volume relationship. The importance of a proper reference point is often overlooked. The level of the right atrium may be difficult to estimate from external landmarks, especially in patients with an abnormal chest wall.

Central venous pressure is also commonly used to monitor intravenous fluid administration on the assumption that a sharp rise in this pressure will warn of a dangerous increase in pulmonary venous pressure and thus permit the fluid administration to be stopped before pulmonary edema develops. The implicit assumption is that increase in pulmonary venous pressure is accompanied by an increase in right atrial pressure. Swan has examined this problem by the use of a special flotation catheter which permits measurement of pulmonary artery and pulmonary wedge pressure in desperately ill patients. He has demonstrated conclusively that central venous pressure may at times not be a reliable indicator of left atrial pressure. Marked elevation of pulmonary venous pressure may occur in left ventricular failure in the presence of a normal right atrial pressure. Shubin and Weil admit that direct measurement of pulmonary vascular pressure is a much more reliable index of left ventricular function than measurement of right atrial pressure.

What is the appropriate use of central venous pressure measurement in the management of the acutely ill patient? Both authors agree that the measurement may have value in acutely ill patients with circulatory failure if evaluated in the context of the total clinical picture. A low central venous pressure which fails to increase with administration of small amounts of fluid strongly suggests hypovolemia and the need for adequate fluid replacement. On the other hand, if measurement of central vascular pressure is to be used to avoid pulmonary edema resulting from administration of excessive amounts of fluid, then the measurement of pulmonary vascular pressure with a flotation catheter has much merit.

I do not believe either author intended to leave the impression that the use of the flotation catheter and measurement of pulmonary vascular pressure was necessary for routine monitoring of intravenous fluid administration. Usually the amount of fluid necessary can be estimated from the fluid losses and daily requirements. In difficult and complicated problems, the measurement may be exceedingly helpful and justify the small risk inherent in any invasive procedure.

RICHARD V. EBERT

8

Prevention of Atherosclerosis

Sugar and Coronary Disease
   by John Yudkin

Prevention of Atherosclerosis by Dietary Control of Hyperlipidemia
   by William Dock

A Fat Controlled Diet for All
   by Haqvin Malmros

Control of Hyperlipidemia by Surgery
   by Henry Buchwald and Richard L. Varco

A Skeptical View of a National Diet Program
   by Norton Spritz

Comment
   by Donald S. Fredrickson

Sugar and Coronary Disease

JOHN YUDKIN

University of London

Many important discoveries have sprung from observations made by scientists who at the time did not appreciate their potential significance. We nevertheless recognize the merit of these early workers, and justifiably we praise them. As only one example, we recall that the revolution in many spheres of science that was marked by the introduction of modern chromatographic techniques is rarely mentioned without a tribute to Tswett's discoveries at the turn of this century.[1]

It is right that we should praise the pioneers who did not foresee the important avenues of discovery that were opened up by their work. I sometimes wonder then whether it would not be a logical corollary of this that we should blame those pioneers who did not foresee the byways and diversions and blind alleys that were opened up by *their* work. If we did this, we should especially have to censure Liebermann and Burchard, who, 80 or so years ago, were responsible for devising and improving the methods by which we can now so readily assay the levels of cholesterol in blood plasma.[2,3]

The Cholesterol Obsession

The existence of these methods has resulted in a vast literature concerned with the possible role of this substance in the pathogenesis of coronary heart disease (CHD). It has resulted in a state of mind, not only in hundreds of scientific workers but in millions of lay persons, that assumes a direct and causative relationship between the level of cholesterol and the risk of developing CHD. Any agent that causes a rise in this level is at once assumed to increase the chances of developing the disease; any agent that causes a reduction in cholesterol level is assumed to decrease the chances of developing the disease. The result has been a diversion of huge resources in time and people and money from other and more plausible areas of research, so that, after nearly 20 years of intensive chasing of this chimera, we still have no real understanding of what causes CHD, nor of the way the disease develops. There is much to be said for the view of Dr. M. D.

Altschule that the level of cholesterol is a biochemical measurement in search of clinical significance.[4]

These remarks should not be taken to imply that I believe that the cholesterol content of the blood will ultimately be shown to have nothing whatever to do with the disease process. But what I do believe is that we do not yet know for certain whether this substance in any way itself determines the disease process, and if so to what extent. Secondly, I believe that our obsession with cholesterol levels has made many of us forget that CHD is a disease of considerable complexity, and that an abnormality in cholesterol level is only one of the large number of disturbances that we find in the disease. I might even say that we are wrong to look for a biochemical cause for CHD; it is much more likely to have a hormonal cause. I hope to justify this somewhat oversimplified statement later in this paper.

I begin by stating precisely what I do believe in relation to the role of dietary sugar (sucrose) in the etiology of CHD. This is necessary, not because I have hitherto failed to express my views, but because these are so often misrepresented. First, I believe that the causes of coronary disease are many. There is the genetic factor; there are also the environmental factors. These include stress, cigarette smoking, lack of physical activity, overeating in general, and the consumption of high levels of sugar. I do not believe we can entirely separate these factors; Dr. Meyer Friedman's Types A and B may owe their different proneness to the disease both to a genetic factor that may largely determine their personality, and to the environmental factor that produces the stressful situation to which their personality reacts.

Secondly, I am speaking not of carbohydrate in general, nor of any sort of monosaccharide or disaccharide usually listed under the heading of simple sugars; I am speaking specifically of sucrose. About 50 per cent of the calories taken in the diets of people in the Western countries comes from carbohydrate. The relative contribution of the different types of carbohydrate is something like 50 per cent from starch; 40 per cent from sucrose from the sugar cane or sugar beet; 5 per cent from lactose, and 5 per cent from other sugars, mostly glucose, fructose, and sucrose from fruits and vegetables.[5]

My hypothesis then is that one of the etiologic agents in CHD is sucrose, which contributes nearly 20 per cent to the average dietary calories in countries like the United States and the United Kingdom.

The evidence for this hypothesis is of varying significance and comes from various sources; it is the sum of the evidence from these sources that in my view now makes it impossible to dismiss the hypothesis as being less plausible than that for any other of the suggested causative agents of CHD.

Sucrose—A New Food

As a nutritionist I have always felt that we would do well to look to the sorts of diets consumed by early man and his immediate ancestors if we wish to have some idea of the food to which we have, as a species, became adapted during the course of evolution. Just as we are likely best to preserve the health of wild animals in our zoological gardens by feeding them their "natural" diets, so we would do best ourselves if we adhered as much as we could to the sorts of foods we ate when we too were wild. It is less than 10,000 years since men began to become food producers, and this enormously changed the food eaten. Before that time, and for at least some millions of years, meat contributed largely to men's diets, and they ate not only the flesh but all the fat they could get, including that from bones that were cracked open in order to get at the fatty marrow.[6] For this reason, I find it difficult to suppose that animal fat has much to do with coronary disease.

Compared with animal fat, the inclusion of sugar from the cane and later from the beet (together technically called centrifugal sugar) is a very recent introduction indeed. We in Britain were among the earliest people to have it in any quantity because of our involvement in the slave trade between West Africa and the Caribbean. Our consumption at the beginning of the eighteenth century was something like four pounds per person per year; it is now about 120 pounds.[7] Increasingly we take it in manufactured foods like ice cream and soft drinks. There thus seems to be a changing pattern of consumption. Children take more and more, while older people, worried chiefly about their expanding waist lines, take less and less. It is widely believed that environmental factors play a more important part in causing CHD when they act during childhood than when they act in later life. If this is so, the constant average intake of sugar in the United States during the past 30 or 40 years would still be consistent with an increasing effect in heart disease if this constancy were hiding an increase in younger persons.

If sugar consumption is a cause of coronary disease we should find a relationship between the amount consumed and the prevalence of the disease. This can be examined in several ways. One way is to look at the increase of prevalence in a given population in relation to an increase in the consumption of sugar, as I have just indicated. A second way is to look at the relative prevalence in different populations in relation to their consumption. Thirdly, we can look at the consumption of sugar within one population, comparing those who develop the disease with those who do not develop the disease. In general, we may say that these three lines of epidemiological evidence—from historical studies, interpopulation studies, and intrapopulation studies—show a positive relationship between sugar consumption and coronary disease.[8]

We must not, however, expect too close a relationship for a number of reasons. First, average consumption tells us nothing about the distribution of consumption within a population. As we saw, a constant average can conceal a changing pattern of consumption, with children taking more and adults taking less. Again, a high average can derive equally well from a few individuals with a very high consumption and a majority with a low consumption, or a large number with a moderate consumption and a fair number with a low consumption. If we assume that there is a threshold level below which the disease is not produced, then the country in the first example will have fewer cases than that in the second example, even though they have the same average consumption. Second, while it is not difficult to get reliable information about average sugar consumption in most countries, information about coronary deaths is of very varying reliability, both because of the varying sophistication of the medical services, and because of the varying criteria of diagnosis and methods of recording causes of death. Third, if as is likely the disease takes many years to develop, we need to know the consumption of sugar over a long period; this is much more difficult to ascertain than it is to ascertain the consumption at a given time. Fourth, and most importantly, we cannot predict coronary proneness from sugar consumption unless we are sure that we know what are the other causative factors, the size of these factors, and the importance of each of them in relation to the others.

The Limitation of Epidemiology

The best we can expect from epidemiologic studies is an indication of the factors that are involved: a clue as to hypothesis so that we know the direction in which our further research should proceed. And of course we must inject a little common sense into the interpretation of the results of our epidemiologic studies. The historical rise in the prevalence of CHD in many Western countries in the last 50 years or so runs parallel not only with an increase in dietary sugar but also with the number of people who have radios or motor cars.[9] It is unlikely that the chances of developing coronary disease are increased simply because one possesses a radio; it is, however, likely that they are increased if one possesses a motor car, since this implies that one will be physically less active, and most workers believe that there is a relationship between sedentariness and proneness to coronary disease.

A too complete reliance on epidemiologic evidence can lead to an obsessional attachment to a hypothesis and to an irrational response to any alternative suggestion; read, for example, an article published in 1971 by Dr. Ancel Keys.[10] His adherence to the theory that saturated fat is a dominant factor in atherogenesis and coronary heart disease derives from his early observation that in six countries there was a relationship between fat intake and coronary mortality. I have pointed out that, if we took *all* the published information, relating to 15 countries, there was a better relationship with sugar.[9] I am now told that this does nothing to support the sugar hypothesis, for Finland's sugar consumption was lower than that of Sweden, although its coronary mortality was higher; no mention is made by Dr. Keys that the same is true for animal fat.

Here is one more example, again from the article by Dr. Keys, of the absurd position in which one can find oneself by leaning too heavily on epidemiologic evidence for the support of an entrenched hypothesis. As long ago as 1964 I showed that the average sugar consumption of populations was closely related to their average fat consumption.[11] Clearly then from this alone one can say either that fat in the diet is a cause of heart disease with sugar related coincidentally, or conversely that sugar is a cause with fat related coincidentally. One needed other sorts of evidence, I pointed out, in order to distinguish beween these two hypotheses. But now Dr. Keys draws attention to some recent work that he and his colleagues have completed, in which they have discovered (more correctly, rediscovered) the relationship between fat and sucrose in several countries. This, we are told, *demonstrates* that it is fat that is involved in the etiology of coronary disease; any relationship between the disease and sugar must be purely coincidental, it is said, and derives simply from the association between sugar consumption and fat consumption.

In one of our early studies we found that persons suffering from their first known coronary attack had been eating substantially more sugar than had control subjects without the disease.[12] We confirmed this a year or two later in a second study; on both occasions we pointed to the importance of ensuring both that the coronary subjects were examined immediately after their first known attack, and that the control subjects were well matched with those having the disease.[13] Several other studies have since been published, and many of them do not confirm our findings. The reasons for this are very clear; they have not heeded our insistence on the care with which both coronary subjects and control subjects must be chosen.

Even better than the retrospective studies such as those I have just mentioned would be prospective studies. Only one study has been reported concerning sucrose consumption and subsequent development of manifest coronary disease;[14] in this a relationship was found between sugar intake and disease. On the other hand, there was no relationship found, in this or in any other study, between fat intake and the development of the disease. It is sometimes said that if there is a relationship between sugar intake and coronary disease, it is coincidental because of the relationship between sugar intake and smoking. If this were so, it is even more interesting that fat intake is not related to the disease, since this too is related to smoking.[15] All in all, the evidence points rather better to an association of CHD with sugar consumption than with fat consumption.

At this point let me repeat that epidemiologic evidence alone cannot be expected to give us more than a clue as to etiology. We must now look for other evidence. One field in which we can look is in the field of experiment. Manipulation of the diet, or of any other environmental circumstance, can be designed either to induce the condition that we are studying, or to prevent it, or to cure it once it has occurred.

Prevention of the disease has been studied by changing the diet in apparently healthy individuals to see whether this reduces the chances that they develop CHD. As for cure, the nearest that investigators have come to studying this is in attempting to reduce the risk of recurrence in subjects who have already had, and obviously have survived, one or more attacks of myocardial infarction. Both of these approaches, usually called primary prevention and secondary prevention, have most commonly studied the effects of manipulation of dietary fat, in which the content of saturated fat in the diet has been reduced and that of polyunsaturated fat increased. I do not propose to join the interminable discussion as to the interpretation of the results obtained so far in preventive trials, except to make three brief points. One is that in at least two of the trials often quoted as demonstrating the benefits of changing the dietary fat, there was also a difference in dietary sucrose between the experimental group and the control group.[16, 17] The second point is that a far larger number of subjects than has been used so far is needed in order to establish unequivocally that a reduced risk of new or renewed CHD follows dietary change.[18] Third, if a large increase in dietary polyunsaturated fat really does reduce the risk of developing CHD, and does so without producing any ill-effects—neither of which has been demonstrated—it would not necessarily prove that deficiency of polyunsaturated fat caused the disease. Bacterial endocarditis may be cured by penicillin, but it is not caused by deficiency of penicillin.

In regard to the production of the disease, it is clearly out of the question that we attempt to do this in man; a further restraint in our research is that the condition as we know it in man cannot be induced in the experimental animals that we usually use in our laboratory. We are thus virtually restricted, in both man and animals, to attempt to induce changes that are associated with the human disease rather than the disease itself.

Experiments with Sucrose

Here let me summarize some of the effects that are produced by sucrose in conditions in which two diets are compared that are as similar as possible except that one contains starch as the sole or major carbohydrate and the other, sucrose.

In rats sucrose has been found always to induce an increase in plasma triglycerides, and sometimes an increase in cholesterol.[19] There is a very rapid and considerable increase in lipogenic enzymes in the liver, and a decrease in the enzyme activities in adipose tissue.[20] There is a reduction in glucose tolerance and in plasma insulin level, an increase in liver and kidney weight, and an increase—sometimes a considerable increase—in liver fat. The enlargement of the liver is accompanied by hyperplasia as well as by hypertrophy. It occurs in young animals within two or three weeks of the addition of sucrose to the diet and continues into adult life. Sucrose also causes an enlargement of the adrenal glands in young animals, but this does not continue; the effect of sucrose here appears to be to induce premature maturation of the adrenal glands.

Aortic atheroma has been reported in rats fed sucrose.[21] However, we have not been able to induce it in any of the three strains of rats that we have used by changing either the fat or the sucrose in the diet. Nevertheless, with dietary sucrose (although not with dietary fat) we have succeeded in increasing the level of cholesterol and triglyceride in the wall of the aorta.[22]

Sucrose caused an increase in the level of plasma triglycerides and of insulin in pigs. In cockerels it caused a rise chiefly in plasma cholesterol. In one strain it produced an accumulation of sudanophil material in the aorta; the area of the intima that was stained varied considerably and was proportional to the level of plasma cholesterol. In another strain of cockerels sucrose again produced variable changes in the aorta; in some animals there was obvious atheromatous deposit while in other animals the aortas appeared normal. None of the control cockerels, however, showed atheromatous lesions.

In young men, we have examined a number of parameters before and after the substitution of part of the starch in the diet by sucrose.[23] In all of our experiments, sucrose increased the level of plasma triglyceride; in some it has also increased the level of plasma cholesterol. About 30 per cent of our subjects showed a number of additional changes, including an increase in body weight and in platelet stickiness. In these subjects the platelets also showed a paradoxical response to ADP, in that their electrophoretic mobility was increased by a small concentration of added ADP, but not by a higher concentration.[24] The same subjects show an increase of some 50 to 100 per cent in plasma insulin, and of 300 to 400 per cent in 11-hydroxycorticosteroid.[25] We have suggested that it is only in those subjects that are susceptible to the atherogenic action of sucrose in whom sugar produces the increase in hormones and the associated changes that I have described.

Let us avoid at this point entering into a discussion of such still unsolved problems as the exact role that the stickiness or electrophoretic behavior of platelets plays in the pathogenesis of CHD. All that need concern us just now is that these abnormalities, together with reduced glucose tolerance, a rise in plasma lipids (more commonly in triglycerides than in cholesterol), a rise in plasma insulin, an enlargement of the liver, and of course atheroma, often if not always accompany CHD in man. All these changes can be seen when sucrose is included, or increased, in the diet of experimental animals or man.

We may now turn to a different sort of evidence concerning the etiology of CHD; this is a combination of epidemiologic and experimental evidence. There are several diseases that, in greater or lesser degree, are related to CHD. These include obesity, diabetes mellitus, duodenal ulceration, and perhaps gout. There is evidence, again of varying strengths, that dietary sucrose is involved in the production of each of these conditions. As regards obesity, animal experiment has demonstrated that sucrose increases lipogenesis.[26] As regards diabetes, dietary sucrose has been shown to diminish glucose tolerance both in man and in experimental animals.[27]

It is relevant here to refer to the recent work of A. M. Cohen of Jerusalem on the relationship between diet and genetics in the experimental production of diabetes. By separating rats according to the extent to which dietary sucrose reduces glucose tolerance, Cohen, Teitelbaum, and Saliternik[28] were able to breed a strain in which sucrose-fed animals developed blood glucose levels of 250 mg./100 ml. during an oral glucose tolerance test. When fed on sucrose-free diets, the blood glucose level reached the same level of 120 mg./100 ml. as had the parent strain. Two conditions were thus necessary in order to produce a considerable impairment of glucose tolerance: the rats had to have both the appropriate genetic predisposition and the appropriate dietary stimulus, sucrose.

Recently we have shown that the symptoms of patients with chronic dyspepsia due to duodenal ulcer or a variety of other causes are frequently improved by diets low in carbohydrate and especially in sucrose.[29] We have also given test meals to normal subjects before and after two weeks on diets high in sucrose and shown that they develop an increase in gastric acidity and especially in pepsin activity. Finally, CHD is associated with hyperuricemia, and experiments have shown that the level of blood uric acid is increased by fructose.

The Multiple Manifestations of Coronary Heart Disease

One possible explanation for these observations is that each is caused by several factors, of which one is a high intake of sucrose. We may say that factor A or B or sucrose can cause diabetes, and factor C or D or again sucrose may cause

CHD. Then, depending on their genetic makeup, persons with a high sugar intake might develop either diabetes or CHD, or they might show signs of neither, or of both diseases. Those subject to factor A, however, could develop diabetes but not CHD, and those subject to factor C could develop CHD but not diabetes. The result would be the sort of partial association between the two diseases that in fact exists.

The complex and manifold changes that are seen in CHD make it highly unlikely that it comes about by some simple biochemical perversion of fat metabolism that results in an increased level of cholesterol in the blood. A much more plausible hypothesis is that the primary disturbance is an alteration in the secretion of one or other hormone. There is much to be said, for example, for the view that the disease begins with an increase in the level of circulating insulin. The administration of insulin to the rat causes an increase in the content of cholesterol in the aortic wall.[30] Several of the conditions associated with CHD, such as cigarette smoking, maturity onset diabetes, obesity, and peripheral vascular disease, frequently exhibit a raised level of plasma insulin, as CHD itself often does. On the other hand, increased physical activity and the reduction of obesity, both of which are associated with a decreased risk of CHD, show a fall in the level of plasma insulin. Thus we might suppose that sucrose causes coronary disease in those subjects in which it produces elevation in plasma insulin.

After we observed that sucrose causes an even greater rise in corticosteroids than it does in insulin, and that in rats it leads to a premature development of the adrenal glands, I am now less insistent that the primary stage in atherogenesis and CHD is likely to be its effect on insulin. Since the body's hormones are known to interact in an elaborate and complex manner, it may well be that the changes observed in insulin level are secondary to changes in another hormone, and that this may perhaps be a corticosteroid.

At present, however, we are clearly aware of only a small part of the changes induced by sucrose, or by any other known or suspected agent in the sequence of events that leads to CHD in man. It would thus be profitless to pursue these ideas until we have much more information. But we shall be hampered in obtaining this information so long as we continue to confine our attention to lipid metabolism in general, or to plasma cholesterol levels in particular.

My purpose in writing this paper was twofold. First, it was to stress that CHD in man has many manifestations, and these can best be explained by an alteration in hormone activity. Secondly, it was to suggest that, apart from the strong evolutionary, historical, and epidemiologic evidence that dietary sucrose is one of the important factors causing the disease, we now have evidence that it profoundly affects at least two hormones of the body. I am convinced that it is by studying these sorts of effects that we shall best learn to understand and then to control the coronary epidemic.

References

1. Tswett, M.: Adsorptions Analyse und chromatographische Methode. Anwendung auf die Chemie des Chlorophylls. Ber. Deutsch. Bot. Ges. *24*:384, 1906.

2. Liebermann, C.: Über das Oxychinoterten. Ber. Deutsch Chem. Ges. *18*:1803, 1885.
3. Burchard, H.: Beiträge zur Kenntnis des Cholesterins. Chem. Zbl. *61*:I, 25, 1890.
4. Altschule, M. D.: Medical Counterpoint. January, 1970.
5. Yudkin, J.: Evolutionary and historical changes in dietary carbohydrates. Amer. J. Clin. Nutr. *20*:108, 1967.
6. Ardrey, R.: *African Genesis*. New York, Atheneum Press, 1961.
7. Yudkin, J.: *In* Yudkin, J., Edelman, J., and Hough, L. (eds.): *Sugar*. London, Butterworth & Co., Ltd., 1971.
8. Yudkin, J.: Why blame sugar? Chem. Ind. 1464, 1967.
9. Yudkin, J.: Diet and coronary thrombosis. Hypothesis and fact. Lancet *2*:155, 1957.
10. Keys, A.: Sucrose in the diet and coronary heart disease. Atherosclerosis *14*:193, 1971.
11. Yudkin, J.: Dietary fat and dietary sugar in relation to ischaemic heart disease and diabetes. Lancet *2*:4, 1964.
12. Yudkin, J., and Roddy, J.: Levels of dietary sucrose in patients with occlusive atherosclerotic disease. Lancet *2*:6, 1964.
13. Yudkin, J., and Morland, J.: Sugar intake and myocardial infarction. Amer. J. Clin. Nutr. *20*:503, 1967.
14. Paul, O., Lepper, M. H., Phelan, W. H., Dupertius, G. W., MacMillan, A., McKean, H., and Park, H.: A longitudinal study of coronary heart disease. Circulation *28*:20, 1963.
15. Bronte-Stewart, B.: Cigarette smoking and ischaemic heart disease. Brit. Med. J. *1*:379, 1961.
16. Rinzler, S. H.: Primary prevention of coronary heart disease. Bull. N.Y. Acad. Med. *44*:936, 1968.
17. Turpeinen, O., Miettinen, M., Karvonen, M. J., Roine, P., Pekkarinen, M., Lehtosuo, E. J., and Alivirta, P.: Dietary prevention of coronary heart disease. Long term experiment. Amer. J. Clin. Nutr. *21*:255, 1968.
18. American Heart Association. Monograph 18, 1969.
19. Qureshi, R. U., Akinyanju, P. A., and Yudkin, J.: The effect of an "atherogenic" diet containing starch or sucrose upon carcass composition and plasma lipids in the rat. Nutr. Metab. *12*:347, 1970.
20. Bruckdorfer, K. R., Khan, I. H., and Yudkin, J.: Dietary carbohydrate and fatty acid synthetase activity in rat liver and adipose tissue. Biochem. J. *123*:7P, 1971.
21. Chevillard, L., Portet, R., Combescot, Ch. and Senault-Bournique, S.: Effets physiopathologiques des sucres et des lipides du régime chez les rats adaptés à 5° ou 30° C. (Communication non publiée au Symposium du groupe Lipides-Nutrition, 1968.) (Quoted by Tremolières, J., and Lavau, M.: Cah. Nutr. Diet. *4*:83, 1969.)
22. Bruckdorfer, K. R., Khan, I. H., and Yudkin, J.: The lipid content of the aortas of rats fed sucrose. Proc. Nutr. Soc. *31*:9A, 1972.
23. Szanto, S., and Yudkin, J.: The effect of dietary sucrose on blood lipids, serum insulin, platelet adhesiveness and body weight in human volunteers. Postgrad. Med. J. *45*:602, 1969.
24. Szanto, S., and Yudkin, J.: Dietary sucrose and platelet behaviour. Nature (London) *225*:467, 1970.
25. Yudkin, J., and Szanto, S.: Hyperinsulinism and atherogenesis. Brit. Med. J. *1*:349, 1971.
26. Bruckdorfer, K. R., Kari-Kari, B. P. B., Khan, I. H., and Yudkin, J.: Activity of lipogenic enzymes and plasma triglyceride levels in the rat and the chicken as determined by the nature of the dietary fat and dietary carbohydrate. Nutr. Metab. *14*:228, 1972.
27. Cohen, A. M., Teitelbaum, E., Balogh, M., and Groen, J. J.: Effect of interchanging bread and sucrose as main source of carbohydrate in a low fat diet on the glucose tolerance curve of health volunteer subjects. Amer. J. Clin. Nutr. *19*:59, 1966.
28. Cohen, A. M., Teitelbaum, E., and Saliternik, R.: Genetics and diet as factors in development of diabetes mellitus. Metabolism *21*:235, 1972.
29. Yudkin, J., Evans, E., and Smith, M.G.M.: The low-carbohydrate diet in the treatment of chronic dyspepsia. Proc. Nutr. Soc. *31*:12A, 1972.
30. Stout, R. W.: Insulin stimulated lipogenesis in arterial tissue in relation to diabetes and atheroma. Lancet *2*:702, 1968.

Prevention of Atherosclerosis by Dietary Control of Hyperlipidemia

WILLIAM DOCK

Veterans Administration Hospital, New York

Genesis of Atheromas: Infiltration of Plasma Proved to Cause Atheromas and Xanthomas in Man

Many physicians and their patients would probably agree that the diet on which they grew up is ideal and should never be changed. This is why physicians sometimes seem to seek to escape the conclusion that our leading cause of death, obstructive vascular disease, is the result of diets which keep our plasma lipids at levels far higher than those of many other populations whose incidence of gallstones and atherosclerosis is almost nil, and whose serum cholesterol rarely rises above 170 mg. per 100 ml. and often averages under 150. Seventy-five years ago William Osler discussed the importance of food, drink, tobacco, and personal and occupational stresses as factors contributing to "angeiosclerosis."[1] More recently softness of drinking water, autoimmune reactions, arterial hypertension, and lack of exercise have been added to the list. Mural thrombosis,[2] intimal synthesis due to impaired mitochondrial respiration,[3] and intimal infiltration of lipids from plasma abnormally rich in lipoproteins have been suggested as the mechanisms causing atheromas. There is valid statistical support for all the suggested factors except intimal synthesis, and there are innumerable experiments on animals and birds in support of the intimal infiltration theory.

The opponents of the infiltrative hypothesis reject the experimental evidence because different species vary greatly in the effects of diet on their plasma lipids and their arteries. Many species show little or no arterial disease after being fed diets rich in cholesterol or in saturated fats. Similar objections were raised to the theory of a dietary origin of scurvy, which could only be evoked in guinea pigs, and to the dietary origin of beriberi, supported only by experiments on pigeons. The opponents of the lipid infiltration theory fail to note that men with Fredrickson's Type II hyperlipidemia[4] are almost as sensitive to ingestion of cholesterol as were Anitschkow's rabbits, or that men with Type V hyperlipidemia are almost as sensitive to saturated fats as were Bragdon's squirrels.[5] Families of men vary as much as species of animals in the effects of diet on their plasma lipids and the incidence of atherosclerosis.

Before 1970 all the statistical and experimental evidence favoring any theory of atherogenesis could be dismissed as "purely circumstantial," but by 1972 three studies published in the Journal of Clinical Investigation had provided direct evidence of lipid infiltration of men's arterial walls when plasma lipids were high,[6] and of the regression of atheromas when very high plasma lipid levels were reduced to those found in populations free of gallstones and obstructive vascular disease.[7] This new evidence proved that atheromas are intimal xanthomas, and that all we have learned about atherogenesis in animals is relevant to the human condition.

In one study[6] the electron microscope played the same role as the light microscope had played in revealing the causes of malaria, anthrax, tuberculosis, and puerperal sepsis. Biopsies of the xanthomas erupting in the skin of untreated diabetics were compared with biopsies of lesions, initially identical, as they rapidly regressed after low fat diets had cleared the patients' plasmas of chylomicrons. In a typical case, plasma lipid fell from 5000 mg. per 100 ml. to 700, and cholesterol from 1250 mg. to 240.[6] Biopsies of the erupting xanthomas showed innumerable droplets in the basal lamina of arterioles and in the perivascular spaces. The droplets were identical, under the electron microscope, with the chylomicrons in similar preparations of the patients' milky plasma. Pericytes adjacent to endothelial cells and macrophages near the blood vessels were filled with these droplets. Biopsies taken 10 to 20 days after the plasma cleared showed no droplets in the basal lamina or the pericytes, and only a few in perivascular spaces and in the macrophages, which were shrunken and had scalloped, infolded borders and contained vacuoles filled with cholesteryl esters.

On fractional lipid analysis the initial biopsies showed a high content of triglyceride, with the ratios of cholesteryl esters and phospholipid much like those of the chylomicrons. As the lesions regressed triglyceride content fell while the ratio of cholesteryl esters rose.[6] After a few weeks the lipid analyses of regressing lesions approached the values found in the fatty streaks of early aortic atherosclerosis.[8] The electron microscopic appearance of initial biopsies is similar to that seen in arteries of suckling rats;[9] in later biopsies the lesions resemble the structures seen in early atheromas.[10] The conventional fat-stained sections of the xanthomas resembled those made from aortas of suckling rabbits[11] and from human sucklings.[12] The "cholesterolosis" seen in the arteries of all suckling mammals, the early lesions of human or experimental atherosclerosis, and the erupting xanthomas are morphologically and chemically identical. They all appear to be due to infiltration by macromolecules and chylomicrons from hyperlipemic plasma. The studies of xanthomas show how rapidly the triglycerides can be broken down and eliminated. Cholesteryl esters of saturated fatty acids are more refractory than those of the unsaturated variety and form 95 per cent of the lipid material separated from atheromas by homogenization and centrifugation.[13]

The identity of xanthomas and atheromas, as infiltrates from the plasma, was demonstrated in a series of hyperlipemic patients given a single intravenous dose of isotope-tagged cholesterol.[13a] For 50 to 70 weeks the decay of specific activity of serum cholesterol was followed, and during the study specific activity of cholesterol in xanthomas removed by biopsy was measured. Serum activity fell exponentially, while xanthoma activity increased, exceeding serum levels after eight to 30 weeks and then falling very slowly. In a patient who died 53 weeks after isotope injection, the content of isotope-tagged cholesterol, per gram, was 30 times greater in xanthomas, and 10 times greater in atheromas, than in the liver or any other tissue of the body, including the uninvolved aortic wall. In apparently normal aortic wall, specific activity of cholesterol was as high as in the atheromas, but cholesterol content was only one tenth as high. In the brain, cholesterol content was six times that of normal aortic wall, but specific activity only 6 per cent as high. This study confirms the infiltrative origin of atheromas and xanthomas in quantitative terms.

The cholesterolosis of sucklings and the atheromas of experimental origin in animals regress, like the xanthomas, when plasma lipids fall on weaning or on removal from the atherogenic diet. Atheromas also regress in men with wasting diseases,[14] but relatively rapid regression of severe arterial narrowing in an individual had not been demonstrated before studies were made on patients with Type III hyperlipidemia. These patients have eruptive xanthomas which regress on a regimen of diet and drugs. Zelis and his colleagues at the National Institutes of Health have shown that the regimen which lowers the plasma lipids and clears xanthomas also markedly improves the flow of blood to limbs threatened by obstructing atheromas.[7] In six patients, a proper diet and 2 gm. of chlorphenylisoxybutyrate per day lowered mean serum cholesterol from 380 to 180 mg. per 100 ml., triglyceride from 540 mg. to 110. After four months on this regimen the maximal blood flow to the legs, after five minutes of total ischemia, rose from 20 ml. per 100 ml. of leg tissue before treatment to 32 ml., while there was no rise, in comparable periods of time, in the reactive flow rates of 29 untreated hyperlipemic patients. The initial flow rates in the treated group were lower than in any control subjects of the same age, but they rose into the normal range in five of the six within the four-month period of study.[7] It seems reasonable to conclude from this meticulously conducted study that the atheromas which had narrowed the arteries to the legs had regressed just like the xanthomas. This permitted a 60 per cent increase in the maximal blood flow during reactive hyperemia.

This direct evidence of the relation of high plasma lipid to lipid infiltration of arterial walls does not prove that the rate of atherogenesis may not also be accelerated by the many factors obvious to physicians for nearly a century. These factors can act by raising plasma lipids or arterial pressure. Local factors explain how infiltration can cause severe coronary lesions with minimal disease elsewhere, or severe disease of the distal aorta as compared with that in the ascending part.[15] Of these aggravating factors, the most significant is the level of intravascular pressure.

Atheromas never occur in veins, nor in the pulmonary arteries of those dying with severe aortic and coronary lesions but no evidence of pulmonic arterial hypertension. Pulmonary atheromas are observed in some patients with mitral stenosis or other conditions raising pressure in the pulmonary arteries above 50 mm. Hg. This seems to be the critical pressure at which lipid infiltration can lead to visible lesions. In man, and in experimental studies of animals, hypertension accelerates atherogenesis at any level of hyperlipemia. The observations on localization are incompatible with the view that atherogenesis is initiated by mural thrombosis. The veins are the favorite site for mural thrombosis but never have atheromas. The pulmonary arteries have emboli attached to their intima far more often than do the systemic arteries, yet are relatively free of atheromas. There is, however, abundant evidence that hyperlipidemia does retard fibrinolysis and that coronary disease and thromboembolic disease show parallel trends in populations, fall together during periods of low fat, low calorie diet, and rise together when the usual diet is resumed. Thrombosis in atherosclerotic arteries frequently completes the obstruction which causes the clinical evidence of vascular disease. But the chylomicronemia which accelerates thrombosis in veins or in damaged arteries is eliminated, together with atherogenesis, by diets which keep the serum cholesterol plus triglyceride below 300 mg. per 100 ml.

The preferred sites of atheroma formation do not fit the recent theory that excessive local synthesis of cholesterol, due to impaired respiration of intimal cells, causes these lesions.[3] Abundant in systemic arteries, where the oxygen tension is the highest in the body, atheromas are absent in the veins and in pulmonary arteries where intimal cells are constantly exposed to hypoxia. The experiments cited in support of the hypothesis of local synthesis[16,17] do fit the infiltrative theory. Rabbits exposed to hypoxia or carbon monoxide while on cholesterol feeding have plasma cholesterol levels 20 to 30 per cent higher than controls on the same diet,[16,17] and this could account for their more severe atherosclerosis. Rabbits on normal diets have no rise in plasma cholesterol, no atherogenesis, when exposed to hypoxia. It would be most unfortunate if physicians accepted the existence of the hypothesis about mural thrombosis or the local synthesis by mitochondria as justification for ignoring the evidence that atherosclerosis is a reversible form of lipid infiltration, and diet is a critical factor in causation.

The levels of chylomicronemia are very high, and the rates of deposition of lipids in the skin and in the intima can be very fast in uncontrolled diabetics and in Type III hyperlipoproteinemia. The lesions formed as a result are succulent and hyperemic. There is little fibrosis, but a high content of easily disposable triglyceride. As in sucklings on weaning, such patients can have rapid regression of their lesions when plasma lipids are reduced to normal. In the slowly developing and fibrotic atheromas of most adults regression undoubtedly is slow, with scars and calcium deposits remaining after all lipid has been resorbed.[14] But even slow regression permits a collateral circulation to develop, with remission of symptoms. It also reduces the risk of more marked obstruction which might cause massive necrosis in legs, brain, or the heart if such lesions had progressed.

The observations on xanthomas of diabetics suggest that only chylomicrons or the macromolecules of beta lipoprotein are trapped in the tissues after filtering through the arterial endothelium, while the alpha lipoprotein molecules move more rapidly, with albumin and gamma globulins, into the lymph and venules. Plasma lipids show a continuous spectrum of particle sizes, from chylomicrons (0.5 to 0.08 μ in diameter) through pre-beta (0.08 to 0.03 μ), beta (0.02 μ), and down to alpha lipoproteins which are ovoid and 0.03 by 0.005 μ.[4] The concentration of cholesterol rises, that of triglyceride falls, as one moves from chylomicrons to beta lipoproteins.[4] In patients with Type II hyperlipidemia and in rabbits fed cholesterol, triglyceride levels remain low and the plasma free of chylomicrons. Rabbits develop atheromas in weeks, and Type II patients have precocious coronary occlusion. This suggests that while chylomicrons are important in causing cholesterolosis of sucklings and the eruptive xanthomas of adults, the beta lipoprotein molecules, smaller and much richer in cholesterol, are the most effective agents in causing atheromas and the xanthelasmas of the eyelids.

The process of deposition and transformation of lipids in arterial walls begins in all mammals when they are being nourished on maternal milk. They all show cholesterolosis of the arterial walls from the first weeks of life until after being weaned.[9, 11, 12] A diet rich in fat, cholesterol, and phospholipids is essential for rapidly growing vertebrates and is provided in the egg yolk of birds, reptiles, amphibia, and fishes. In hens' eggs the ratio of cholesterol to protein is 10 times as high as in cow's milk; in egg yolk it is 30 times as high. Apparently the need for exogenous cholesterol falls during growth from very high levels in the embryo to zero in the hatched or weaned creatures. The milk diet of the suckling is like that of the nomad herdsmen, but the caloric needs of a 4-kg. infant are two and a half times as great, per kg. per hour, as those of a 70-kg. adult. This can only be met by an intake which gives suckling mammals milky plasma with a relatively low cholesterol content. The active response of the pericytes and macrophages prevents formation of atheromas as the result of the intimal infiltration evident histologically, and leads to disappearance of this lipid after weaning. Some species of animals and most men cannot maintain low plasma lipid when they are on diets rich in calories, cholesterol, or saturated fats. Alcohol, per gram, is a more potent cause of hyperlipidemia than saturated fat or sucrose.[18] When the rate of intimal infiltration exceeds the capacity of foam cells to eliminate cholesteryl esters, grossly visible lesions appear and may lead to obstruction. The demonstration that these lesions undergo resolution when plasma lipids return to normal levels is the most encouraging finding in the recent clinical investigations.

Relative Importance of Cholesterol, Saturated Fats, and Carbohydrates in Raising Plasma Lipids

An exaggeration of the importance of dietary cholesterol in atherogenesis was an unfortunate consequence of the use of rabbits in the pioneer experiments. Squirrels, like men, are omnivorous and do not develop atherosclerosis when cholesterol is added to their food, but they do have a rise in plasma lipids and develop atheromas when their diets are supplemented with peanuts, free of cholesterol but rich in starch and saturated fat.[5] Saturated fat, carbohydrate, and alcohol in the diets of men play a much larger role than cholesterol in raising plasma lipid and cholesterol levels.[19, 20] This has been made strikingly evident in studies of pastoral African tribes. These people maintain blood cholesterol levels of 135 to 180 mg. per ml. while living exclusively on milk.[21-24] Each of them ingests about half a gram of cholesterol daily, the equivalent of that in two eggs. They have a low carbohydrate intake (15 per cent of total calories) and a high intake of protein. They also may have relatively high intakes of polyunsaturated fatty acids, since the free-living African herbivores, eating leaves as well as grass, have up to 30 per cent of their fat in polyunsaturated forms, while giraffes, browsing only on leaves, have 40 per cent. In hay-fed giraffes this falls to 2 per cent, as in our cattle and their milk.[25] Leaves of shrubs and trees are rich in polyunsaturated fats and these provide much of the food of the nomadic herds.[24] In most types of hyperlipidemia, plasma cholesterol falls when polyunsaturated fatty acids replace saturated fats in the diet.[26] Thus, it is probable that the milk-drinking pastoral nomads have an almost ideal diet.

The Masai also maintain, as adults, a relatively high level of suppression of endogenous synthesis of cholesterol when cholesterol is added to their diet.[23] This could be a genetic trait in tribes which were carnivorous for thousands of years before they became herdsmen. They never had the low cholesterol, high carbohydrate diets of farmers living on cereal and beans. Such diets may sensitize to cholesterol feeding. But all infants have low plasma cholesterol levels, the mean rising from 80 mg. per 100 ml. at birth to 140 to 180 mg. at the time suckling ends. Thus, it is possible that suppression of cholesterol synthesis when on milk diets, like the production of enteric lactase, is gradually lost when babes are weaned onto diets low in cholesterol, but persists, like lactase production, if they merely change from mother's milk to animal milk as main source of calories. The milk-drinking tribes continue, as adults, to absorb lactose[27, 28] and to suppress endogenous synthesis of cholesterol.

When a normal man suddenly increases his carbohydrate intake from 1 gm. per kg. of body weight per day to 7 gm., his serum triglyceride level rises within five to eight days to a peak of 250 to 400 mg. per 100 ml. above the control level, and then falls somewhat over the next few weeks. Those whose levels rise to more than 400 mg. are said to have carbohydrate-induced hyperlipidemia.[20] Although serum cholesterol rises slightly with the triglycerides when we are on carbohydrate-rich diets, this is minimal as long as there is a low cholesterol intake and an adequate supply of the essential (polyunsaturated) fatty acids. This is the usual dietary pattern in populations living on rice and soybean oil, or on maize and beans. Most of these people do hard physical work, while the victims of atherosclerosis are relatively sedentary and, hence, need to exercise more and restrict their caloric intake to achieve normal levels of plasma lipids.

In our population there are a few people with metabolic machinery capable of holding plasma lipids at relatively safe levels in spite of an excessive intake of carbohydrates and saturated fats. There are many of all races who develop aortic atheromas but only minimal coronary narrowing when on rich diets for a few years. Those who are overweight and have serum cholesterol levels over 200 mg. per 100 ml. vary in sensitivity to diets rich in carbohydrates or saturated fats, but most of them will have atherosclerosis before they are 30. Diabetics run the greatest risk of obstructive vascular disease, both in their arteries and arterioles, when they consume the average United States diet. Diabetics in other lands do not develop any of these lesions when they live on diets poor in cholesterol and saturated fat but relatively rich in essential (polyunsaturated) fatty acids.[29] It is wrong to place the blame for atherogenesis mainly on the carbohydrate intake, just as it was to make cholesterol in the diet the most deadly factor. Moderation and balance are the key elements in making up a safe and appetizing diet.

The Management of Patients—Diet and Drugs

There can be no improvement in the prognosis of patients with evident or latent vascular disease until physicians accept the authoritative evidence, from the study of man, that hyperlipidemia is the critical factor in initiating and sustaining atherogenesis and that no aggravating factor can produce these lesions in human beings who have a plasma cholesterol plus triglyceride constantly under 300 mg. per 100 ml. The physician must also realize that plasma lipids can be reduced to a safe level in most people by diet alone—and by diets as varied as those of Eskimos living solely on seafood, Asiatic peasants living mainly on vegetables, and Africans or Arabs living mainly on milk.

Drugs may be essential to manage those cases of endogenous hyperlipidemia with levels of cholesterol over 180 mg. per 100 ml. and triglyceride over 120 mg. in spite of several months of optimal dietary control. These drugs—nicotinic acid, dextrothyroxine, clofibrate, or cholestyramine—may be the physician's main weapons in dealing with those who cannot or will not modify their diets.

No patient should be considered properly managed merely because his cholesterol comes down to 220 mg. per 100 ml. and his xanthomas melt away, for atheromas can continue to grow slowly at even lower levels. Eruptive xanthomas rarely appear until serum cholesterol is over 400 mg. and triglyceride over 500 mg. Unfortunately physicians and their patients soon realize that all the effective drugs either are unpleasant to take or have unpleasant side effects in the dosage necessary to control hyperlipidemia without the proper diet. Such a diet may provide 40 per cent of the needed calories from carbohydrate, even in the most "carbohydrate sensitive" subjects, or may be too rich in fat at 20 per cent of calories from corn oil in patients deficient in lipoprotein lipase (Type I). Just as an antibiotic effective for one infection is often useless for another, the diet and drug combination effective in one type of hyperlipidemia may be useless or harmful in another type. Management which controls a patient in the hospital may be a failure when he returns home and resumes his usual intake of four ounces of whiskey a day.[19]

Men who reject proper dietary control may be reminded that before the sixteenth century the greatest minds and the greatest warriors were content with diets very similar to the ones we recommend today. These admired and powerful men knew nothing of potatoes, sugar, or drinks stronger than wine or beer. Today, faced with every type of atherogenic temptation, what the patient needs most is the philosophy General Eisenhower expressed after he had followed doctors' orders to stop smoking: "It's not bad as long as you don't get sorry for yourself." This philosophy, and the dietary advice appropriate for each patient, cannot be imparted effectively by obese and flabby physicians, eager to prove that diet and smoking are not important in the causation of arterial obstruction.

Reduction in the vascular death rate depends on re-education of both physicians and the public. The experience with bronchogenic cancer and cigarette smoking shows how difficult it is to implement such a program of re-education. People suffer if they have to change their diets—they may starve rather than switch from rice to wheat, or wheat to rice. The obese hypertensive patients will seek out reassuring physicians to tell them they do not need to cut down on salt, or alcohol, or calories.

There are patients, including some very fine physicians, who accept the facts of atherogenesis and the necessity for dietary control but see no reason to do without the foods they enjoy merely in expectation of doing without them for a longer time. They prefer, like Stevenson, "to go rushing full-bodied over the precipice rather than dwindle away in sandy deltas." However, there is a large population of patients with dependents, or with devoted spouses, for whom optimal control of atherosclerosis is a social obligation which they are not tempted to evade. There are also many people who take pride in keeping fit as they age. The physician must learn how to guide all these patients, or rather how best to guide each patient, depending on the type of lipid disturbance, the customary diet and way of life, and the personal and family problems which may arise in relation to a desirable change in diet. The physician's task is complicated by the fact that most of his colleagues do not believe any progress has been made in our knowledge of these problems in the two centuries since Jenner recognized that coronary obstruction caused angina pectoris. Now that there is direct evidence that human atheromas are due to hyperlipidemia and can be reversed by optimal therapy, we can hope for a gradual change in this professional attitude, but the history of scurvy, rickets and other nutritional disorders reminds us how reluctant physicians are to accept a dietary explanation of disease. We should be neither surprised nor indignant if it takes two or three generations for our present knowledge of atherogenesis to effect a real decrease in the death rate from obstructive vascular disease.

Summary

Recent studies of men have shown that atheromas and xanthomas are histologically and chemically identical during the early phases of their development. Both arise from the infiltration of chylomicrons and beta lipoproteins during periods of hyperlipidemia. Both regress, with disappearance of the lipids, when plasma lipids remain normal; that is, when the serum cholesterol plus triglyceride does not exceed 300 mg. per 100 ml.

Cholesterol added to a vegetarian diet was first shown to be a potential cause of atherosclerosis, but alcohol, saturated fats, and carbohydrates, taken in excessive amounts, have also been shown to produce hyperlipidemia and can thus lead to atherosclerosis. Different species of animals and different individuals vary in their sensitivity to each of these dietary factors. Other factors, such as hypertension, accelerate atherogenesis and mural thrombosis on the diseased intima. Biochemically and psychologically each hyperlipidemic person presents a unique therapeutic problem in dietary management and in the selection of drugs to decrease absorption or endogenous synthesis of lipids.

References

1. Osler, W.: *Lectures on Angina Pectoris and Allied States.* New York, D. Appleton and Company, 1897.
2. McLetchie, N. G. B.: *Coronary Atheroma: A Diary of Discovery.* Springfield, Ill., Charles C Thomas, 1970.
3. Whereat, A. F.: Is atherosclerosis a disease of intramitochondrial respiration? Ann. Intern. Med. 73:125–127, 1970.

4. Bagdade, J. D., and Bierman, E. L.: Diagnosis and treatment of blood lipid disorders. Med. Clin. N. Amer. 54:1383–1398, 1970.
5. Bragdon, J. H.: Hyperlipemia and atherosclerosis in a hibernator. Circ. Res. 2:520–524, 1954.
6. Parker, F., Bagdade, J. D., Odland, G. F., and Bierman, E. L.: Evidence for the chylomicron origin of lipids accumulating in diabetic eruptive xanthomas: A correlative lipid, biochemical, histochemical and electron-microscopic study. J. Clin. Invest. 49:2172–2187, 1970.
7. Zelis, R., Mason, D. T., Braunwald, E., and Levy, R. I.: Effects of hyperlipoproteinemias and their treatment on the peripheral circulation. J. Clin. Invest. 49:1007–1015, 1970.
8. Insull, W., Jr., and Bartsch, G. E.: Cholesterol, triglyceride and phospholipid content of intima, media and atherosclerotic fatty streak in human thoracic aorta. J. Clin. Invest. 45:513–523, 1966.
9. Suter, G. I., and Franch, J. E.: Passage of lipid across vascular endothelium in newborn rats. J. Cell Biol. 27:163–177, 1965.
10. Balis, J. V., Haust, M. D., and More, R. H.: Electron-microscopic studies in human atherosclerosis: Cellular elements in aortic fatty streaks. Exp. Molec. Path. 3:511–525, 1964.
11. Bragdon, J. H.: Spontaneous atherosclerosis in the rabbit. Circulation 5:641–646, 1952.
12. Kube, N., and Ssolowjew, A.: Über die Lipoidablagerung in der Aorta von Kindern in frühen Sauglingsalter. Frankfurt Z. Path. 40:302–311, 1930.
13. Lang, P. D., and Insull, W., Jr.: Lipid droplets in atherosclerotic fatty streaks of human aorta. J. Clin. Invest. 49:1479–1488, 1970.
13a. Samuel, P., Perl, W., Holtzman, C. M., Rochman, N. D., and Lieberman, S.: Long term kinetics of serum and xanthoma cholesterol radioactivity in patients with hypercholesterolemia. J. Clin. Invest. 51:266–278, 1972.
14. Wilens, S. L.: Resorption of arterial atheromatous deposits in wasting disease. Amer. J. Path. 23:793–804, 1947.
15. Dock, W.: Why are men's coronary arteries so sclerotic? J.A.M.A. 170:152–156, 1959.
16. Astrup, P., Kjelden, K., and Wanstrup, J.: Enhancing influence of carbon monoxide on the development of atheromatosis in cholesterol-fed rabbits. J. Atheroscler. Res. 7:343–354, 1967.
17. Kjelden, K., Wanstrup, J., and Astrup, P.: Enchancing influence of hypoxia on the development of atheromatosis in cholesterol-fed rabbits. J. Atheroscler. Res. 8:845–854, 1968.
18. Feigl, J.: Neue Untersuchungen zur Chemie des Blutes bei akuter Alkoholintoxikation-Untersuchungen zur Kenntnis der Entwicklung und des Aufbaues von Lipaemien. Biochem. Z. 92:294–315, 1918.
19. Amatuzio, D. S., and Hays, L. J.: Dietary control of essential hyperlipemia: Effect of dairy foods, phospholipid, coconut oil and alcohol. Arch. Intern. Med. 102:173–178, 1958.
20. Lees, R. S., and Frederickson, D. S.: Carbohydrate induction of hyperlipemia in normal man. Clin. Res. 13:327, 1965.
21. Lapiccirella, V., Lapiccirella, R., Ablione, F., and Liotta, S.: Enquéte clinique, biologique et cardiographique parmi les tribes nomades de la Somalie qui se nourrissent seulement de lait. Bull. WHO 27:681–697, 1962.
22. Shaper, A. G., Jones, K. W., Jones, M., and Kyobe, J.: Serum lipids in three nomadic tribes of northern Kenya. Amer. J. Clin. Nutr. 13:135–146, 1963.
23. Biss, K., Ho, K. J., Mikkelson, B., Lewis, L., and Taylor, C. B.: Some unique biologic characteristics of the Masai of East Africa. New Eng. J. Med. 284:694–699, 1971.
24. Shaper, A. G.: *Current Developments in Atherosclerosis Studies in Africa. Atherosclerosis.* Proceedings of the Second International Symposium. New York, Springer-Verlag, 1970, p. 314–320.
25. Crawford, M. G.: Fatty-acid ratios in free living and domestic animals. Possible implications for atheroma. Lancet 1:1329–1333, 1968.
26. Spritz, N., and Mishkel, M. A.: Effects of dietary fats on plasma lipids and lipoproteins. J. Clin. Invest. 48:78–86, 1969.
27. Bolin, T. D., Davis, A. E., Seah, C. S., Chua, K. L., Yong, V., Kho, K. M., Siak, C. L., and Jacob, E.: Lactose intolerance in Singapore. Gastroenterology 59:76–84, 1970.
28. Kretchsmer, N., Ransome-Kuti, O., Hurwitz, R., Dungy, C., and Alakija, W.: Intestinal absorption of lactose in Nigerian ethnic groups. Lancet 2:392–395, 1971.
29. Snapper, I.: *Chinese Lessons to Western Medicine.* 2nd ed. New York, Grune & Stratton, 1965, pp. 362 and 378.

A Fat Controlled Diet for All

HAQVIN MALMROS

University of Lund, Sweden

A sine qua non for effective prevention of a disease is knowledge of its cause. Concerning atherosclerosis, it is often asserted that the etiology of the disease is not known with certainty and is probably multifactorial. Statistical analysis of data obtained in mass health surveys of persons free from clinical evidence of atherosclerotic disease has shown that such factors as high blood pressure and cigarette smoking favor the development of coronary heart disease. Since unanimity has not been achieved on the relative importance of such risk factors, many investigators feel that the cause of atherosclerosis is so controversial that it is at present impossible to recommend any radical nationwide preventive measures. This negative attitude to the problem of atherosclerosis is regrettable because it is one of the commonest and most serious human diseases. In some parts of the world, particularly in the more economically developed countries, atherosclerosis is almost universal, and atherosclerotic complications in the heart and in the brain are the commonest cause of death.

But have we only vague ideas and no factual knowledge about the cause of atherosclerosis? Is there no firm ground on which to base effective prophylaxis? In the debate on the etiology and prevention of atherosclerosis a clear distinction must be made between atherosclerosis and the complications that may occur in its wake. In other words, atherosclerosis cannot be equated with coronary heart disease and myocardial infarction. It is true that atherosclerotic lesions are practically always present in the coronary arteries in patients with myocardial infarction, but the cause of the acute episode with complete occlusion of a coronary branch may be quite different from the cause of the basic disease, i.e., atherosclerotic plaques in the vessel wall. It is therefore not possible to use the relapse rate of myocardial infarction in an experimental group as an indicator of the efficacy of any particular regimen, such as a certain diet intended to prevent the development of atherosclerosis.

It is indeed very difficult to study the development of atherosclerosis in man because atherosclerotic lesions cannot be visualized directly during life, but only at autopsy. We must therefore resort to experiments on animals. A large number of such investigations have been performed in recent years and valuable observations have been made, which might prove of interest also in the problem of atherosclerosis in man. In experimental investigations it is possible to study the effect of one variable at a time. It ought therefore to be possible in animal experiments to ascertain whether the etiology of atherosclerosis is unifactorial or multifactorial.

Cholesterol as the True Causal Agent of Atherosclerosis

As early as some 60 years ago Anitschkow[1] showed that it is possible to induce atherosclerosis in rabbits by feeding them a diet containing cholesterol dissolved in sunflower seed oil. Later investigations have shown that such a diet can produce atherosclerosis in other animals, including omnivorous species. Patho-anatomic investigations of the aorta and other arteries in experimental animals fed a high cholesterol diet have revealed an increased amount of cholesterol, particularly esterified cholesterol, in the atherosclerotic plaques. Relatively large amounts of cholesterol have also been found in human atherosclerotic lesions, both in children—in fatty streaks—and in adults.

Cholesterol is a naturally occurring component of all cells and of blood plasma in animals and humans. It may therefore appear strange that deposition of cholesterol in vessel walls is capable of irritating the tissue and inducing atherosclerotic plaques. That cholesterol deposits in collagen tissue are by no means indifferent but may be the direct cause of a strong tissue reaction is apparent from the findings by the author in the rabbit experiments illustrated in Figures 1 to 3. In a group of rabbits fed a diet consisting of commercial rabbit pellets with addition of 1 per cent cholesterol, distinct eye changes sometimes occurred in the form of a gray-white margin along the periphery of the cornea. This arcus corneae increased progressively, and after some months the cornea in one of the animals was completely covered by an opaque white layer. At the end of the experiment after one year, microscopic examination of the eye showed that the pannus covering the cornea consisted of collagen tissue with countless needle-like clefts left after dissolution of cholesterol ester crystals. The serum cholesterol level in these

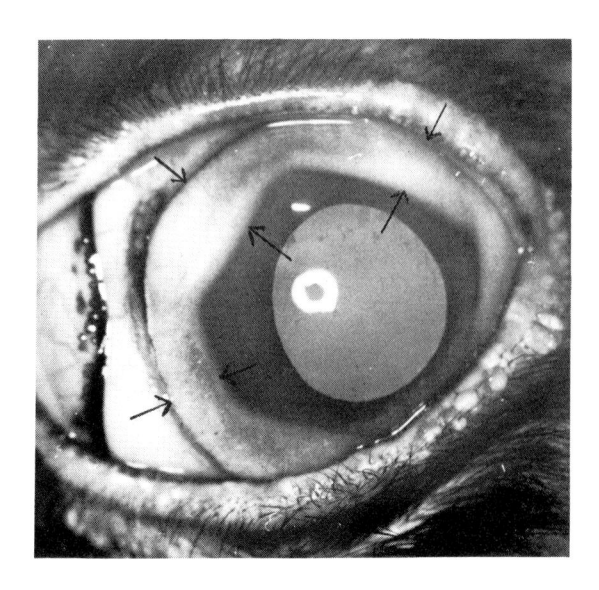

Figure 1. Arcus lipoides corneae (outlined by arrows) in a rabbit fed a diet containing 1 per cent cholesterol.

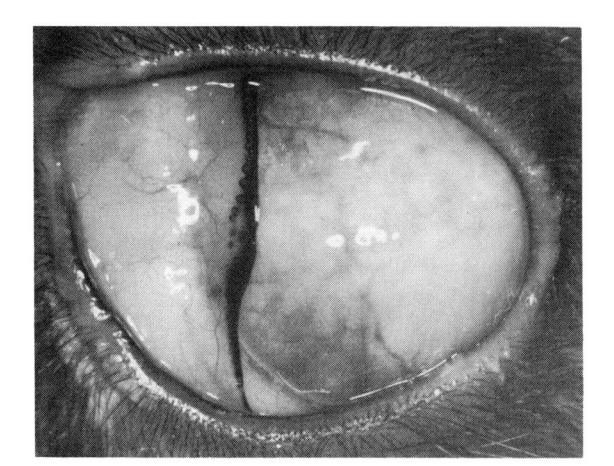

Figure 2. Extensive involvement of the entire cornea, which is covered by a white membrane.

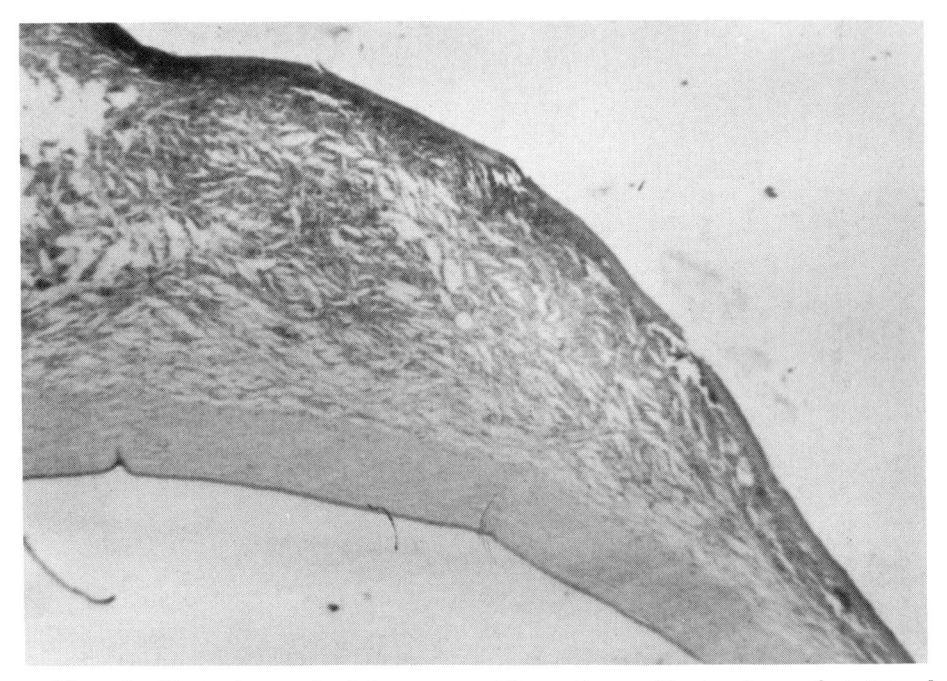

Figure 3. Photomicrograph of the corneae. Fibrous tissue with abundance of cholesterol ester deposits (clefts where cholesterol crystals have been dissolved).

animals was very high. Widespread atherosclerotic changes were also found in the aorta, coronary arteries, and other vascular areas. Microscopic examination of the atherosclerotic plaques showed, as in the cornea, numerous spaces left by cholesterol ester crystals. Similar findings have been found in the atheromatous plaques in other animals with experimentally induced hypercholesterolemia (Fig. 4). This also holds for human atherosclerosis in which, for example, microscopic sections of the aorta show needle-shaped clefts left by dissolved cholesterol ester crystals (Fig. 5).

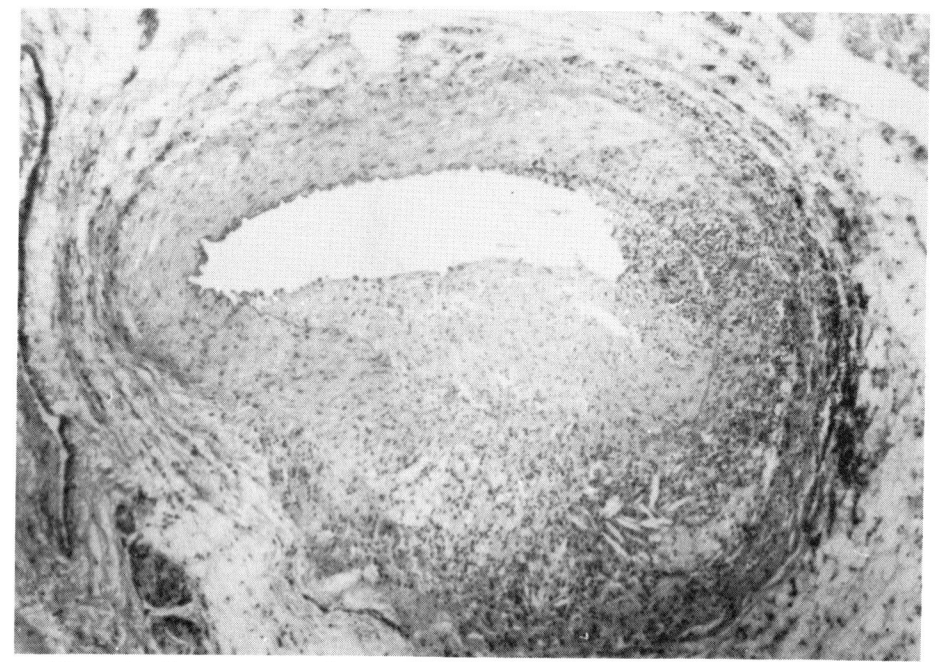

Figure 4. Coronary artery from a dog fed a semisynthetic diet containing hydrogenated coconut fat and cholesterol. Atherosclerotic plaque with cholesterol clefts at the base of the lesion.

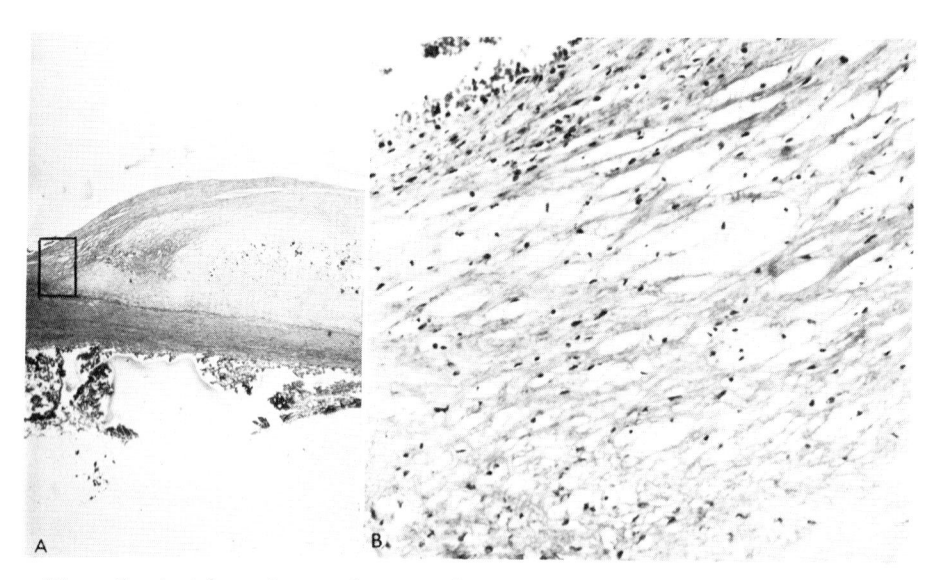

Figure 5. A, Atherosclerotic plaque in the aorta of a man. B, Higher magnification of the verge of the plaque showing numerous cholesterol clefts.

Significance of Hypercholesterolemia

In rabbits hypercholesterolemia is a prerequisite for the deposition of cholesterol in the vessel wall, with the subsequent development of atherosclerotic plaques. These animals are very susceptible to dietary cholesterol, and relatively mild or moderate hypercholesterolemia is sufficient to produce atherosclerotic lesions. A serum level of about 300 mg./100 ml. is thus sufficient, if maintained for some months to one year. Atherosclerosis can be produced in rabbits not only by dietary cholesterol but also by saturated fats, e.g., hydrogenated coconut fat.[2, 3] These diets will likewise produce atherosclerosis only if a distinct hypercholesterolemia is maintained for a relatively long time.

Dogs have long been believed to be insusceptible to dietary cholesterol.[4] Atherosclerosis could be induced only by further addition of thiouracil to the diet. It is, however, possible to produce hypercholesterolemia and atherosclerosis in dogs without thiouracil if saturated fat, e.g., hydrogenated coconut fat, is included in the diet.[5] With a diet containing cholesterol and hydrogenated coconut fat, we have likewise produced hypercholesterolemia and atherosclerosis in cynomolgus monkeys, and in a few cases this diet even resulted in myocardial infarction.[6, 7] Such a diet has also been shown to induce hypercholesterolemia and atherosclerosis in several other species of experimental animals. It has not, however, proved possible to produce atherosclerosis without raising the serum cholesterol to abnormal levels. Clinical observations and postmortem findings definitely suggest that hypercholesterolemia also plays an important role in the development of human atherosclerosis. Premature severe atherosclerosis is, for example, often observed in familial hypercholesterolemia (Type II according to Fredrickson).

Effect of Saturated and Polyunsaturated Fats

Numerous quantitative dietary investigations in healthy volunteers and in patients with known atherosclerosis have unequivocally shown that saturated fat enhances, and polyunsaturated fat depresses, the serum cholesterol level. In such investigations it has not been possible to obtain direct evidence of a possible atherogenic effect of a given sort of fat. Neither has it been possible to follow for any length of time the isolated effect of various triglycerides containing different kinds of fatty acids; however, this is possible in rabbit experiments.[8] Of the saturated fatty acids studied, we found lauric acid (C12) and myristic acid (C14) to have the strongest enhancing effect on the cholesterol level and also to have the strongest atherogenic effect. Stearic acid (C18) produced hardly any elevation of the cholesterol level. Linoleic acid (C18:2) was found to suppress the serum cholesterol level and to counteract the enhancing effect of saturated fatty acids on the serum cholesterol. But such counteraction required, for example, at least 15 gm. of linoleic acid to compensate the effect of 10 gm. of lauric acid. Liquid vegetable oils with a high content of linoleic acid produced no increase in the serum cholesterol or any atherosclerotic lesions, even when the experiments were continued for a long time. Such an experiment with corn oil was continued for three years and postmortem examination revealed no atheromatous plaques or other pathological changes in the internal organs.

An analogous experimental model has also proved useful in the investigation of the important question of whether replacement of saturated fat by polyunsaturated fat can reverse manifest atheromatosis in rabbits.[9] In such experiments it was found that atheromatous lesions in the aorta regressed when hydrogenated coconut oil fat was replaced by an equivalent amount of corn oil. It was also found that the total amount of cholesterol in the carcass became almost normal after replacement of the dietary saturated fat by polyunsaturated fat. These rabbit experiments do not warrant any far-reaching conclusions, especially as rabbits are herbivorous animals. Experimental investigations on monkeys have, however, produced similar results. Armstrong[10,11] has shown that dietary measures can produce a regression of already formed atherosclerotic changes in monkeys. He also found a much lower cholesterol content of the coronary arteries in monkeys treated with a cholesterol-free diet containing corn oil.

Comparative studies of the effect of saturated fat, polyunsaturated fat, and dietary cholesterol in man and in some of our most common experimental animals, such as rabbits, dogs, cockerels, and monkeys, have shown that the serum cholesterol level will rise in all experimental animals as well as in man if the diet contains both cholesterol and saturated fat. Such a diet, which corresponds to what most people eat every day, will induce atherosclerotic lesions within a short time in animals. Saturated fat without supplementary cholesterol causes hypercholesterolemia in rabbits and in man. If the saturated fat is replaced by polyunsaturated fat, the serum cholesterol becomes normal in rabbits and in human beings. Cholesterol, even when dissolved in oil rich in linoleic acid, e.g., corn oil, markedly enhances the serum cholesterol in rabbits. Human beings using a cholesterol-free diet with corn oil will also react with a certain increase in the serum cholesterol on addition of cholesterol, e.g., in the form of yolk of eggs.[12] Human beings are less susceptible to dietary cholesterol than rabbits, but rather susceptible to saturated fat. For that reason the major part of the population in North America, Western Europe, and Northern Europe, i.e., people consuming abundant saturated fat, have abnormally high serum cholesterol levels.

The "Normal" Serum Cholesterol Level

Opinions differ on the normal range of variation of serum cholesterol. Many investigators still regard 300 mg. per 100 ml. as the upper limit of the normal range. Though such high cholesterol values have often been found in mass health surveys of apparently healthy persons in economically well developed countries, such levels cannot be regarded as "normal," for in these countries most adults who feel healthy have atherosclerotic lesions in the aorta and often also in the coronary arteries. Only newborn infants can be regarded as really normal in such populations, i.e., completely free from atheromatosis.

In newborns the serum cholesterol concentration is generally about 75 mg. per 100 ml.; newborn African and European infants have similar levels.[13] It would thus appear that we all have good initial values. The cholesterol level rises rapidly during the first three days of life and continues to rise slowly so that by the end of the first year it is about 150 mg. per 100 ml., i.e., twice that at birth.[14] The level of the serum cholesterol during the first year of life is, however, dependent on the infant's diet. The linoleic acid content of breast milk varies considerably with the mother's diet.[15] The amount of saturated fat and of polyunsaturated fat in commercially available baby foods also varies considerably. If the diet of the weaned baby contains only very small amounts of saturated fat, the serum cholesterol level will not rise but, rather, tend to fall.

In people living on a high carbohydrate and very low fat diet, e.g., the natives of New Guinea, the serum cholesterol is low even in adults, about 130 mg. per 100 ml.[16] In numerous experiments on healthy volunteers, both young medical students and elderly men with widely varying occupations, we have found that the serum cholesterol falls to about 200 mg. per 100 ml. or to a still lower level within the first week if saturated fat in the diet is replaced by polyunsaturated fat, e.g., corn oil or sunflower seed oil, and if they cease to consume eggs and other substances rich in cholesterol.[17,18] In children and in youths (<20 years) using an ordinary diet the cholesterol level is, as a rule, at the most 200 mg. per 100 ml. Later in life the cholesterol level rises, and values of 250 to 300 mg. per 100 ml. or more are not uncommon. But much suggests that values above 200 mg. per 100 ml. should not be regarded as normal for man.

In comparative investigations of the population in various countries, Keys and co-workers[19,20] as well as other investigators have found much lower serum cholesterol levels in those countries where the consumption of saturated fat is low and that of polyunsaturated fat relatively high. The five-year experience of mortality in the International Cooperative Study conducted under the supervision of Keys, and comprising 12,770 men aged 40 to 59, showed that the death rates in coronary heart disease were closely related to the mean serum cholesterol levels and equally closely related to the mean percentages of calories supplied by saturated fatty acids in the diets. Deaths from all causes were also notably lower in those countries where the mean cholesterol levels of the populations were low.

It is clear from these investigations and many others that the diet, and particularly the fat content and the qualitative composition of the fat, strongly affect the serum cholesterol concentration in all people. Modification of the diet, with a considerable reduction of the amount of saturated fat and replacement of part of the fat by polyunsaturated fat and a reduction of dietary cholesterol, will usually produce a considerable reduction of serum cholesterol. Clinical data and comparative investigations of populations in different parts of the world suggest that a reduction of the serum cholesterol should be useful in the prevention of atherosclerosis. Several long-term dietary trials on survivors of myocardial infarction and groups of men without previously known heart disease also argue in the same direction.[21-24] In animal experiments it has been clearly shown that hypercholesterolemia causes atheromatosis and that such changes can regress if the serum cholesterol is reduced by modification of the diet, e.g., replacement of saturated fat by polyunsaturated fat or exclusion of dietary cholesterol. It thus appears that dietary prevention of atherosclerosis is possible when one is well motivated.

Who Should Change the Fat Composition of the Diet?

It is widely believed that it is difficult to change deeply rooted dietary habits and that it is hardly worthwhile to try to do so, except in special cases, such as in patients with myocardial infarction and severe hyperlipemia; in other words, only in patients or possibly in persons with a strong family history of atherosclerotic heart disease, where it is a question of dietary treatment under medical supervision. It is true that persons with manifest hyperlipemia require dietary treatment and possibly also suitable drugs to achieve normal lipid levels. But such a program will embrace only a very small proportion of the many persons prone to develop coronary heart disease or other complications of atherosclerosis.

In some quarters a further step has been taken; for example, mass surveys of 40 to 50 year old men have been carried out to detect those particularly susceptible to coronary disease. The examinations have usually included not only determination of the serum cholesterol and triglyceride levels, but also measurement of the blood pressure, electrocardiography, and notes about smoking habits and signs, if any, of diabetes, adiposity, and certain personality characteristics. Such health surveys for detecting "coronary prone" adults require the services of many physicians and technicians as well as large sums of money. Even in economically highly developed countries it is difficult to mobilize sufficient personnel and to raise sufficient funds for such surveys, except for examination of limited groups of the population. Moreover, such expensive projects can hardly be expected to produce any useful results for the simple reason that it is too late to start preventive measures at the age of 40 to 50 years. At such an age practically all men have atherosclerotic lesions in the aorta and many also in the coronary arteries.

At what age, then, should preventive measures be started if they are to ward off atherosclerosis which is the basic disease? Extensive postmortem studies have shown that the initial signs of atherosclerosis can be detected early in life. Thus, Holman et al.[25] in New Orleans found intimal fatty streaks in the aorta in every case three years of age or older. Strong and McGill[26] found fatty streaks in the coronary arteries in many cases in the second decade; thereafter practically all cases had coronary lesions. Fibrous plaques in the coronary arteries began to appear in the second decade.

Data from the International Atherosclerotic Project (IAP) have shown that lesions in the coronary arteries seem to be related to serum cholesterol and dietary fat when populations are compared.[27] As already pointed out, the serum cholesterol level tends to rise continuously throughout childhood and adolescence in those countries where the diet contains abundant saturated fat. If a serious attempt is to be made to prevent atherosclerosis, it would therefore appear necessary to start such measures so early that a marked rise of the serum cholesterol level is prevented. In other words, a prudent diet should be used from infancy.

In What Respect Should the Diet Be Changed?

A program to reduce blood cholesterol levels by dietary measures should include:

1. A marked reduction of the saturated fat content.

2. Replacement of the saturated fat by polyunsaturated fat, when possible.

3. Reduction of the consumption of foods rich in cholesterol, e.g., egg yolk.

The total consumption of fat should be kept reasonably low, particularly by people with a tendency to adiposity and by people with low calorie requirements (less than 2000 calories a day). But one should not aim at prescribing a "low fat diet" in which most energy is derived from foods high in carbohydrates. People soon tire of such a diet, and experience has shown that it does not in the long run clearly lower the serum cholesterol level.

Replacement of saturated fat by polyunsaturated fat in various food products requires the help of the food industry, which, at least in highly industrialized countries, occupies a key position as far as the composition of the diet is concerned. In recent years tremendous advances have been made in food technology. The dairy and margarine industry now have numerous possibilities to improve their products by changing the composition of the fat content. For example, in Sweden it is now possible to buy butter which has been made rich in linoleic acid by addition of 20 per cent sunflower seed oil, and which has the same consistency as "refrigerator margarine." But there are still many products whose fat composition is unsuitable in spite of the fact that this is neither necessary nor very advantageous from an economic or technical point of view. Thus, coconut fat, which has the strongest atherogenic effect of all fats, is still widely used in the manufacture of margarine, cream substitutes, filled milk, ice cream, and most baby foods. In such products, as well as in baked goods and salad dressings, one might suitably use a linoleic-rich vegetable oil, such as sunflower seed oil, corn oil, or safflower oil. Such oils should not, however, be regarded as medicines and taken by the spoonful, for such a practice will often result in too high a consumption of fat and, what is more, in a dislike for all food prepared with such oil. Vegetable oils are often hydrogenated, which gives them a harder consistency but at the same time renders them less suitable from a nutritional point of view. One should therefore not unnecessarily hydrogenate oils rich in linoleic acid.

Existing laws and regulations should be revised so as not to hinder the production of valuable fat-modified products. On the other hand, the labeling and advertising of such products should be controlled; e.g., the fat composition of a given product should be clearly stated on the label, and use of the term "vegetable fat" should be forbidden because coconut fat may masquerade under this name.

It is also important to consider the fat composition of other foods and to make available leaner meats and processed meats with a low content of saturated fats. The climate permitting, farmers should be encouraged to grow oil plants whose seeds have a high content of linoleic acid, e.g., sunflower seed oil. The import of sunflower seeds to those countries where the plant cannot be cultivated should be facilitated. Since fish contain polyunsaturated fatty acids with a cholesterol-depressing effect, attempts ought to be made to encourage people to eat more fish by subsidizing the fishing industry. On the other hand, the consumption of egg yolk should be diminished, and the public should be dissuaded from eating eggs and bacon regularly for breakfast.

It is often difficult to change deeply rooted dietary habits, and therefore it is important to devise a readily understandable education program and to begin to use it now in the elementary schools. Especially as far as children are concerned, a reduction in the consumption of saturated fat should not be compensated by an increase in the consumption of sugar in the form of jam, marmalade, honey and biscuits, and so forth. It is better to replace part of the saturated fat by polyunsaturated fat than by sugar, which gives only empty calories and which may have an injurious effect on the teeth. "Fat-modified" products should thus contain as little saturated fat as possible, and part of the saturated fat should be substituted by polyunsaturated fat. The cholesterol content of the products should be kept as low as possible.

Owing to double bonds in the carbon chain, polyunsaturated oil is more sensitive to high temperatures and to light. Therefore, when such oil is used for frying, care should be taken that it is not heated to such a temperature as to cause it to fume. It is also important that oils rich in linoleic acid contain sufficient tocopherol.

Many peoples, such as the Italians, have for centuries used olive oil for preparing their food and have shown that dishes made with oil can be both appetizing and palatable. Such oil has not been found to have any carcinogenic or other undesirable effect. This also holds for sunflower seed oil, which is rich in linoleic acid and which is widely used in Southeast Europe. In Bulgaria, for example, the consumption of sunflower seed oil per capita is 12–16 kg. a year. Very little saturated fat is used—1.7 kg. butter, 1.3 kg. lard, and no margarine. The mortality from ischemic heart disease is low in Bulgaria—163—and also the mortality from malignant neoplasm—134 per 100,000 in 1969.[28] Even in other countries with a high consumption of sunflower seed oil, the mortality from neoplasms is lower than in countries where more saturated and less polyunsaturated fat is used. In the U.S.S.R. the mortality from malignant neoplasms is 125 and in Rumania, 122 per 100,000. These figures do not suggest that a high consumption of polyunsaturated fat favors the development of cancer.

References

1. Anitschkow, N.: Uber die Veränderungen der Kaninchenaorta bei experimentellen Cholesterinsteatose. Beitr. Path. Anat. 56:379, 1913.
2. Wigand, G.: Induction of atherosclerosis in rabbits by cholesterol-free diet containing 8% hydrogenated coconut oil. (Entry for Ciba Foundation awards for basic research relevant to the problems of ageing, 1957.)
3. Wigand, G.: Production of hypercholesterolemia and atherosclerosis in rabbits by feeding different fats without supplementary cholesterol. Acta Med. Scand., suppl. 166, 1959.
4. Steiner, A., and Kendall, F. E.: Atherosclerosis and arteriosclerosis in dogs following ingestion of cholesterol and thiouracil. Arch. Path. 42:433, 1946.
5. Malmros, H., and Sternby, N. H.: Induction of atherosclerosis in dogs by a thiouracil-free semisynthetic diet containing cholesterol and hydrogenated coconut oil. Progr. Biochem. Pharmacol. 4:482, 1968.
6. Malmros, H., and Wigand, G.: Experimental hypercholesterolemia and hypertriglyceridemia in cynomolgus monkeys fed saturated fat and cholesterol. J. Atheroscler. Res. 5:474, 1965.
7. Malmros, H., Wigand, G., Sternby, N. H., and Arvidson, G.: Atherosclerosis and myocardial infarction in cynomolgus monkeys fed hydrogenated coconut fat and cholesterol. To be published.
8. Malmros, H., and Wigand, G.: Atherosclerosis produced in rabbits by cholesterol-free diet. In Speranskij, I. I.: *Modern Problems of Cardiology*. Papers dedicated to Professor A. Miasnikov, Moscow, 1960, p. 113.

9. Malmros, H.: Reversibility of atherosclerotic lesions in rabbits. To be published.
10. Armstrong, M. L.: Regression of coronary atheromatosis in rhesus monkeys. Circ. Res. 27:59, 1970.
11. Armstrong, M.: Can regression of atherosclerotic lesions occur and at what stage? Paper read at the International Symposium on Atherosclerosis, Toronto, 1971.
12. Malmros, H.: Importance of dietary cholesterol and fat in the pathogenesis of atherosclerosis. Paper read at the 4th International Congress of Dietetics, Stockholm, 1965.
13. Bersohn, I., and Wayburne, S.: Serum cholesterol concentration in new-born African and European infants and their mothers. Amer. J. Clin. Nutr. 4:117, 1956.
14. Rafstedt, S., and Swahn, B.: Studies on lipids, proteins and lipoproteins in serum from newborn infants. Arch. Pediat. 43:221, 1954.
15. Saito, K., et al.: Studies in human milk. Report of research laboratory No. 69, Snow Brand Milk Product Co. Ltd., Tokyo, 1965.
16. Whyte, H. M., and Yee, I. L.: Serum cholesterol levels of Australians and natives of New Guinea from birth to adulthood. Aust. Ann. Med. 7:336, 1958.
17. Malmros, H., and Wigand, G.: The effect on serum cholesterol of diets containing different fats. Lancet 1:8, 1957.
18. Malmros, H.: The effect of dietary fats on serum cholesterol. In Sinclair, H. M. (ed.): *Essential Fatty Acids.* London, Butterworths Scientific Publications, p. 150.
19. Keys, A.: Coronary heart disease in seven countries. American Heart Association, Monograph No. 29, 1970.
20. Keys, A.: Epidemiology of atherosclerosis, Concluding remarks. In Jones, R. J. (ed.): *Atherosclerosis.* New York, Springer-Verlag, 1970, p. 399.
21. Leren, P.: The effect of plasma cholesterol lowering diet in survivors of myocardial infarction. Acta Med. Scand., suppl. 466, 1966.
22. Turpeinen, O., Miettinen, M., Karvonen, M. J., Roine, P., Pekkarinen, M., Lehtusuo, E. J., and Alivirta, P.: Dietary prevention of coronary heart disease: Long-term experiment. Amer. J. Clin. Nutr. 21:55, 1968.
23. Dayton, S., Pearce, M. L., Hashimoto, S., Dixon, W. J., and Tomiyasu, U.: A controlled clinical trial of a diet high in unsaturated fat. American Heart Association, Monograph No. 25, 1969.
24. Christakis, G., Rinzler, S. H., Archer, M. S., Winslow, G., Jampel, S., Stephenson, J., Friedman, G., Fein. H., Kraus, A., and James, G.: The anti-coronary club. A dietary approach to the prevention of coronary heart disease; a seven-year report. Amer. J. Pub. Health 56:299, 1966.
25. Holman, R. L., McGill, H. C., Jr., Strong, J. P., and Geer, J. C.: The natural history of atherosclerosis. The early aortic lesions as seen in New Orleans in the middle of the 20th century. Amer. J. Path. 34:209, 1958.
26. Strong, J. P., and McGill, H. C., Jr.: The natural history of coronary atherosclerosis. Amer. J. Path. 40:37, 1962.
27. Strong, J. P., and Eggen, D. A.: Risk factors and atherosclerosis. In Jones, R. J. (ed.): *Atherosclerosis.* New York, Springer-Verlag, 1970, p. 355.
28. Mortality Statistics, Demographic Yearbook 1970. New York, United Nations, 1971.

Control of Hyperlipidemia by Surgery

HENRY BUCHWALD and
RICHARD L. VARCO

The University of Minnesota Medical School

Unfortunately there are still those who classify diseases as "medical" or "surgical." As we have seen over the years, the treatment of processes such as Hodgkin's, congenital heart defects, Crohn's, and so forth, may pass from the care of one group to that of another. Rationally, internists and surgeons may find that their best results can come from a united effort. We shall attempt to present sufficient data to convince the objective reader that the surgical approach has a complementary role with diet and drugs in the control and understanding of the hyperlipidemias.

Historical Background

It is proper to start our historical resumé with the publication of Kremen, Linner, and Nelson[1] in 1954 that explored elective nutritional deprivation by upper and lower small intestinal exclusion procedures. In 1956 Payne[2] performed his first jejuno-ileal bypass for management of obesity; in 1962 Lewis, Turnbull, and Page,[3] in a fine metabolic clinical study, showed that blood cholesterol levels were reduced after jejuno-ileal bypass. In 1963 the Minnesota program of distal small intestinal bypass, or partial ileal bypass specifically for management of the hyperlipidemias, was initiated.[4] The partial ileal bypass operation is similar to the much more extensive jejuno-ileal bypass operation only in its ability to lower serum lipids. The primary purpose of jejuno-ileal bypass is to achieve a caloric deficit and, hence, weight loss; the partial ileal bypass operation does not cause weight loss and is selective in its induction of beneficial malabsorption of cholesterol and bile acids.

"Metabolic" surgery, as a rule, is the product of an extensive laboratory background, and its development depends on a dialogue with the laboratory over the years. Briefly, laboratory studies that form the basis for our clinical program have shown that partial ileal bypass causes reduction of serum cholesterol in normal and hypercholesterolemic adult rabbits, that the same is true for infant rabbits, that the operation prevents atherosclerosis in mature and in young rabbits, and that atherosclerosis arrest, healing of plaques, and possible reversal of lesions (in association with a quantitative reduction in plaque cholesterol) is seen after bypass in mature and in young rabbits.[5, 6] We have also been able to demonstrate reduction of serum cholesterol in the pig.[7] Other animal studies include those of Dr. H. William Scott and his associates, who have shown that partial ileal bypass reduces serum cholesterol in dogs[8] and in the rhesus monkey.[9] Ileal bypass is also responsible for prevention, and possibly reversal, of atherosclerosis in dogs[8] and in rhesus monkeys,[9] and has a superior protective effect against hyperlipidemia-atherosclerosis when compared with high doses of cholestyramine in rhesus monkeys.[10] The research team of Okuboye and associates[11] confirmed our cholesterol findings of arrest and partial reversal of atherosclerosis in the rabbit. An interesting experiment by Gomes and coworkers[12] on white Carneau pigeons, a species that has naturally occurring atherosclerotic disease, demonstrated prevention and reversal of atherosclerosis by partial ileal bypass, without changes in growth or weight.

Technique and Rationale

A carefully measured 200 cm. of the distal small intestine or one third of the small bowel, whichever is larger, is bypassed in the operation as we perform it (Fig. 1). Only in the case of a seven year old child have we ever bypassed less than 200 cm. We believe, for clinical comparison between our technique and that of any group utilizing a related operative approach, that this feature of minimal bypass length should be precisely the same. Our insistence on this is based on the negative clinical report of the Rockefeller Institute[13] in which a 100 cm. bypass was used, and on the carefully documented animal findings of Scott et al.[9, 14] demonstrating that there was a statistically significant difference in the reduction of serum cholesterol engendered by a 25 per cent intestinal bypass if compared to a one third intestinal bypass. To prevent future intussusception, the closed proximal end of the bypassed loop is attached to adjacent viscera; we have never experienced postoperative loop intussusception. We also take care in closing all rotational and divisional mesenteric defects to prevent an internal hernia.

The primary rationale of the partial ileal bypass operation is partial interference with the enterohepatic cholesterol and the enterohepatic bile acid cycles. Normally cholesterol enters the small intestine via the bile, by secretion directly through the intestinal wall, and in ingested food. Cholesterol is primarily absorbed and reabsorbed back into the circulation from the distal small intestine.[15] The enterohepatic bile acid mechanism is extremely efficient, so that essentially the same bile acids are used for emulsification of breakfast, lunch, and dinner. Following the operation there is interference with these cycles, with an increase in the

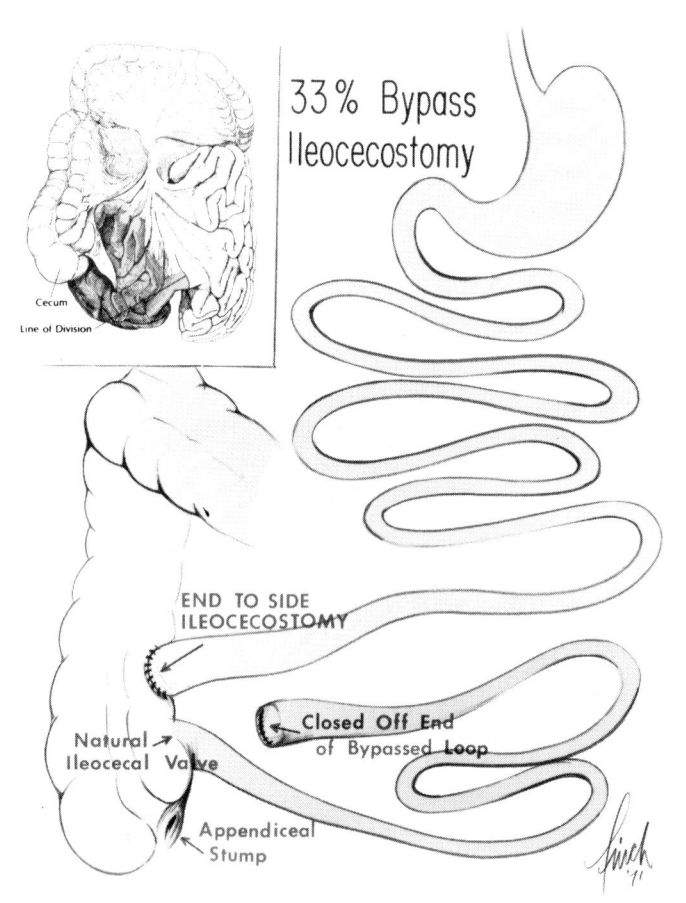

Figure 1. Partial ileal bypass consists of division of the bowel at 200 cm. or one third the small intestinal length, whichever is longer. Bowel continuity is restored by end-to-side anastomosis of the proximal small intestine to the cecum; the closed end of the bypassed segment is attached to the anterior taenia of the cecum, and the rotational mesenteric defect is closed.

loss of cholesterol and bile acids (the metabolic end-product of cholesterol metabolism) in the stool, resulting in (1) a direct loss of cholesterol from the body, and (2) an indirect drain on the cholesterol pool by the forced conversion of cholesterol to bile acids.

Over the past years we have carried out studies to substantiate the above premise and to quantitate the changes in cholesterol metabolism brought about by partial ileal bypass. In summary there is, as expected, a marked reduction in cholesterol absorption; on the average the preoperative absorptive capacity is reduced by 60 per cent.[7] There is a concomitant increase in fecal steroid excretion of 380 per cent, with the major increase in this excretion occurring in the bile acid fraction, accompanied by a significant increase in neutral sterol excretion.[16, 17] There is a 450 per cent compensatory increase in cholesterol synthesis and an associated 300 per cent increase in cholesterol turnover.[16, 17] The serum lipid changes in association with these rather marked upheavals in cholesterol dynamics will be reviewed later; it should be remembered at this time that the circulating cholesterol content is only a small fraction of the total body cholesterol pool. Our studies have shown that the total miscible body cholesterol pool is markedly reduced after bypass; namely, 35 per cent from the preoperative base line. This reduction takes place both in the freely miscible component, reflected by the circulating, liver, and intestinal mucosal cholesterol and in the less rapidly miscible cholesterol pool, consisting of cholesterol contained in muscle, connective tissue, and other body sites, including atherosclerotic plaque lesions.[16, 17]

Effect on Circulating Lipids

We now have nine years of clinical experience with the partial ileal bypass operation and have operated upon 120 patients. To date 94 patients have been followed for at least six months, and these 94 patients have been used for the development of the following data: There are 63 males and 31 females in this group. The average age of the males prior to operation was 41.5 years and the average age of the females was essentially identical at 41.3 years; the youngest patient in the group was seven years old at the time of operation and there are eight prepubertal youngsters in this series. With respect to hyperlipidemia, 65 of the patients are classified as Type II, one is a Type III, 17 patients are Type IV, six are classified as a mixed hyperlipoproteinemia; five of the earliest patients were not classified. Forty-one per cent of the patients were angina pectoris negative prior to operation and 59 per cent were positive. Fifty-four per cent of the patients had a negative resting electrocardiogram, and 48 per cent had a negative exercise electrocardiogram before bypass. Forty-six per cent had a positive resting electrocardiogram, with 26 of these 43 patients showing evidence of a previous myocardial infarction, and 40 per cent had a positive exercise electrocardiogram before operation. Eleven had no exercise electrocardiogram before their surgery. Coronary arteriography, in those patients in whom the procedure was carried out (early in our series no coronary arteriography was performed), was positive 81 per cent of the time. And, finally, in 76 patients (81 per cent) the operation was carried out therapeutically, and in 18 patients (19 per cent) the operation was carried out prophylactically, i.e., in hyperlipidemic individuals with no clinical, electrocardiographic, or arteriographic evidence of atherosclerotic disease.

Figure 2 illustrates the average serum cholesterol level response according to lipoprotein type for three months and one year following bypass; the five unclassified lipoprotein type patients have not been included in this bar graph. The preoperative base line average values, to which the postoperative values are compared, represent the maximum reduction achieved by diet alone, and at times by the combined use of diet and drugs, in these patients. In the Type II patients, excluding the homozygous patients, there was an average reduction of the serum cholesterol at one year of 37 per cent; in the one Type III patient we have only a three-month value—a 48 per cent reduction; in the Type IV patients there was an average serum cholesterol level reduction of 47 per cent at one year; and in the mixed type there was an average reduction of 40 per cent at one year. If we com-

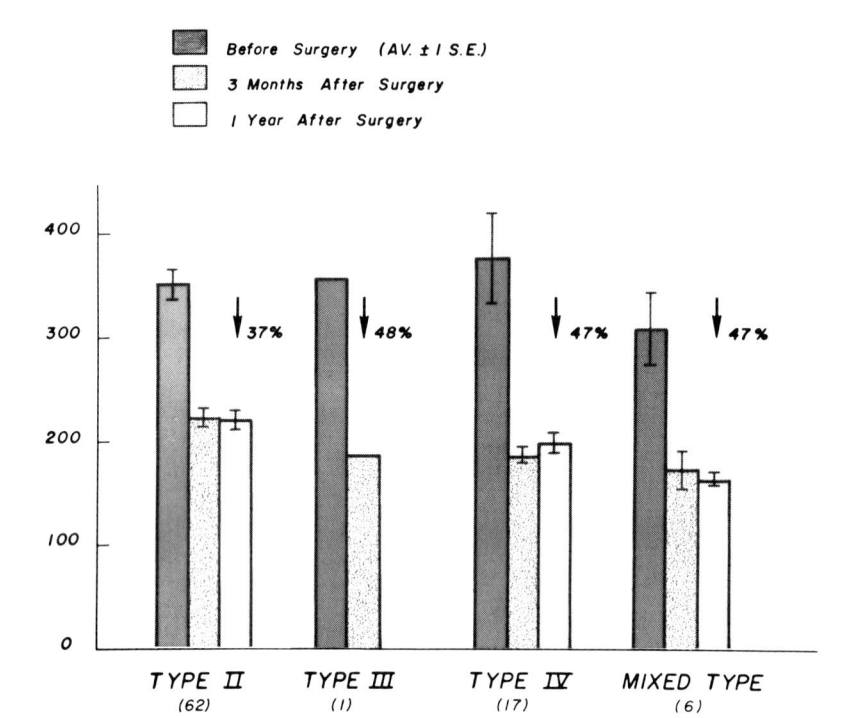

Figure 2. Average serum cholesterol response according to lipoprotein type with the exclusion of three homozygous Type II patients; the preoperative base lines represent the average cholesterol level after type specific dietary management.

bine all lipoprotein type patients (except the homozygous subgroup) and look at an overall plot of average serum cholesterol levels extended for seven years (Fig. 3), we see that the reduction in serum cholesterol varies from a maximum of 43 per cent to a minimum of 36 per cent, with an average persistent reduction over the years of 40 per cent from the preoperative postdietary base line determination.

Three of the Type II patients were classified as homozygous for the trait and their cholesterol reduction from base line was moderate at best, with average one-year reductions of 13, 19, and 15 per cent; the response of the homozygous Type II patient definitely falls in a different range from the cholesterol reduction that we have come to expect from the heterozygous patient. Unfortunately in the homozygous individual the partial ileal bypass, though the most effective single means of therapy currently available, does not provide for an acceptable lipid reduction.

We were able to study a subgroup of 24 heterozygous Type II patients prior to dietary management, postdiet and preoperatively, and again after bypass. In this cohort an 11 per cent reduction in serum cholesterol was achieved by dietary management alone (423 mg. per cent to 377 mg. per cent), and subsequent to bypass the total reduction from the premanagement base line was 53 per cent (423 to 224 mg. per cent), essentially a halving of the serum cholesterol level (Fig. 4).

Examining the change in the average serum triglyceride level, (where accu-

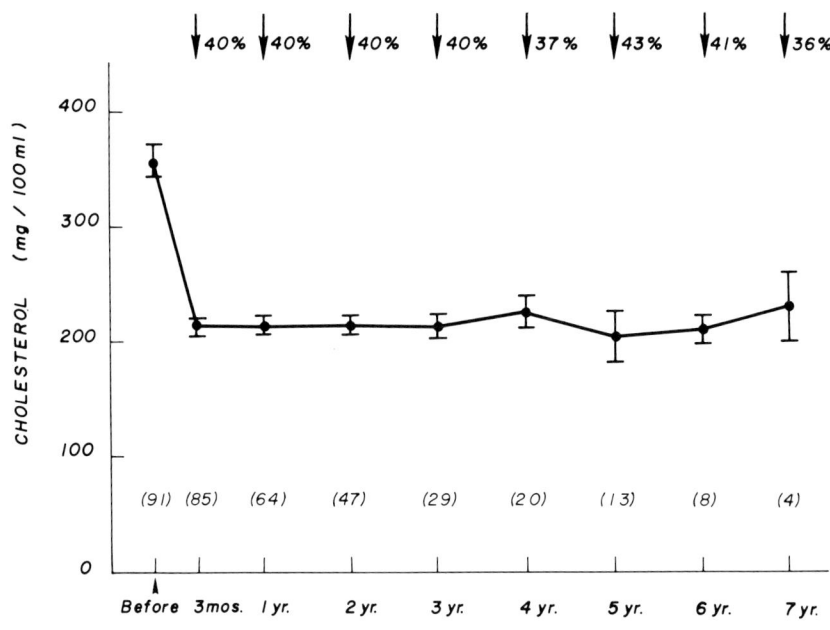

Figure 3. Cumulative plot of cholesterol response of patients in entire follow-up group, excluding three homozygous individuals.

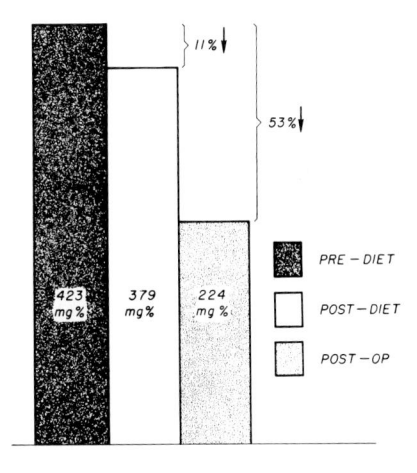

Figure 4. Twenty-four patients subgroup plot, illustrating response to diet and subsequently to partial ileal bypass.

rate pre- and postoperative triglyceride concentrations were available) again by lipoprotein type, we found no change in average triglyceride in the Type II patients, a slight (6 per cent) increase in triglyceride in our one Type III patient at three months, a 68 per cent one-year triglyceride lowering in the Type IV patients (compared to the preoperative post-type specific dietary management base line), and a 23 per cent reduction in triglyceride at one year in the mixed group (Fig. 5). In certain of the Type II patients with low serum triglyceride prior to surgery (below 160 mg. per cent or the so-called Type IIA patient) a paradoxical increase in serum triglyceride into the 200 to 300 mg. per cent range was seen.

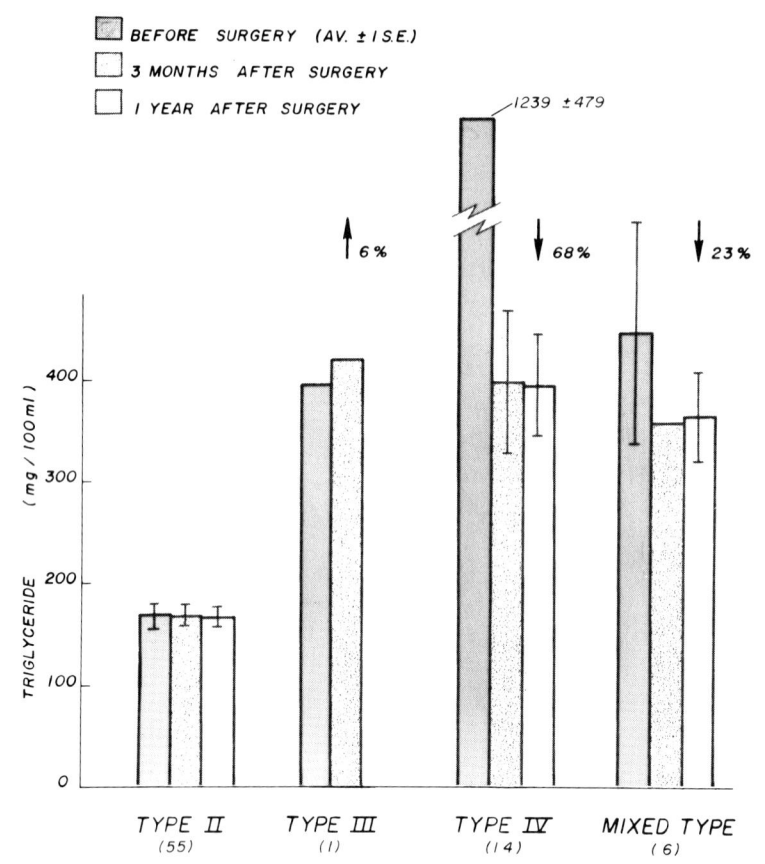

Figure 5. Average serum triglyceride response according to lipoprotein type; the preoperative base lines represent the average triglyceride level after type specific dietary management.

Clinical Results

Let us now turn to our clinical findings: mortality, morbidity, complications, and side effects, as well as clinical symptomatology, physical findings, electrocardiographic changes, and arteriographic data. Nine patients have died since their operative procedure. Only one patient died in hospital following the operation; he succumbed to an acute myocardial infarction sustained four days after his procedure; he had experienced three previous myocardial infarctions. Thus, our in-hospital operative mortality has been less than one per cent. The other eight patients died at varying time intervals following the operation, and six of these patients died of acute myocardial infarctions. Complications directly related to surgery consist of three episodes of bowel obstruction due to the development of adhesions, two of the proximal and functioning segments of the small intestine and one of the distal bypassed segment. We have not had any episodes of obstruction due to internal hernia formation or, as previously stated, any occurrence of intussusception of the closed end of the bypassed loop.

On the basis of a patient questionnaire, postoperative bowel habits have been cataloged. Better than half the patients stated that they had some problem with the frequency of bowel evacuations. Approximately 90 per cent of the patients, at one year following the operation, have less than five stools per day on minimal to no bowel control medications. There seems to be some increase in firmness in the consistency of the stools with the passage of time, going from what was termed loose stools to soft, partially formed stools. As previously stated, there is no weight loss associated with this limited bowel bypass. There has been no change in serum electrolytes and serum proteins. Since it is well known that vitamin B_{12} is exclusively absorbed in the distal small intestine,[18] all our patients are given 1000 μgm. of Vitamin B_{12} intramuscularly every two months. We have never seen the development of an anemia, macrocytosis, or any of the symptoms of pernicious anemia.

As our study progressed we became more and more aware that our patients volunteered that they had an improvement in their symptoms of angina pectoris. Of the 94 patients summarized in this report, 39 were angina pectoris negative prior to operation and 100 per cent of these patients showed no change, i.e., they did not develop angina pectoris. Fifty-five patients were angina pectoris positive, and of these, 7 per cent stated they were worse, 24 per cent had no change, 25 per cent reported a moderate improvement as determined by a reduction in their use of nitroglycerin, 18 per cent stated that they had marked improvement as determined by a reduction in the use of nitroglycerin and a significant increase in exercise capacity, and 26 per cent stated that they had complete remission in association with increased activity. Thus, 69 percent of all patients with angina pectoris present prior to surgery experienced some degree of improvement. Perhaps this is the result of psychotherapy, or perhaps it stems from increasing myocardial oxygen availability secondary to marked reduction of circulating lipid. We are currently conducting a rheological and hemodynamic research program to quantify the basis for this clinical finding. At times there was an improvement in exercise capacity on the treadmill electrocardiogram associated with the reduction in angina symptoms; however, this pattern was not consistent.

Our postoperative patients are seen three months following their procedure and then at the yearly anniversary of their operation. During these interval examinations a complete historical, physical, and laboratory (including lipid profile) evaluation, as well as electrocardiographic testing, are carried out. Our study is unique in obtaining serial follow-up coronary and aorto-iliac arteriograms in all our patients at two- to three-year time intervals. By a method of point for point discrimination of luminal size and measurement of lesions, performed by Dr. Kurt Amplatz of our Department of Radiology, we have demonstrated no essential change in nine technically comparable aorto-iliac arteriograms. Twenty-one patients have had technically comparable coronary arteriograms, and of these 14 showed no change, three showed new occlusions, one showed progression of an atherosclerotic plaque, and three patients revealed larger diameter vessels. It is interesting to compare this series with that of the Peter Bent Brigham Hospital,[19] which showed a 50 per cent progression rate in nonlipid-managed patients with comparable disease over the same length of time; combining the number of patients with new lesions or occlusions, our documented progression rate is 19 per cent.

A Census of the Clinical Experience of Others

We have attempted to ascertain, after reviewing available information sources, the experience of other investigators with the use of partial ileal bypass in the management of the hyperlipidemias. We have compiled both positive and negative results.

Rowe and associates[20] report a series of eight patients with a cholesterol reduction comparable to our own; however, they reject the operation because they noted a progression of arterial disease on repeat coronary arteriography. Strishower and co-workers[21] performed the procedure in two patients, with a 40 per cent cholesterol reduction but they, too, gave up the operation and offer as reasons for this rejection the perseverence of diarrhea and severe weight loss. We have not found significant weight loss in any instance of more than 100 cases. Did these workers possibly bypass much more than one third of the intestinal length? The British group of Johnston and associates[22] report one patient with only a transient cholesterol reduction; this patient was a homozygous Type II child. Grundy et al.[13] report on four patients, two of whom were homozygous. They achieved a cholesterol reduction in their heterozygous patients. They do not recommend the procedure, since they failed to obtain more significant cholesterol lowering then they were able to achieve with cholestyramine. We point out again that they bypass only 100 cm. Finally, Lees and Wilson[23] in a summary article discredited ileal bypass on the basis of diarrhea, an episode of bowel obstruction in one of five patients, and because (they stated) the results were no better than for drug therapy. We are somewhat at a loss to comment on these findings, since these authors failed to provide any data to substantiate their conclusions; indeed, there is no indication that they cite personal experience.

Lewis et al.[24] have operated upon two patients, one of whom was carefully followed for an extended period of time. They report an average cholesterol lowering of 40 per cent and no prorgession of atherosclerotic lesions by coronary arteriography. Morgan and Moore[25] have five patients in their series and report an average cholesterol reduction of 40 per cent. Streuter,[26] with seven patients, found an average cholesterol response of 40 per cent as well. He reported difficulty with diarrhea in one patient. Fritz and Walker[27] report one patient with a 46 per cent cholesterol reduction who had only transient diarrhea, a reduction in his angina pectoris, and an increase in his weight. Swan and McGowan[28] have operated upon four patients, with an average cholesterol reduction of 40 per cent; their patients have adjusted to the postoperative bowel pattern and state that they have experienced a decrease in angina pectoris symptomatology. Miettinen and associates[29] have operated upon 19 patients, with a cholesterol reduction ranging between 30 to 40 per cent after maximum dietary management; these authors state that their average reduction value is reduced by inclusion in their data of a homozygous patient, who responded relatively poorly. Helsingen and Rootwell[30] report nine patients, with an average cholesterol reduction of 43 per cent; they state that their patients have a tendency toward moderate diarrhea. They also report some diminution in symptoms of angina pectoris and no clinical evidence of progression of atherosclerosis. And, finally, Sodal et al.,[31] with nine patients and an average 40 per cent cholesterol reduction, report no difficulty with postoperative diarrhea.

Conclusions

Comparison of the average serum cholesterol levels of our partial ileal bypass patients to the average cholesterol concentrations found in comparably age and sex matched groups in the United States statistical survey of 1967[32] indicates that our patients are in the upper 5 to 10 per cent of the distribution curves preoperatively and well below the means postoperatively. Plotting the average preoperative cholesterol concentration on the Cornfield Framingham[33] risk curve, the patients in our series fall well above the 200 per cent risk level (100 per cent equal normal risk) preoperatively and are at about 75 per cent of normal risk postoperatively. Only the future and the completion of a randomized study can add statistical validity to these predictions.

At present we conclude that the advantages of partial ileal bypass in management of the hyperlipidemias are: (1) maximum effectiveness, (2) maintenance of lipid reduction, (3) safety, and (4) the obligatory nature of the procedure. The data clearly show that diet and drug therapy, singly or in combination, cannot approach the lipid reduction feasible by partial ileal bypass. Contrary to the results of drug therapy, the cholesterol lowering effect of partial ileal bypass is lasting, and there has been no report of response escapes. Patients may or may not adhere to a diet, may or may not take pills, but once the operation is performed its therapeutic effects are maintained and obligatory.

References

1. Kremen, A. J., Linner, J. H., and Nelson, C.: An experimental evaluation of the nutritional importance of proximal and distal small intestine. Ann. Surg. 140:439, 1954.
2. Payne, H. J., DeWind, L. T., and Commons, R. R.: Metabolic observations in patients with jejunocolic shunts. Amer. J. Surg. 106:273, 1963.
3. Lewis, L. A., Turnbull, R. B., Jr., and Page, I. H.: "Short-circuiting" of the small intestine. J.A.M.A. 182:187, 1962.
4. Buchwald, H.: A surgical operation to lower circulating cholesterol. Circulation 28(II): 649, 1963.
5. Buchwald, H.: The effect of ileal bypass on atherosclerosis and hypercholesterolemia in the rabbit. Surgery 58:22, 1965.
6. Buchwald, H., Moore, R. B., Bertish, J., and Varco, R. L.: Effect of ileal bypass on cholesterol levels, atherosclerosis and growth in the infant rabbit. Ann. Surg. 175:311, 1972.
7. Buchwald, H., and Gebhard, R. L.: Effect of intestinal bypass on cholesterol absorption and blood levels in the rabbit. Amer. J. Physiol. 207:567, 1964.
8. Scott, H. W., Jr., Stephenson, S. E., Jr., Younger, R., Carlisle, R. B., and Turney, S. W.: Prevention of experimental atherosclerosis by ileal bypass: 20% cholesterol diet and I^{131} induced hypothyroidism in dogs. Ann. Surg. 163:795, 1966.
9. Scott, H. W., Jr., Stephenson, S. E., Jr., Hayes, C. W., and Younger, R. K.: Effects of bypass of the distal fourth of small intestine on experimental hypercholesterolemia and atherosclerosis in rhesus monkeys. Surg. Gynec. Obstet. 125:3, 1967.
10. Younger, R. K., Shepard, G. H., Butts, W. H., and Scott, H. W., Jr.: Comparison of the protective effects of cholestyramine and ileal bypass in rhesus monkeys on an atherogenic regimen. Surg. Forum 20:101, 1969.
11. Okuboye, J. A., Ferguson, C. C., and Wyatt, J. P.: The effect of ileal bypass on dietary induced atherosclerosis in the rabbit. Canad. J. Surg. 11:69, 1968.
12. Gomes, M. M. R., Kottke, B. A., Bernatz, P. E., and Titus, J. L.: Effect of ileal bypass on aortic atherosclerosis of white Carneau pigeons. Surgery 70:353, 1971.
13. Grundy, S. M., Ahrens, E. H., Jr., and Salen, G.: Interruption of the enterohepatic circulation of bile acids in man: Comparative effects of cholestyramine and ileal exclusion on cholesterol metabolism. J. Lab. Clin. Med. 78:94, 1971.

14. Shepard, G. H., Wimberly, J. E., Younger, R. K., Stephenson, S. E., Jr., and Scott, H. W., Jr.: Effects of bypass of the distal third of the small intestine on experimental hypercholesterolemia and atherosclerosis in rhesus monkeys. Surg. Forum *19*:302, 1968.
15. Buchwald, H.: Lowering of cholesterol absorption and blood levels by ileal exclusion: Experimental basis and preliminary clinical report. Circulation *29*:713, 1964.
16. Moore, R. B., Frantz, I. D., Jr., and Buchwald, H.: Changes in cholesterol pool size, turnover rate, and fecal bile acid and sterol excretion after partial ileal bypass in hypercholesteremic patients. Surgery *65*:98, 1969.
17. Moore, R. B., Frantz, I. D., Jr., Varco, R. L., and Buchwald, H.: Cholesterol dynamics after partial ileal bypass. *In* Jones, R. J. (ed.): Proceedings of the Second International Symposium on Atherosclerosis, 1970, p. 295.
18. Buchwald, H.: Vitamin B_{12} absorption deficiency following bypass of the ileum. Amer. J. Dig. Dis. *9*:755, 1964.
19. Bemis, C. E., Eber, L. M., Kemp, H. G., and Gorlin, R.: Cine-arteriographic progression of coronary disease: Clinical and metabolic correlates. Circulation *44*(II):47, 1971.
20. Rowe, G. G., Young, W. P., and Wasserburger, R. H.: The effects of reduced serum cholesterol on human coronary atherosclerosis. Circulation *40*(III):22, 1969.
21. Strishower, E. W., Kradjian, R., Nichols, A. V., Coggiola, E., and Tsai, J.: Effect of ileal bypass on serum lipoproteins in essential hypercholesterolemia. J. Atheroscler. Res. *8*:525, 1968.
22. Johnston, I. D. A., Davis, J. A., Moutafis, C. D., and Myant, N. B.: Ileal bypass in the management of familial hypercholesterolemia. Proc. Roy. Soc. Med. *60*:16, 1967.
23. Lees, R. S., and Wilson, D. E.: The treatment of hyperlipidemia. New Eng. J. Med. *284*:186, 1971.
24. Lewis, L. A., Brown, H. B., and Page, I. H.: Ten years treatment of hyperlipidemia. Circulation *38*(IV):128, 1968.
25. Morgan, F., and Moore, F. B.: Personal communication.
26. Streuter, M.: Personal communication.
27. Fritz, S. H., and Walker, W. J.: Ileal bypass in the control of intractable hypercholesterolemia. Amer. Surgeon *32*:691, 1966.
28. Swan, D. M., and McGowan, J. M.: Ileal bypass in hypercholesterolemia associated with heart disease. Amer. J. Surg. *116*:22, 1968.
29. Miettinen, T.: Proceedings of the Second International Symposium on Atherosclerosis, 1970, p. 304; also personal communication.
30. Helsingen, N., Jr., and Rootwelt, K.: Partial ileal bypass for surgical treatment of hypercholesterolemia. Nord. Med. *7*:1414, 1969.
31. Sodal, G., Gjertsen, K. T., and Schrumpf, A.: Surgical treatment of hypercholesterolemia. Acta Chir. Scand. *136*:671, 1970.
32. Health, Education and Welfare: Serum cholesterol levels of adults: U.S.A. 1960–1962. Vital and Health Statistics Series 11, #22, 1967.
33. Cornfield, J.: Joint dependence of risk of coronary heart disease on serum cholesterol and systolic blood pressure. A discriminant function analysis. Fed. Proc. *21*(II):58, 1962.

A Skeptical View of a National Diet Program

NORTON SPRITZ

New York University School of Medicine

Considerable indirect evidence suggests that the occurrence of atherosclerotic disease could be decreased in the United States were we to institute changes in the pattern of national food intake. This body of evidence has led to several recommendations for extensive alterations of the nation's diet. Such large scale changes in a nation's diet have serious economic and biological implications and require for their justification at least three conditions: the disease process to be prevented has to represent an extreme risk to the population; a role for diet in its genesis or as a preventative measure has to be established by a convincing body of consistent evidence; and finally, the nature of the dietary deletions and/or additions likely to produce the desired effect has to be clearly established. In considering these criteria for a national diet policy for the prevention of atherosclerotic disease, the first requirement is certainly met. In my view, however, sufficient doubt exists concerning the other two to make unwarranted at this time a recommendation on a national scale.

One type of information that supports the idea that if we ate differently we would have less vascular disease derives from comparisons of dietary intake among population groups with different rates of atherosclerotic disease. The most recently published study[1] of this type is a carefully executed survey of the eating patterns and other environmental factors among men in seven population groups that have a wide variation in the occurrence rate of coronary heart disease. As has been less rigorously shown in other studies, there is a significant association between the per cent of dietary intake as saturated fat, the plasma cholesterol concentration, and the prevalence and incidence of cardiovascular disease among these seven groups. Deaths from all causes, however, showed a far less clear association with dietary patterns. The Japanese, Italian, and American groups had comparable overall death rates, but their intake of saturated fat varied from 3 to 18 per cent of total calories—essentially the entire range of the seven groups under study.

In addition to uncertainties about the relationship between diet and overall death rates among nations, there are other questions about the relevance of studies of different populations to recommendations for dietary change in a single population. Recommendations based on this type of information are based on the assumption that environmental factors that are important in atherogenesis in one culture are equally important in another. Direct evidence exists that this, indeed, may not be the case. For example, the striking importance of cigarette smoking as a risk factor for coronary artery disease has been repeatedly established in the United States.[2, 3] Yet in many other countries with both low and high incidences of vascular disease, smoking is unrelated to such disease.[1] This discrepancy among nations remains unexplained but provides serious reservations about the validity of altering an environmental factor as a preventative measure in one country on the basis of its correlation with vascular disease among different population groups.

Even more direct evidence exists that dietary factors, which may correlate among nations with their rates of vascular disease, are not important determinants of disease within a single country. Differences in dietary intake as a correlative factor with the risk of vascular disease have not been identified within any single population group. For example, in a prospective study of the diets of approximately 1000 people in Framingham, Massachusetts,[4] neither cholesterol content, the amount or type of fat, nor total calories were different in those who did and did not develop coronary heart disease during the eight-year prospective study. In sum, this and similar studies fail to support the idea that dietary intake plays an important role in determining either the level of plasma lipids or risk of vascular disease.

This conclusion has been attacked on the basis that all members of populations like that of Framingham have a similar and excessively high intake of cholesterol and saturated fat and, for that reason, a selective effect of diet cannot be established. While this contention may be true, there is within that population a wide range of plasma cholesterol concentrations (from approximately 150 to 300 mg. per cent), with an associated three-fold difference in risk of developing coronary heart disease between those with the highest and lowest levels. This wide variation in cholesterol concentration, with its concomitant variation in risk of heart disease, forms the very basis for the recommendation to lower plasma cholesterol. Yet, the best information today indicates that this variation in cholesterol concentration results from factors other than diet and does not provide support for the idea that a cholesterol-lowering diet would affect the occurrence of vascular disease.

Of all sources of information, perhaps most pertinent to the question of a national diet recommendation is the group of investigations in which diets have been manipulated in order to determine whether such alterations affect the occurrence of vascular disease. I should like to focus consideration in this discussion on three such studies, each of which has been carefully carried out over a long period, and each of which is generally considered to support the idea that diet alterations will prevent vascular disease. In at least two of the three, those of Dayton et al. in Los Angeles[5] and Leren in Norway,[6] a similar pattern emerges —subjects receiving the cholesterol-lowering diet had an apparently lower incidence of new vascular disease, but with no significant effect (for eight and 11 years in the two studies, respectively) on total mortality.

For several reasons, mortality, rather than incidence of new manifestations of atherosclerotic disease, is the critical determinant when one considers these studies in relationship to the question of a national dietary recommendation. Apparent effects of the dietary manipulation on parameters other than mortality are more subject to uncertainties that derive from differences in experimental design and diagnostic criteria. This problem in interpretation of morbidity data is pointed up by distinct qualitative differences in the protection afforded by the diet in the treatment of groups in the two studies under consideration. In the Norwegian study the occurrence of angina was lower in the treatment group and provided the bulk of data supporting the idea that diet protected against heart disease. In the Los Angeles study, on the other hand, there was no effect on this manifestation of heart disease. In the Norwegian study protection was shown in subjects who had had a myocardial infarction prior to their entry into the study; in the Los Angeles study those with prior vascular disease obtained no protection from the diet. In fact, the most clearly similar finding between these two studies, which together involved a total of over 1000 men followed for from eight to 11 years, was that at no time in either study was the death rate in the treated group significantly less than that in controls.

The most recently published study[7] is of a different design in that the study groups were institutionalized in two hospitals and the cholesterol-lowering diet was administered to the patients in one hospital, and then after six years, the other. Comparisons were then made for each hospital between its control and experimental period. Whereas in this study the incidence of new coronary heart disease and mortality from heart disease were found to be lower during the experimental periods, total mortality was not affected at all in women and insignificantly in men.

The inability to convincingly alter total mortality in the large number of persons involved in these studies requires very careful consideration before making a national diet recommendation. In two of these studies the subjects were middle-aged and older men with and without evidence of ischemic heart disease—a group in which any significant effect on atherosclerotic disease should have been reflected by decreased mortality at some time during the study. In the study in Los Angeles the deaths from vascular disease that were apparently prevented by diet were offset by an increase in deaths from neoplastic disease. This observation was not borne out in a compilation of five studies in which dietary alterations had been carried out,[8] but the compilation also showed that, even when large numbers are analyzed together, a significant effect of the cholesterol-lowering diet on mortality is not seen.

The uncertain effects of diet alteration on total mortality stands in contrast to studies in which other risk factors, notably smoking and hypertension, have been manipulated. Essentially without exception, examinations of overall mortality in ex-smokers shows their rates to be lower than those in current smokers and similar to those who have never smoked.[9] The differences in mortality between the smokers and nonsmokers are severalfold and are independent of blood pressure or plasma cholesterol concentration. Similarly, in a study of the effect of treatment for five years on moderate hypertension involving 380 men, total mortality in the untreated group was more than twice that in the treated group.[10]

Like those concerning cholesterol-lowering diets, the studies of changes in smoking and blood pressure may not be considered conclusive. They do, however, provide considerably more evidence than do the studies on diet that programs on a national scale aimed to decrease smoking and to treat hypertension would result in favorable effects on mortality. It is certainly possible that more studies in which diet is manipulated would provide a similarly stronger basis for a national diet policy. Even more likely, diet alterations instituted earlier in life might have an important effect on death rate. Yet, given the data available today, at the very least it is evident that recommendations to the population that they stop smoking cigarettes and that they participate in a program to detect and treat hypertension can be made with considerably more assurance than those concerning diet.

Interpretation of diet studies and considerations of a national diet recommendation are confounded further by uncertainties about the composition of an ideal diet. Decrease in saturated fats, increase in polyunsaturated fats, decrease in cholesterol in the diet can all be shown to decrease plasma cholesterol concentration. In general, available evidence suggests that the diet changes are additive in their effect on plasma cholesterol concentration. In the diet studies cited previously, all these alterations were utilized in the experimental diet. Present recommendations focus on decrease in saturated fat and a decrease in dietary cholesterol, with only modest increase in polyunsaturated fats. This decrease in cholesterol-lowering potential in the presently recommended diet from that used in diet trials makes these trials an even less certain basis for the proposed national diet recommendations. The elimination of recommended changes in polyunsaturated fats as a part of a lipid-lowering dietary program derives from the fact that high polyunsaturated fat intake is not the dietary pattern of any large population group and its safety in the long term is yet to be established. While this precaution represents sound policy, it also weakens the cholesterol-lowering effect of diet programs and concomitantly, at least in theory, its potential for the prevention of atherosclerotic disease. The effects on heart disease and overall mortality of diets with low cholesterol and decreased saturated fat (with only minor manipulation of the polyunsaturate content) are unestablished, since well controlled studies specifically designed to investigate this question have not been carried out.

The magnitude of the fall in plasma cholesterol that would be seen as a result of a national program is also an important uncertainty. In most of the investigations in which small study groups have been given cholesterol-lowering diets in a controlled trial, decreases of 15 to 20 per cent have been achieved in the treatment group. The quantitative effect of the removal of large amounts of polyunsaturated fat from the diet program remains unknown. In a large study designed to establish the feasibility of diet change on a large scale in a healthy population,[11] degree of change in plasma cholesterol was considerably smaller than in those considered previously, even with diets with high polyunsaturated content as well as low cholesterol and saturated fat intake. In fact, in that study, weight loss per se had an effect almost equivalent to that produced by qualitative changes in diet. The subjects receiving cholesterol-lowering diets whose weights did not change during the year of diet trial had only an 8.2 per cent fall in cholesterol compared to 5.4 per cent fall for those given a control diet, but in whom weight loss did occur. This study, which involved several thousand participants, provides little basis for a diet recommendation on a large scale for the lowering of plasma cholesterol other than a decrease in total caloric intake.

Finally, the focus of recommendations for an alteration in the national diet has been limited to plasma cholesterol without consideration of the importance of plasma triglyceride. Although the data have more uncertainties, it now seems clear that higher levels of triglyceride,[12] at least as frequently as those of cholesterol, are associated independently with increased risk of vascular disease.[13] The presently recommended cholesterol-lowering diets are quite different from those that would be recommended to the nation or to an individual were lowering triglyceride the goal of the dietary intervention.[14] Decrease in total calories without specific qualitative changes might be the most important part of a program directed to the lowering of triglyceride. Carbohydrate restriction, either in toto or by the interdiction of specific sugars, has been shown to lower triglyceride[14] and, although a controversial issue, deserves further trial as a tool for the management of hypertriglyceridemia and the prevention of vascular disease.

It is tempting to conclude that, in spite of all the uncertainties outlined in this discussion, the established statistical association between plasma cholesterol concentration and vascular disease and the ability to lower cholesterol by dietary means, provide together sufficient basis for a national diet recommendation even in the absence of a more direct basis for such a decision. One needn't look beyond the area of prevention of atherosclerotic disease, however, for a recommendation, based on similarly convincing indirect evidence, that appears to be incorrect as more information has been accumulated. The higher incidence of vascular disease in men than in women, and the loss of this differential in women after menopause and the favorable effect of estrogens on lipoprotein patterns, taken together, provided a seemingly unassailable basis for recommendations for the widespread administration of estrogens to both men and postmenopausal women in order to prevent vascular disease. Some of the early trials of estrogen therapy produced data consistent with this recommendation. Yet in the past two decades further support for that idea has not been obtained and, indeed, estrogen administration has produced apparent increase in vascular disease[15, 16] such that present recommendations caution *against* its use in patients at high risk for coronary heart disease.

This discussion should not be interpreted as a plea for inaction in the area of prevention of atherosclerotic disease. On the contrary, a major objection to the institution of a complex and expensive effort to change food intake and to alter patterns of food production on a national scale without adequate experimental support is that such an effort will divert and dilute efforts that should be expended on programs more likely to make an important impact. Such programs should include extensive campaigns to decrease cigarette consumption; to detect and treat higher levels of blood pressure; and to identify persons in whom elevations of cholesterol and/or triglyceride constitute major risk factors and to institute diet or drug therapy appropriate for their specific lipid abnormality.

References

1. Keyes, A. (ed.): Coronary Heart Disease in Seven Countries. American Heart Association. Monograph No. 29, 1970.
2. Doyle, J. T., Dawloen, T. R., Kannell, W. B., et al.: The relationship of cigarette smoking to coronary heart disease. J.A.M.A. *190*:886, 1964.
3. Smoking and Health: Report of the Advisory Committee to the Surgeon General of the Public Health Service. Washington, D.C., U.S. Dept. of Health, Education, and Welfare, Public Health Service Document No. 1103, 1964.
4. Kannell, W. B., and Gordon, T.: U.S. Dept. of Health, Education and Welfare. The Framingham Study. Section 24, The Framingham Diet Study: Diet and the Regulation of Serum Cholesterol, 1970.
5. Dayton, S., Pearce, M. L., et al.: A controlled clinical trial of a diet high in unsaturated fat. Circulation *40*(Suppl.II), 1969.
6. Leren, P.: The Oslo Diet-Heart Study: Eleven year report. Circulation *42*:935, 1970.
7. Miettinen, M., Turpeinen, O., et al.: Effect of cholesterol-lowering diet on mortality from coronary heart disease and other causes. Lancet *2*:835, 1972.
8. Ederer, F., Leren, P., et al.: Cancer among men on cholesterol-lowering diets. Lancet *2*:203, 1971.
9. Kahn, H. A.: The Dorn study of smoking and mortality among U.S. Veterans: Report on 8½ years of observation. *In* Haenszel, M. (ed.): Epidemiological Approaches to the Study of Cancer and Other Diseases. National Cancer Institute, Monograph No. 19, 1966.
10. Veterans Administration Cooperative Study Group on Antihypertensive Agents: Effects of treatment on morbidity in hypertension. II Results in patients with diastolic pressure averaging 90 through 114 mm Hg. J.A.M.A. *213*:1143, 1970.
11. National Diet-Heart Study Research Group: Final Report. Circulation *37*(Suppl.1), 1968.
12. Albrink, M. J., and Man, E. G.: Serum triglycerides in coronary artery disease. Arch. Intern. Med. *103*:4, 1958.
13. Heinle, R. A., Levy, R. I., and Fredrickson, D. S.: Lipid and carbohydrate abnormalities in patients with angiographically documented coronary artery disease. Amer. J. Cardiol. *24*:178, 1969.
14. Julley, S. B., Wilson, W. S., et al.: Lipid and lipoprotein responses of hypertriglyceridemic outpatients to a low carbohydrate modification of the A.H.A. fat-controlled diet. Lancet *2*:55, 1972.
15. The Coronary Drug Project Research Group: The coronary drug project initial findings leading to modification of its research protocol. J.A.M.A. *214*:1303, 1970.
16. Bailar, J. C., III, and Byar, D. P. (VA Cooperative Urological Research Group): Estrogen treatment for cancer of the prostate: Early results with three doses of diethylstilbestrol and placebo. Cancer *26*:257, 1970.

Comment

Prevention of Atherosclerosis

The Editors have tempted me to comment on the accompanying views about prevention of atherosclerosis. The space allotted will do nicely for airing a few prejudices; the reader will not confuse them with reasoned arguments. I am in agreement with Yudkin's minor thesis that causation of coronary heart disease is polyvalent and that a monotonous fare of fats and sterols is unhealthful for experimentalists and theorists alike. But I am inclined to think his "sucrose hypothesis" is too simply concocted and lacking in substance. The available evidence linking insulin, sugar and steroid hormones to vascular decay cannot match the weight of experimental support for the "lipid infiltrative theory." Dock, a steadfast prophet of the latter faith, finds confirmation in signs that will not convert all skeptics. I am not sure, for example, that chylomicrons and low density lipoproteins have comparable effects on the intima. With no offense meant to valued co-workers, I also feel that the design of the Zelis experiments in Type III patients was not sufficient to prove the regression of atheromas. But like Dock, I believe that lipoprotein concentration is a prime determinant of the rate of atheroma formation, that hyperlipidemia should therefore be controlled, and by means that are not the same for all patients. Buchwald and Varco insist that therapy for some of these patients should be surgery; and I say, amen, for *some*.

Among most of us, then, there is shared a conclusion that the evidence is sufficient to encourage the testing of radical diets, or drugs, or intestinal bypasses, provided the subjects are middle-aged, with coronary artery disease and supra-average cholesterols. Spritz articulates well the cautions against allowing the spirit of intervention to lead us into tampering with the diets of the young and still healthy. They are the orthodox views, made tolerable by the promise of definitive knowledge to come. I am afraid, however, that the experiment that removes all doubt about the efficacy of changing the national menu probably will never be done. My prejudices lie with Malmros, although I would excuse infants from his prescription until we learn that filled milks are as good for the brain as the arteries. Since the rest of the children already know all about the birds and the bees, I think it's time we told them about the corn and the cow. Perhaps, after "health steak" (New Engl. J. Med. 288:415, 1973) is on every menu, and the aggravation of the intima by lipids has been brought to a communal minimum, we can get down to the real cause(s) of atherosclerosis.

DONALD S. FREDRICKSON

9

The Place of IPPB in the Management of Chronic Obstructive Lung Disease

IPPB Is a Useful Modality in the Treatment of Chronic Obstructive Lung Disease
   by Robert L. Mayock

The Dangers and Limitations of IPPB in Managing Diseases Affecting Ventilation
   by R. Drew Miller and Norman G. G. Hepper

Comment
   by Richard V. Ebert

IPPB Is a Useful Modality in the Treatment of Chronic Obstructive Lung Disease

ROBERT L. MAYOCK

Hospital of the University of Pennsylvania, Cardio-Pulmonary Division

The use of intermittent positive pressure breathing (IPPB) in chronic obstructive pulmonary disease (COPD) has been controversial since its original introduction in 1947 by Motley et al.,[1] and this controversy has continued until today. IPPB is accepted universally in certain areas of therapy since it is the method that characterizes most of the ventilators in current use for total respiratory support, as well as those used for the treatment of chronic bronchitis, emphysema, and asthma. No one would seriously challenge its role in respiratory failure, but many question its value in the diseases mentioned above. To appraise its usefulness fairly one must first define what is meant by IPPB and then evaluate the evidence for and against its use in COPD.

Intermittent positive pressure breathing is defined as the use of positive pressure to inflate the lungs regularly during either inspiration or apnea. This technique has been employed for ventilation in respiratory arrest and hypoventilation; to support the chest wall in crush injuries; to promote deep breathing in patients after surgery when pain, anesthesia, or sedation may cause limitation of motion and disappearance of sighing; to rest fatigued respiratory muscles in asthma or when lungs are stiffened as a result of pulmonary edema or fibrosis; to increase available air for coughing in patients with paradoxical rib cage motion and flat diaphragms; and to limit fluid transudation in pulmonary edema. In addition to the foregoing mechanical functions, it is also used to deliver aerosols of water, saline, catecholamines, mucolytic agents, and other drugs, as well as to give varied concentrations of oxygen.

IPPB, literally defined, includes mouth-to-mouth resuscitation and "bagging" with hand-squeezed bags for ventilation, as well as ventilation by standard respirators. By usage, however, it is usually limited to the mechanical demand type techniques (Bird, Bennett, Mine Safety Apparatus (MSA) Ventilators) or hand operated ventilators (Hand-E-Vent).

IPPB must be considered separately from positive-negative respiration, in which a negative phase is added during expiration, and continuous positive pressure breathing (CPPB) and positive end-expiratory breathing (PEEP), in which some positive pressure is also maintained during expiration. Positive end-expiratory pressure (PEEP) is used to supplement IPPB, producing continuous positive pressure breathing (CPPB), thus extending our methodology for the therapy of widespread pneumonia, shock lung, pulmonary edema, and other disseminated pulmonary diseases. IPPB, with its more sophisticated developments in the form of ventilators and anesthesia machines, has enabled us to treat many pulmonary conditions formerly not amenable to therapy.

The machines in use today are the result of extensive experimentation, beginning in the 1930's and continuing during World War II and the postwar period. The physiological studies of Rahn, Fenn, Chadwick and Otis,[2-4] who defined the pressure-volume relationships of the lung, and the work of Cournand, Motley, Werko and Richards[5] delineating the hemodynamic effects of IPPB, have laid the physiological groundwork for the technology required to develop this technique.

In presenting my rationale for using IPPB in chronic lung disease, I would like first to review the physiological background of IPPB and the abnormalities present in COPD. I will then discuss the therapeutic approaches that are commonly used to correct these abnormalities and consider the role of IPPB in therapy of COPD. Since complications can occur with this form of therapy and since technique of administration is important for proper results as well as to avoid complications, these topics will be reviewed also.

Physiological Background

Normal tidal respiration is accomplished by the contraction of the muscles of the thorax and diaphragm, reducing the mean negative intrapleural pressure of -5 cm. of water to -10 cm. of water. This increase in gradient causes the flow of tidal volume into the lungs and increases venous return and output of the right heart. Because of opening of lung capillaries, less blood goes to the left heart so that the output of the left heart and systemic blood pressure fall for several beats. During expiration the passive recoil of the thorax causes the intrathoracic pressure to rise, resulting in expiration of the tidal volume, less venous return, decreased output of the right heart, and the emptying of the blood from the lung vessels into the left heart. This causes an increased output of the left heart and rise in systemic blood pressure for several beats.

With increased tidal volumes, airway obstruction, and stiffening of the lungs, greater muscle action during inspiration and active and forceful contraction during expiration are required. The work of breathing is dependent on the degree of activity of the muscles of inspiration and expiration.

IPPB markedly changes and modifies the above patterns. In the relaxed individual, the positive pressure in the airways is transmitted to the alveoli and intrathoracic contents during inspiration, resulting in a flow of air and decreased venous return to the right heart, fall in output of the right heart, and rise in peripheral venous pressure. When the pressure is cycled off, the intrapulmonary and intrathoracic pressures fall with flow of air from the lungs and flow of blood into the thoracic cavity. The air flow is due to elastic recoil of the lungs, which is usually passive, even in patients with COPD. Thus, little muscle effort is ordinarily required in properly administered IPPB.

The amount of pressure required to produce ventilation depends on the volume sought, the degree of airway obstruction, and the compliance (distensibility) of the lungs. Pressure measurements in IPPB are made and regulated at the mask. When airway obstruction is high or the lungs are stiff, the mask pressure may be much higher than the intrathoracic pressure because a large part of the pressure is dissipated in overcoming frictional air flow resistance in obstructive disease and viscous tissue resistance in stiff lungs. Thus, in airway obstruction the circulatory effects are considerably less than might be anticipated since the intrathoracic pressure changes may be relatively small compared to those that occur normally.[6] However, if the positive pressure is sustained, cardiac output falls as a result of the continued high intrathoracic pressure, which results in decreased venous return. Cournand et al.[5] found the best cardiac return was present when the mask and intrabronchial pressures built up gradually, the peak dropped rapidly to ambient levels after cycling, and expiration was maintained as long as inspiration.

When combined with expiratory pressure elevation, the circulatory effects described above may be aggravated with a marked and often serious drop in blood pressure. This formerly major limiting complication of IPPB used with positive expiratory pressure is now relatively easy to overcome by increasing the blood volume with colloid or blood products, thus producing an increased venous pressure with an adequate gradient from the peripheral veins to the right heart, permitting flow with satisfactory filling.

The ventilators commonly used are either "pressure-cycled" or "volume-cycled." In the former, the machine shuts off when a preset mask pressure is reached; in the latter, when a predetermined volume of gas is delivered. The pressure-cycled respirators are more satisfactory in the conscious patient, who is thus permitted to change his breathing pattern without too great discomfort. The volume-cycled respirators are most effective in intubated patients in coma or precoma, since the patient will receive the preset volume, irrespective of his own pattern of breathing and the level of airway resistance. Most of the present respirators can be "time-cycled" also, in that they may be operated on patient demand or at a variety of rates from two per minute to 60 per minute.

An important feature of respirators is "flow control." It can be shown theoretically[7] and experimentally[8] that rapid rates of flow (100 L./min. or more) result in poor delivery of gas to airways with partial obstruction because of increased turbulence at the areas of narrowing, which produces slowing of flow to these areas. Slower flow rates (15 L./min. or less), produce less turbulence and better gas distribution in partially obstructed airways. Theoretically the slowest flow tolerated produces the best distribution, the major limiting factor being the length of time required before the patient requires the next breath.

INSPIRATORY PRESSURE

Measurement of the pressure of inspiration is made at the mask as stated and does not represent intrathoracic pressure or even pressure lower in the airways. Ordinarily pressures of 10 to 20 cm. of water produce an augmented tidal volume without abnormal sensation and with no apparent lung damage. Higher pressures are sometimes used, usually with intubated patients and in patients with markedly increased resistance and respiratory failure. Pneumothorax may occur if the pressure is much in excess of 40 cm. of water; beyond 20 cm. of water, the patient also may have frightening sensations.

With these pressure levels, little inspiratory muscle activity is ordinarily required, and by having the patient concentrate on expiration, the hyperinflation that sometimes occurs can be avoided.

The ventilators usually deliver compressed gas, which is dry and will result in mucosal desiccation and irritation unless humidified. Humidification has been achieved by a variety of nebulizers that add water and medication as desired to the air stream. The nebulizers are highly efficient and may provide one of the major benefits of IPPB therapy, since they begin with the first air movement and provide continuous medication during the entire inspiratory cycle in such a way that there is little the patient can do advertently or inadvertently to thwart delivery of the nebulized solution.

The gas used to ventilate the patient usually is composed either of air or air with varying percentages of oxygen up to 100. These concentrations are difficult to vary in some machines, and in others the concentrations are very unreliable, going far beyond the stated range, thus making the patient susceptible to oxygen toxicity.

The sensitivity of the machine must be set to allow the patient's negative pressure of inspiration to trigger the machine easily, yet not have the machine start unexpectedly, causing anxiety.

Thus, the effects of IPPB on the individual patient depend technically on the type of machine employed, the sensitivity of triggering, flow pattern and flow rate, mask pressure, per cent oxygen, nebulized solutions and medications, and use of expiratory positive pressure.

PATIENT AND HIS DISEASE

The patient and his disease also have major effects on the physiological consequences. The state of consciousness, presence or absence of apprehension, willingness to cooperate, ability to relax, presence of bronchial secretions, presence of bronchospasm, presence of bronchial narrowing and collapse, presence of lung stiffening and edema, paradoxical chest wall and diaphragmatic motion—all have important effects on the patient's therapeutic response. Many of the disparities in the reported results of therapy could conceivably be due to these variables either in technique or patient selection.

Patient's Mental State

As stated, there is general acceptance of the value of IPPB in ventilating the unconscious or comatose patient who cannot be encouraged to breathe spontaneously. Patients with chronic obstructive lung disease who are in precoma can often be ventilated reasonably well by IPPB with proper attention on the part of the therapist. A major factor in the production of hypoventilation in many of these patients is muscular fatigue brought on by high airway resistance. If the patient is able to relax properly, muscle rest can be achieved during the period of ventilation. If the machine is used 15 minutes out of each hour, enough rest will usually be provided for muscle recovery from fatigue. In the presence of anxiety, marked increase in metabolic rate results in increased CO_2 production and oxygen demand, with an overall unfavorable response to therapy. If the patient actually resists or opposes the action of the machine, a dramatic worsening may occur.[9] In patients with psychological problems, the use of the nose clip, placing of the mouthpiece, sound of the gas and sensation of inflation of the mouth, chest, and eustachian tubes may all produce anxiety with rejection of therapy. IPPB, therefore, requires a considerate, patient, and verbal therapist, who is able to demonstrate and explain the technique he is employing before starting, and who can avoid or manage patient concern.

Pathophysiological Abnormalities in COPD

Before consideration of the effects of IPPB on chronic obstructive lung disease, it will be necessary to outline briefly the principal abnormalities found in this condition. The term "COPD" has been applied[10] to a group of patients who in reality represent a composite of several clinical pictures, having in common the presence of airway obstruction without proved allergy or other specific infectious or chemical cause. The presence or absence of a bronchitis with cough and/or sputum serves to separate the patients into three groups. One may see bronchitis alone, bronchitis with emphysema, and emphysema with little or no bronchitis. All three groups show an obstructive picture clinically and by pulmonary function testing. A better therapeutic response would be anticipated and is found in the patients with bronchitis since many elements of bronchitis are treatable and have reversible pathophysiological abnormalities. Emphysema with none of the elements of bronchitis has been found to have fewer abnormalities and less of an ability to respond to any modality of therapy.

The presence of an allergic component also has functional and therapeutic implications. At times patients who appear to have chronic obstructive lung disease will respond dramatically to sympathomimetic drugs and corticosteroids, suggesting an unrecognized allergy that might either serve as the primary cause or act as an additional pathogenetic mechanism in these patients.

In discussing the pathophysiological abnormalities that are present in chronic obstructive pulmonary disease, it is helpful to consider them in terms of the findings in bronchitis and of those associated with emphysema.

Chronic bronchitis is by definition a chronic daily cough that is present a minimum of three months in a year for not less than two successive years.[10] Early in its course there may be scant or moderate sputum production, and as the disease progresses the cough becomes more productive, with evidence of airway obstruction such as wheezing and shortness of breath on exercise. Physical signs of bronchial, bronchiolar, and pulmonary infection such as coarse rales, fine rales, and changes in breath and voice sounds may be found as the disease progresses.

With increasing bronchiolar involvement, destruction of neighboring alveoli, more obstruction, and ventilation-perfusion abnormalities with hypoxia and hypercarbia may result. As the obstructive component progresses, hypoventilation may occur, due at least in part to the greatly increased work of breathing with muscular fatigue. The "blue bloater" group appears to have less ventilatory response to increased carbon dioxide tension and decreased oxygen concentration and allows these abnormalities to develop with relatively few symptoms of respiratory distress. Cor pulmonale with right heart failure is seen earlier in this group because of the effect of the abnormal blood gases on the pulmonary vasculature, producing spasm of the pulmonary arterial tree. Spread of infection to the pulmonary parenchyma, bronchiectasis, and atelectasis are common late occurrences in these patients.

The patient with pure emphysema essentially has destruction of the alveoli with loss of bronchiolar support, beginning with little or no clinical evidence of bronchitis. The prototype of this condition is that of emphysema seen in association with alpha-1 antitrypsin deficiency, which usually begins insidiously with shortness of breath on exercise as its primary manifestation of airway obstruction and progresses to marked dyspnea even at rest and eventual death of the patient with cor pulmonale. Bronchitis is usually seen terminally when the patient becomes unable to clear the tracheobronchial tree satisfactorily because of the obstructed airways, and infection supervenes.

Many of these individuals preserve a good response to hypoxia and hypercarbia and will ventilate adequately in spite of greatly increased work of breathing. This type of fighting response in patients has earned them the title of "pink puffers." The pathophysiological changes in the patients with relatively pure emphysema are those of loss of lung tissue with few important reversible components.

An unanticipated response to bronchodilators is seen at times in these patients; it might be explained by the release of bronchial tone that is present, even in normal individuals, thus improving air flow. However, patients with this type of COPD usually respond poorly or not at all to all the modes of therapy employed.

One should hasten to note that the vast majority of patients present with some combination of the elements of bronchitis and emphysema with enough of a bronchitic component to make therapy worthwhile.

Therapeutic Approaches in COPD

The elements of both conditions susceptible to improvement by modern therapy are: (1) bronchial irritation of a physiochemical nature due to smoke, dust, fumes, and gases which results in edema, spasm, and mucus production; (2) bronchial infection with mucosal edema, bronchospasm, bronchial erosion, and excessive secretions; (3) hypoxia caused by ventilation-perfusion abnormalities and hypoventilation; (4) hypercarbia from the same processes as hypoxia; (5) cor pulmonale secondary to hypoxia and hypercarbia; (6) muscular fatigue from a chronic or acute increase in the work of breathing; and (7) polycythemia from hypoxia. In addition, if one accepts an allergic component in some of these patients, (8) bronchial allergy must be added to the treatable aspects of chronic lung disease.

It is possible to employ a wide variety of therapeutic modes for patients with this diverse group of pathophysiological abnormalities. It should be noted that it is rare for any patient to present with a single abnormality that responds to a single mode of therapy, so that since one is faced with multiple abnormalities, most of the patients require a regimen of several modes of therapy. The setting up of controlled studies of IPPB therapy has been difficult, in large part owing to the varied associated measures that are concomitantly employed by the various investigators.

I would like to consider the modes of therapy in common use for the above abnormalities.

Bronchial irritation. Removal of all air pollutants, particularly use of or exposure to tobacco. It is particularly important to avoid all smoke and smoking since the effect of one cigarette on increasing airway resistance can be demonstrated for four hours. Also, as with alcohol, few people are able to confine themselves to an "occasional" use. Use of air conditioning, proper humidification, and dust and pollen removal are important.

Bronchial infection. Control of infection by use of antibiotics based on cultures. Prevention of infection by chemoprophylaxis with broad spectrum antibiotics (tetracycline and ampicillin).

Mucosal edema. Shrinkage of mucosal edema with vasoconstrictors (epinephrine, phenylephrine) given by nebulizer (hand, gas, or propellant operated) or given by IPPB.

Excessive secretions. These are often most difficult to remove. Physical therapy, IPPB, nasotracheal suction, bronchoscopy, nasotracheal intubation, or tracheostomy with suction have all been employed. Mucolytic agents (N-acetylcysteine) have been used to aid in the liquefaction of mucus, and enzymes (pancreatic dornase) have been given to liquefy purulent secretions.

Bronchial spasm. This may be attacked with oral ephedrine and oral, rectal, or intravenous theophylline, as well as the commonly employed nebulized catecholamines given by nebulizer or IPPB.

Ventilation-perfusion abnormalities. These respond to some extent to general improvement in the airways. IPPB improves distribution of gas by promoting deeper breathing, by aiding in bronchodilatation and by helping with removal of secretions. Physical therapy is also used to promote deep breathing and to aid in removal of secretions.

Hypoxia. Hypoxia usually can be accurately corrected by administering the proper concentration of inspired oxygen. Since oxygen toxicity is a major threat, inspired concentrations should be limited to those that produce a physiological blood gas level (PO_2 65 to 80 mm. Hg). Controlled oxygen therapy can be administered by Venturi mask, nasal catheter, nasal prongs, or IPPB.

Hypercarbia. Hypercarbia can be corrected only by improving the state of the airways and concomitantly the V'Q abnormality or by hyperventilation employing breathing exercises, IPPB, or intubation with ventilation.

Cor pulmonale and right heart failure. These respond best to treatment of blood gas abnormalities, but diuretics, low salt diet, and digitalis compounds also help.

Muscle fatigue. This ordinarily requires mechanical assistance to rest the muscles of respiration. Some form of IPPB is necessary if the other pathophysiological abnormalities causing fatigue (i.e., increased airway resistance or decreased compliance) cannot be corrected rapidly.

Polycythemia. Polycythemia may respond to improvement in blood oxygen tension or can be treated by phlebotomy.

Allergy. Steroid therapy is effective in relieving the allergic component if such exists and, in addition, should reduce inflammatory edema and exudation from infection.

Evaluation of the Role of IPPB in Therapy of COPD

From the foregoing it can be seen that IPPB should rarely be used alone, but rather in conjunction with other forms of therapy. The results obtained with IPPB in the individual patient are dependent on the type of disease the patient has, the machine employed, the settings used, the type of nebulized solutions and medications employed, the skill of the therapist, the proper use of supplemental oxygen, and the associated therapy employed. Patient selection is of major importance. It might be predicted that the patient with moderately severe emphysema with little or no cough or sputum and no evidence of bronchospasm by pulmonary function testing would do very poorly unless muscular fatigue, secondary infection, or respiratory discoordination has developed.

Evaluation of therapy for COPD has been difficult for many reasons. Of the studies performed, none are comparable in patient selection, controls, method of therapy, type of adjuvant therapy, and types of equipment employed. As Gaensler and Graham note,[11] subjective improvement is a particularly unreliable criterion because these patients with chronic, progressive disabling disease respond favorably to encouragement, moral support, and frequent care. Controlled studies with placebo or sham therapy result in subjective response. They also emphasize that the diurnal, daily, and seasonal variation in these patients is extremely large because of infections, allergic, and cardiac components. Two extensive reviews[12, 13] of the experimental basis for IPPB are available and both emphasize the extreme variability of the findings of the various investigators. It would be quite easy to present a battery of scientific reports defending this mode of therapy, as well as attacking it. Unfortunately any "definitive" article on the role of IPPB in COPD sought by the general internist and house officer, either pro or con, has been contradicted shortly by articles presenting an opposing point of view.

Which of the therapeutic actions of IPPB have acceptance and what is the basis of this acceptance?

Administration of Nebulized Bronchodilator and Vasoconstrictor Medications

One of the most important therapeutic effects of IPPB results from its ability to deliver aerosolized medications. Sheldon[12] has reviewed the reports from the literature which present evidence in favor of, or which are opposed to, this form of nebulization compared to various other forms. He concluded that in those reports of failure to obtain more satisfactory results from IPPB, the authors used high flow rates, or failed to dilute medications so as to avoid systemic side effects and chemical bronchitis. In those reports in which these technical problems were not present, IPPB appeared to deliver aerosols in a manner superior to other methods.

Delivery of nebulized solutions using IPPB is more reliable, especially in the senile or confused patient who needs constant instruction for the use of a patient-operated nebulizer, which requires synchronization with inspiration. Once the patient is placed on the machine properly, nebulization begins at the onset of each breath and continues throughout that breath in a way that is impossible for the patient to avoid unless he removes the mouthpiece from his mouth.

Effects on Ventilation

There is little argument today that IPPB can affect respiratory depth and minute volume in COPD.[14, 15] The increased ventilation occurs whether the patient has been intubated or breathes with a mask or oral tube. In the obstructed patient this increase may require a high inspiratory pressure with its potential effect on the circulation, but ordinarily results in better alveolar ventilation, with removal of carbon dioxide and better oxygenation. In patients with flattened diaphragms and paradoxical rib motion, IPPB reverses the inspiratory retraction of the lower thoracic cage and produces more effective ventilation in this area.

Following use of the ventilator, the patient will return to his former pattern of respiration unless other benefits of the therapy have resulted, such as improved cerebration from better arterial PO_2 and PCO_2, bronchodilation, and return of muscle strength as a result of rest. Better distribution of air has been reported with IPPB,[16] but this results from the greater depth of respiration rather than from the pressure per se. Improved distribution reduces right to left shunting of blood and improves oxygenation, and the deeper breathing also should combat the fall in compliance and right to left shunting seen with small tidal volumes ("microatelectasis").

Flow rate control has been found to be critical in producing adequate ventilation in patients with obstructive lung disease. Untoward effects were noted,[9, 17] with failure to improve tidal volume, respiratory rate, oxygen saturation, PCO_2, and pH when patients were ventilated with high flow rates. These same effects were not reported when using lower flow rates.[13] Both in acute and chronic studies,[14, 15] IPPB given with slow flow, without bronchodilators, and using compressed air was able to produce lowering of PCO_2 in patients with COPD.

Airway resistance can be improved by IPPB in animals and normal subjects, probably by dilatation from the positive pressure,[18] but only if thoracic volume is increased by the treatment.[19] Since airway obstruction is the major feature of COPD, all patients show a high resistance to rapid air flow, probably as a result of turbulence developing in the areas of narrowing, secretions, and spasm. Airway resistance is also dependent on the rate at which lungs are changing volume. Mead et al.[8] have shown that rapid breathing increased resistance and caused a drop in compliance. They also demonstrated that, with slower flow rates, airway resistance was markedly less. Thus, slow flow is a most important aspect of the use of IPPB.

Respiratory fatigue

In COPD the muscular work required to produce a given rate of flow is much greater than in normals[8, 20] because of the obstructive phenomena previously noted. Positive pressure may replace the energy required from the muscles of respiration not only for the extra work but also for part of the normal work of breathing. If a greater inflation is achieved, expiration will begin at a larger lung volume, which increases the force of retraction of the lung and chest wall and decreases airway resistance, thus reducing expiratory work also.[20, 21] In a relaxed, normal individual, the work of breathing during IPPB approaches zero; however, some oxygen utilization may occur as a result of the basal metabolism of the muscles of respiration and the effect of stretching on muscle. The bulk of evidence seems to indicate that IPPB can cause marked reduction of the work of breathing in COPD in the relaxed, cooperative patient, with correctly adjusted pressure and flow settings. This patient attitude may be difficult to achieve and requires skill on the part of the therapist. The work of breathing can be increased to the point of patient exhaustion[22] if either the therapy is incorrectly performed or the patient does not relax.

Many of the therapeutic failures are the result of adverse reactions to IPPB, and correct use of this therapy must involve understanding of these problems.

Adverse Responses to IPPB

Carbon dioxide narcosis. This has been induced with oxygen-driven machines in patients with severe COPD, disappearing when therapy was stopped or air employed as the energy source. The increased oxygen tension reduces chemoreceptor drive to respiration, thus contributing to hypoventilation and producing increased PCO_2. For this reason air is the best gas to use unless some form of monitoring is employed to ensure physiological blood gas levels. If supplemental oxygen is needed, blood gases should be measured to ensure the effectiveness of the inspired concentrations.

Decreased cardiac output. Decreased cardiac output with production of shock can largely be avoided by the use of ventilators with a sufficiently long expiratory cycle to permit intrathoracic pressure drop and right heart filling and by the use of plasma expanders when indicated, as previously discussed.

Pneumothorax. Pneumothorax occurs rarely if inspiratory pressures are kept in the 10 to 20 cm. of water range. The intra-alveolar pressure may not be greatly increased because of frictional loss in overcoming flow resistance noted above. The risk is greatly increased during intubation with inspiratory mask pressures of 40 cm. of water or more that may be needed with high airway resistance or low compliance.

Sympathomimetic effects. Sympathomimetic effects of the various bronchodilators (isoproterenol, epinephrine) and vasoconstrictors (phenylephrine, epinephrine) may cause major symptoms and cardiac responses. Nervousness, tachycardia, tremor, and CNS stimulation cause patient anxiety, with increased oxygen consumption and CO_2 production. Such reactions oppose any therapeutic benefits of the medications and are aggravated when the patient is on other medications with similar actions (theophylline, ephedrine) during therapy with sympathomimetic amines with or without IPPB. Dysrhythmias are commonly seen in these patients with hypoxia and hypercarbia when given sympathomimetic amines, especially with cor pulmonale and in older patients with arteriosclerosis. The dose of these drugs should be adjusted to avoid this reaction.

Mucosal drying and irritation. This may occur if the inspiratory gas is not adequately humidified or if local irritation occurs from medication. *Bronchospasm* may result from the use of N-acetylcysteine or saline used for humidification without a concomitant bronchodilator.

Marked increase in dyspnea with IPPB. This may be the result of a high inspiratory flow rate. Such rates produce increased turbulence and may actually decrease flow in areas of spasm, edema, and secretions so that no air enters these areas and peripheral pressure builds up, causing the machine to cycle to expiration. This results in further anoxia with increased dyspnea.

This situation requires a decrease in flow rate as the first step for correction. If this fails to decrease dyspnea and no other technical abnormality is noted, therapy should be discontinued.

Nosocomial pneumonia. Nosocomial pneumonia has been reported seconary to bacterial contamination of the equipment and solutions. Contamination of solutions is related to the amount of ambient air bubbled through them, with the mainstream nebulizer being one of the worst offenders. Gram negative bacilli are frequently cultured when sterility precautions have not been properly maintained. Proper, frequent sterilization of equipment with the use of acetic acid or copper ion usually results in control of this particularly frightening complication.

Respiratory alkalosis. This can easily occur in patients with less severe disease and no respiratory acidosis. The marked increase in alveolar ventilation with drop in PCO_2 may produce symptoms and signs of neurological irritability with numbness, tingling, and increased reflexes going to convulsions when not recognized. This has been reported even in patients with advanced respiratory failure.[23] In the alert patient this hyperventilation causes frightening sensations capable of producing anxiety and neutralizing any benefit that might otherwise occur. A trained therapist can detect this by questioning the patient for symptoms, and can treat it by interrupting therapy and allowing the patient to reaccumulate CO_2.

Hypokalemia. Hypokalemia can occur with prolonged ventilation secondary to the rise in pH in a patient who is already depleted of total body potassium secondary to prolonged acidosis and, often, diuretic therapy. Improvement in ventilation and loss of CO_2 requires concomitant monitoring of the serum electrolytes.

Oxygen toxicity. Oxygen toxicity with damage to alveoli is directly related to the inspiratory PO_2 and the duration of therapy. It has been noted during periods of continuous ventilation and has been particularly pronounced in machines using a Venturi oxygen-air mixer that may give high concentrations of oxygen in the presence of high airway resistance or low compliance. However, there is no report to my knowledge showing oxygen toxicity using the 10- to 15-minute treatments ordinarily employed in COPD.

Increased secretion of ADH. This occurs with IPPB as a result of the stimulation of volume receptors in the atria via vagal afferent fibers. Although the possibility of electrolyte imbalance is present with continuous IPPB therapy, no major problems should occur in patients given therapy on a more interrupted basis (10 to 15 minutes every two to eight hours).

A more rapid deterioration of lung function. This deterioration, as shown by decrease in FEV_1, has been reported by Curtis et al.[24] in the chronic use of IPPB in home therapy. However, these authors stated that the respirators were helpful during acute exacerbations of bronchitis or bronchospasm. It is interesting to note "almost all patients stated that IPPB treatment helped them open their air passages and raise secretions." It may be that with repeated inflation, already damaged alveolar septa were further injured by mechanical stretching.

Indications for IPPB Therapy in COPD

IPPB is most likely to be of value and should be tried in those patients with COPD who have one or more of the following abnormalities: bronchitis with secretions, hypoventilation, muscular fatigue, ventilation-perfusion abnormalities, and paradoxical lower costal cage motion. A therapeutic response is less likely in those patients who have mild disease, little or no clinical evidence of bronchitis, normal blood gases, no muscular fatigue, and no evidence of reversibility after bronchodilators shown by pulmonary function testing. However, IPPB should be only part of a therapeutic regimen designed to reverse the many abnormalities that have been described in this condition.

Results of Therapy

Response to treatment may be immediate, with the coughing up of previously retained secretions, decrease in wheezing, improvement in PO_2 and PCO_2, less dyspnea at rest, loss of sense of fatigue, and clearing of obtundation. Therapy may also provide the long-term results of improved exercise tolerance, improvement in cor pulmonale and right heart failure, and loss of chronic respiratory acidosis.

References

1. Motley, H. L., Werko, L., Cournand, A., and Richards, D., Jr.: Observations on the clinical uses of intermittent positive pressure. J. Aviation Med. 18:417, 1947.
2. Otis, A. B., Fenn, W. O., and Rahn, H.: Mechanics of breathing in man. J. Appl. Physiol. 2:592, 1950.
3. Rahn, H., Otis, A. B., Chadwick, L. E., and Fenn, W. O.: The pressure-volume diagram of the thorax and lung. Amer. J. Physiol. 146:161, 1946.
4. Fenn, W. O.: Mechanics of respiration. Amer. J. Med. 10:77, 1951.
5. Cournand, A., Motley, H. L., Richards, D. W., and Werko, L.: Physiological studies of the effects of intermittent positive pressure breathing on cardiac output in man. Amer. J. Physiol. 152:162, 1948.
6. Ambiavager, M., Jones, E. S., and Roberts, D. V.: Intermittent positive pressure ventilation in severe asthma. Anaesthesia 22:134, 1967.
7. Lyager, S.: Influence of flow pattern on the distribution of respiratory air during intermittent positive-pressure ventilation. Acta Anaesth. Scand. 12:191, 1968.
8. Mead, J., Lindgren, I., and Gaensler, E. A.: The mechanical properties of the lungs in emphysema. J. Clin. Invest. 34:1005, 1955.
9. Jones, R. H., MacNamara, J., and Gaensler, E. A.: The effects of intermittent positive pressure breathing in simulated pulmonary obstruction. Amer. Rev. Resp. Dis. 82:164, 1960.
10. Chronic bronchitis, asthma, and pulmonary emphysema. A statement by the Committee on Diagnostic Standards for Non-Tubercular Respiratory Diseases, H. W. Harris, Chairman. Amer. Rev. Resp. Dis. 85:762, 1962.
11. Gaensler, E. A., and Graham, G. B.: Treatment of emphysema. Fact or fancy? In Ingelfinger, F. J., Relman, A. S., and Finland, M. (eds.): *Controversy in Internal Medicine.* Philadelphia, W. B. Saunders Company, 1966, p. 399.
12. Sheldon, G. P.: Pressure breathing in chronic obstructive lung disease. Medicine 42:197, 1963.
13. Pierce, A. K.: Assisted respiration. Ann. Rev. Med. 20:431, 1969.
14. Jameson, A. G., Ferrer, M. I., and Harvey, R. M.: Some effects of mechanical respirators upon respiratory gas exchange and ventilation in chronic pulmonary emphysema. Amer. Rev. Resp. Dis. 80:510, 1959.
15. Fraimow, W., Cathcart, R. T., and Goodman, E.: The use of intermittent positive pressure breathing in the prevention of the carbon dioxide narcosis associated with oxygen therapy. Amer. Rev. Resp. Dis. 81:815, 1960.
16. Torres, G., Lyons, H. A., and Emerson, P.: The effects of intermittent positive pressure breathing on intrapulmonary distribution of inspired air. Amer. J. Med. 29:946, 1960.
17. Cullen, J. H., Brum, V. C., and Reidt, W. U.: An evaluation of the ability of intermittent

positive pressure breathing to produce effective hyperventilation in severe pulmonary emphysema. Amer. Rev. Tuberc. 76:33, 1957.
18. Kilburn, K. H.: Dimensional responses of bronchi in apneic dogs to airway pressure, gases and drugs. J. Appl. Physiol. 15:229, 1960.
19. Maloney, J. V., Jr., Otis, A. B., Fenn, W. O., and Whittenberger, J. L.: The effect of positive pressure breathing on air flow resistance of the tracheobronchial tree. J. Clin. Invest. 29:832, 1950.
20. Fry, D. L., Ebert, R. V., Stead, W. W., and Brown, C. C.: The mechanics of pulmonary ventilation in normal subjects and in patients with emphysema. Amer. J. Med. 16:80, 1954.
21. Ayres, S. M., Kozam, R. L., and Lukas, D. S.: The effects of intermittent positive pressure breathing on intrathoracic pressure, pulmonary mechanics, and the work of breathing. Amer. Rev. Resp. Dis. 87:370, 1963.
22. Kamat, S. R., Dulfano, M. J., and Segal, M. S.: The effects of intermittent positive pressure breathing (IPPB/I) with compressed air in patients with severe chronic nonspecific obstructive pulmonary disease. Amer. Rev. Resp. Dis. 86:360, 1962.
23. Rotheran, E. B., Jr., Safar, P., and Robin, E. D.: CNS disorder during mechanical ventilation in chronic pulmonary disease. J.A.M.A. 189:993, 1964.
24. Curtis, J. K., Liska, A. P., Rasmussen, H. K., and Cree, E. M.: IPPB therapy in chronic obstructive pulmonary disease. J.A.M.A. 206:1037, 1968.

The Dangers and Limitations of IPPB in Managing Diseases Affecting Ventilation

R. DREW MILLER and
NORMAN G. G. HEPPER

Mayo Clinic and Mayo Foundation

"There is that glorious Epicurian paradox uttered by my friend the historian in one of his flashing moments, 'Give us the luxuries of life and we will dispense with its necessities.'"

O. W. Holmes, The Autocrat of the Breakfast Table

Debate over the benefits of a given mode of treatment usually revolves around objective versus subjective changes, the potential or real hazards or side effects, and the type of patients or clinical conditions in which the controversial treatment is most appropriate. More recently, with spiraling costs of health care causing public and governmental furor, cost/effectiveness of treatment has entered as still another consideration. All these are pertinent to the polemics surrounding intermittent positive pressure breathing (IPPB). It is crucial in this discussion to consider the debate on IPPB as part of the overall program of rehabilitation of the patient with chronic diffuse obstruction of the airways. The treatment of chronic obstructive pulmonary disease (COPD) encompasses a number of components, including the protection of the airways from irritants, adequate hydration, combating infection, use of various bronchodilators, breathing training, general muscle conditioning, and other efforts at rehabilitation, including low flow oxygen in selected cases.

The thesis of this presentation will be that IPPB in the inspiratory phase, except in ventilatory assistance in various hypoventilatory states, is a luxury that often causes the patient and his physician to forget the aforementioned important necessities.

Instrumental Development

Research and development of pressure breathing equipment of various types were spurred particularly during World War II for use by aviators exposed to low oxygen tensions in unpressurized aircraft. The unfavorable circulatory effects of constant positive pressure systems led to the development of ingenious, subject-cycled IPPB apparatus providing pressure at the upper airway only during inspiration.[1-4] This resulted in less pronounced circulatory impairment owing to lower mean intrathoracic pressure. Furthermore, the intermittent pressure applied to the upper airways provided ventilatory assistance to patients with respiratory pump failure and relatively normal airways seen in depression of the central nervous system, muscular weakness, or flail chest, where tank or other external respirators had previously been the only ventilators available.[5] In the early designing of the instruments, careful attention was given to the rate of increase of pressure in the inspiratory phase and the abruptness of release of pressure at the onset of expiration. Of equal importance was the relative timing of expiration to inspiration, particularly when treatment for COPD was anticipated. Apparatus producing a slowly developing pressure through inspiration and the rapid release of pressure at the onset of expiration proved most suitable.[1] In addition, further protection of the cardiac output was reported by use of positive-negative pressure equipment.[6] The ventilatory advantage of this latter type of instrument was less apparent, and for other technical reasons the positive-negative type ventilators did not gain wide acceptance.

While the more sophisticated and automated IPPB units became steadily more expensive, a new generation of simpler, more compact, and more economic hand-held devices became available as an equally functioning alternative to those physicians and patients wanting some type of IPPB.[7]

In further contrast to these innovations, there came into use several simple, commercially available hand-bulb nebulizers, which could deliver reasonably fine uniform aerosols of desired drugs to the major and small airways and which cost $5 or less.

IPPB as a Method of Delivering Aerosols

The routine use of IPPB to deliver bronchodilator aerosols to ambulatory patients with chronic obstructive pulmonary disease probably has the least supportive objective evidence and yet it is widely used at considerable expense—units cost several hundred dollars, but are ultimately set aside or used only sporadically. Early reports on chronic obstructive pulmonary disease with clinical trials of IPPB with aerosolized bronchodilator did not include the control feature of IPPB or aerosol bronchodilator alone. At the Mayo Clinic first efforts were made to measure these factors separately.[8,9] In ambulatory patients with moderate to moderately severe COPD, the change in ventilatory measurements immediately after treatment was identical, whether the bronchodilator was delivered by a hand-bulb nebulizer or with IPPB. IPPB without the bronchodilator resulted in no significant change of vital capacity (VC) or maximal breathing capacity (MBC) immediately after 15 to 20 minutes of therapy, while both measurements increased 20 to 40 per cent above pretreatment levels after aerosol bronchodilator with or without IPPB.

Leslie and associates[10] reached the same conclusions in a similar study in which administration of aerosol bronchodilators with and without IPPB was compared on twice daily treatment over four to eight weeks. Goldberg and Cherniack[11] found no difference between beneficial effects of bronchodilator delivered with IPPB or a hand nebulizer. In most cases, airway conductance improved if corrected for lung volume. Since most subjects breathed at a lower functional residual capacity (FRC) after aerosol bronchodilator, the actual airway conductance was the same as that at pretreatment higher lung volumes.

The long-term effects and survival with these two forms of aerosol administration were demonstrated by Curtis and associates,[12] who obtained an average four-year follow-up on patients who were indoctrinated in a comprehensive program for home treatment of COPD. Of 187 patients in their series, 50 who were not using IPPB were matched with 50 patients using IPPB on the basis of objective pulmonary function data at the onset of treatment. The forced expiratory volume in one second (FEV_1) or one-second vital capacity deteriorated more rapidly in the group using IPPB (99 ml./yr.) than in the controls (44 ml./yr.). Survival in the two groups was similar. In a recent short-term controlled study, Lefcoe and Carter[13] reached conclusions similar to those in five studies reported previously. They compared "sham" IPPB at 2-cm. water pressure to 20-cm. water pressure. In addition, isoproterenol and saline solution also were controlled in this double-blind study. Interestingly, of the four groups, only the group receiving sham IPPB and isoproterenol showed a significant reduction in arterial carbon dioxide tension (P_{CO_2}), both groups receiving IPPB at 20-cm. water pressure being unchanged. It is not surprising that IPPB is of questionable inherent value in generating aerosols for ambulatory patients with COPD since it has been shown that their respiratory muscle strength is normal. They can develop normal to supernormal intrathoracic positive and negative pressures.[14] The "respiratory pump" does not need assistance except in patients with fatigue states or serious complicating infections.

Wu and associates[15] showed that patients without excessive bronchopulmonary secretions responded as well objectively to nebulizer-generated bronchodilator as to IPPB with bronchodilator. They described patients with excess secretions or inability to coordinate the nebulizer treatment in whom IPPB with aerosol bronchodilator resulted in greater and more prolonged objective response.

If we consider administration of IPPB to patients with more advanced chronic obstructive pulmonary disease, the objective evidence still shows variable results. Segal and associates[16,17] have reported extensive studies both on the benefits of IPPB and on its limitations and untoward side effects. In a detailed study of 18 severely disabled patients with COPD, they found 16 were tired after IPPB and five became exhausted. In only seven of 36 patients did the arterial P_{CO_2} decrease; in fact, it actually increased in 13. Alveolar ventilation decreased 20 per cent on the average and dead space ventilation increased in most instances. Cohen and Hale,[18] who measured airway resistance by the volume displacement body plethysmograph, found no difference between the response to isoproterenol aerosol administered via three different vehicles or diluents and the response to IPPB. The best response occurred with simple aerosol of isoproterenol with phenylephrine in that the decay of the response was delayed longer. The administration of 0.4 mg. of isoproterenol produced a decrease in airway resistance that was not decreased significantly by IPPB even after giving as much as 5.0 mg. of the drug.

The careful study of patients with COPD by Payne and associates[19] stressed the well known day-to-day variability in base-line measurements and the varying response to a given mode of therapy; however, they did not compare the response to aerosol dilators with and without IPPB. Thus, the response of each patient to any mode of therapy must be observed by the physician or a well trained paramedical person on his team and as much objective data as clinically reasonable recorded. Objective measurements provide the most reliable guide to continued effective clinical management.

Since we have often found patients using nebulizers in a manner less than optimal, it is appropriate to outline our instructions, which are given to ambulatory patients by the technician in the Emphysema Clinic. This technique is similar to that described by Miller[20] and used by others. A simple routine for use of a hand-bulb nebulizer will assure the patient of maximal benefit from the bronchodilating aerosol. The dose of bronchodilator should be diluted with normal saline or distilled water to a volume of 20 to 30 drops. The nebulizer should be held with its orifice within the open mouth and directed over the tongue. With inspiration of a resting tidal volume, the patient compresses the bulb once. This is repeated three times. Then the patient exhales to near residual volume and as he inhales to near total capacity, he squeezes the bulb several times. At full inspiration he holds his breath for a few seconds and then exhales to repeat the cycle of three inhalations of resting tidal volume followed by a deep breath. He should rest periodically to avoid fatigue and hyperventilation. Such treatment, leisurely carried out, requires 10 to 15 minutes. The purpose of the repeated, deep, sustained inhalations is to obtain maximal distribution of the drug into the less well ventilated units of the lung and thereby to obtain maximal benefit from the bronchodilator. If a hand-bulb nebulizer is used in this manner, it seems impossible that administration of a bronchodilator by IPPB can achieve better drug distribution in this type of patient.

IPPB in Ventilatory Failure

The strongest case for the use of IPPB can be made in the treatment of patients with acute ventilatory failure. The patient with COPD may no longer be able to use a nebulizer effectively for the administration of bronchodilators because of fatigue, weakness, a disturbed sensorium, or just because he is so ill. An aerosol may be administered effectively by IPPB under these circumstances. When intubation is deemed necessary in the treatment of acute ventilatory failure because of impaired sensorium, worsening of the symptoms despite best efforts at treatment without intubation, or failure of the ventilatory apparatus as in muscle weakness, one of the modes of IPPB is usually necessary. If the patient can relax and allow the machine to do the work of ventilating the lung, the metabolic production of CO_2 by the respiratory muscles can be reduced[21] and the elevated P_{CO_2} lowered.[22] However, as will be pointed out again later, if the patient resists the efforts of the machine, the work of breathing will be increased. Then sedation and even muscular paralysis induced with curare may be necessary to improve ventilation. Even in the arena of emergency care, however, opinions conflict as to the indications for intubation and controlled ventilation.

Kettel and associates[23] reported their experiences using tracheal intubation and controlled ventilation in a less prominent perspective. Of 62 patients treated in 87 episodes in which the P_{CO_2} exceeded 55, the survival rate was 71 per cent on a comprehensive program of cardiopulmonary therapy where controlled ventilation was used on only 15 occasions. Of this group requiring transtracheal ventilation, only 26 per cent survived, suggesting that once the more aggressive treatment is needed the die has already been cast and the salvage rate is low. Eldridge and Gherman[24] also emphasize the value of the Barach[25] low flow oxygen technique in managing most cases of respiratory acidosis.

Asmundsson and Kilburn[26] reported on the treatment of 239 episodes among a somewhat more heterogeneous group of patients; continuously controlled ventilation was used in 23 per cent of them with a similar low percentage of immediate survival. Even more interesting was the long-term follow-up, with 20 per cent survival after 30 months among those requiring controlled ventilation. Chronic bronchitics, and especially obese bronchitics, survived the longest.

The most challenging indictment of the use of IPPB in patients with respiratory failure is that of Jones and associates,[27] who reported an extensive clinical experience at Boston City Hospital. They, like Segal's group, found that the condition of half their patients deteriorated during intensive care with IPPB. They constructed a mechanical model of the Starling resistor type to analyze in more detail changes in COPD that negate the potential or theoretic benefits of IPPB. They concluded that mechanical work of ventilation could actually increase with IPPB. Sukumalchantra and associates[28] in New York also reported that IPPB failed to reduce arterial P_{CO_2} in 60 per cent of recorded episodes. By pressure-volume work loops, they demonstrated how patients who do not understand the use of IPPB increase the work of breathing and endogenous production of CO_2. The next commonest cause of IPPB failure, they observed, was the increase in dead space ventilation beyond that found in voluntary hyperventilation, a phenomenon described by Briscoe and Cournand.[29]

Complications

The use of IPPB and the ancillary inhalation therapy equipment in the treatment of patients with respiratory failure is not without some attendant risk. Pneumonia, usually caused by *Pseudomonas*, accounted for 40 per cent of the fatal complications in the report by Asmundsson and Kilburn.[30] Pierce and associates[31] studied the high incidence (8 per cent) of necrotizing pneumonia due to *Pseudomonas* in all autopsies in their hospitals in 1963, a tenfold increase in 11 years. The most significantly related conditions were reservoir nebulization, broad spectrum or gram positive-specific antibiotic agents, and, less predominantly, shock and anemia.[32-35] Inoculation of large numbers of gram negative bacilli by contaminated aerosol is an ancillary risk of this form of therapy. It must be appreciated that inhalation therapy equipment will be the source of nosocomial infections unless this equipment is diligently cared for by people knowledgeable in the sometimes complex methods of sterilization and proper maintenance.

Intubation and IPPB, "To Do or Not To Do?"

Tulou[36] recently confirmed earlier reports of decreased cardiac output in patients during IPPB, with concomitant failure to require the high arterial P_{CO_2}. His normal subjects, by contrast, showed less reduction of cardiac output and at the same time had a lower arterial P_{CO_2} while on IPPB. It is in this area of ventilatory control in COPD that IPPB is clearly indicated for therapeutic trial under critical observation.[37]

The expertise of the personnel in intensive respiratory care units and the capabilities of these teams in supporting ventilation and life are well established. In some cases such life-sustaining measures should not be employed. We must now define the criteria for such cases. The most agonizing complication for patient, physician, and family is the patient who is kept alive by controlled ventilation but who cannot be weaned from the machine. He can never be even minimally self-sufficient, and medical and hospital bills may approach the cost of his home and his life savings. Thus, it is important to avoid this complication, which is often difficult to foresee, even though the alternatives are immediately more difficult to choose.

Asmundsson and Kilburn's[26] survival data, representative of that of many authors, and suggestions of Jessen and associates[38] indicate which types of patients will be productively benefited by controlled transtracheal ventilation. The latter reported that the patients who required controlled tracheal ventilation but who had been chronically confined to their homes or rooms before hospitalization had a 50 per cent hospital mortality and a 10 per cent one-year survival; the patients who had been unable to work but who had managed minimal self-care and could occasionally go outside had only a 35 per cent one-year survival; the patients who had worked prior to sudden respiratory failure had a 62 per cent one-year survival, clearly calling for heroic measures of treatment. The wide variety of methods to maintain life of severe respiratory cripples requires exceptional judgment by the physician in counseling the patient and his family.

The Role of IPPB in the Postoperative State

A final controversial area in which IPPB is extensively used is the postoperative period. After early descriptions of methods[39] and favorable comments[40] in uncontrolled studies, several groups did alternate case studies in routine abdominal or thoracic operations in patients without regard to presence of pulmonary impairment.[41-43] They noted no difference in postoperative complications of pneumonia or atelectasis. No indication is apparent for routine use of IPPB after operation in all patients. Anderson and associates[44] showed a significant reduction (from 19 to 2.5 per cent) of postoperative complications by IPPB if patients had a preoperative maximum breathing capacity (MBC) of less than 60 per cent of predicted normal. Preoperative preparation has been advocated particularly to instruct dyspneic patients in use of IPPB in case it is used in the early postoperative period. Some patients recovering from extracorporeal circulation for cardiovascular surgery have IPPB controlled ventilation in the surgical intensive care units during the altered consciousness period with considerable benefit to overall management. These patients usually have relatively normal airways which pose no impedance to assisted ventilation.

Some Misconceptions About IPPB

It is sometimes said that IPPB "pushes" the medicine to the underventilated parts of the lung. In fact, the flow down an airway is a function of the pressure gradient along that airway, the related airway and the tissue resistance, and of other mechanical properties that determine the time constants of various pulmonary units. A pleural pressure of −15 cm. of water gives *essentially* the same distribution of flow as +15 cm. of water applied at the mouth if the subject is relaxed. The rate of increment of pressure gradient, the respiratory rate, and the pauses at inspiration or expiration influence distribution of gas and aerosol. The alert patient with indoctrination in breathing control can administer an effective aerosol bronchodilator to himself. Likewise, the same patient, well instructed in utilizing an IPPB instrument, will receive a good aerosol treatment, but there is nothing inherent in this which is not available in the simpler method in this type of clinical situation.

Frequently patients are advised to go to a hospital unit or to an outpatient facility several times a week for IPPB treatments which, at best, have a measurable effect for one to three hours. If an aerosol treatment is worth doing, it should be used several times a day, with or without IPPB, and the latter is more trouble-free.

Some physicians have said, "I don't have time to train my patient to use a nebulizer. IPPB is quicker for me." In fact, the patient requires as much or more instruction to use IPPB effectively if it is actually to assist respiration. A patient can actually increase the work of breathing by attempting to lead or fight the machine or cycle it too rapidly. The concept of paramedical personnel participating in therapy and instruction invalidates the "too much time" excuse.

Conclusion

Numerous commercially available devices provide mechanical ventilatory assistance for patients with respiratory pump failure related to oversedation, neuromuscular paralysis, flail chest, or respiratory muscle fatigue. Diffuse obstructive pulmonary disease, however, presents complex problems that render the role of IPPB questionable in most instances. It has no inherent value in generating an aerosol for alert, well instructed patients who can use a hand nebulizer costing less than five dollars.

Ventilatory failure of chronic obstructive pulmonary disease, heralded by rising arterial P_{CO_2} despite low flow administration of oxygen and a battery of conservative measures, warrants an objective, monitored trial of mechanical ventilation. Even in this situation, IPPB poses the threat of lowered cardiac output and nosocomial infection with necrotizing pneumonia.

References

1. Cournand, A., Motley, H. L., Werko, L., et al.: Physiological studies of the effects of intermittent positive pressure breathing on cardiac output in man. Amer. J. Physiol. 152:162–174, 1948.
2. Carr, D. T., and Essex, H. E.: Certain effects of positive pressure respiration on the circulatory and respiratory systems. Amer. Heart J. 31:53–73, 1946.
3. Fenn, W. O., Otis, A. B., Rahn, H., et al.: Displacement of blood from the lungs by pressure breathing. Amer. J. Physiol. 151:258–269, 1947.
4. Motley, H. L., Cournand, A., Werko, L., et al.: Intermittent positive pressure breathing: A means of administering artificial respiration in man. J.A.M.A. 137:370–383, 1948.
5. Engström C-G: Treatment of severe cases of respiratory paralysis by the Engström Universal Respirator. Brit. Med. J. 2:666–669, 1954.
6. Maloney, J. V., Jr., Elam, J. O., Handford, S. W., et al.: Importance of negative pressure phase in mechanical respirators. J.A.M.A. 152:212–216, 1953.
7. Petty, T. L., and Broughton, J. O.: A new, simple IPPB device for hospital and home use. J.A.M.A. 203:871–874, 1968.
8. Fowler, W. S., Helmholz, H. F., Jr., and Miller, R. D.: Treatment of pulmonary emphysema with aerosolized bronchodilator drugs and intermittent positive-pressure breathing. Mayo Clin. Staff Proc. 28:743–751, 1953.
9. Miller, R. D., Fowler, W. S., and Helmholz, H. F., Jr.: The treatment of pulmonary emphysema and of diffuse pulmonary fibrosis with nebulized bronchodilators and intermittent positive pressure breathing. Dis. Chest 28:309–326, 1955.
10. Leslie, A., Dantes, A., and Rosove, L.: Intermittent positive-pressure breathing: Appraisal of use in bronchodilator therapy of pulmonary emphysema. J.A.M.A. 160:1125–1129, 1956.
11. Goldberg, I., and Cherniack, R. M.: The effect of nebulized bronchodilator delivered with and without IPPB on ventilatory function in chronic obstructive emphysema. Amer. Rev. Resp. Dis. 91:13–20, 1965.
12. Curtis, J. K., Liska, A. P., Rasmussen, H. K., et al.: IPPB therapy in chronic obstructive pulmonary disease: An evaluation of long-term home treatment. J.A.M.A. 206:1037–1040, 1968.
13. Lefcoe, N., and Carter, P.: Intermittent positive-pressure breathing in chronic obstructive pulmonary disease. Canad. Med. Ass. J. 103:279–281, 1970.
14. Byrd, R. B., and Hyatt, R. E.: Maximal respiratory pressures in chronic obstructive lung disease. Amer. Rev. Resp. Dis. 98:848–856, 1968.
15. Wu, N., Miller, W. F., Cade, R., et al.: Intermittent positive pressure breathing in patients with chronic bronchopulmonary disease. Amer. Rev. Tuberc. 71:693–703, 1955.
16. Segal, M. S., Salomon, A., Dulfano, M. J., et al.: Intermittent positive pressure breathing: Its use in the inspiratory phase of respiration. New Eng. J. Med. 250:225–232, 1954.
17. Kamat, S., Dulfano, M. J., and Segal, M. S.: The effects of intermittent positive pressure breathing (IPPB/I) with compressed air in patients with severe chronic nonspecific obstructive pulmonary disease. Amer. Rev. Resp. Dis. 86:360–380, 1962.
18. Cohen, A. A., and Hale, F. C.: Comparative effects of isoproterenol aerosols on airway resistance in obstructive pulmonary diseases. Amer. J. Med. Sci. 249:309–315, 1965.

19. Payne, C. B., Jr., Chester, E. H., and Hsi, B. P.: Airway responsiveness in chronic obstructive pulmonary disease. Amer. J. Med. 42:554–566, 1967.
20. Miller, W. F.: A consideration of improved methods of nebulization therapy. New Eng. J. Med. 251:589–595, 1954.
21. Birnbaum, M. L., Cree, E. M., Rasmussen, H., et al.: Effects of intermittent positive pressure breathing on emphysematous patients. Amer. J. Med. 41:552–561, 1966.
22. Jameson, A. G., Ferrer, M. I., and Harvey, R. M.: Some effects of mechanical respirators upon respiratory gas exchange and ventilation in chronic pulmonary emphysema. Amer. Rev. Resp. Dis. 80:510–521, 1959.
23. Kettel, L. J., Diener, C. F., Morse, J. O., et al.: Treatment of acute respiratory acidosis in chronic obstructive lung disease. J.A.M.A. 217:1503–1508, 1971.
24. Eldridge, F., and Gherman, C.: Studies of oxygen administration in respiratory failure. Ann. Intern. Med. 68:569–578, 1968.
25. Barach, A. L.: Physiological methods in the diagnosis and treatment of asthma and emphysema. Ann. Intern. Med. 12:454–481, 1938.
26. Asmundsson, T., and Kilburn, K. H.: Survival of acute respiratory failure: A study of 239 episodes. Ann. Intern. Med. 70:471–485, 1969.
27. Jones, R. H., MacNamara, J., and Gaensler, E. A.: The effects of intermittent positive pressure breathing in simulated pulmonary obstruction. Amer. Rev. Resp. Dis. 82:164–185, 1960.
28. Sukumalchantra, Y., Park, S. S., and Williams, M. H., Jr.: The effect of intermittent positive pressure breathing (IPPB) in acute ventilatory failure. Amer. Rev. Resp. Dis. 92:885–893, 1965.
29. Briscoe, W. A., Cournand, A.: The degree of variation of blood perfusion and of ventilation within the emphysematous lung, and some related considerations. In de Reuck, A. V. S., and O'Connor, M. (eds.): Ciba Foundation Symposium on Pulmonary Structure and Function. Boston, Little, Brown and Company. 1962, pp. 304–326.
30. Asmundsson, T., and Kilburn, K. H.: Complications of acute respiratory failure. Ann. Intern. Med. 70:487–495, 1969.
31. Pierce, A. K., Edmonson, E. B., McGee, G., et al.: An analysis of factors predisposing to gram-negative bacillary necrotizing pneumonia. Amer. Rev. Resp. Dis. 94:309–315, 1966.
32. Phillips, I., and Spencer, G.: Pseudomonas aeruginosa cross-infection: Due to contaminated respiratory apparatus. Lancet 2:1325–1327, 1965.
33. Nash, G., Blennerhassett, J. B., and Pontoppidan, H.: Pulmonary lesions associated with oxygen therapy and artificial ventilation. New Eng. J. Med. 276:368–374, 1967.
34. Reinarz, J. A., Pierce, A. K., Mays, B. B., et al.: The potential role of inhalation therapy equipment in nosocomial pulmonary infection. J. Clin. Invest. 44:831–839, 1965.
35. Joffe, N.: Roentgenologic aspects of primary *Pseudomonas aeruginosa* pneumonia in mechanically ventilated patients. Amer. J. Roentgenol. 107:305–312, 1969.
36. Tulou, P. P.: Cardiac output and arterial CO_2 response during intermittent positive pressure breathing with oxygen: A comparison of patients with chronic airflow obstruction and controls. Thorax 26:33–38, 1971.
37. Sheldon, G. P.: Pressure breathing in chronic obstructive lung disease. Medicine 42:197–227, 1963.
38. Jessen, O., Kristensen, H. S., and Rasmussen, K.: Tracheostomy and artificial ventilation in chronic lung disease. Lancet 2:9–12, 1967.
39. Noehren, T. H., Lasry, J. E., and Legters, L. J.: Intermittent positive pressure breathing (IPPB/I) for the prevention and management of postoperative pulmonary complications. Surgery 43:658–665, 1958.
40. Rudy, N. E., and Crepeau, J.: Role of intermittent positive pressure breathing postoperatively. J.A.M.A. 167:1093–1096, 1958.
41. Becker, A., Barak, S., Braun, E., et al.: The treatment of postoperative pulmonary atelectasis with intermittent positive pressure breathing. Surg. Gynec. Obstet. 111:517–522, 1960.
42. Sands, J. H., Cypert, C., Armstrong, R., et al.: A controlled study using routine intermittent positive pressure breathing in the post-surgical patient. Dis. Chest 40:128–133, 1961.
43. Baxter, W. D., and Levine, R. S.: An evaluation of intermittent positive pressure breathing in the prevention of postoperative pulmonary complications. Arch. Surg. 98:795–798, 1969.
44. Anderson, W. H., Dossett, B. E., Jr., and Hamilton, G. L.: Prevention of postoperative pulmonary complications: Use of isoproterenol and intermittent positive pressure breathing on inspiration. J.A.M.A. 186:763–766, 1963.

Comment

The Place of IPPB in the Management of Chronic Obstructive Lung Disease

Obstructive lung disease associated with chronic bronchitis and emphysema is a common and vexing problem. Patients with this illness are uncomfortable and face progressive limitation of their activity and an early death. Although the disease could be effectively prevented by abolition of cigarette smoking, treatment is for the most part ineffective. Nevertheless, the patient is driven to seek whatever help he can obtain and physicians in their desperation are willing to try every conceivable therapy. In this setting the subjective response to treatment is difficult to evaluate.

IPPB has been used in three ways to treat patients with chronic obstructive lung disease. The first is to assist the delivery of a bronchodilator to obstructed portions of the lung. As pointed out by Miller and Hepper, there is very little objective data to support the use of IPPB for this purpose. The delivery of a nebulized solution containing a bronchodilator without IPPB appears equally effective in most patients. There remain a few patients who because of fatigue or difficulty in coordination require IPPB for effective use of a nebulizer.

The second use is to reduce the work of breathing and to allow the fatigued patient respite from the excessive muscular activity necessary to maintain breathing. Many patients have difficulty in relaxing and allowing the ventilator to take over. In these patients the work of breathing may not be reduced and at times may be increased.

The third use is in patients with increasing hypoxia and hypercapnia related to an exacerbation of obstructive lung disease. Most of these patients are best treated with inhaled oxygen at a tension slightly above that of the atmosphere together with avoidance of sedatives, encouragement to cough, bronchodilators, and antibiotics. A few have progressive increase in carbon dioxide tension in the arterial blood and require assisted respiration. IPPB is used to increase alveolar ventilation in these persons. Most require tracheal intubation and use of a cuffed tube for effective therapy.

Thus, IPPB has a modest place in the therapy of chronic obstructive lung disease. How then do we explain the growth of a multimillion dollar industry based on the use of these machines and the rapid expansion of inhalation therapy units in hospitals? We must admit that IPPB therapy is often used in an uncritical manner. Is this a manifestation of the growing faith in technology as the solution to the problems of medicine?

RICHARD V. EBERT

10

Management of Acute Pulmonary Insufficiency

The Advantages of an Aggressive, Prophylactic Approach
    by Morley M. Singer

The Indications for Artificial Ventilations Are Limited
    by Peter T. Macklem

Comment
    by Richard V. Ebert

The Advantages of an Aggressive, Prophylactic Approach

MORLEY M. SINGER

San Francisco Medical Center, University of California

A dramatic forward leap in the understanding and treatment of acute respiratory failure (ARF) has occurred in the past decade. The high incidence of ARF in a broad spectrum of medical and surgical patients has been recognized, and the vital role of ventilatory support is now commonly accepted. Only a few years ago the institution of such support was regarded as a "last resort" form of therapy which invariably preceded a fatal outcome. This reversal results in large part from the establishment of intensive care units, with a team approach to the management of ARF allowing effective application of the meticulous care necessary to avoid the complications of therapy.

We propose that patients with (1) ARF, (2) impending respiratory failure (IRF), and (3) acute restrictive pulmonary disease with impaired respiratory reserve (IRR) (vital capacity (VC) less than 10 ml./kg.), be treated aggressively by endotracheal intubation and intermittent positive pressure ventilation (IPPV). This proposal requires some definitions, some amplification, and some qualification.

At one end of the spectrum of disorders of respiratory function, and excluded from the groups listed above, are those patients with *impaired oxygenation* of the arterial blood, i.e., an arterial oxygen tension (PaO_2) less than normal while inspiring ambient air, but normal or low arterial carbon dioxide tension ($PaCO_2$). Vital capacity exceeds 15 ml./kg., respiratory frequency is less than 35 per minute, subjective respiratory distress is minimal, and radiologic infiltrates, if present, are usually localized. These patients do not require ventilatory support, and impaired oxygenation can be corrected by standard methods of O_2 administration. Examples of this group would be patients with lobar atelectasis, or pleural effusions, or small pneumonic infiltrates.

At the other end of the spectrum of disorders of respiratory function are those patients with hypercarbia (which, of course, is accompanied by hypoxemia if the patient is breathing ambient air). Acute respiratory failure may be defined as an acute rise in $PaCO_2$ to over 55 torr (in the absence of metabolic alkalosis), and it is doubtful whether any would disagree that this constitutes a medical emergency requiring immediate intervention with endotracheal intubation and IPPV. ARF may result from central depression of respiratory drive (drug overdose, cerebral trauma), from failure of the neuromuscular apparatus of respiration, or from major loss of parenchymal lung function (adult respiratory distress syndrome).

The introduction into clinical practice of readily available arterial blood gas and pH analysis was invaluable in defining the entities just described. Excessive attention to the value of arterial blood gas measurements, however, has led to a restricted view of the therapeutic approach to acute impairment of respiratory function, particularly by those whose main clinical experience is in the realm of chronic pulmonary disease. The emphasis on arterial blood gas analysis in diagnosis has unfortunately led some physicians to feel that patients do not require ventilatory support until hypercarbia is manifest. It is most important that the reader be convinced that while arterial blood gas analysis is essential for a precise diagnosis, and while hypercarbia is the sine qua non of ARF, *arterial blood gas analysis alone does not exclude impending respiratory failure.* The limitations of arterial blood gas values may be illustrated by the following: An arterial blood gas sample showing $PaO_2 = 50$ torr, $PaCO_2 = 30$ torr, pH = 7.48 might have been drawn from (1) a healthy mountaineer recently arrived at 12,000 feet altitude, capable of carrying a 40-pound pack for a day's hike; (2) a patient with a mild asthmatic attack; (3) a patient in severe, life-threatening status asthmaticus; (4) a patient with mild pulmonary edema; or (5) a patient with upper airway obstruction—in extremis and in urgent need of ventilatory support. These values result from the important fact that *as long as the respiratory center is intact and functioning normally, the patient "wants" to keep $PaCO_2$ normal (or lower) and will utilize the motor apparatus of respiration at whatever level of exertion is required to do so.* Hypercarbia is therefore a late sign of respiratory failure and once present, progresses rapidly.

In the absence of hypercarbia the appropriate criteria for institution of endotracheal intubation and IPPV are a collection of clinical, laboratory, and radiologic findings which constitute the syndrome of IRF, combined with awareness of the natural history of primary disease. These findings have been documented elsewhere. The most important are:

1. Vital capacity <10 ml./kg.
2. An alveolar-arterial PO_2 difference >350 torr (or inability to maintain PaO_2 > 70 torr with O_2 administered by standard methods).
3. Respiratory frequency >35 per min. in adults.
4. Increasing dyspnea.
5. Increasing radiologic infiltrates.

Extensive experience in close monitoring of these functions has made it abundantly clear that many instances of acute cardiopulmonary collapse and acute hypercarbia have been preceded by this syndrome. What appears to be an "acute" problem, however, is in fact the end result of insidious impairment of ventilatory function. Measurements of arterial blood gas values during this slow deterioration will invariably reveal some degree of hypoxemia (if the patient is inspiring ambient air), but normal or low $PaCO_2$. To wait until hypercarbia develops in such patients is akin to allowing a drowning man, struggling to keep his head above water, to submerge and lose consciousness before attempting to rescue him. Recognition of the signs of IRF should lead to early intervention with endotracheal intubation and IPPV, preventing the inevitable progression to hypercarbia and its consequences. A parallel example which may be more familiar to some readers is the recognition of the signs of ventricular irritability which usually precede ventricular fibrillation in patients monitored in coronary care units. The incidence of cardiopulmonary resuscitation required for ventricular fibrillation has been reduced by aggressive prophylactic treatment of the early signs of ventricular irritability.

It seems logical and appropriate to us to extend aggressive management to patients with severely impaired respiratory reserve. The most typical example of this group would be patients with neurologic disease such as Guillain-Barré syndrome or myasthenia gravis. Though arterial blood gas values for O_2 and CO_2 may be normal, and the patient in no subjective distress, the patient is at risk when vital capacity decreases to 15 ml./kg. and should be intubated and ventilated when it approaches 10 ml./kg. When the maximum power of the respiratory muscles approaches the power required for normal ventilation, atelectasis tends to occur owing to shallow respiration, cough becomes ineffective, and acute decompensation is a frequent and catastrophic event. Also included in this group would be postsurgical patients with a predictably high potential for ARF. A typical example would be the elderly, debilitated, obese patient with pre-existing pulmonary disease, undergoing thoracic or upper abdominal surgery. Postoperative pain and immobilization and the predictable adverse effects of such surgery on vital capacity and cough effectiveness combine to decrease respiratory reserve. Aggressive management consisting of IPPV via an endotracheal tube left in place at the termination of surgery assures adequate gas exchange, prevents atelectasis, and allows good tracheobronchial toilet while the patient recovers from the acute effects of surgery.

This aggressive approach to ARF, IRF, and IRR must be qualified in several respects:

First, this applies specifically to the management of *acute* situations and not to patients with chronic hypercapnia secondary to chronic lung disease. The latter group are frequently in a steady state of hypercapnia, compensated such that arterial pH is near normal. Conservative management with controlled oxygen therapy is adequate in most of these patients. However, in the small percentage in whom conservative therapy is inadequate, the syndrome of IRF, interpreted against the patient's steady state circumstances, may indicate the need for more aggressive therapy.

Another important qualification is that endotracheal intubation and IPPV should never substitute for definitive treatment of the primary pathology leading to respiratory distress. An analogy to acute renal failure might be made. Renal failure resulting from a variety of etiologic factors is treated in identical fashion, i.e., dialysis, once the organ failure is established. Though such supportive care is effective and frequently successful, prevention is more appropriate. Thus, if aggressive therapy of impaired respiratory function can be avoided by *specific* therapy such as diuresis to remove interstitial pulmonary edema, or reversal of airway obstruction by bronchodilators in the asthmatic, these maneuvers are obviously appropriate. However, even in these situations, if conservative therapy does not result in rapid improvement, or if the patient is judged to be in immediate life-threatening circumstances, intubation and IPPV may be necessary supportive measures until further definitive treatment can be applied.

A further qualification is that intubation and IPPV must be executed in an environment, such as an ICU, under continuous supervision of a physician and staffed by personnel familiar with all aspects of respiratory care. It is only in such an environment that morbidity can be held to the minimum necessary to justify the aggressive approach advocated.

What are the disadvantages of aggressive therapy? Endotracheal intubation is not without hazard. Acute complications include trauma to the upper airway, hypoxemia during difficult tube insertion, and obstruction and displacement of the tube. Late complications include laryngeal scarring and tracheal stenosis. With attention to detail and awareness of the hazards, it is rare to see serious problems arise during intubation. Late complications are infrequent when intubation is required for less than 24 to 48 hours. Many patients requiring aggressive therapy can be extubated within this time period. If prolonged care is anticipated, tracheostomy is usually substituted for endotracheal intubation.

The many hazards of IPPV (acute circulatory depression, atelectasis, pneumothorax, infection, oxygen toxicity, pulmonary interstitial edema) can be prevented or minimized by caring for the patient in specialized units in which close monitoring is available and personnel are familiar with these hazards. Indeed, patients with respiratory failure have been successfully ventilated in such units for months and even years without complications.

What are the advantages of the aggressive approach?

1. Acute major impairment of gas exchange with severe hypoxemia and hypercarbia with secondary deleterious effects on central nervous system, myocardial, and other organ function is avoided. The importance of this cannot be overemphasized. Initially successful resuscitation of patients with severe hypoxemia and hypercarbia cannot be applauded should the patient later succumb from inadequate myocardial function or survive with permanent cerebral damage.

2. Airway closure may be reduced or prevented by use of large tidal volumes (12–15 ml./kg.) and/or use of positive end-expiratory pressure. It seems likely that prevention or early reversal of atelectasis or low regional lung volume is more easily accomplished than reinflation of lung units which have been closed for a more prolonged period.

3. Pulmonary lesions may be prevented from progressing to atelectasis, consolidation, interstitial hemorrhage, and edema. This advanced pathology, once established, usually requires IPPV with high inflation pressures and high inspired oxygen concentrations which, in turn, may cause further pulmonary damage.

4. Effective tracheobronchial toilet via the endotracheal tube may clear retained secretions and yield good sputum specimens for more precise diagnosis of pulmonary infection. Cultures from sputum expectorated or aspirated from the pharynx in nonintubated patients frequently do not represent the organism infecting the lower airway or lung parenchyma.

The advantages of the prophylactic aggressive approach have been long recognized and applied in selected groups of patients, in whom the benefits have been unequivocal. Following complex cardiac surgery it has become common practice to continue IPPV via an endotracheal tube until the morning following surgery. Dramatic decrease in the mortality from myasthenia gravis and from thymectomy for that disease resulted from the effective application of prophylactic ventilatory support when respiratory *reserve* was diminished—not by waiting for gross ARF to occur. A similar approach to ascending polyneuritis has proved effective. The adverse effects of peritonitis on ventilary function and gas exchange are so predictable that tracheostomy and IPPB should be instituted promptly when this diagnosis is established.

What of the fact that it seems inevitable that some patients will be subjected to endotracheal intubation and IPPV who would have managed adequately without it? That question might also be asked regarding surgery for suspect appendicitis. It is necessary to do some negative surgical exploration to avoid the complications of nonintervention. In the case of ARF, IRF, or IRR it is our opinion that the hazards of nonintervention, i.e., the patient progressing to late respiratory failure with severe hypoxemia and hypercarbia, greatly outweigh the hazards of the aggressive approach.

Institution of treatment in these circumstances might be likened to dialysis for acute renal failure. One does not wait for the late signs of uremia to become manifest before instituting dialysis. We maintain that erosion of ventilatory reserve and its potential consequences can be recognized with the same confidence as increasing uremia can be predicted in patients without renal function. In light of this confidence and predictability we maintain that aggressive therapy is desirable and beneficial.

The Indications for Artificial Ventilations Are Limited

PETER T. MACKLEM

Respiratory Division, McGill University Clinic, Royal Victoria Hospital, Montreal

In general, internal medicine is heavily overburdened with a dogmatism which we religiously boil down to lists of rules and regulations, leaving little room for flexibility and judgment. We tend to memorize and apply, willy-nilly, indications for this and contraindications for that without taking the contingencies of particular cases into account.

This situation is particularly apparent in the treatment of respiratory failure. For example, a recent review lists the following indications for intubation, tracheotomy, and artificial ventilation:

"1. Respiratory rate greater than 35/min.
2. Vital capacity less than 15 ml./kg.
3. Inspiratory force less than 25 cm. H_2O.
4. Alveolar-arterial oxygen tension difference of greater than 350 mm. Hg breathing 100 per cent oxygen.
5. Arterial partial pressure of oxygen of less than 70 mm. Hg on mask oxygen.
6. Dead space, tidal volume ratio greater than 0.6.
7. Arterial partial pressure of carbon dioxide greater than 60 mm. Hg except in chronic hypercapnia."[1]

On the surface these may seem to be reasonable indications, particularly as the authors emphasize the trend in these measurements, but I would like to know where they came from and what evidence there is in their support? Are they merely an arbitrary list, or have these rules been tested scientifically? Why should a normoxic and normo- or hypocapnic patient whose respiratory rate is 40 per min. undergo the hazards of intubation and/or tracheostomy and artificial ventilation? It is generally stated that such patients will become exhausted and develop CO_2 retention, but this has rarely been documented adequately. Who established that an inspiratory "force" of greater than 25 cm. H_2O is necessary for adequate ventilation? This measurement is notoriously difficult to make in a sick patient as it requires breath holding, an airtight seal between the patient's airway and the pressure measuring device, and (contrary to the author's opinion) patient cooperation. A slightly confused, uncooperative patient who does not understand what is required of him may indeed pay for his sins. Why should a patient whose arterial PO$_2$ is 68 mm. Hg when breathing oxygen by mask be artificially ventilated? For a normal oxyhemoglobin dissociation curve the arterial blood is about 90 per cent saturated at this PO$_2$. With a normal cardiac output and hemoglobin concentration, the oxygen delivery to the tissues is perfectly adequate. Indeed, central cyanosis does not appear until the PO$_2$ has fallen to a considerably lower level, and lactic acidosis (which indicates a failure of tissue oxygenation) does not occur until the arterial PO$_2$ is less than 35 mm. Hg.[2] What good will be accomplished by artificial ventilation in a patient with multiple pulmonary emboli whose dead space : tidal volume ratio is greater than 0.6? Is a PCO$_2$ in excess of 60 mm. Hg a sufficient reason to institute artificial ventilation in a patient with chronic obstructive pulmonary disease if he is wide awake and alert?

It is evident that many of these indications for artificial ventilation are prophylactic. Artificial ventilation is thus recommended to prevent a catastrophe, which is assumed to be inevitable if artificial ventilation is not instituted. But this is an extraordinary situation. I am all in favor of preventive medicine, but should heroic therapy be based upon an unproved assumption?

Quite clearly, artificial ventilation is not without hazard. The incidence of serious complications following tracheostomy and intubation is not negligible.[1, 3] A single instance of laryngeal stenosis following intubation is enough to discourage one forever from unnecessary insertion of the endotracheal tube. Artificial ventilation, particularly with positive end-expiratory pressure, may decrease cardiac output so that, in spite of the fact that the arterial PO$_2$ is increased, oxygen delivery to the tissues may be decreased.[4] Finally, positive pressure ventilation eliminates two-way verbal communication with the patient which is so essential in assessing the condition of someone seriously ill. Surely careful patient observation with frequent monitoring of arterial blood gas tension is preferable to this heroic form of prophylaxis.

The reader should not misunderstand my position. I am not necessarily adamantly opposed to the indications listed previously or to the growing use of prophylactic artificial ventilation, but I need to be convinced by scientific data that demonstrate their value.

What can one expect to accomplish by artificial ventilation? Apart from purely prophylactic use, artificial ventilation is instituted to improve CO$_2$ elimination and O$_2$ delivery to the tissues. With respect to CO$_2$ elimination, the situation is clear-cut; the arterial PCO$_2$ is inversely proportional to alveolar ventilation and directly proportional to CO$_2$ production and is given by:

$$\text{Pa}_{CO_2} = 0.863 \frac{\dot{V}_{CO_2}}{\dot{V}_A} \quad \quad \text{Equation 1}$$

where Pa$_{CO_2}$ = arterial partial pressure of CO$_2$, $\dot{V}_{CO_2}$ is the CO$_2$ production, and $\dot{V}_A$ = alveolar ventilation. The graphic solution for this equation is shown in Figure 1 for four different values of $\dot{V}_{CO_2}$. The graph illustrates how effective relatively small increases in alveolar ventilation are in reducing Pa$_{CO_2}$ when this value is initially high. Above a Pa$_{CO_2}$ of 40 mm. Hg one encounters diminishing returns

Figure 1. Graphical solution of the equation:
$$PaCO_2 = 0.863 \frac{\dot{V}_{CO_2}}{\dot{V}_A}$$
for different values of $\dot{V}_{CO_2}$
Pa_{CO_2} = partial pressure of CO_2 in arterial blood
$\dot{V}_A$ = alveolar ventilation
$\dot{V}_{CO_2}$ = CO_2 production

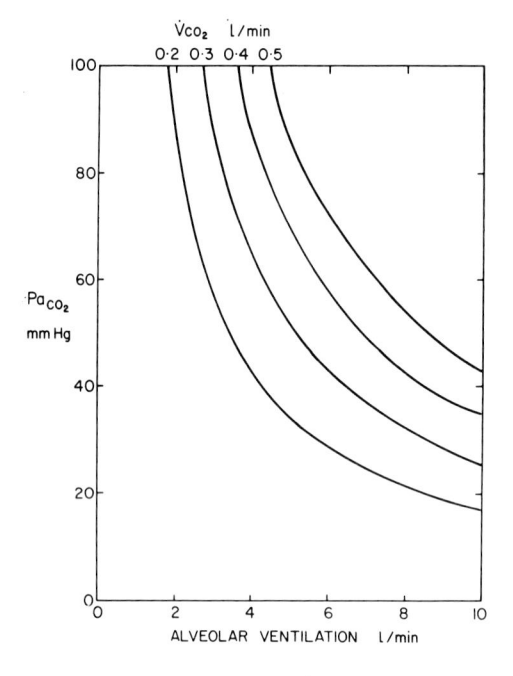

for further increases in $\dot{V}_A$ but, of course, it is unnecessary to reduce the Pa_{CO_2} below this value. Thus, in terms of Pa_{CO_2}, artificial ventilation is most effective over the range of Pa_{CO_2} where it is most needed. This then is the prime indication for artificial ventilation—to reduce the Pa_{CO_2} when this value is abnormally high; but it is not an absolute indication.

The decision to administer artificial ventilation rather than more conservative therapy depends on the degree, cause, and duration of the hypercapnia as well as the condition of the patient. I trust that no physician today would recommend artificial ventilation for a patient with chronic compensated respiratory acidosis, although in the early days of positive pressure ventilation this was commonly done because we lacked understanding of blood gas derangements. Even a patient with acute or acute chronic respiratory acidosis with chronic obstructive lung disease may not require artificial ventilation if he is wide awake and alert. As Campbell has pointed out, death by hypoxia will occur before death by hypercapnia in this condition, so that enhancement of the inspired oxygen tension by controlled oxygen therapy is much more vital to the patient's management.[5] It is only when hypercapnia is progressive, or the patient becomes confused and somnolent in spite of controlled oxygen therapy that artificial ventilation should be instituted. The situation is less clear in patients with acute or acute chronic respiratory failure who do not have chronic obstructive lung disease. The underlying cause may be pneumonia, pulmonary edema, asthma, neurologic disease, or a variety of other conditions. It has long been wondered if hypercapnia under these conditions is an indication of impending doom, and in the absence of information to the contrary, it has seemed reasonable to assume that it is. In the past two or three years, however, we have successfully treated several such patients with controlled oxygen therapy without artificial ventilation. It is my impression, although it has not been scientifically demonstrated, that Campbell's teaching applies to conditions other than chronic obstructive lung disease. Clearly more knowledge is needed in this crucial area.

Can artificial ventilation improve oxygen delivery to tissues? Two mechanisms could operate to accomplish this: First, artifical ventilation can increase alveolar PO_2 so that for a given alveolar arterial oxygen tension difference the arterial PO_2 would increase. Secondly, artificial ventilation might decrease the alveolar arterial oxygen tension difference so that for a given alveolar PO_2, arterial PO_2 would increase.

The relationship between alveolar PO_2 and alveolar ventilation is given by:
$$PA_{O_2} = PI_{O_2} - 0.863 \frac{\dot{V}_{O_2}}{\dot{V}_A} \qquad \text{Equation 2}$$
where PA_{O_2} = alveolar partial pressure of O_2, PI_{O_2} is the inspired partial pressure of oxygen, $\dot{V}_{O_2}$ is the oxygen uptake and $\dot{V}_A$ is alveolar ventilation. Three variables control the PA_{O_2}; i.e., PI_{O_2}, $\dot{V}_{O_2}$ and $\dot{V}_A$. Although the most important is the inspired O_2 tension, the alveolar PO_2 can be increased by increasing alveolar ventilation. In considering the effect of artificial ventilation on oxygen delivery, the important variable is not the arterial PO_2 but the volume of oxygen carried per unit volume of blood. The relationship between the two is the oxyhemoglobin dissociation curve which, in turn, is influenced by P_{CO_2} and pH. Figures 2 A and B illustrate the influence of alveolar ventilation and arterial P_{CO_2}, respectively, on the oxygen content of arterial blood for various differences between alveolar and arterial PO_2. These curves illustrate that the improvement of oxygen delivery by increasing alveolar ventilation is of most benefit when the initial values of arterial P_{CO_2} are high and those of alveolar ventilation are low. Under these circumstances improving alveolar ventilation alone can be lifesaving. Even with an arterial alveolar oxygen tension difference as large as 60 mm. Hg on air, an adequate oxygen delivery can be maintained with an arterial P_{CO_2} of 30 mm. Hg without enriching the inspired air with oxygen.

When initial values of arterial P_{CO_2} are normal or low, and alveolar ventilation is high, increasing the ventilation still further does little to improve oxygen delivery. Under these circumstances artificial ventilation is not indicated, except perhaps if it acts through the second mechanism, i.e., by decreasing the alveolar arterial oxygen tension differences.

Although dramatic improvement in oxygen delivery can be accomplished by increasing alveolar ventilation under the circumstances outlined above, it is rarely necessary to resort to this measure, as even more dramatic improvements may be accomplished by enriching the inspired gas with oxygen. This is evident from Equation 2 and is further illustrated in Figure 3, which is the graphic solution of this equation. The left-hand panel shows the relationship between inspired oxygen concentration and alveolar PO_2 for a constant alveolar ventilation and oxygen uptake. The right-hand panel shows the relationship between alveolar ventilation and alveolar PO_2 for constant values of inspired oxygen concentration and oxygen uptake. Quite clearly, increasing inspired oxygen concentration is vastly more effective than increasing alveolar ventilation. By doubling the inspired oxygen concentration from 20 to 40 per cent (an inspired oxygen concentration which can be tolerated with impunity indefinitely), the alveolar PO_2 increases by over

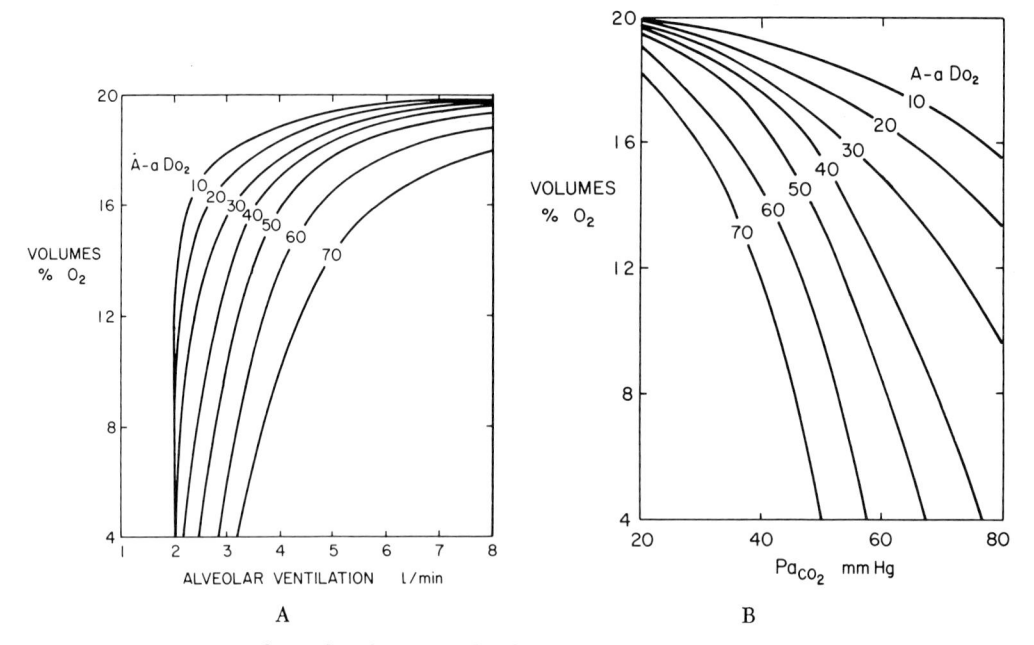

Figure 2. A, Relationship between alveolar ventilation and oxygen content of arterial blood expressed as volumes per cent of O_2 for different values of alveolar arterial oxygen tension difference $(A-aD_{O_2})$.

B, Relationship between arterial partial pressure of CO_2 (Pa_{CO_2}) and oxygen content of arterial blood expressed as volume per cent of O_2 for different values of alveolar arterial oxygen tension differences.

These graphs were constructed assuming a Hb concentration of 15 gm. per cent, oxygen uptake of 250 ml./min., and CO_2 production of 200 ml./min. Equations 1 and 2 were solved for arterial P_{CO_2} and alveolar PO_2 for different values of alveolar ventilation. Arterial PO_2 was calculated by subtracting the appropriate alveolar arterial oxygen tension difference from the alveolar PO_2. Knowing the arterial partial pressures of O_2 and CO_2, the oxygen content was calculated using the Dill Henderson nomogram.[6,7]

140 mm. Hg. Under most circumstances this is more than enough to correct hypoxia due to hypoventilation, ventilation perfusion imbalance, and diffusion defects. However, as Campbell has pointed out, an increase in inspired oxygen concentration of this degree may be dangerous if the patient has lost his sensitivity to P_{CO_2} and depends upon a hypoxic stimulus to maintain ventilation. Under these circumstances adequate oxygenation may frequently be achieved by administering 25 to 35 per cent O_2.[5]

Under apparently increasing circumstances, increasing the inspired oxygen concentration to 40 per cent does not result in a satisfactory delivery of oxygen to the tissues. In order to define these circumstances one needs first to define satisfactory oxygen delivery. This is a thorny and complicated problem. For a given oxyhemoglobin saturation, the oxygen delivery to the tissues depends upon the cardiac output, the Hb concentration, the blood volume, the distribution of perfusion and the oxygen demands of the tissues. Unfortunately this information is not available. In its absence one can only draw up rough guidelines as to what constitutes a satisfactory oxygen delivery, with the realiza-

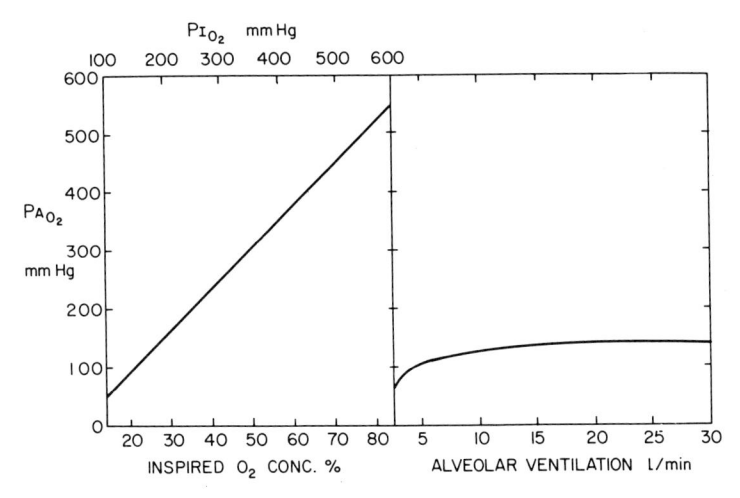

Figure 3. Graphical solutions of the equation:
$$P_{A_{O_2}} = P_{I_{O_2}} - \frac{0.863 \dot{V}_{O_2}}{\dot{V}_A}$$
where $\dot{V}_{O_2}$ = O_2 uptake = 250 ml./min.
$P_{A_{O_2}}$ = alveolar partial pressure of O_2
$P_{I_{O_2}}$ = inspired partial pressure of O_2
$\dot{V}_A$ = alveolar ventilation

Left-hand panel is the relationship between inspired O_2 concentration and alveolar P_{O_2} for a constant alveolar ventilation. Right-hand panel is the relationship between alveolar P_{O_2} and alveolar ventilation for a constant inspired O_2 concentration (air).

tion that the unmeasured and/or unmeasurable factors listed previously may modify these guidelines substantially.

The demonstration of arterial lactic acidosis in the presence of a reduced oxygen delivery indicates hypoxic tissue damage, and under these circumstances improvement of tissue oxygenation must be accomplished rapidly. However, the degree of hypoxemia required to produce lactic acidosis in the presence of a normal cardiac output and Hb concentration is severe (arterial PO_2 less than 35 mm. Hg).[2] In the presence of shock, lactic acidosis occurs much more readily, so that the combination of hypoxemia and reduced tissue perfusion is particularly lethal.[2]

With these considerations in mind I maintain that, in general, it is unnecessary to maintain the arterial PO_2 above 80 mm. Hg, and that values between 60 and 80 are adequate. When the arterial PO_2 is in the 50's, oxygen delivery is still adequate, but the patient is in a very delicate situation. Further deterioration of gas exchange will result in a precipitous fall in oxygen delivery, so that he needs to be watched with great care. For levels of arterial PO_2 below 50 (unless this is chronic) it is usually mandatory to improve tissue oxygen delivery.

Sometimes this can be achieved by increasing the inspired oxygen concentration above 40 per cent. In general, a loose-fitting mask will not deliver an O_2 concentration greater than 40 per cent even with high flow. A more tightly fitting mask fitted with a Hans-Rudolph valve at the inlet, to separate inspiratory and expiratory flow, with a reservoir bag on the oxygen inflow line will provide an inspired oxygen concentration greater than 40 per cent. Even if this improves oxygen delivery satisfactorily, it may lead to oxygen toxicity if administered over a period of days. More information is badly needed about the time it takes for oxygen toxicity to develop with a given inspired oxygen concentration. In the absence of this information one needs to weigh the possible dangers of oxygen toxicity against the hazards of artificial ventilation.

If a high oxygen concentration is inadequate or if it is necessary to administer it for prolonged periods, artificial ventilation may be used to increase oxygen delivery by the second mechanism previously described, namely, to decrease the alveolar-arterial oxygen tension difference. The rationale for this use of artificial ventilation is to convert lung units in which there is perfusion but no ventilation (ventilation perfusion ratio=zero) to units with a finite ventilation perfusion ratio, that is, to convert shunts in the lungs to ventilated air spaces. Lung shunts occur in diseases which lead to filling of alveoli with liquid or to alveolar instability and atelectasis (pulmonary edema, pneumonia, respiratory distress syndrome, and so forth). Because of surface tension between the air liquid interface in the lung, it may require high pressures to inflate these alveoli. Under these circumstances continuous positive pressure ventilation is usually necessary, with the added hazards of pneumothorax, interstitial and mediastinal emphysema, and decreased cardiac output. Additionally increasing the inspired PO_2 is usually necessary to minimize the effect on arterial O_2 content of units with low ventilation perfusion ratios. (Parenthetically it should be stated that the common practice of maintaining continuous positive pressure by adding a resistance to the expired line is less useful than placing the expired line under a water seal to the desired depth. In the former instance the end-expiratory pressure will vary according to the end-inspiratory pressure, the expiratory time, total respiratory flow resistance, and total respiratory compliance. The latter method depends only upon the depth at which the expiratory line is placed below the water seal). It is becoming abundantly clear that continuous positive pressure ventilation may prove lifesaving when other efforts at reversing life-threatening hypoxia fail. One must remember, however, that it is likely to succeed only when there are lung shunts. Hypoxia due to low ventilation perfusion ratios, diffusion defects, and hypoventilation does not require this form of therapy. Hypoxia resulting from intracardiac shunts cannot be reversed by any of these means.

In summary, artificial ventilation to improve hypoxia is indicated only under two circumstances:

1. When it is also indicated for hypercapnia and alveolar hypoventilation.

2. To convert lung shunts into units with a finitive ventilation perfusion ratio. Here continuous positive pressure ventilation with enrichment of inspired gas with oxygen is also necessary.

It is difficult if not impossible to establish a long list of indications and contraindications for artificial ventilation on the basis of present knowledge. The decision must be based on the careful assessment of each individual patient with as much understanding as possible of the underlying pathophysiology. Artificial ventilation for prophylactic reasons requires better documentation of its value before these heroic means are justified to prevent deterioration.

References

1. Pontoppidan, H., Laver, M. B., and Geffin, B.: Acute respiratory failure in the surgical patient. In Welch, C. (ed.): *Advances in Surgery.* Vol. 4. Chicago, Year Book Medical Publishers, Inc., 1970, pp. 163–254.
2. Oliva, P. B.: Lactic acidosis. (Review.) Amer. J. Med. *48:*209, 1970.
3. Bendixen, H. H., Egbert, L. D., Hedley-Whyte, J., Laver, M. B., and Pontoppidan, H.: *Respiratory Care.* St. Louis, The C. V. Mosby Co., 1965, pp. 118–119.
4. Lenfant, C.: Revival of an old battle: Intermittent vs continuous positive-pressure breathing. (Editorial.) New Eng. J. Med. *283:*1463–1464, 1970.
5. Campbell, E. J. M.: Respiratory failure. Brit. Med. J. *1:*1451, 1965.
6. Dill, D. B., Talbott, J. H., and Consolazio, W. V.: Blood as a physicochemical system. Man at rest. J. Biol. Chem. *118:*649, 1937.
7. Henderson, L. J.: *Blood, a Study in General Physiology.* New Haven, Yale University Press, 1928.

Comment

Management of Acute Pulmonary Insufficiency

Medicine has its fashions and enthusiasms as does every other aspect of human activity. A current one is the use of tracheal intubation and positive pressure ventilation in a variety of acute pulmonary illnesses. No one questions that maintenance of pulmonary ventilation by this means can be lifesaving. The controversy concerns the indications for the application of this drastic therapy. Singer presents the views of the enthusiasts and Macklem those of the conservatives. Both emphasize the dangers inherent in the method. These include injury to the larynx and trachea, obstruction from improper placement or plugging of the tube, and damage to the lung. The latter problem is most commonly seen with prolonged use of the respirator in association with high concentrations of oxygen.[1] The benefit to be derived from respirator therapy must be balanced against these hazards.

There is surprising agreement between the authors on the management of chronic obstructive lung disease. Both recommend the management of the great majority of these patients with controlled oxygen therapy. The rationale for this approach has been lucidly presented by Campbell. It is dependent on retention of the hypoxic stimulus to ventilation while avoiding danger to tissues from severe hypoxia. In applying this method of therapy it is essential that drugs such as sedatives or tranquilizers that depress ventilation should be assiduously avoided.

There is also little difference of opinion that progressive increase in the carbon dioxide tension of the arterial blood in disorders such as drug overdosage or acute neurologic disease is an indication for ventilatory assistance. The disagreement is in regard to the use of this therapy in patients with acute respiratory illnesses without hypercapnia. Singer has used the term "impending respiratory failure" to designate this group of patients. The assumption underlying his approach is that, without ventilatory assistance, these patients will ultimately develop respiratory failure with progressive increase in $PaCO_2$. As Macklem points out, there is no reason to assume that all or even the majority of these patients will pursue this course or that the early use of assisted respiration is beneficial. Well designed clinical studies are not available.

Most important is the need to consider each illness and each patient separately. The indications for ventilatory assistance are quite different in the patient who is recovering from recent cardiac surgery and a patient with extensive pneumonia. A patient with myasthenia gravis and marked weakness of respiratory muscles may benefit from assisted respiration, and yet the procedure may not be indicated in a patient with multiple pulmonary emboli.

As pointed out by Macklem, there has been recent interest in the use of positive end expiratory pressure to alter the pulmonary lesion in patients with pulmonary edema from a variety of causes.[2] A specific indication is failure to correct hypoxia by inhalation of oxygen. It is believed that positive end-expiratory pressure prevents terminal air space collapse, thus restoring ventilation to previously nonventilated but perfused lung units. Continued study of this type of therapy should better define the indications.

Measurement of the tension of oxygen and carbon dioxide in arterial blood has become commonplace in most hospitals. Associated with this development is a belief that is important to maintain the PaO_2 at normal levels. Adherents to this concept should read carefully the discussion by Macklem. He points out that the oxygen content of the arterial blood is more important than the oxygen tension. The aim of therapy should be to maintain an adequate oxygen tension in the tissue. Oxygen transport to the tissue will depend not only on the tension of oxygen in the arterial blood, the hemoglobin content of the blood, and the oxyhemoglobin dissociation curve, but also on the cardiac output and the local blood flow to the tissue.

References

1. Nash, G., Blennerhassett, J. B., and Pontoppidan, H.: Pulmonary lesions associated with oxygen therapy and artificial ventilation. New Eng. J. Med. 276:368–374, 1967.
2. Kumar, A., Falke, K. J., Geffin, B., et al.: Continuous positive-pressure ventilation in acute respiratory failure. Effects on hemodynamics and lung function. New Eng. J. Med. 283:1430–1436, 1970.

RICHARD V. EBERT

11

Treatment of Massive Pulmonary Embolism

The Effectiveness of Thrombolytic Therapy
  by Richard D. Sautter

The Advantages of Embolectomy
  by Robert L. Berger

Comment
  by Richard V. Ebert

The Effectiveness of Thrombolytic Therapy

RICHARD D. SAUTTER

Marshfield, Wisconsin

"And never a saint in heaven took pity on my soul in agony."
Coleridge, Ancient Mariner

There is no need to trace the historical background of pulmonary thromboembolism. All physicians who have spent time on the medical-surgical wards have seen, though not always recognized, this sometimes insidious and other times suddenly catastrophic disease.

While prevention is perhaps the most important consideration, it is not the subject of this paper, and until methods of prevention are much more effective than at present, it is important to plan a therapeutic approach which will not be more hazardous than the disease itself. This essay will deal principally with the various forms of therapy, presented in a highly editorialized fashion. It would indeed be presumptuous of me to recommend the precise therapy for massive pulmonary emboli, because of its dependence upon the facilities and resources available to the physician, as well as his particular abilities. Because complete answers to some questions are not yet available, the physician's choice of therapy may also in part depend upon his prejudices. The controversy concerning management of massive emboli revolves about when or if pulmonary embolectomy is indicated. A controlled study pitting embolectomy against nonoperative management would end this controversy.

I, at present, hold the biased position, as a cardiothoracic surgeon, that embolectomy is rarely indicated. This opinion is based on the results reported in the literature, and on my personal experience with 22 pulmonary embolectomies and the nonoperative management of the patient with massive pulmonary embolization. The following pages will explain this position. The important areas to consider that relate to therapy for massive pulmonary emboli are: (1) natural history, (2) experience with thrombolytic therapy, and (3) experience with pulmonary embolectomy.

Natural History

The tributaries of the inferior vena cava are almost invariably the source of major pulmonary emboli. The iliofemoral channel is by far the single most common source, with a few major emboli originating from the leg veins.[1] This has important implications when planning the prevention of pulmonary embolic disease.

Although mechanical blockade of the pulmonary artery by emboli does not completely explain *all* the deaths related to this disease, or its entire pathophysiology, it is by all odds the most important factor in determining survival. The amount of embolic obstruction that causes death is variable, seldom does less than 50 per cent obstruction cause death, and seldom do patients survive more than 75 per cent obstruction. There is little evidence to suggest that humoral mechanisms play a role in causing death from pulmonary embolism in man; however, such evidence does exist relative to certain experimental animals.[2]

The majority of patients suffering a massive embolus do not succumb. For those patients who do ultimately succumb, the interval between massive embolus and death is quite important when contemplating specific therapy. Nearly half the patients who die will do so in the first 15 minutes; 60 per cent or more will be dead in 30 minutes; and only one fourth to one third will live an hour.[3] The mortality rate after one hour drops precipitously, with only one half of the remaining patients dead at six hours. Of those who succumb, some do so as a result of the second or third episode of embolization, indicating that more attention should be given to the "herald" embolus.[4]

There are several questions concerning the ultimate fate of pulmonary thromboemboli. Do thromboemboli resolve spontaneously? Is resolution complete? When and how often? Does a major pulmonary artery recanalize following complete obstruction? There are no complete answers to these questions, but available information contains the answer to whether pulmonary embolectomy is ever indicated for the preservation of pulmonary function.

Without question, the intrinsic fibrinolytic system spontaneously lyses pulmonary emboli. The rate of lysis varies and depends on a variety of factors including: (1) the age of the thromboemboli (fresh thrombi lyse more easily and more quickly than old thrombi); (2) the size, location, and perfusion of the thromboemboli (thromboemboli lyse slower where obstruction is complete than where it is incomplete); and (3) the potential of the intrinsic fibrinolytic system.

By means of serial pulmonary arteriography we have demonstrated that lysis can occur in as short a time as 24 hours.[5] Also, as have several other authors,[6-9] we have seen this process take several weeks or months. In some circumstances it likely takes more than four months, as suggested by Lord Brock.[10]

The completeness of lysis is critical. Using conventional tests of pulmonary function, we studied 14 patients who survived for one year following massive embolus. Eight of the patients had minimal deficits easily explained on the basis of pre-existing cardiorespiratory disease. None of these patients complained of compromised pulmonary function or showed clinical evidence of it. Although most patients have considerable pulmonary reserve, and conventional tests do leave some restriction of pulmonary function undetected, restriction of any significant magnitude should most certainly be apparent clinically. If it is not, does failure of resolution really represent a problem?

The reader must remember that I am discussing single acute episodes of massive embolization; these remarks do not apply to recurrent embolization.

The Urokinase Pulmonary Embolism Trial (UPET) has provided additional, although somewhat controversial, information.[11] Of 105 patients who had pulmonary scans one year following the initial embolic episode, 19 had a perfusion deficit of 1 per cent or less. Mean perfusion deficit in the entire group was 5.2 per cent. Perfusion deficit exceeded 10 per cent in 17 patients, nine of whom received urokinase and eight of whom received heparin. The greatest residual deficit was 32.6 per cent, and the average deficit in these 17 patients was 17.2 per cent. Six of the 17 had a history of previous pulmonary embolus, and 14 had massive emboli. Two of the 17 had recurrent pulmonary emboli during the first two weeks of observation. How many had recurrent emboli afterward is unknown. Presumably the perfusion deficit at one year was in the same area as the initial one, but this has not been confirmed.

These data would have been much more meaningful had the 17 patients with deficits of 10 per cent or more been evaluated by pulmonary arteriography and pulmonary function studies. This is especially true in the light of work by Isawa et al.,[12] who showed that, in pulmonary scans made following an acute embolic episode, the sequential changes are best explained by the changes in pulmonary arterial pressure and resistance in parallel circuits. By positioning the patient, he has shown normal perfusion (by pulmonary scan) in areas of previous deficit. It is important to emphasize that in the 17 patients with residual deficits of 10 per cent or more at one year, six had suffered a previous embolus; the number who had recurrent emboli in the 50 weeks before the last pulmonary scan is unknown.

Mr. Paneth[13] and others, who believe that major pulmonary arteries rarely recanalize following complete obstruction, have not followed such patients long enough, and they ignore the autopsy data. The only evidence of previous old emboli that the prosector usually finds is fibrous plaques, atheromatous foci, bands, and cords. Only *rarely* is a major vessel completely obstructed.[14, 14a]

Although not conclusive, the evidence seems to indicate that acute pulmonary emboli usually spontaneously resolve, leaving little clinical pulmonary deficit.

Diagnosis

When dealing with a catastrophic, massive pulmonary embolus, speed and diagnostic accuracy are invaluable. Because an absolutely positive diagnosis is essential before definitive treatment can be instituted, the only method of obtaining a specific diagnosis is by pulmonary angiography. No patient is too ill for this procedure if massive embolization is suspected. Pulmonary arteriography can be safely done in critically ill patients.[15]

Experience with Thrombolytic Therapy

There are numerous reports in the literature concerning the use of lytic agents in the treatment of pulmonary embolism.[16-23] The largest and most significant study is Phase I of the UPET.[11] This was a multi-institutional, rigidly controlled study pitting a 12-hour infusion of urokinase against conventional heparin sodium therapy. Patients receiving urokinase were given a loading dose of 2000 CTA units per pound body weight, followed by a constant infusion of the same amount of drug per hour for a 12-hour period. Patients receiving heparin received a loading dose of 75 units per pound body weight, followed by a constant infusion of 10 units per pound body weight for a 12-hour period. All patients received heparin sodium intravenously for a minimum of five days before oral anticoagulant therapy was instituted.

Independent panels with no knowledge of assigned therapy evaluated the data from the initial and 24-hour pulmonary arteriograms, serial radioisotope pulmonary scans, and the initial and 24-hour right heart and pulmonary arterial pressure. At 24 hours the improvement in each of these parameters was definitely superior in the urokinase-treated group as compared to the heparin-treated group. The most dramatic improvement was seen in the small group of patients with massive emboli who were in shock.

The results of this study demonstrated unequivocally that:

1. Urokinase accelerates lysis of pulmonary emboli, *especially massive pulmonary emboli*.

2. Compared with heparin sodium therapy, urokinase exposes the patient to a twofold higher incidence of bleeding.

3. Urokinase does not affect the recurrence rate of pulmonary embolization.

Exactly when a significant lysis occurs after the initiation of lytic therapy is yet to be determined, but it probably takes several hours. This is under study in Phase II of the Urokinase-Streptokinase Pulmonary Embolism Trial (USPET). Our experience in the pilot phase (pre-Phase I UPET) using urokinase to treat pulmonary embolism was variable, but in general the pulmonary artery pressure fell near the end of the eight-hour urokinase infusion. Presumably this was secondary to lysis of the embolus. One patient who sustained a massive embolus and was in profound shock, requiring support with vasopressors, became normotensive without vasopressors two hours after the initiation of urokinase therapy. This same patient showed significant lysis of emboli when the initial arteriogram was compared with the arteriogram done immediately following the cessation of urokinase therapy (eight hours).[23]

For the purpose of the UPET study, massive embolization was defined as an obstruction or filling defect present in two or more lobar arteries or their equivalent. This group was further divided into those who had persistent shock and those who did not. Shock was defined as a systolic arterial blood pressure of less than 80 mm. Hg (or less than 100 mm. Hg if a previously well documented history of systolic hypertension existed) by multiple sphygmomanometer readings at one-minute intervals for at least 10 minutes. There were 89 patients with massive emboli admitted to the trial, 11 of them in shock.

While this group (the patients entered with massive embolization and shock) is small, it bears close inspection. Of these 11 patients, seven received urokinase and four received heparin sodium. *Not one patient died as a result of the massive embolus.* There were, however, two deaths, both in the urokinase-treated group; one patient died of respiratory arrest secondary to central nervous system metastasis of a malignant melanoma. The second death occurred 12 hours after the cessation of urokinase infusion as a result of bleeding from multiple gastric stress ulcers. A poll of the participating institutions indicated five embolectomies were done during the conduct of the trial. There was one survivor. It does appear that the patients submitted to embolectomy may have been more seriously ill than those admitted to the trial.

There seems to be some confusion by Dr. Attar[24] and perhaps others concerning patients entered in the study who were in shock but had submassive emboli (three patients). All died, not as a result of pulmonary embolization, but rather of their underlying disease process.

A 66 year old female admitted to the study with massive embolization and shock is of particular interest. Because of rapid deterioration and difficulty supporting her blood pressure with vasopressors, she was placed on partial cardiopulmonary bypass by femoral-femoral cannulation; local anesthesia was used. Heparin sodium was the drug assigned for therapy, and during the infusion she was intermittently supported by partial cardiopulmonary bypass over an eight-hour period. Bleeding from repair of the venotomy-arteriotomy after the cessation of bypass was troublesome. However, this patient is a long-term survivor who, incidentally, has no decrease in pulmonary reserve demonstrated by conventional pulmonary function tests.

Bleeding complications in the study were defined as moderate if estimated blood loss was 500 to 1500 ml., or if the hematocrit fell five to 10 points, or if the patients received two or less units of blood. The complications were considered severe if any of these upper limits were exceeded. The bleeding in almost every instance was the result of an invasive procedure, such as venous cutdown, or arterial or venous puncture. Forty-five per cent of the patients who received urokinase had moderate or severe bleeding complications; 20 per cent of those treated with heparin sodium suffered this complication. The bleeding attributed to urokinase appears early and clearly coincides with the period of infusion. At first glance this complication is somewhat frightening, but it is important to explain that for the purposes of the UPET study many invasive procedures were required. Testimony to this fact is that 27 of the patients who experienced severe bleeding received only heparin sodium. During the pilot period, we treated 25 patients with urokinase; none lost more than 500 cc. of blood. Also, the incidence of moderate or severe bleeding at this institution during Phases I and II was less than 13.5 per cent (five of 37). One institution, presently in Phase II of the USPET, which did not employ arterial punctures, has treated 32 patients with lytic agents without a single severe bleeding complication.[25] Bleeding complications from clinical use of the drug can be reduced to an acceptable level if meticulous attention is paid to invasive procedures.

The contraindications for the use of lytic agents are, of course, directly related to the hazards of bleeding. These are well described in the paper reporting Phase I of the UPET. In general, the contraindications are the same as for anticoagulant therapy, with the strongest contraindication being the violation of a major body cavity in the 10 days preceding contemplated therapy. These contraindications also include diagnostic invasive procedures, such as biopsy of the liver or kidney, lumbar puncture, and thoracentesis. In the pilot study preceding Phase I, we did treat a patient who had had cholecystectomy only five days before the urokinase infusion. Although this patient did not suffer a bleeding complication, that hazard was present. Certainly patients who sustain a life-threatening massive embolus and who have undergone only surface surgery, where bleeding in the operative area would be readily apparent, might be considered for lytic therapy prior to the 10th postoperative day. More experience is necessary to determine exactly when in the postoperative period lytic agents can be safely administered.

The recurrence rate of embolization during the first two weeks of observation between the urokinase and heparin sodium-treated groups is 15 and 19 per cent, respectively. This cannot be regarded as hard data, as recurrent embolization was considered proved if the radioisotope lung scan and the clinical signs were positive, and considered probable if either was present. The vagaries of the radioisotope pulmonary scan, and more importantly the subjective interpretation of the patient's symptoms, do not provide as reliable information as had pulmonary arteriography-confirmed re-embolization.

Experience with Pulmonary Embolectomy

Perhaps no other surgical procedure has so long a controversial history as pulmonary embolectomy. Since described by Trendelenburg 64 years ago,[26] the worth of this worn courtesan of surgery has involved some of the leading practitioners of our art. One of the reasons she continues in favor is the theatrical setting provided and thereby the dramatic opportunity for the heroic surgeon to pit his skills against nearly insurmountable odds.

In 1944 Ochsner, in an attempt to lay this procedure to rest, addressed the American Surgical Association: "I hope we will not have any more papers on the removal of pulmonary emboli before this organization." And now, 28 years later, I, although most humbly, recommend nearly the same course, and so the circle closes for yet the second time.

Several methods for removing emboli from the pulmonary artery have been described. The Trendelenburg procedure requires the ultimate in luck, skill, and a superaggressive attitude. However, by all odds the safest and easiest method of performing this relatively simple procedure is to employ cardiopulmonary bypass. This may be established best by peripheral cannulation using local anesthesia. Because successful induction of general anesthesia without severe hypotension or cardiac arrest suggests either a superlative anesthesiologist or, more likely, sufficient pulmonary reserve to obviate embolectomy, the support offered by partial cardiopulmonary bypass allows the surgeon to proceed in an orderly and deliberate manner to remove the emboli. One of the most striking observations made during our experience with embolectomy was the immediate and pronounced improvement seen in patients with massive embolization once supported by partial cardiopulmonary bypass. It is likely that, since the development of membrane oxygenators, this support may be allowed to continue for days. Sufficient improvement in cardiopulmonary reserve may be established by the intrinsic fibrinolytic processes during this period of support.

Perhaps the commonest indication for embolectomy now in vogue is 50 per cent or more obstruction of the pulmonary artery and the presence of shock. This indication would seem to ignore the 11 patients admitted to the UPET that fit this description, none of whom died of pulmonary emboli after receiving "nonaggressive expectant type of therapy."[27]

In discussing mortality from pulmonary embolectomy, it is important to recall that half the patients who succumb will do so within the first 15 minutes, 60 per cent in 30 minutes; and only one third survive an hour following the onset of symptoms. If pulmonary embolectomy is performed several hours after the onset of symptoms, survival should, in most cases, be expected. The interval between onset of symptoms and embolectomy is the most likely explanation for the wide variability in the mortality statistics, some surgeons reporting 80 per cent survivors[28] and others reporting 80 per cent deaths.[29] At one time early in our experience, our reaction time from onset of symptoms to embolectomy was one half hour, which for the most part explains our dismal survival rate (four out of 22). Eight of these patients suffered cardiac arrest and were brought to the operative suite with resuscitative measures in progress. Since one patient in this category survived, it is feasible to resuscitate such patients; however, they may not require embolectomy. Of interest are the six patients submitted to embolectomy because of rapid deterioration during induction of anesthesia for contemplated caval ligation. This emphasizes the delicate balance of the cardiorespiratory system in patients with massive embolism, so that any caval interruptive procedure should be done using local anesthesia. We at present use femoral vein plication or the vena caval umbrella to prevent recurrent pulmonary emboli. Both these procedures can be done using only local anesthesia.

The patient's age has a definite effect on the survival and is related to the degree of cardiopulmonary reserve present at the time of embolization. We observed one young person who was normotensive despite 70 per cent obstruction of his pulmonary circulation. Conversely, 50 per cent (or occasionally less) obstruction in elderly patients, especially those with serious pre-existing cardiopulmonary disease, causes shock and extremely rapid deterioration. The suggestion of Makey and Bliss[30] that this operation be confined to younger patients who have no chronic disease would indeed decrease the mortality rate, as it would confine the embolectomy to those patients most likely to survive without it.

For those who are incurably surgically oriented, the Trendelenburg procedure, or a modification[31, 32] thereof should be the logical choice of therapy for those patients who will die before cardiopulmonary bypass can be established.

Particular circumstances are required if this surgical approach is to save more patients than it kills. A very skillful surgeon, with appropriate assistance and instruments, must be in close proximity to the patient who is to have the massive, fatal embolus. This surgeon must possess almost supernatural abilities (1) to know instantly those patients who will not survive without embolectomy, and (2) to instantly make a positive diagnosis on only clinical evidence (myocardial infarction is eight times as common as pulmonary embolism and both cause cardiovascular collapse). These circumstances have been reported less than 100 times in the last 64 years. Of more importance is the unknown number of patients who have succumbed from this procedure who would have lived without it, or who were operated upon for a mistaken diagnosis. The suggestion by Murley[4] that training for urgent embolectomy is necessary in all hospitals, combined with his statement that the Trendelenburg-type procedure, despite its high mortality, is the "only operation possible in many cases," and the delight he expressed at the formation of a mobile embolectomy team, could make simple fainting a fatal disease in the hospitals of England.

The experience in the literature and my personal experience with massive pulmonary embolism lead me to the following opinions:

First, pulmonary embolectomy never was nor is now indicated except as a lifesaving maneuver; that is, the patients not in shock never were and never are candidates for the procedure. To suggest that this procedure is indicated for the preservation of pulmonary function on the basis of presently available information is absurd. I implore any who have demonstrated persistent obstruction of a major pulmonary artery by arteriography one year after the initial embolic episode uncomplicated by re-embolization to report this experience.

Second, if there are, indeed, candidates for embolectomy, it must be performed quickly, preferably within one hour or less after the onset of symptoms, as this is the period of time in which the highest mortality occurs. To be significant, all future reports of pulmonary embolectomies must state the time from onset of symptoms to embolectomy, for after one hour the survival rate without surgery, or for that matter any form of therapy, improves greatly (remember the 11 patients in the UPET with massive embolization and shock, none of whom succumbed from pulmonary embolism).

Third, cardiopulmonary bypass alone will resuscitate many patients without the added hazard of embolectomy. Cardiopulmonary bypass utilizing membrane oxygenators can likely be continued for days.

Fourth, embolectomy is perhaps indicated in those *rare* instances when there is an absolute contraindication to long-term heparin sodium therapy which would prevent long-term support with cardiopulmonary bypass.

Lastly, because cardiopulmonary reserve is restored more quickly by thrombolytic agents than by the natural intrinsic process, and because these agents are particularly effective against massive emboli, they will likely evolve as the treatment of choice for massive acute emboli. Although bleeding may be formidable, a cautious trial of such agents is indicated for patients being supported by cardiopulmonary bypass.

The controversy, however, will continue until a trial pits embolectomy against nonoperative management. The individual physician will treat the individual patient according to his own persuasion and, until the facts are at hand, this is how it should be.

Because I have never had to say in retrospect concerning any patient I have seen with massive emboli, "I wish I had done an embolectomy," my prejudice will remain until the completion of such a trial.

References

1. Mavor, G. E., and Galloway, J. M. D.: The iliofemoral venous segment as a source for pulmonary emboli. Lancet 1:871–874, 1967.
2. Thomas, D. P., Tanabe, G., Khan, M., and Stein, M.: Humoral factors mediated by platelets in experimental pulmonary embolism. In Sasahara, A. A., and Stein, M. (eds.): Pulmonary Embolic Disease. New York, Grune & Stratton, 1965, pp. 59–64.
3. Soloff, L. A., and Rodman, T.: Acute pulmonary embolism. II. Clinical. Amer. Heart J. 74:829–847, 1967.
4. Murley, R. S.: Massive pulmonary embolism: What can be done to improve survival? Brit. J. Surg. 57:771–775, 1970.
5. Sautter, R. D., Fletcher, F. W., Ousley, J. L., and Wenzel, F. J.: Extremely rapid resolution of a pulmonary embolus. Report of a case. Dis. Chest 52:825–827, 1967.
6. Fred, H. L., Axelrad, M. A., Lewis, J. M., and Alexander, J. K.: Rapid resolution of pulmonary thromboemboli in man. J.A.M.A. 196:1137–1139, 1966.
7. Dalen, J. E., Banas, J. S., Brooks, H. L., Evans, G. L., Paraskos, J. A., and Dexter, L.: Resolution rate of acute pulmonary embolism in man. New Eng. J. Med. 280:1194–1199, 1969.
8. Secker Walker, R. H., Jackson, J. A., and Goodwin, J.: Resolution of pulmonary embolism. Brit. Med. J. 4:135–139, 1970.
9. Sautter, R. D., Fletcher, F. W., Emanuel, D. A., Lawton, B. R., and Olsen, T. G.: Complete resolution of massive pulmonary thromboembolism. J.A.M.A. 189:948–949, 1964.
10. Brock, L., Nabil, H., and Gibson, R. V.: Case of late pulmonary embolectomy. Brit. Med. J. 4:598–599, 1967.
11. Cooperative Study: Urokinase pulmonary embolism trial, phase 1 results. J.A.M.A. 214:2163–2172, 1970.
12. Isawa, T., Wasserman, K., and Taplin, G. V.: Variability of lung scans following pulmonary embolization. Amer. Rev. Resp. Dis. 101:207–217, 1970.
13. Paneth, M.: Surgical treatment of massive pulmonary embolism. Trans. Med. Soc. London, Vol. 85, 1969.
14. Hume, M. Sevitt, S., and Thomas, D. P.: Venous Thrombosis and Pulmonary Embolism. Cambridge, Harvard University Press, 1970, Chap. 11, pp. 212–213.
14a. Edwards, J. E.: Personal communication, 1973.
15. Dalen, J. E., Brooks, H. L., Johnson, J. W., Meister, S. G., Szucs, M. M., Jr., and Dexter, L.: Pulmonary arteriography in acute pulmonary embolism, indications, technique and results in 367 patients. Amer. Heart J. 81:175–185, 1971.
16. Tow, D. E., Wagner, H. N., and Holmes, R. A.: Urokinase in pulmonary embolism. New Eng. J. Med. 277:1161–1167, 1967.
17. Hirsh, J., McDonald, I. G., O'Sullivan, E. F., and Jelinek, V. M.: Comparison of the effects of streptokinase and heparin on the early rate of resolution of major pulmonary embolism. Canad. Med. Ass. J. 104:488–491, 1971.
18. Hirsh, J., et al.: Streptokinase in the treatment of major pulmonary embolism: Experience with 25 patients. Aust. Ann. Med. 19(Suppl. 19):54–59, 1970.
19. Kakkar, V. V., and Raftery, E. B.: Selection of patients with pulmonary embolism for thrombolytic therapy. Lancet 2:237–241, 1970.
20. Sasahara, A. A., Cannilla, J. E., Belko, J. S., Morse, R. L., and Criss, A. J.: Urokinase therapy in clinical pulmonary embolism. New Eng. J. Med. 277:1168–1173, 1967.
21. Miller, G. A., Sutton, G. C., Kerr, I. H., Gibson, R. V., and Honey, M.: Comparison of streptokinase and heparin in the treatment of isolated acute massive pulmonary embolism. Brit. Med. J. 2:681–684, 1971.
22. Hirsh, J., Hale, G. S., McDonald, I. G., McCarthy, R. A., and Cade, J. E.: Resolution of

acute massive pulmonary embolism after pulmonary arterial infusion of streptokinase. Lancet 2:593–597, 1967.
23. Sautter, R. D., Emanuel, D. A., Fletcher, F. W., Wenzel, F. J., and Matson, J. I.: Urokinase for the treatment of acute pulmonary thromboembolism. J.A.M.A. 202:215–218, 1967.
24. Attar, S.: In discussion of Sautter, R. D., Myers, W. O., and Wenzel, F. J.: Implications of the Urokinase study concerning the surgical treatment of pulmonary embolism. J. Thorac. Cardiov. Surg. 63:54–59, 1972.
25. Bell, W. R., and Wagner, H. N.: Personal communication.
26. Trendelenburg, F.: Ueber die operative behandlung der Embolie der Lungenarterie. Arch. Klin. Chir. 86:686–700, 1908.
27. Cooley, D. A., and Beall, A. C., Jr.: Embolectomy for acute massive pulmonary embolism. Surg. Gynec. Obstet. 126:805–810, 1968.
28. Berger, R. L.: Pulmonary embolectomy for massive pulmonary embolism. Amer. J. Surg. 121:437–441, 1971.
29. Sautter, R. D., Myers, W. O., and Wenzel, F. J.: Implications of the Urokinase study concerning the surgical treatment of pulmonary embolism. J. Thorac. Cardiov. Surg. 63:54–59, 1972.
30. Makey, A. R., and Bliss, B. P.: Pulmonary embolectomy, review of five cases with three survivals. Lancet 2:1155–1158, 1966.
31. Wieberdink, J.: Trendelenburg's operation for pulmonary embolism with modified technique. J. Int. Coll. Surgeons 34:380–385, 1960.
32. Vossschulte, K., Stiller, H., and Eisenreich, F.: Emergency embolectomy by the transsternal approach for acute pulmonary embolism. Surgery 58:317–323, 1965.

The Advantages of Embolectomy

ROBERT L. BERGER

Boston University School of Medicine and Boston City Hospital

Pulmonary embolectomy for massive embolization was conceived and reared in an atmosphere of adversity and it was not allowed to grow to full maturity. The disease is sudden in onset; it is quickly lethal and presents a desperate clinical picture. In an attempt to meet such a lethal threat, equally desperate measures were deemed acceptable for therapy. Trendelenburg's operation represents such a last ditch and almost hopeless effort. The procedure consists of removal of the clot through an incision in the pulmonary artery without cardiopulmonary bypass. It was doomed from the start except in rare situations in which circumstances were miraculously favorable for the operation. The procedure was introduced in 1908, Trendelenburg himself never had a survivor, and it took almost 20 years before Kirschner reported the first success. Because of the poor record, only terminal and dying patients were regarded as candidates for embolectomy. They were beyond salvage, the number of operative deaths increased, and pulmonary embolectomy acquired a poor reputation.

The second phase in the development of pulmonary embolectomy coincided with the employment of the heart and lung machine during the performance of embolectomy. The results were far more gratifying than the experience with the Trendelenburg operation; however, the salvage was still only in the vicinity of 50 per cent. Some of the failures were related to the developmental problems of open heart surgery, but many more patients were lost because of irreversible circulatory collapse during induction of anesthesia and exposure of the heart.[1] The potential of the pump oxygenator as a life-sustaining device during this critical preoperative period was not fully appreciated. However, with increasing experience the need for mechanical circulatory support in the preoperative stages became apparent, and with the addition of this new dimension significant improvement in survival rates was obtained. The use of the heart and lung machine for preoperative support as well as intraoperative bypass ushered in the third phase in the development of pulmonary embolectomy. By the time this effective method evolved it was too late to dispel a firmly entrenched sentiment against the operative approach, and therefore "modern" pulmonary embolectomy has not received fair evaluation. The lack of an appropriate trial is most unfortunate, since pulmonary embolectomy is conceptually most attractive and there are indications that in practice it can be extremely rewarding.

Natural History and Results of Therapy

Pulmonary embolectomy is reserved for massive embolization, defined as acute occlusion of more than one half of the pulmonary vascular tree resulting in sustained or profound shock. (Lesser degrees of embolization are not considered as "massive" in this discussion.) The establishment of an angiographic diagnosis and preparations for the operation consume approximately two hours, and only patients who survive this period are candidates for the procedure. In an autopsy study of 63 fatal massive embolizations, 57 per cent of the patients died within two hours of the attack. The remaining 43 per cent survived the immediate episode only to die subsequently (two hours to 12 weeks), either from the initial embolus or from recurrent bouts of embolization.[2] Thus, slightly less than one half of patients who died of massive pulmonary emboli were potential operative candidates. Survival figures with medical management were obtained from a retrospective clinical study. The mortality was 100 per cent with supportive therapy, 78 per cent with heparin alone, and 60 per cent with heparinization and venous interruption.[3] These observations resemble the findings of other authors, provided only patients with truly massive embolization (greater than 50 per cent obstruction and sustained shock) are included in the series. The results of embolectomy in 28 institutions were surveyed by Cross and Mowlem.[4] They reported a 43 per cent survival rate in 137 pulmonary embolectomies. The large majority of these operations were performed without preoperative circulatory support during the developmental phases of open heart surgery when problems with perfusion were many and so common that mortality with any type of open intracardiac procedure was rather high.

In our own experience with 17 embolectomies with the almost routine use of preoperative peripheral cannulation for circulatory assistance, 13 patients survived and four died (Table 1). The first fatality occurred in a patient who had a sudden and unexpected circulatory collapse while convalescing after a mitral valvulotomy. The clinical picture was consistent with massive pulmonary embolization. Time did not permit angiography and the patient was rushed to the operating room for circulatory support and embolectomy. After cannulation of the femoral artery and vein and institution of cardiopulmonary bypass the sternum was split and the heart was exposed. The pulmonary artery was soft, without any clots. The patient died, and at autopsy a recent myocardial infarction was found. This experience emphasizes the importance of a definitive diagnosis prior to embolectomy, and the most reliable method is pulmonary angiography. Except under most unusual circumstances pulmonary embolectomy should not be performed without contrast visualization of the pulmonary vasculature. A second patient exsanguinated from a tear in the inferior vena cava during ligation of the vessel and following a successful pulmonary embolectomy. The third fatal case sustained cardiac arrest a few minutes after massive pulmonary embolization. He

Table 1. *Embolectomy in Massive Pulmonary Embolization*

CASE NO.	AGE (YR.) AND SEX	ASSOCIATED DISEASES	TIME* (HR.)	ANGIO- GRAPHY	PREOPERATIVE PERIPHERAL CANNULATION†	PREOPERATIVE MECHANICAL CIRCULATORY SUPPORT†	PROCEDURE	COMMENT
1	71, M	Postprostatectomy	6½	Yes	Yes	No	Embolectomy; IVCL‡	Survived
2	56, M	Post mitral valvotomy	½	No	Yes	Yes	Exploration	No pulmonary embolism, but myocardial infarction; died
3	58, M	Guillain-Barré syndrome	8	Yes	Yes	No	Embolectomy, IVCL	Survived
4	64, M	Postcolectomy	½	No	Yes	Yes	Embolectomy, IVCL	Late death
5	38, F	? Pill	5	Yes	Yes	No	Embolectomy, IVCL	Survived
6	64, F	Postcholecystectomy	2	Yes	Yes	Yes	Embolectomy, IVCL	Survived
7	63, F	Postcolectomy	1½	No	Yes	No	Embolectomy	Survived
8	67, M	? "Flu"	3	Yes	Yes	Yes	Embolectomy, IVCL	Survived
9	68, F	Phlebitis	8	Yes	Yes	Yes	Embolectomy, IVCL	Survived
10	53, F	Diabetes	5	Yes	Yes	Yes	Embolectomy	Caval tear, died
11	61, M	Cerebrovascular accident	28	Yes	No	Late	Embolectomy	Died
12	58, M	Phlebitis	5	Yes	Yes	No	Embolectomy, IVCL	Survived
13	45, M	None	7	Yes	Yes	Yes	Embolectomy, IVCL	Shock during induction for IVCL; survived
14	38, M	Paraplegia, empyema	8	Yes	Yes	Yes	Embolectomy, IVCL	Cardiac arrest during IVCL; survived
15	77, F	Phlebitis	24	Yes	Yes	Yes	Embolectomy, Femoral Vein Ligation	Survived
16	59, F	Pituitary adenoma—postop	6	Yes	Yes	Yes	Embolectomy, IVCL	Survived
17	60, F	Postgastrectomy	6	Yes	Yes	No	Embolectomy, IVCL	Survived; hypotension during IVCL

* Between embolization and operation.
† Preoperative peripheral cannulation refers to the mere insertion of peripheral catheters for connection with the pump oxygenator. Preoperative mechanical circulatory support indicates that hypotension or cardiac arrest was encountered during induction of anesthesia or thoracotomy, necessitating the prompt institution of partial cardiopulmonary bypass.
‡ Inferior vena cava ligation.

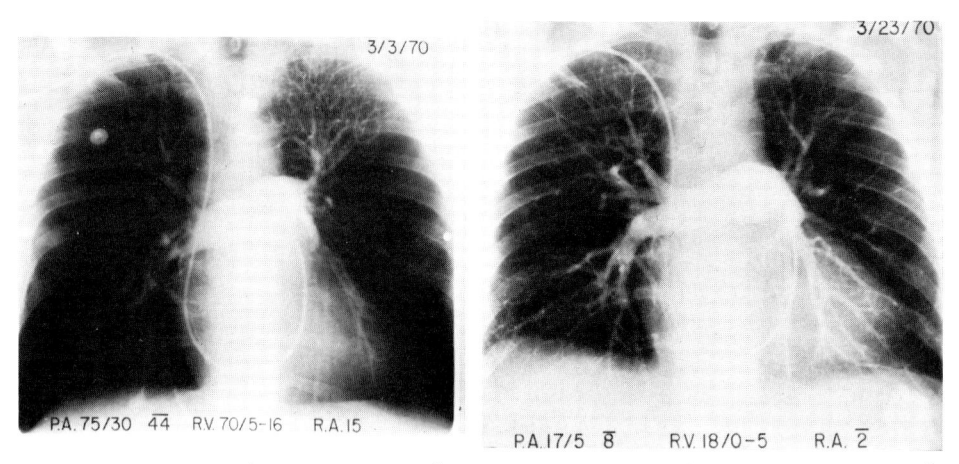

Figure 1. Pre- and postoperative pulmonary angiogram on Case No. 13. P.A. = pulmonary artery; R.V. = right ventricle; R.A. = right atrium. The unit employed is mm. of Hg.

was rushed to the operating room while cardiac massage was applied. Embolectomy was performed, satisfactory cardiorespiratory function returned but the patient remained in deep coma. Mechanical ventilation was discontinued 10 days following the operation. In retrospect it seems almost certain that the cerebral injury was sustained prior to the operation. In a fourth man, preoperative mechanical circulatory support was not employed and a refractory cardiac arrest was precipitated by induction of anesthesia. The postoperative course in the surviving 13 patients was surprisingly smooth. Repeat catheterization in three patients within 20 days of the embolectomy revealed a normal pulmonary angiogram and normal pressures in the right side of the heart (Fig. 1).

Discussion

Massive pulmonary embolization with shock implies a grave prognosis and poses a therapeutic dilemma. The choice is between drug therapy (heparin or thrombolytic agents) and pulmonary embolectomy. The objective is to select the modality which promises the highest rate of survival. The selection is difficult since available information on the efficacy of these two methods is conflicting. Usually the reported results appear on the surface more favorable with medical approach. In our own experience, however, heparinization with or without venous interruption has been an utter failure and has carried an extremely high mortality.[2,3] Consequently we turned to the operative approach in the hope of improving upon these results. The surgical experience has been gratifying and has prompted a review of the entire problem in an attempt to elucidate on the reasons for this apparent contradiction.

The term pulmonary embolization refers to a broad spectrum of cardiorespiratory insults ranging from a small single embolus manifested by fleeting chest pain to massive embolization with profound circulatory collapse. A classification or staging of the severity of the embolization has not been developed, and when the results are reported the extent of the obstruction is frequently not specified; hence, it is difficult to obtain meaningful information from the literature on the impact of treatment on the disease. This is especially true of drug therapy since it is employed in the entire spectrum of the disease, and when the results of medical management are lumped together for all patients regardless of the extent of the thrombotic occlusion, it is most difficult to evaluate the yield in the massive form of the disease. Furthermore, failure of intensive and prolonged medical efforts represents the most frequently employed indication for the operative approach. Thus, the severe and highly lethal embolizations are weeded out from the medical groups and added to the surgical experience with obvious distortion of the operative statistics. Documentation for this is ample in the literature: ". . . the best indication for an emergency operation is a patient in extremis with sustained peripheral hypotension"[5]; ". . . patients who deteriorate on medical treatment will be submitted to pulmonary embolectomy"[6]; ". . . restrict embolectomy to patients who suffered cardiac arrest. . . ."[7] With such case selection, comparable series with medical and surgical therapy are unavailable. If these terminal embolectomy patients were retained in the medically managed population the mortality in this group would approach 100 per cent, whereas if embolectomy were performed in the less severe forms, and earlier, surgical survival figures would improve dramatically. Thus, any comparison of the efficacy of the two forms of therapy based on available literature tends to be invalid.

An additional source of error in evaluating the potential of pulmonary embolectomy has been failure to recognize recent advances in surgical technique, and viewing the results of the older operative experience. The crucial role of pre-embolectomy mechanical circulatory support with the pump oxygenator has been recognized only in the last few years, and many deaths in the earlier series were due to cardiac arrest during induction of anesthesia and exposure of the heart without provision of mechanical circulatory assistance. These deaths are preventable with the more advanced techniques.

The series of pulmonary embolectomies reported in this paper deserves a closer look since it is by no means unique but, rather, representative of other groups in which similar indications and techniques were employed.[8] In this series, three of the four deaths, i.e., an error in diagnosis, irreversible brain death prior to embolectomy, and technical error during vena cava ligation, were not due to embolectomy and would have resulted in certain death with medical management. In the fourth instance, preoperative mechanical circulatory support was not employed because of an error in judgment. Thus, in this series of embolectomies the true operative mortality was one in 17 or less than 10 per cent. This experience strongly suggests that with strict adherence to the protocol outlined in this discussion, i.e., preoperative use of circulatory support and avoidance of unduly long exposure to shock, the results presented here are reproducible. This is not surprising since early in the course of embolization the major if not the sole pathology is mechanical obstruction to right ventricular outflow and right ventricular stress. Operative extraction of the clots corrects this deficit and restores normal hemodynamics. The operation is usually well tolerated and survival can be offered, with a low mortality. However, as the patient is exposed to prolonged shock, right heart failure is compounded by the metabolic derangements of a low flow state. At this late stage, removal of the obstruction by embolectomy corrects the cardiac deficit but it may not be sufficient to reverse the biochemical changes of prolonged shock at the cellular level. Thus, the high surgical mortality is due not to the operation itself but rather to the adverse changes produced by longstanding shock. These derangements are highly lethal regardless of the method of management; therefore, effective therapy should be instituted early.

Drug therapy for massive pulmonary embolization sufficiently severe to produce sustained shock is associated with a high mortality. When it is effective the complication rate is significant. Moderate to severe bleeding is encountered in 25 to 40 per cent of the patients.[6] Recurrent embolization, a highly lethal event in an already heavily occluded pulmonary vasculature, is not prevented and the incidence is between 15 and 35 per cent. Actually, a case report is on record in which thrombolytic therapy was thought to have precipitated a fatal recurrent embolus by lysis of a fresh but adherent iliofemoral thrombus.[9] Vena cava ligation is the most effective prophylaxis against recurrent embolization, but in the presence of a massive pulmonary vascular obstruction with marginal cardiorespiratory reserve, the procedure without embolectomy carries a higher mortality than embolectomy performed under the protective umbrella of mechanical circulatory support. Administration of anesthesia may relax compensating and life-sustaining vasoconstriction sufficiently to produce circulatory collapse regardless of the nature of the operative procedure. We have encountered three patients who sustained deep hypotension or cardiac arrest during vena cava ligation for massive embolization. This is a well recognized hazard and, therefore, in our institution the pump oxygenator is kept on a standby basis whenever inferior vena cava ligation is performed for massive embolization. If cardiac arrest or deep hypotension is precipitated during the operation, mechanical circulatory support is provided by cannulation of the femoral artery and vein, the embolectomy is performed, and the vena cava is ligated. Three such operations have been performed, with survival of all three patients.

Another potential disadvantage of medical management relates to the fate of the thrombus in the pulmonary vasculature. Spontaneous or drug-induced lysis of the clot has been documented, but the process is by no means universal or complete.[10] Organization with chronic obstructions and development of pulmonary hypertension have been described and may be more common than hitherto recognized. With pulmonary embolectomy the clots are extracted and the potential source of pulmonary hypertension is removed.

The ultimate goal in massive pulmonary embolization is to select a form of therapy which offers the greatest chance of survival. Medical management of massive embolization with shock will result in successful treatment, but the outcome in the individual patient is unpredictable and the overall mortality rate is high. Embolectomy performed early in the course of the disease, with preoperative circulatory support, subjects the patient to the stress of a surgical procedure, but the operation removes the source of the pathology and consequently it offers an extremely high survival rate with little morbidity. A critical analysis of available experience indicates that the treatment of choice for massive pulmonary embolization associated with shock is pulmonary embolectomy, while anticoagulants and thrombolytic agents should be reserved for lesser degrees of embolization and for situations in which an operation is contraindicated by other associated diseases.

References

1. Stansel, H. C., Jr., Hume, M., and Glenn, W. L.: Pulmonary embolectomy. New Eng. J. Med. 276:717, 1967.
2. Berger, R. L., Gibson, H., and Ferris, E. J.: A reappraisal of the indications for pulmonary embolectomy. Amer. J. Surg. 116:403, 1968.
3. Berger, R. L.: Pulmonary embolectomy for massive embolization. Amer. J. Surg. 121:437, 1971.
4. Cross, F. S., and Mowlem, A.: A survey of the current status of pulmonary embolectomy for massive pulmonary embolism. Circulation 35(Suppl.):1, 1967.
5. Riccitelli, M. L.: Pulmonary embolism: Modern concepts and diagnostic techniques. J. Amer. Geriat. Soc. 18:714:1970.
6. Miller, G. A. H.: Massive pulmonary embolism. Brit. Med. J. 2:777:1970.
7. Sautter, R. D., Myers, W. O., and Wenzel, F. J.: Implications of the Urokinase Study concerning the surgical treatment of pulmonary embolism. J. Thorac. Cardiov. Surg. 63:54:1972.
8. Safur, A.: Discussion. J. Thorac. Cardiov. Surg. 63:59:1972.
9. Gajewsky, J.: Thrombolytic therapy and fatal massive pulmonary emboli. Ann. Intern. Med. 74:450:1971.
10. Dalen, J. E., Banas, J. S., Jr., Brooks, H. L., Evans, G. L., Paraskos, J. A., and Dexter, L.: Resolution rate of acute pulmonary embolism in man, New Eng. J. Med. 280:1194:1969.

Comment

Treatment of Massive Pulmonary Embolism

In the past few years there has been a surge of interest in the management of pulmonary embolism. The use of pulmonary scanning after the injection of radioactive albumen aggregates and the development of pulmonary angiography have made accurate diagnosis possible. Improved modes of therapy include the use of thrombolytic agents such as urokinase and streptokinase, the use of cardiopulmonary bypass, and the development of the umbrella method of interrupting the inferior vena cava.

The goal of therapy in patients with small and moderate-sized pulmonary emboli should be prevention of recurrence. This is usually done by the use of anticoagulants, with interruption of the vena cava being reserved for those instances in which anticoagulant therapy fails or a special problem exists. The results of the Urokinase Pulmonary Embolism Trial (UPET) gave no evidence that thrombolytic agents prevent recurrent pulmonary emboli.

The management of massive pulmonary embolism with shock remains controversial. This is because time has not permitted the evaluation of newer forms of therapy and because of the paucity of controlled studies. As pointed out by Sautter, the UPET gave unequivocal evidence that urokinase hastens the lysis of emboli and lowers the pulmonary arterial pressure in patients with massive pulmonary emboli. Thus, fibrinolytic therapy seems a reasonable adjunct to the conservative management of massive pulmonary emboli. Unfortunately, a hemorrhagic state is produced which renders immediate surgery hazardous.

As pointed out by both authors, most deaths associated with massive emboli occur in the first few hours. The action of fibrinolytic agents may not be sufficiently rapid to prevent these deaths. Both authors suggest the use of partial cardiopulmonary bypass to sustain life in these patients. Cannulation of peripheral vessels can be performed, using local anesthesia. Sautter would continue these patients on bypass with a membrane oxygenator until improvement occurs as a result of action of the intrinsic fibrinolytic system. Berger would proceed to embolectomy, providing the angiogram demonstrates a massive embolus. The dilemma lies in selecting those patients who will die without some type of surgical intervention. It is apparent that the indications for surgery used by the two authors are quite different and that more data will be required before a firm conclusion can be drawn. Further studies are also needed to determine whether fibrinolytic therapy can be combined with the use of a membrane oxygenator without an unacceptable risk of hemorrhage.

RICHARD V. EBERT

12

Prophylaxis Against Tuberculosis

ROUTINE CASE FINDING AND APPROPRIATE CHEMOTHERAPY
DESERVE TO BE CONTINUED
   by Phyllis Q. Edwards

ADVANTAGES OF SELECTIVE USE OF BCG
   by Sol Roy Rosenthal

COMMENT
   by Maxwell Finland

Routine Case Finding and Appropriate Chemotherapy Deserve To Be Continued

PHYLLIS Q. EDWARDS

Center for Disease Control, Atlanta

The controversy about isoniazid chemoprophylaxis, if in fact there is one, probably stems from differing opinions on when to treat, and when not to treat, an asymptomatic tuberculin-positive person in whom there is no evidence of active tuberculosis. Why preventive treatment? Because living tubercle bacilli in human beings carry the potential for producing active tuberculosis, and that potential can be reduced by isoniazid.

The crux of the matter lies in assessing the chance that active disease will develop, and setting that against the effectiveness of preventive treatment, its cost in time, money, and inconvenience, and the risk of drug-related complications. Benefit versus cost: every physician weighs such questions each time he makes a diagnosis and writes out a prescription.

Tubercle bacilli in the pulmonary secretions of a patient with active disease may be passed on to anyone who is in the right place at the right time to inhale a viable bacillus that will reach the fertile soil of an alveolus. Implantation, multiplication, and lymphohematogenous dissemination follow in rapid order. Secondary foci are established in favored sites: bone, kidneys, apices of lungs. Immunologic response halts further growth. Some of the bacillary foci may be extinguished; others may become walled off; still others may have reduced numbers of bacilli but with a few "persisters" that are able to remain dormant until some change takes place in the patient's physical status. Reactivation of latent foci in the apices and subapical areas of the lungs accounts for most of the cases of active tuberculosis seen in this country today.[1]

These latent foci are generally inapparent, so their presence cannot be detected by chest roentgenography. By the same token, if a latent focus were extinguished, there would be no way to know it had happened. The problem is that no test has yet been developed, serologic or otherwise, to detect the presence of living tubercle bacilli in a person's body. We need such a test. It would then be possible to pick out just those who harbor living bacilli for preventive treatment. Lacking that capability, we have little choice but to assume that the presence of reactivity to tuberculin signifies the presence of sufficient antigenic stimulus to maintain cutaneous hypersensitivity. In other words, tuberculin reactivity is taken as evidence of living bacilli, actively multiplying or dormant. And it is among the known tuberculin reactors that we find most of today's cases of tuberculosis, and tomorrow's cases as well.

Latent foci can and do reactivate, touched off by several known factors and probably by a variety of subtle and not-so-subtle but still unknown factors. Immunosuppressive therapy, immunologic deficiency states, lymphoproliferative disorders, and uncontrolled diabetes are among the conditions recognized as increasing the chances of reactivation. Silicosis and gastric resection are also thought to be contributing factors. Tenuous but suggestive evidence points to stress as a triggering mechanism; and by stress is meant such physically traumatic events as loss of economic or emotional support, an intolerable domestic situation, death of a close relative or friend, or fear or apprehension of an impending change in job, environment, or personal relationships. Stress in another sense may be an expression of endocrine dysfunction, steroids, adolescence, pregnancy, and the like.

Risk of Developing Disease

Risk of developing active disease has been shown to differ widely under a variety of conditions,[2-5] although, not surprisingly, clinical impression had earlier indicated that certain kinds of persons are more likely to develop disease than others. Heading the list is the patient with an abnormality on the chest x-ray suggestive of inactive tuberculosis but not shown to be inactive. History of a previous episode of active disease either before the chemotherapeutic era or treated inadequately by present-day standards supports the presumption of high risk. How high? Around 1 to 3 per cent per year, on average, the risk varying with the nature of the earlier disease, such as time interval elapsed since clinically active, type of treatment (if any), and response; and the nature of the patient himself—age, immunologic status, concurrent medical problems, and perhaps his ability to handle stressful situations. Thus, a mark of high risk is an old lesion on the chest roentgenogram, the kind that used to be called a "fibrotic lesion of no clinical significance"; another is a history of tuberculosis.

The tuberculin reactor with normal chest roentgenographic findings and no known condition likely to compromise his immunologic integrity lies at the other end of the risk spectrum. His risk is about 1 per 1000 per year, perhaps somewhat lower. This is at least tenfold less than for the person with an inactive untreated lesion but, on the other hand, it is at least tenfold more than for one who has never been infected.

The highest risk category of all is the newly infected person, one who was known to be tuberculin negative and now has become positive. The appearance of tuberculin sensitivity, commonly called "tuberculin conversion," signals the onset of the immune response to *Mycobacterium tuberculosis* and is usually the only sign that infection has taken place. The bacteremia that occurs during the "incubation period" probably escapes notice because symptoms are usually minimal, transient, and unspecific. Persistent symptoms signal progressive clinical disease, which occurs in 3 to 4 per cent of the newly infected during the first year and in another 1 to 2 per cent during the second year. Thus, the person whose skin test has recently converted from negative to positive stands at a high risk of developing clinical tuberculosis within the next few years.

Effectiveness of Isoniazid Chemoprophylaxis

The effectiveness of isoniazid as an antituberculosis agent was recognized in the early 1950's, and the drug has remained the mainstay of first-line treatment regimens ever since that time. The first departure from its strictly therapeutic use was taken by the U. S. Public Health Service in 1955, in a controlled study of the possibility that administration of isoniazid to children with asymptomatic primary tuberculosis might reduce the frequency of serious complications—progressive pulmonary disease, miliary tuberculosis, and tuberculous meningitis.[2]

In the mid 1950's, incredible though it seems to us now, more than 15 years later, primary tuberculosis was not treated with chemotherapy but was watched carefully for signs of the complications that appeared most often within the first year. The study provided an isoniazid umbrella for the year following diagnosis. A comparable group of randomly selected controls received a placebo. The trial was double blind: neither patients nor clinicians could distinguish between the two kinds of pills.

Results showed a striking 80 per cent reduction in the frequency of complications among the children who took isoniazid compared with those on a placebo. It was therefore decided to extend the follow-up observations for a second year, in case the year on medication served only to postpone the development of complications, as some believed possible. Reduction during the second year was 65 per cent. This suggested an effect on disease potential that persisted after the year on medication—an intriguing possibility inviting further scrutiny.

Another larger controlled study was therefore initiated in 1957 among household contacts of newly diagnosed cases of active disease.[2] The rationale in selecting family contacts was recognition of the high risk of additional cases during the first year after diagnosis of a case in the household. Again randomly selected controls were given a placebo instead of isoniazid to provide a comparison group for assessing the effect of isoniazid. Disease incidence was reduced in the isoniazid group by 80 per cent during the year of medication; and over the next nine years the incidence was reduced by 60 per cent, with only minor fluctuations from year to year. After 10 years' observation of 28,000 participants, altogether 215 cases had developed in the placebo group, 86 in the isoniazid group.[6] Even during the eighth through tenth years of observation, 14 cases occurred among initially positive tuberculin reactors in the placebo group, compared with only two in the corresponding isoniazid group.

Effectiveness of isoniazid in preventing development of disease was not affected by age of the participants in the trial: in all age groups the annual incidence of tuberculosis was reduced by about 60 per cent during the 10-year period of observation.

The encouraging early results of these and other trials of isoniazid for preventive treatment of new infections opened the way for the next question: Could isoniazid affect inactive disease to reduce the chance of reactivation? Similar isoniazid-placebo double-blind trials designed to examine this question have shown an average reduction of about 60 per cent during, as well as after, the treatment year. Results range from little effect in poor pill-takers to a reduction in active tuberculosis ranging between 80 and 90 per cent in those who took at least 40 per cent of the recommended one-year course of isoniazid. Regardless of age and sex, the reduction during six years of follow-up observation in one study group ranged from 79 per cent for those classed as inactive "primary" to 87 per cent for "reinfection" type untreated inactive tuberculosis.[7]

The fact that isoniazid not only reduces the amount of disease developing during the treatment year but also during the subsequent years indicates some kind of significant change in the potential for a latent focus to reactivate at some later date. One can only speculate on the nature of the change brought about. Perhaps the focus is eradicated entirely, even though tuberculin reactivity is rarely affected, most persons remaining tuberculin positive. Perhaps the size of the bacterial population is reduced below its capacity to overcome the natural defenses of the host. Perhaps some entirely different mechanism is at play. We do not know *how* it works, only that it *does* work in significant numbers of persons.

It is quite possible that isoniazid is a far more effective drug for preventive treatment than it appears to be. Indications from several studies as well as clinical observations point toward nearly complete protection against developing active tuberculosis among those at risk who ingest enough isoniazid spread out over a sufficient period of time. How much is "enough," and how long is "sufficient"? Studies are presently under way to help to provide better information on these points. But there can be little doubt today that a dose of 300 mg. isoniazid, if taken daily or almost daily, for a year or almost a year, can be close to 100 per cent effective in preventing development of tuberculosis among those at risk—the infected, converters as well as "old positives."

Cost of Preventive Treatment

The cost of chemoprophylaxis must be reckoned in terms of what it takes to assure one year of treatment: the value in time, energy, and resourcefulness of one or more persons responsible for the administration of isoniazid and surveillance of the patient; and the direct cost of the drug itself. These costs have been variously estimated at around $50 on average, but ranging widely from as low as $5 to as much as $500, depending on the time, place, procedures, and persons involved.[8, 9] The drug itself costs about $2.

What are the costs in terms of adverse reactions, from transient side effects to fatal complications? Side effects are difficult to evaluate, largely because of their nonspecific nature. Their frequency can best be estimated from double-blind trials, in which half the participants received isoniazid and half received placebo; and in which neither the patients nor the clinic staffs could distinguish one type of medication from the other.[2] Between 2 and 7 per cent of the patients in two of our Public Health Service trials complained of such symptoms as gastric distress, rash, fever, dizziness, headache, numbness, "feel sick," and "feel tired." In comparing isoniazid with placebo groups, only 1 to 3 per cent of the symptoms could presumably be caused by isoniazid. Reactions were more common in women than in men with both isoniazid and placebo, although gastrointestinal complaints were more common in men. Neurologic reactions showed the greatest difference in frequency between isoniazid and placebo groups. Some patients noted feelings of light-headedness and euphoria—the "two-martini syndrome"—during the first few days or weeks of treatment.

Hypersensitivity reactions are potentially the most serious adverse effect. Skin rash was seen in 0.1 to 0.4 per cent of the patients in the Public Health Service trials. Jaundice was seen even less often: in 0.1 per cent of patients. The highly publicized 19 cases of isoniazid-associated hepatitis, including two deaths, which developed during a chemoprophylaxis program started in February, 1970, among 2300 Capitol Hill employees, were wholly unexpected for several reasons.[10] A rate of nearly 1 per cent hepatitis in that group was far higher than ever seen before. The cases appeared over a period of nine months, not clustered in the early months as suggested by previous observations of serum glutamic oxaloacetic transaminase levels in healthy persons taking isoniazid chemoprophylaxis.[11] The isoniazid product used for the Capitol Hill program was from a domestic manufacturer who supplies a large number of pharmaceutical firms in this country. No impurity was identified. Cases of isoniazid-associated hepatitis have been reported subsequently from several treatment centers and health department clinics, in some localities approaching a frequency of 1 per cent, and only rarely in other geographic areas. Thus, several questions still remain to be answered, the most critical being the frequency and cause of isoniazid-associated hepatitis. Studies presently under way are designed to provide information on these and other questions, such as possible interactions with other medications, including nonprescription items; time interval before appearance of clinical hepatitis after starting treatment; time changes in serum transaminase levels; and comparison of different methods of making the determinations.

An Advisory Committee to the Center for Disease Control has recommended that all patients receiving isoniazid be monitored at monthly intervals for possible signs or symptoms of hepatitis, so that the drug can be stopped and the patient evaluated.[12] The Committee emphasized that monitoring treatment with SGOT determinations is not recommended since the significance of most changes is not understood. Moreover, they concluded that the development of liver disease is not predictable in the individual patient. It appears to be an expression of delayed hypersensitivity to isoniazid and occurs more frequently in older persons than in children. Nor can this type of hepatitis be differentiated from viral hepatitis either pathologically or clinically.

The question is sometimes raised about the possibility of drug resistant organisms if, sometime after the year of isoniazid alone for preventive treatment, a person develops active pulmonary tuberculosis. This concern probably stems from confusion over the need for multiple drug therapy in the presence of a large bacterial population, where organisms naturally resistant to isoniazid can be expected at a rate of about 1 in 100,000; whereas candidates for preventive treatment have far fewer organisms and, hence, the probability is low of significant numbers of resistant organisms. Experience has borne this out. In most of the cases of active disease which have developed in persons who presumably took isoniazid prophylaxis, the cultures showed isoniazid-sensitive organisms. Ever since the introduction of isoniazid in 1952 about 3 per cent of strains from new active cases, not previously treated, have been called "resistant" in vitro by laboratory tests. Presumably if a population of tuberculin reactors is selected for chemoprophylaxis, no more than 3 per cent might have isoniazid-resistant bacilli before treatment is started. It would be reasonable to assume isoniazid prophylaxis would not alter their chances of breakdown, and that if they did develop active disease, their bacilli would be isoniazid-resistant, not because of prophylaxis but because they were resistant *before* prophylaxis.[2, 13]

Carcinogenicity and teratogenicity of isoniazid have been reported from animal experiments characteristically at very high doses of the drug. Neither effect has been found in human beings. As to teratogenic effects, in three controlled Public Health Service trials of isoniazid prophylaxis in humans, there was no difference between the number of live births or the birth weight of children born to parents who were or were not receiving isoniazid when conception occurred. Similarly, careful examination of death certificates has shown no evidence of excess mortality from cancer in the Public Health Service trial participants who received isoniazid, compared with those given placebo.[2]

Rationale for Preventive Treatment

The case for isoniazid chemoprophylaxis rests, it might seem, more on a commitment to preventive medicine than to clinical medicine. But I believe the compelling reason for chemoprophylaxis lies in plain view of all: 640 persons are being reported each week as new active cases of tuberculosis; this week, last week, next week—and by the end of this year some 33,000 new cases will have been diagnosed and reported. Added to this will be an estimated 5000 reactivated cases, plus an unknown number of new cases which are simply not reported. Tuberculosis has not exactly disappeared in this country; not yet, at least, and its present rate of decline would hardly suggest that another 10 years will see its extinction.

Most cases of tuberculosis are symptomatic by the time they are diagnosed. Most are moderately or far advanced in terms of extent of disease. Most are likely to have become infectious and to have transmitted tubercle bacilli to at least one other person. Twenty years ago we believed tuberculosis could be found early, while still only minimal, asymptomatic, and not infectious. Mass x-ray surveys were developed for that purpose; and all adults were urged to have a routine check-up every year "to prevent tuberculosis." It didn't work. Most of the new cases are still moderately or far advanced, symptomatic, and capable of transmitting infection. Annual chest x-rays have not prevented the development of tuberculosis, nor have they improved the early detection rate. The reason is that the disease usually progresses rapidly to reach the advanced, symptomatic form within a matter of several weeks to several months. All but a small fraction of today's new patients have been tuberculin positive for some years. Their disease arises characteristically in the subapical areas where dormant foci have remained invisible since the time of the initial infection.[1]

Is the use of isoniazid for such dormant foci considered prophylaxis or treatment? The question may be debatable, but the reason for giving isoniazid is clear. We recognize that the tuberculin-positive person is at risk of developing active pulmonary disease, and this is an *annual* risk that varies from 0.07 to 3 per cent or more, depending on other factors mentioned earlier. Take, for example, the healthy young adult man with a positive tuberculin test and normal chest roentgenogram. If he was tuberculin negative a year ago, he has been infected within the past 12 months. As a converter he stands a 3 to 4 per cent chance of developing clinical tuberculosis within the coming year. Tubercle bacilli are presumed to be actively multiplying and readily accessible during this early period of the initial infection. Treatment with isoniazid for one year is therefore considered mandatory. The risk of adverse reactions to isoniazid is plainly offset by the greater risk of disease.

Suppose this same healthy, tuberculin-positive young man with a normal chest roentgenogram has been a positive reactor for at least five years. Should he have isoniazid chemoprophylaxis? His risk of disease is probably about 0.07 per cent per year; his risk of isoniazid-associated hepatitis is likely not more than 0.8 per cent during the year of isoniazid. The risk of disease is continuous, year after year; the risk of hepatitis occurs only during the treatment year and can be reduced by monitoring the patient for early symptoms of liver dysfunction.

Although such an individual may not, himself, be considered a prime candidate for preventive treatment ("I've been a tuberculin reactor for years, and I'm still perfectly healthy, so why INH now?"), he and the millions like him who make up the reservoir of infection contribute the bulk of the new cases of tuberculosis that emerge each year. In contrast, the other young man who is a recent converter, and the few thousand others like him, contribute only a small portion of the annual number of new cases.

Here, I believe, is the crux of the controversy in TB chemoprophylaxis: the conflict between the clinical and the public health view on preventive treatment. Clinically the patient most likely to develop disease is at the top of the priority list for chemoprophylaxis because of the expected benefit to the health of *the individual*. But the health of *the community* is far more threatened by the large numbers of cases developing in the vast pool of positive tuberculin reactors who as individuals are at much lower levels of risk. Some among this infected reservoir may be picked out as constituting a special potential threat to some segments of the community, should they develop infectious disease; and here one would consider persons providing child care, schoolteachers and school bus drivers, hospital and nursing home employees who provide patient care, and other such persons.

The question of chemoprophylaxis probably lies in a difference in orientation, clinical versus public health. Should there really be a difference?

In summary, let it first be said that in discussing chemoprophylaxis it was not my intention to minimize the urgent importance of prompt, effective multiple-drug treatment of a patient with active or presumed active tuberculosis. Good initial treatment is the key to preventing reactivation in the future. It is also the key to preventing spread of infection in the present.

Prompt, effective treatment of the infected is likewise the key to preventing the development of active disease in the future. Single-drug treatment with isoniazid alone, 300 mg. once daily for one year, is currently recommended for all but children (10 mg./kg., 300 mg. maximum). Shorter periods of treatment are now being evaluated in several different countries.

Priority groups for preventive treatment have been listed in a joint statement recently issued by the American Thoracic Society, the National Tuberculosis and Respiratory Disease Association, and the Center for Disease Control.[14] First priority is given to newly infected persons—household contacts and converters of any age; next are persons diagnosed as having inactive tuberculosis with a history of active disease; tuberculin-positive persons with abnormal findings on chest roentgenogram; and positive tuberculin reactors under 20 years of age, in special clinical situations, and, finally, all other positive reactors.

The Public Health Service chemoprophylaxis trials have included a wide variety of persons of both sexes and all ages; different races; different geographical areas; newly infected, long-time reactors; high as well as low risk of disease—in every situation far fewer cases of tuberculosis have developed in those taking isoniazid, not only during the treatment year but throughout the post-treatment years of follow-up. These findings point inescapably, I believe, to the conclusion that isoniazid acts on a tuberculosis infection to reduce its potential for ever progressing to clinically active disease. If this is so, then the benefit of preventive treatment lasts not only for the treatment year but presumably for a lifetime during which the chance of a second infection is rare, and becoming rarer.

References

1. Pinner, M.: *Pulmonary Tuberculosis in the Adult; Its Fundamental Aspects.* Springfield, Ill., Charles C Thomas, 1947.
2. Ferebee, S. H.: Controlled chemoprophylaxis trials in tuberculosis. A general review. Bibl. Tuberc. 26:28, 1970.
3. Grzybowski, S., McKinnon, N. E., Tuters, L., Pinkus, G., and Philips, R.: Reactivations in inactive pulmonary tuberculosis. Amer. Rev. Resp. Dis. 93:352, 1966.
4. Horwitz, O., Wilbek, E., and Erickson, P. A.: Epidemiological basis of tuberculosis eradication. 10. Longitudinal studies on the risk of tuberculosis in the general population of a low-prevalence area. Bull. WHO 41:95, 1969.
5. Palmer, C. E., and Edwards, L. B.: Identifying the tuberculous infected. The dual-test technique. J.A.M.A. 205:167, 1968.
6. Tuberculosis Branch, Center for Disease Control: Unpublished data.
7. Comstock, G. W., and Ferebee, S. H.: Preventive treatment of untreated nonactive tuberculosis in an Eskimo population. Arch. Environ. Health (Chicago), 25:333, 1972.
8. A modern attack on an urban health problem; report of the task force on tuberculosis in

New York City. Commissioner of Health, Health Services Administration, The City of New York, 1968.
9. Moulding, T.: Chemoprophylaxis of tuberculosis: When is the benefit worth the risk and cost? Ann. Intern. Med. 74:761, 1971.
10. Garibaldi, R. A., Drusin, R. E., Ferebee, S. H., and Gregg, M. B.: Isoniazid-associated hepatitis: Report of an outbreak. Amer. Rev. Resp. Dis. 106:357, 1972.
11. Sharer, L., and Smith, J. P.: Serum transaminase elevations and other hepatic abnormalities in patients receiving isoniazid. Ann. Intern. Med. 71:1113, 1969.
12. Isoniazid and liver disease; Report of an ad hoc committee on isoniazid and liver disease. (Center for Disease Control, Department of Health, Education, and Welfare, March 17–18, 1971.) Amer. Rev. Resp. Dis. 104:454, 1971.
13. Horwitz, O., Payne, P. G., and Wilbek, E.: Epidemiological basis of tuberculosis eradication. 4. The isoniazid trial in Greenland. Bull. WHO 35:509, 1966.
14. Preventive treatment of tuberculosis; a joint statement of the American Thoracic Society, the National Turberculosis and Respiratory Disease Association, and the Center for Disease Control. Amer. Rev. Dis. 104:460, 1971.

Advantages of Selective Use of BCG

SOL ROY ROSENTHAL

*Department of Preventive Medicine,
Institution for Tuberculosis Research,
University of Illinois, Medical Center
and Research Foundation*

BCG (bacillus Calmette and Guérin) is an attenuated viable bovine tubercle bacillus that has proved to be highly effective in increasing the body's resistance against tuberculosis both experimentally and clinically. The organism was first isolated in 1908 from the udder of a tuberculous cow. Its attenuation was achieved fortuitously by repeated transfer on bile potato media. Its attenuation and proved effectiveness in animals was not achieved until 1921 when the vaccine was applied clinically in an infant born of a tuberculous mother. Since that time there have been more than 500,000,000 human vaccinations performed all over the world, including every continent. In many countries BCG vaccination is mandatory by law (France, West and East Germany, Norway, Russia, Poland, Brazil, and Japan). In other countries (Sweden, Denmark, the United Kingdom, Canada, and India, for example) it is universally practiced on a voluntary basis. As far back as 1955 Geoffrey Edsall, then editor of the *Journal of Immunology*, stated: "However, it is interesting to note that more convincingly statistically significant evidence has been accumulating for the efficacy of such bacterial vaccine, as for example the BCG strain of *Mycobacterium tuberculosis*, or pertussis vaccines, than it has been possible to collect even for diphtheria or tetanus toxoids; this is not said to imply that toxoids are not highly effective."[1] Yet BCG has had but limited use in the U.S.A. as a vaccine against tuberculosis. Ironically enough it has been more widely accepted and used in the treatment of cancer and leukemia.[2] Workers in the field of oncology have been aware of its highly potent properties as a stimulator of immune mechanisms through the reticuloendothelial system.[3,4] They have not been cognizant of the prejudices or been subjected to the pressures from official sources that have curtailed the use of BCG in the tuberculosis field.

In a conference on "The Laboratory Evaluation of Immunization Against

Tuberculosis" sponsored by the Office of International Research, National Institutes of Health, in cooperation with the American Thoracic Society, and the National Tuberculosis Association, November 16–19, 1966 (in Washington, D.C.), where all available nonviable and viable vaccines against tuberculosis were compared, D. Koch-Weser, the Chairman of the conference, summarized the reports as follows: "Almost all the reported materials demonstrated immunogenic activity in some but none in all of the very many test systems. Effective in almost all systems were only the whole living organisms." The keynote address stated: "Wise men should realize that for the time being they should use the available weapons against tuberculosis as effectively as possible. This still includes intensive case-finding, chemotherapy and, when indicated, chemoprophylaxis. It most certainly includes the wide employment of BCG which, with up to 87 per cent protection, is not such a bad weapon after all."[5]

Recently two groups of investigators vaccinating rhesus monkeys intravenously or by an aerosol method followed by aerosol challenge with virulent human tubercle bacilli demonstrated practically complete protection in these animals. The controls not vaccinated had extensive tuberculous pneumonia, with cavitation as well as extensive lymph node involvement.[6, 7]

Clinically D'Arcy Hart, past President of the Medical Research Council of the Tuberculosis Vaccine Clinical Trials Committee, selected six clinical studies from around the world which, in his judgment, were well controlled and would bear statistical analysis. It can be noted in Table 1 that, except for the two U.S.P.H.S. studies, the reduction in the incidence of tuberculosis in vaccinated subjects, as compared to the nonvaccinated, was from 60 to 80 per cent, which is statistically significant.[8] The reduced incidence in the vaccinated subjects was not only against primary disease but against chronic pulmonary disease and pleurisy with effusion; miliary tuberculosis and tuberculous meningitis were completely eliminated.[9]

The poor results obtained by the U.S.P.H.S. Tuberculosis Section[10, 11] were the prominent factor which influenced the thinking of this agency and which have been prejudicial toward the wider use of the vaccine in the U.S.A.

What are the reasons for the wide differences in the results between the

Table 1. *Six Controlled Trials with BCG Vaccine**

POPULATION GROUP	REFERENCE	VACCINE	OBSERVATION PERIOD (YEARS)	EFFICACY OF BCG (%)
North American Indians	Aronson, 1958	Phipps	20	80
Chicago infants	Rosenthal, 1961	Tice	12 to 23	74
Puerto Ricans	Palmer, 1958 (U.S.P.H.S.)	N.Y. State	6 to 7	31
Georgia/Alabama residents	Comstock and Palmer, 1958 (U.S.P.H.S.)	Tice	7	36†
British urban schoolchildren	Medical Research Council, 1963, 1966	Danish	12½	79
South Indian villagers	Frimodt-Moller, 1964	Madras	2 to 7	60

* Modified from Hart, P. D'A.: Brit. Med. J. *1*:587, 1967.
† At 14 years, 14 per cent.

U.S.P.H.S. and other well controlled studies? One prominent difference was in the choice of those to be included in the study based on their reactions to tuberculin. For the studies other than the U.S.P.H.S., a nonreactor was considered as one having 0 to 4 mm. induration to 100 TU. The U.S.P.H.S. considered a nonreactor as one not reacting to 5 TU. Thus, a high percentage both in the vaccinated and control groups in the U.S.P.H.S. study reacted to 100 TU. It has been shown by British Medical Research Council studies[9] and by Palmer[12] that those individuals who do not react to 5 TU but do react to 100 TU or have slight reactions to 5 TU (5 to 9 mm.) have an appreciable resistance to tuberculosis. In the British trials the tuberculosis morbidity rate for those not vaccinated who failed to react to 100 TU was 283/100,000/year, whereas among those who reacted to 100 TU it was 122/100,000/year. Palmer, who directed the U.S.P.H.S. (Tuberculosis Division) studies, later admitted that this factor may explain the differences between the British and U.S.P.H.S. results. D'Arcy Hart, in an analysis of the U.S.P.H.S. 14-year follow-up results of the Georgia-Alabama study, in which only a 14 per cent reduction in the morbidity incidence in the vaccinated vs. controls was noted, calculated that if the vaccine were 80 per cent effective, then there should have been a 50 per cent difference instead of the 14 per cent reported. He concluded, therefore, that additional factors might explain the differences in U.S.P.H.S. and British studies. One such factor considered was a vaccine of low potency.[8] It is known, for example, that BCG strains do vary in their potency, and indeed one of the six daughter strains carried by the Tice Laboratory had partially lost its potency.[14-16] Fortuitously, however, vaccine from this strain was never sent to the Georgia-Alabama project,[17] and the vaccine sent to that project was found highly effective both in guinea pigs[18] and in clinical studies.[19, 20] Moreover, the vaccine made by the Tice Laboratory of Chicago has been adopted by the American Thoracic Society for the standard control of other antituberculosis vaccines. Many workers have reported on the Tice BCG vaccines and have found them to be among the most potent in the world.[16, 21-26]

Although a vaccine of inferior potency could not be implicated, the tuberculin reaction rates (greater than 5 mm.) obtained two years after vaccination were low, namely 54 per cent to 5 TU.[11] Three to six months following BCG vaccination among varying age groups (newborns to young adults), approximately 90 per cent should react to 5 TU with an average induration of from 10 to 15 mm. After two years 70 to 85 per cent should still react to 5 TU (greater than 5 mm. induration; average, 10 to 12 mm.).

The explanation for the low tuberculin rates as explained by Rosenthal, consultant to the U.S.P.H.S. on this project, is that the technique of vaccination must have been faulty. In the multiple puncture method used, the instrument of vaccination was a straight sewing type needle.[27] The principle of this method is to deliver the antigen to the upper layers of the cutis (a site of the reticuloendothelial system[20]). This necessitates firm downward pressure, holding the shaft of the needle parallel to the skin and then thrusting the point of the needle forward into the cutis for a distance of 2 mm. Some five individuals on the project were instructed in the method, but on a later routine inspection by Rosenthal it was found that the personnel had been changed, and the newly assigned nurses were using the superficial pressure method as for smallpox vaccination. The two methods differ radically, since in the former the cutis is entered, whereas in the latter the epidermis is lightly pierced as is required for virus multiplication. The breach in technique was brought to the attention of the project directors verbally and later by letter.[17] This history is essential in evaluating the success of BCG vaccination, since in the literature faulty technique has not been adequately considered.

An additional explanation for the differences in the results obtained between the British and American studies is that the risk of infection in the Georgia-Alabama area was very low. For example, no case of primary tuberculosis was detected among the more than 7000 white control subjects under 20 years of age, and only two cases of primary disease were found among the nearly 3500 non-vaccinated black children during the 14 years that this study was underway.[11] In the British study the attack rates were ten times greater than in the Georgia-Alabama study.[8]

Thus, in the U.S.P.H.S. Tuberculosis Division studies in Georgia-Alabama, the area chosen was unfortunate since the risk of infection and the attack rates were low (the tuberculosis mortality rate was lower than that of the U.S.A. as a whole); both the control and vaccinated groups contained individuals who were reactors to 100 TU (53 per cent in both groups) and, therefore, had a certain degree of immunity; and the technique of vaccination was at fault.

The stigma of the poor showing of the U.S.P.H.S. Tuberculosis Division study has built up a deep prejudice by the U.S.P.H.S. against the use of BCG in the U.S.A. The arguments given by this agency are that BCG is not applicable in the U.S.A. because of the low incidence of tuberculosis,[11] that 80 per cent of the new cases of tuberculosis originate from the positive tuberculin reactors (these are not eligible for vaccination), and that the tuberculin test as an epidemiologic tool has limited value.[28]

Morbidity and Mortality of Tuberculosis in the U.S.A.

For the country as a whole there has been a steady drop in the incidence of and death rate for the disease. However, the curve for new active cases has flattened out, and the predicted further decline has not been realized.[29] There were 37,137 new cases of tuberculosis reported in 1970 and 5560 deaths, which certainly does not represent disease control. In provisional reports for mortality there was a 4.1 per cent increase in 1970 over 1969 (5560 vs. 5340).[30] The 1970 case rate for whites was 12.4/100,000 and for nonwhites 59/100,000.[31] Many large metropolises have new case rates in the nonwhite population that are exceedingly high, approaching the overall rates for some of the so-called underdeveloped countries (Table 2). This is also true of certain community areas of large cities. In Chicago in 1970, for example, there were 12 community areas out of 67 with case rates of 100/100,000 or more (range 109.4 to 178.1).[32] Quoting the overall statistics for the U.S.A. is misleading, for my recommendations have always been to vaccinate only in the high U.S.A. incidence areas.[20] In a conference (held in October, 1971), on Immunization in Tuberculosis under the sponsorship of the Surgeon General

Table 2. *1970 New Tuberculosis Case Rates by Race for Cities of 250,000 or More Population**

| CITY | NEW CASE RATE PER 100,000 ||| MULTIPLE |
	Total	White	Nonwhite	Nonwhite to White
Honolulu	52.9	11.8	74.0	6.3
Norfolk	26.3	10.2	63.5	6.2
Rochester, N.Y.	28.4	16.4	84.5	5.2
New York City	32.4	18.1	79.2	4.3
Tampa	29.9	18.0	101.1	4.3
Birmingham	52.8	23.0	93.7	4.1
Miami (Dade Co.)	28.2	19.1	77.5	4.0
Buffalo	35.7	22.2	85.4	3.8
Pittsburgh	39.0	24.7	93.7	3.8
Atlanta (Fulton Co.)	38.8	18.4	70.3	3.8
Philadelphia	38.9	20.9	73.3	3.5
Seattle	27.5	21.1	71.7	3.4
Cleveland	41.3	22.7	70.4	3.1
San Francisco	45.7	29.0	87.5	3.0
Indianapolis (Marion Co.)	30.4	22.6	67.9	3.0
Boston	48.0	34.9	107.4	3.0
Washington, D.C.	48.9	20.5	59.8	2.9
Kansas City, Mo.	28.0	19.7	56.2	2.8
Baltimore	54.4	31.3	80.5	2.6
Chicago	45.6	31.6	72.3	2.3
Detroit	47.6	31.0	68.2	2.2
Los Angeles (Los Angeles Co.)	19.1	16.2	36.0	2.2
Cincinnati	47.3	34.4	80.3	2.2
Dallas	29.4	22.4	49.5	2.2
Houston	35.5	27.9	56.6	2.0

1970 New Tuberculosis Case Rates for United States

Total	White	Nonwhite
18.3	12.4	59.0

* *1970 Tuberculosis Statistics—States and Cities.* Atlanta, Georgia, Center for Disease Control, July, 1971.

of the U.S.A., the recommendations as expressed by William Barclay, its Chairman, were that "for persons at high risk, e.g., residents of inner city ghettos, health personnel, or military personnel serving in high incidence areas of tuberculosis, the benefits of BCG vaccination would be considerable. The use of BCG for such high risk persons would be an adjunct to, not a substitute for, other tuberculosis control measures."[33]

Source of the New Cases of Tuberculosis

The often quoted overall statistic that 80 per cent of the new cases of tuberculosis are derived from the positive reactors[28] needs further elaboration. In a nontuberculosis environment it is true that the positive reactors are most likely to develop tuberculosis because they are the ones who harbor the tubercle bacillus.

Table 3. *Relationship Between Tuberculin Reaction and Development of Tuberculosis in Navy Recruits**

	TOTAL NO. CASES	NO. TB CASES	RATE/100,000/YR.
Negative reactors (0–4 mm. to 5 TU)	61,129	68†	28
Positive reactors (5–9 mm. to 5 TU)	1,715	4	59
Positive reactors (10 mm. and over to 5 TU)	5,910	37	157

* U.S.P.H.S. study.[34]

† 62.4 per cent of actual number of cases of tuberculosis originated in negative reactors (i.e., 68 out of 109 cases).

Note: Total positive reactors = 5 per cent of population

Thus, in navy recruits,[34] who ostensibly lived in a nontuberculosis environment, it was found that for the low dose reactor group (3 to 5 TU) whose reactions were large (10 to 15 mm. or more induration*), the morbidity rate over a six-year period was 157/100,000/year; for those responding with small reactions (5 to 9 mm. induration) to 5 TU, the rate was 59/100,000/year; whereas nonreactors (0 to 4 mm. induration) to 5 TU had a rate of 28/100,000/year (Table 3). Nevertheless 62.4 per cent of the actual cases of tuberculosis developed in the negative reactor group (i.e., 68 out of 109 cases).

On the other hand, in the British study[9] of adolescents and young adults who lived in large, crowded communities and were followed for similar periods of time (two and one half to five years) the rate for high dose reactors (100 TU only) was 122/100,000/year compared to 283/100,000/year for the nonreactors. For low dose (3 TU), large size reactors (15 mm. or more in diameter) the rate was 181/100,000. In high incidence areas the nonreactors had the highest rate of tuberculosis (Table 4). In the U.S.P.H.S. studies of 26,000 students of nursing[12] over a period of seven years it was shown that the tuberculosis rates were 249/100,000/year for nonreactors (5 and 250 TU) and 123/100,000/year for those equivalent to high dose reactors (5 to 9 mm. to 5 TU).[12] The nonreactors had a higher incidence than did the high dose reactors (Table 5). Young adults, as well

---

* Some variations exist in what is considered to be a low dose of tuberculin or a large or small reaction, depending on the reporters. Thus, 3 to 5 TU may be considered a low dose and 100 to 250 TU a large dose. Reactions of 10 to 15 mm. or over to the low dose of tuberculin are considered to be strong reactions, and reactions of 5 to 9 mm. to 5 TU or 5 mm. or more to 100 TU are considered to be small or weak reactions.

Table 4. *Relationship Between Tuberculin Reaction and Development of Tuberculosis in Adolescents**

	TOTAL NO. CASES	NO. TB CASES	RATE/100,000/YR.
Negative reactors (to 100 TU)	12,867	91	283
Positive reactors			
3 TU (5–14 mm.)	8,838	19	86
3 TU (15 mm. and over)	6,866	31	181
100 TU	6,253	19	122

* British study.[9]

Table 5. *Relationship Between Tuberculin Reaction and Development of Tuberculosis in Students of Nursing (26,000 Students)**

	TB RATE/100,000/YR.
Negative reactors > 5 mm. to 250 TU	249
Positive reactors	
5–9 mm. to 5 TU	123
10 mm. or more to 5 TU	398
Total reactors = 13.1%	

* U.S.P.H.S. study.[12]

as children who react to the low doses of tuberculin (5 TU) with reactions of 10 to 15 mm. or more induration may be assumed to have been recently infected, and the course which the infection will take is problematical. Grzybowski and Allen report that the risk of developing tuberculosis in the recently converted is 1:42, whereas with older infections it is 1:1748.[35] Recent converters, therefore, also have a high risk of developing the disease.

Nonreactors and recent converters are the most vulnerable groups. BCG vaccination in high incidence areas *before* infection takes place would, therefore, protect those most likely to develop tuberculosis (80 per cent ±).

Is the Value of the Tuberculin Test Lost?

A distinction must be made between the tuberculin test as an epidemiologic tool and as a means of diagnosis of tuberculosis in a specific case.

In high incidence areas where BCG vaccination is recommended the infection rate is usually high[36] (16 to 40 per cent in four high school populations in Chicago), so that the value of the test as an epidemiologic tool is limited. The tracing of the source cases of the positive reactors has proved to be of limited value and costly. Regular x-ray surveys of such areas are more direct and productive and less expensive. So-called INH prophylaxis in the reactors is not indicated, because it is effective only in recent converters, the cooperation of the parents and subjects is poor, and the procedure is not without danger (hepatitis, autoimmunity, and deaths have been reported[37]).

The tuberculin test is only presumptive evidence that the host has been infected with tubercle bacilli; x-rays and sputum or gastric analysis are more definitive tests.

There are criteria which may distinguish between a tuberculin reactor to BCG and a virulent infection. After BCG vaccination (three to six months) the induration to the Mantoux test (5 TU) is on the average from 10 to 16 mm. (depending upon age when vaccinated) and to the Tine test (5 TU), 2 to 4 mm.[38] There is then a gradual diminution of the size of these reactions with time, so that, for example, one or two years after vaccination the reactions are usually under 15 mm. for the Mantoux test (5 TU) and there is no fusing of the papules of the Tine test. Thus, 15 mm. or more reactions to 5 TU may be considered as presumptive evidence of a virulent infection. Furthermore, if there is an increase of

5 to 10 mm. in the size of the Mantoux test or a fusing of the papules (if not present three to six months after vaccination), this is also presumptive evidence that a virulent superinfection has taken place.

To rule out infection with atypical acid-fast bacilli (which may cause reactions to typical tuberculin), simultaneous testing with atypical tuberculin is indicated. If the reactions to the atypical tuberculins are larger than to the typical tuberculin (2 mm. more or over), an atypical infection may be considered but is not certain.[38, 39]

In high incidence areas BCG vaccination of newborns is the most effective and the least expensive procedure. In the Cook County Hospital experience in Chicago, infants were vaccinated at two or three days of age before they left the hospital. From 1937 to 1955 a strictly controlled study was carried out and the vaccinated and nonvaccinated children were followed regularly in the clinic by tuberculin testing, chest x-ray, and so forth. There was a 75 per cent reduction in morbidity and an 89 per cent reduction in mortality in the vaccinated as compared to the nonvaccinated. (The difference is significant statistically, $p > 0.01$.[20]) Since 1955 BCG vaccination in newborns has been carried out at the Cook County Hospital on a service basis, providing the mother's chest x-ray is negative (within two years—her word is accepted) and there is no history of tuberculosis in the family. Only a small proportion of these children are followed in the clinic, approximately 10 per cent, but the development of tuberculosis in this group is determined by checking against all cases of tuberculosis that develop in the city. There is a highly significant difference ($p > 0.001$) in the morbidity and mortality rates between the vaccinated and the general population coming from similar community areas of high tuberculosis incidence.[38] For these service vaccinated infants the first tuberculin test may be done when the child enters school; if negative, the child is revaccinated. Alternatively one could consider vaccinating for the first time when the child enters school, a procedure that would reveal the infection rate in a given area. Under such conditions all children entering school, whatever their age, should be included for vaccination.

Summary

BCG of known potency and properly administered has been proved to be a highly effective vaccine for increasing the host's resistance to tuberculosis, both experimentally and clinically.

BCG vaccination is indicated and recommended for newborns and for children and adults living in high incidence areas, including tuberculous households, certain hospitals and sanitoriums, medical students and students of nursing, and military personnel likely to be exposed to tuberculosis, especially in foreign countries.

References

1. Edsall, G.: Immunization. Ann. Rev. Microbiol. 9:347, 1955.
2. Rosenthal, S. R.: BCG in cancer and leukemia. Bull. Inst. Pasteur 70:29, 1972.

3. Rosenthal, S. R.: *The General Tissue and Humoral Response to an Avirulent Tubercle Bacillus.* Urbana, Ill., University of Illinois Press, 1938.
4. Mackaness, G. B.: The immunological basis of acquired cellular resistance. J. Exp. Med. *120*:105, 1964.
5. Conference on the Laboratory Evaluation of the Immunization Against Tuberculosis, Airlie House, Washington, D.C., November 16–19, 1966.
6. Schmidt, L., and Good, R. C.: Conference on the Laboratory Evaluation of the Immunization Against Tuberculosis, Airlie House, Washington, D.C., November 16–19, 1966. Ann. N.Y. Acad. Sci. *154*:200, 1968.
7. Barclay, W. B., Busey, W. M., Dalgard, D. W., Good, R. C., Janicki, B. W., Kasik, J. E., Ribi, E., Ulrich, C. E., and Wolinsky, E.: Protection of monkeys against airborne tuberculosis by aerosol vaccination with Bacillus Calmette-Guérin. Amer. Rev. Resp. Dis. *107*:351, 1973.
8. Hart, P. D'A.: Efficacy and applicability of mass BCG vaccination in tuberculosis control. Brit. Med. J. *1*:587, 1967.
9. BCG and vole bacillus vaccines in the prevention of tuberculosis in adolescence and early adult life. Third report of the Medical Research Council. Brit. Med. J. *1*:973, 1963.
10. Palmer, C. E., Shain, L. W., and Comstock, G. W.: Community trials of BCG vaccination. Amer. Rev. Tuberc. *77*:877, 1958.
11. Comstock, G. W., and Palmer, C. E.: Long-term results of BCG vaccination in the southern United States. Amer. Rev. Resp. Dis. *93*:171, 1966.
12. Palmer, C. E.: Symposium on the value of the tuberculin reactions for the selection of cases for BCG vaccination and significance of postvaccination allergy. Bull. Union Int. Tubc. *27*:106, 1957.
13. Palmer, C. E.: BCG in the USA. Southern Med. Bull. *54*:52, 1966.
14. Dubos, R. J., Pierce, C. H., and Schaefer, W. B.: Antituberculosis immunity induced in mice by vaccination with living cultures of attenuated tubercle bacilli. J. Exp. Med. *97*:207, 1953.
15. Jespersen, A., and Weis Bentzon, M. W.: Relationship between tuberculin sensitivity and acquired resistance in guinea pigs vaccinated with BCG of different virulence. Acta Path. Microbiol. Scand. *71*:114, 1967.
16. Willis, H. S., Vandiviere, H. M., Vandiviere, M. R., and Melvin, I. Studies in tuberculo-immunity. Amer. J. Med. Sci. *240*:137, 1960.
17. Palmer, C. E.: Personal communication, June 25, 1968.
18. Seagle, J. B., Karlson, A. G., and Feldman, W. H.: Irradiated antituberculosis vaccine, including comparisons with BCG in experimentally infected guinea pigs. Amer. Rev. Tuberc. *67*:341, 1953.
19. Dickie, H. A.: Tuberculosis in student nurses and medical students at the University of Wisconsin. Ann. Intern. Med. 33:941, 1950.
20. Rosenthal, S. R.: *BCG Vaccination Against Tuberculosis.* Boston, Mass., Little, Brown and Company, 1957.
21. Cohn, M. L., Davis, C. L., and Middlebrook, G.: Comparison of freeze-dried daughter strains of BCG by aerogenic immunization and virulent challenge. Tubercle *47*:263, 1966.
22. Youmans, G.: Personal communication.
23. Barclay, W., and Ribi, E.: Personal communication.
24. Smith, D. W.: Personal communication.
25. Dubos, R. J., and Pierce, C. H.: Tice strain of BCG. Amer. Rev. Tuberc. *75*:62, 1957.
26. Jespersen, A., and Weis Bentzon, M. W.: The virulence of various strains of BCG determined on the golden hamster. Acta Tuberc. Scand. *44*:222, 1964.
27. Rosenthal, S. R.: The multiple puncture method of BCG vaccination. Amer. Rev. Tuberc. *39*:128, 1939.
28. Ferebee, S.: An epidemiological model of tuberculosis in the United States. Bulletin of the National Tuberculosis Association, Jan., 1967, p. 4.
29. The future of tuberculosis control. A report to the Surgeon General of the Public Health Service by a task force on tuberculosis control. Washington, D.C., P.H.S. Pub. No. 1119, 1963.
30. Tuberculosis Statistics—States and Cities, July, 1971. Atlanta, Ga., Center for Disease Control.
31. Reported Tuberculosis Data 1970. Department of Health, Education, and Welfare, Pub. No. (HSM) 72–8096, 1972.
32. Statistical Section, The Tuberculosis Institute of Chicago and Cook County, July 29, 1971.

33. Barclay, W. R.: Status of immunization in tuberculosis in 1971. Report of a Conference on Progress to Date, Future Trends, and Research Needs. Department of Health, Education, and Welfare, Publication No. (NIH) 72-68, p. 245.
34. Palmer, C. E., Jablon, S., and Edwards, P. Q.: Tuberculosis morbidity of young men in relation to tuberculin in sensitivity and body build. Amer. Rev. Tuberc. 76:517, 1957.
35. Grzybowski, S., and Allen, E. A.: The challenge of tuberculosis decline. Amer. Rev. Resp. Dis. 90:707, 1964.
36. Chicago Board of Health, Cook County Hospital and Research Foundation: Unpublished data, 1967.
37. Report of the ad hoc advisory committee on isoniazid and liver disease. Morbidity and Mortality Weekly Report 20: No. 26, July 3, 1971.
38. BCG Vaccination Against Tuberculosis, Biennial Report, 1967–68. Institution for Tuberculosis Research, University of Illinois, Medical Center. Chicago Board of Health, Cook County Hospital, and Research Foundation, June 1, 1970.
39. Palmer, C. E., and Edwards, L. B. Identifying the tuberculous infected. The dual-test technique. J.A.M.A. 205:167, 1968.

Comment

Prophylaxis Against Tuberculosis

In his presentation of the case for BCG vaccination in the United States, Dr. Rosenthal points to the worldwide acceptance of this method for the prevention of tuberculosis, its great efficacy in reducing markedly the rates of disease and of deaths due to tuberculosis wherever it has been adequately applied, its freedom from serious hazards and complications, and its very low cost-benefit ratio. He therefore bemoans what he considers to be the prejudices in "official sources" (presumably referring to the United States Public Health Service) of what he interprets as "pressures to curtail" the use of BCG in the prevention of tuberculosis.

In her elucidation of the indications for chemoprophylaxis and for the efficacy of the use of isoniazid, Dr. Edwards presented her case from two points of view. For the individual who is infected, as evidenced by a positive tuberculin test, it brings about a reduction in the volume of infection, thereby also reducing the risk of manifest and potentially serious disease in that individual. From the point of view of the public health, she stresses the importance of chemoprophylaxis in all individuals who are positive tuberculin reactors, because, being infected with tubercle bacilli, they serve as a potential reservoir for dissemination of the infection to others; in these individuals chemoprophylaxis substantially reduces this reservoir. Since the number of positive reactors is large and widespread, they have a considerably greater potential for infecting larger numbers of other individuals than do the relatively small numbers of cases of overt disease or of those recognized as recently converted to tuberculin-positive reactors.

Both essayists are agreed that the problem is of much smaller magnitude in the United States than in those countries where BCG vaccination is accepted and widely practiced, particularly countries with high density populations, where case rates and death rates for tuberculosis are very high. Presumably both would agree that in the U.S.A. the problem does not arise in communities where tuberculosis has become a rare disease, where case finding is primarily a diagnostic problem, and where therapy or preventive measures can be confined to the rare case and to the contacts of that case. Here there may be some difference of opinion as to whether tuberculin-negative contacts should be vaccinated, whether tuberculin-positive contacts should be treated, or whether both should be kept under surveillance and treated only for evidence of active disease. Even Dr. Rosenthal agrees that universal BCG vaccination of the population is not indicated in the U.S.A.

On the other hand, there are many and increasing numbers of high risk areas in the United States; especially the densely populated, low-income, ghetto areas, where active tuberculosis is frequent and where the risk of acquiring the infection may approach that of the general population of countries where BCG is successfully employed. It is in these circumstances that the controversial problems arise. Even here, some of the problems leave little room for controversy. Certainly prompt and adequate chemotherapy is indicated for all persons with active disease. There is no longer any question that infants and children found to be positive tuberculin reactors should be treated the same as those with early active disease, since the risk of serious, disseminated, and potentially fatal tuberculous disease is very high, and is significantly and substantially reduced by proper chemotherapy. Such infants and children may not have demonstrably active disease, so that their treatment with isoniazid can properly be considered chemoprophylaxis.

What about the contacts of the recent converters? Since the latter are being treated as though they have active and manifest disease, should not the contacts be investigated as possible sources of the infection? Such investigation may uncover persons with active disease, who, of course, would be treated. For the most part, tuberculin tests would reveal positive and negative reactors, some of the former perhaps showing x-ray evidence of inactive disease, but any of the positive reactors may have been the source of a case of active disease or of a converter. From a public health point of view all the positive tuberculin reactors would be considered potential disseminators and, hence, should be given prophylactic chemotherapy with its risks of potential toxic effects. For their own personal welfare and as a public health measure, they should be kept under surveillance for possible development of active disease and they should also be monitored.

The management of the tuberculin-negative contacts of active cases or converters is a real point of controversy. Here BCG vaccination would be considered as offering a simple and prompt solution, with a minimum of cost and hazard. The alternative is to observe these individuals over a period of months for tuberculin conversion or for clinical or x-ray evidence of active disease, either of which would then be treated. BCG vaccination would deprive the tuberculin test of its value as a guide to infection in this circumstance. Surveillance and repeated tests are more costly procedures and are subject to the hazards of failure of compliance. Exempted from vaccination would be individuals with known or suspected immunologic defects, natural or induced, in whom there may be added risk from vaccination. They should be observed closely for tuberculin conversion or evidence of disease.

The major controversy involves essentially "normal" individuals in high risk areas. Is the long range effect in terms of the control of tuberculosis, namely reduction in case rate and death rate, better served by constant surveillance, with chemotherapy for all positive reactors and for all cases of active disease as soon as detected, or by vaccinating all those at risk of infection, namely all negative or probably negative reactors? The latter alternative would involve BCG vaccination of all infants at birth and subsequently all tuberculin-negative persons in the following groups: all children at the time of first entering school, all those entering military service (and perhaps schools and colleges in high risk areas away from home), teachers in high risk areas, and medical and nursing personnel and hospital employees having direct contacts with patients, and possibly others who may be exposed to active cases. The alternative here also is case finding and treatment of converters and of those with disease.

There may also be differences in attitude toward treatment of the person found to be tuberculin positive when first tested. Such an individual is already infected, so that vaccination is not indicated. From the point of view of that individual, the hazards and cost of therapy must be balanced against the potential reduction in the number of viable tubercle bacilli that would be available to produce active disease in that person or in others at some future time. That risk would depend on when that infection was acquired; if it may have been recent, then chemotherapy would be indicated. This could be assumed in all nurses, medical students, military recruits, and other young adults for whom data on previous tuberculin tests are not available. Older persons, with less risk of activating their disease and possibly greater risk of toxicity from isoniazid, may then be selected for surveillance, with therapy offered when active disease is discovered or suspected.

From the point of view of the public health, all positive reactors, except recent recipients of BCG vaccine, are potential sources of dissemination of infection and disease. Those with inapparent infections, that is, without manifest disease, are an important "seedbed of tuberculosis," as shown by the studies of Medlar at Bellevue Hospital more than two decades ago. They include old people with "healed apical lesions." X-rays of the chest may be helpful in delineating such individuals, and the patients would then best be managed by chemotherapy. Their treatment is more for the public good than for their own benefit.

Donald W. Smith[*] summarized the main arguments against BCG vaccination in the United States as follows: (1) the problem is of insufficient magnitude to warrant its use, (2) the vaccine is not safe, and (3) the attendant tuberculin conversion destroys the effectiveness of the tuberculin test as a case-finding tool. He challenges the validity of each of these objections and concludes that BCG vaccination should be recommended for high risk groups. The greater cost of finding and treating cases, the many possibilities of failure at some step in the follow-up (in tuberculin and x-ray case finding), in his view, all support BCG vaccination as the most satisfactory measure. Both he and Rosenthal indicate that the positive tuberculin test in the patient with active infection and disease can be differentiated from that due to the vaccine.

One may therefore appreciate why a physician like Dr. Rosenthal, who for many years has been following children he has vaccinated with BCG and has compared the occurrence of tuberculosis in them and in unvaccinated children, would have some difference in viewpoint from that of the public health worker who considers the problem from the point of view of the general health of the community or of the nation. The former stresses vaccination as protecting the vaccinee at relatively low cost and incidentally reducing the incidence of disease in

---

[*] Smith, D. W.: Ann. Intern. Med. 72:419, 1970.

the community; the latter stresses chemoprophylaxis as reducing the volume of tubercle bacilli available to reinfect the patient and to infect other individuals and thus protecting the "public health." Similar arguments, from the point of view of the population of Great Britain, have been set forth in a recent editorial in the Lancet (2:168, 1972).

MAXWELL FINLAND

13

The Kveim Test

THE KVEIM REACTION IS NOT A SPECIFIC TEST FOR SARCOIDOSIS
    by Harold L. Israel

THE KVEIM TEST IS A RELIABLE MEANS OF DIAGNOSING SARCOIDOSIS
    by Louis E. Siltzbach

COMMENT
    by Maxwell Finland

The Kveim Reaction Is Not a Specific Test for Sarcoidosis*

HAROLD L. ISRAEL

*Jefferson Medical College,
Thomas Jefferson University*

Sarcoidosis is a disease whose extraordinary clinical and immunologic features have fascinated clinicians and investigators alike. One of its most interesting features, first noted by Kveim, is a torpid granulomatous response to intracutaneous injection of lymph node or spleen extracts. This reaction has been widely recommended as a diagnostic test for sarcoidosis, and test materials are provided by the Central Public Health Laboratory to British physicians and by the Commonwealth Serum Laboratories of Australia* to physicians elsewhere. However, neither substance has been approved for import to or distribution in the United States by the Food and Drug Administration. Consequently, although a handful of American investigators have prepared their own test materials, few physicians in the United States have had the opportunity of using the test and only five have published studies of their experience during the past decade (Table 1). This table demonstrates the essence of the controversy concerning the Kveim reaction. How can a test which performs so consistently in sarcoidosis give such divergent results in different hands in other diseases?

Definitions

Sarcoidosis is a systemic granulomatous disease of unknown etiology, in most instances readily distinguished from the infectious granulomatoses by radiologic, immunologic, and pathologic characteristics as well as by its course and response

---

* In November 1972 issue of the antigen was discontinued because "recent investigations made it clear that in a significant number of cases the test material gives a positive reaction not only in sarcoidosis but also in such conditions as lymphoma and pulmonary tuberculosis."[48]

Table 1. *United States Studies of Kveim Reaction 1962 to 1971*
(Frequency of positive tests)

SARCOIDOSIS %	OTHER DISEASES %	TEST MATERIAL	REFERENCE
80	61	Sarcoid spleen*	Daniel and Schneider, 1962
77	0	Sarcoid lymph node†	
90	0	Skin sarcoid†	Kenney and Stone, 1963
56	0	Normal skin†	
82	<1	Sarcoid spleen‡	Siltzbach, 1967
77	0	Sarcoid spleen*	McLean et al., 1967
77	0	Sarcoid spleen‡	
76	50	Sarcoid spleen§	Israel and Goldstein, 1971

*M. Perlich, Department of Health, Cleveland, Ohio.
†Kenney and Stone, Veterans Administration Hospital, New York.
‡Chase-Siltzbach, Rockefeller University, New York.
§Commonwealth Serum Laboratory, Melbourne, Australia.

to corticosteroids. Kooij[6] and Scadding[7] have emphasized the looseness with which the term *specificity* has been used in regard to the Kveim test; the distinction between diagnostic and etiologic specificity has frequently been overlooked.

A truly specific diagnostic test should be positive in all subjects having a disease and negative in all subjects free of the disease. In practice, no test meets this requirement, and many immunologic reactions are regarded as acceptably specific if exceptional behavior is not too frequent. Serologic tests for syphilis, rheumatoid arthritis, typhoid fever, and histoplasmosis, for example, have diagnostic value even though diseases of different etiology may cause cross reactions. Tests for disseminated lupus also have clinical value even though it is recognized that the L. E. syndrome is precipitated by many agents. Diagnostic "specificity" does not require etiologic identity.

Specificity of the Kveim Reaction

Belief in the diagnostic specificity of the Kveim test had been based upon repeated studies which appeared to demonstrate a positive reaction in a majority of patients who exhibited the clinical and histologic features of sarcoidosis, and a great rarity of such reactions in patients or control subjects that did not have sarcoidosis.[8-10] Reports of similar findings in international studies performed by investigators from all parts of the world were construed as evidence that sarcoidosis was a specific disease entity of uniform etiology everywhere.[10-12] From such reports grew the assumption that the Kveim test material contained the etiologic agent of the disease, a concept exemplified in experiments in which the cutaneous reactions were excised and, in turn, used as a test material in other subjects.[3] However, the Kveim reaction might be a "specific" test for a granulomatous pattern characteristic of sarcoidosis, even if sarcoidosis should prove to be a syndrome due to a variety of causes. Some investigators have not made this distinction: the high frequency of positive Kveim tests observed in patients with regional ileitis led to the inference[13] that this disease and sarcoidosis shared a common causal agent.

The belief that the Kveim reaction reflected the presence of a specific etiologic agent was supported by reports which emphasized the frequency of positive Kveim tests in early sarcoidosis,[14] and the absence of reactions in "inactive" sarcoidosis.[15] It was generally assumed but never proved that the Kveim reaction reflected the presence of active granulomatous inflammation owing to the hypothetic etiologic agent of sarcoidosis in any organ or tissue.

Reports[1, 16] of positive Kveim tests in patients with infectious granulomatous disease (mycobacterial or fungal) were attributed to the use of improperly prepared lymph node or splenic suspensions. Confidence in the specificity of properly prepared antigens was enhanced when an English sarcoidal spleen suspension[14] and an Australian one[9] were compared with the Chase-Siltzbach preparation and demonstrated similar behavior in patients with sarcoidosis as well as in normal subjects and patients with other diseases. As a result of these trials, both the English and Australian preparations were designated as "validated."

The first demonstration[13] that a validated test material commonly evoked Kveim reactions in a disease other than sarcoidosis came in 1969. Regional ileitis has certain pathologic resemblances to sarcoidosis, and the demonstration of frequent positive tests in regional ileitis by two groups of investigators employing two validated antigens[17, 18] was interpreted as evidence that a single causal agent was responsible for both diseases. This assumption could no longer be accepted, however, when it was demonstrated that one or both of these validated test materials evoked typical Kveim reactions in patients with glandular tuberculosis (Table 2), chronic lymphatic leukemia,[5] disseminated lupus erythematosus,[21] ulcerative colitis, and celiac disease.[22]

Clearly these disparate diseases do not have the same immunologic or pathologic patterns of response, and it is extremely unlikely that they have the same cause. Thus, both of these validated antigens appear to lack diagnostic as well as etiologic specificity.

Recent reports of in vitro studies of the response of lymphocytes to Kveim antigen have shown no greater specificity than in vivo reactions.[23-25] The observations and conclusion of one recent investigation[23] deserve quotation: "Specific inhibition of leucocyte migration in vitro by a sarcoid spleen suspension has been

Table 2. *Kveim Reaction in Glandular Tuberculosis*

NUMBER TESTED	NUMBER POSITIVE	TEST MATERIAL	REFERENCE
45	0	*	Hirsch et al., 1971
Unspecified	50%	†	Mikhail and Mitchell, 1971
20	9	†, ‡	Karlish, 1971
9	9	‡	Israel, unpublished data

*Chase-Siltzbach, Rockefeller University, New York.
†Central Public Health Laboratory, London.
‡Commonwealth Serum Laboratories, Melbourne.

demonstrated in four out of ten patients with celiac disease and sixteen out of seventeen with dermatitis herpetiformis. . . . The evidence provided by these in vitro findings lends further emphasis to the need for revaluation of the Kveim reaction itself."

Mechanism of the Kveim Reaction

Proponents of the diagnostic and etiologic specificity of the Kveim reaction regard some component of the sarcoid granuloma to be the substance evoking a response in patients who have active sarcoidosis, but little evidence has been adduced to support this belief. For example, it has never been demonstrated that patients with sarcoidal granulomas in lung, liver, lymph nodes, spleen, or bone respond alike to the Kveim test.

On the contrary, Goldstein and I noted that patients with extensive and active osseous, cutaneous, and hepatic sarcoidosis are frequently Kveim negative.[5] All investigators recognize that a negative Kveim test does not exclude the presence of active sarcoidal granulomatosis: a majority of patients with Stage III sarcoidosis are Kveim-negative. The failure of such patients to react has been attributed to chronicity of the disease, but Kveim reactivity does not wane even after decades in patients with longstanding adenopathy due to sarcoidosis.[5]

It has been suggested that Kveim reactions may detect persons with subclinical sarcoidosis or those having a constitutional predisposition to the disease. This possibility was suggested by the demonstration that subjects who failed to develop tuberculin sensitivity after repeated vaccination with BCG frequently manifested Kveim reactions.[26] It seems unlikely, however, that the reaction is indicative of a *terrain sarcoidique*, for loss of Kveim reactivity on repeated testing has been reported.[3] In a study of patients who had recovered from sarcoidosis, Kveim tests were negative, although impairment of delayed hypersensitivity persisted.[27]

Recent observations indicate that several factors are involved in Kveim reactivity in sarcoidosis. One is demonstrated by the response of patients with chronic asymptomatic hilar adenopathy; of 34 such patients tested, 33 have reacted strongly. Mikhail et al.[28] observed positive Kveim tests in patients whose mediastinal nodes had become grossly fibrotic, suggesting that granulomatosis is not essential to persistent Kveim reactivity. In contrast, we have observed that patients with massive but transient (disappearing in less than six months) hilar lymphadenopathy usually fail to react. However, reactions are frequent in patients with transient adenopathy *and* erythema nodosum.

One of our patients demonstrates that the occurrence of positive Kveim tests in patients with erythema nodosum is unrelated to the duration of the sarcoidosis. In 1969 when she had a normal chest x-ray and hepatic and cutaneous granulomatosis, the Kveim reaction was negative. In 1971 erythema nodosum appeared, and the Kveim reaction was strongly positive. It appears inescapable that several antigens exist in Kveim suspensions, in some instances related to adenopathy and in others to erythema nodosum. These factors may be present in various concentrations in different lots and result in divergent (*but not senseless*) patterns of response.

Nature of the Test Material

The belief that the antigen or antigens involved are confined to granulomatous lymph nodes or spleens is open to question. Typical Kveim reactions in sarcoidosis have been elicited by suspensions of normal cow spleen,[29] the spleen of a patient with Banti's syndrome,[30] leukemic lymph nodes,[31] and even the typhoid-paratyphoid vaccine employed in World War II![32] Nelson[33] prepared extracts from 12 normal spleens; two of these elicited typical reactions in sarcoidosis. Kenney and Stone[2] in a double-blind study obtained weak but positive reactions with five of 14 normal skin suspensions. Sarcoidal tissues undoubtedly give a higher yield of potent test materials but, on the other hand, extracts of sarcoidal glands and spleens frequently lack potency and specificity. The differences among these various tissues in suitability as a source of Kveim antigen are those of degree. It is not essential that the source be sarcoid tissue. Although many preparations of sarcoid lymph nodes or spleens and a few of skin have been shown to produce reactions in patients with sarcoidosis, no materials prepared from other sarcoid tissues have been tested. Antigens contained in the organ as well as in the granuloma may be responsible for the inconsistencies which have been documented. It has not yet been determined whether the antigenic substances are single or multiple, of body origin, or of environmental origin.

Conflicting Data

A review of the literature reveals only a single instance in which directly conflicting observations regarding the behavior of the Kveim reaction have been reported. This was in respect to the development of Kveim reactions in subjects who failed to develop tuberculin sensitivity after repeated BCG vaccination. The three groups of investigators involved used the same test material.[26,27,34] The failure of two to confirm the results obtained by the first presumably reflects unrecognized differences among the subjects studied. *In no other instance have different investigators used the same lots of test material in comparable clinical material and reported divergent findings.* Contradictory results have occurred only when different preparations have been used as test materials. The predominant role of test material variability in the divergent observations recently reported is demonstrated by the findings in regional ileitis (Table 3). Positive reactions in this disease were frequent in three studies, absent or rare in three others. Of three lots prepared from spleen K_{12} in the same laboratory with presumably the same technique, two gave negative results and one gave positive results.[40] The authors offer no satisfactory explanation for these disparate findings, and it can only be concluded that the procedures recommended for preparation of Kveim test materials do not yield uniform products.

Table 3. *Kveim Reaction in Regional Ileitis*

TEST MATERIAL	PERCENTAGE POSITIVE	REFERENCE
C.S. lot 10*	0	Siltzbach et al., 1971
Spleen K_{12} lot 5†	46	Mitchell et al., 1970
Spleen K_{12} lot 1†	0	Siltzbach et al., 1971
Spleen K_{12} lot 15†	6	Chapman et al., 1971
Sarcoid lymph node ‡	0	Hannuksela et al., 1971
Spleen C.S.L. lot 004§	63	Mitchell et al., 1970
Spleen C.S.L. lot 004§	53	Karlish et al., 1970
Spleen C.S.L. lot 004§	87	Bartnik and Zych, 1972

*Chase-Siltzbach antigen, Rockefeller University, New York.
†Central Public Health Laboratory, London.
‡Helsinki, Finland.
§Commonwealth Serum Laboratories, Melbourne.

Conflicting Interpretations

Proponents of the specificity of the Kveim test are forced to argue that the positive reactions in diseases other than sarcoidosis are due to presence of foreign materials in some batches of validated test materials[35] or to deficiencies in histologic interpretation resulting from inexperience.[36]

THE TEST MATERIAL

An attempt has recently been made to dismiss the positive reactions in glandular tuberculosis, chronic lymphatic leukemia, and inflammatory gut disease as the result of contamination of test materials by hypothetic foreign matter.[35]

The strong reactions which have been observed in other diseases cannot be due to inclusion of nonspecific foreign body reactions, because each of these reports includes categories in which the Kveim test has been consistently negative. Willoughby and Mitchell[22] found no positive Kveim tests in primary biliary cirrhosis and we have found Kveim tests negative in 20 of 22 patients with sarcoidosis who had normal chest x-rays. Moreover, if foreign materials or errors in interpretation are invoked to explain the frequency of reactions in the diseases just enumerated, how can the same investigators with the same products get satisfactory results in sarcoidosis itself?

I have used the validated British and Australian preparations in duplicate tests in 48 patients. Occasional discordance was found in other diseases, but complete conformity was observed in 37 patients with sarcoidosis, both tests being positive in 28 and both negative in nine. This makes it most improbable that a foreign contaminant is present. Because of the allegation that a minor change in filtration procedure had altered the antigen, the Commonwealth Serum Laboratories prepared a new lot, batch 006, employing precisely the same procedure as in the original batches. Two of 10 cases with lymphoma and seven of 10 with tuberculosis tested in Melbourne[48] and three of four cases with glandular tuberculosis tested in Philadelphia gave positive reactions. As a result of these observations, the Commonwealth Serum Laboratories no longer felt justified in recommending the antigen as a specific diagnostic reagent and ended its distribution.

Histologic Interpretation

Double-blind comparisons of histologic readings have been made and, as might be anticipated, there is some observer variation[4, 41-43] particularly in the minority of reactions with poorly defined granuloma formation. Drury estimated significant observer variation to be about 5 per cent.[43] Differences in histologic interpretation must surely make only a minor contribution to the divergent findings reported by experienced investigators.

Objection has been made[11] that R. A. Goldstein and I failed to take biopsies in the absence of palpable or visible reactions. Our practice in this respect was based on the fact that a study in which biopsies were taken of injection sites that did not have macroscopic reactions revealed only 6 per cent to be microscopically positive.[45] Since the scars which follow biopsy are distasteful to many patients, especially those who develop keloids, it appears to be unjustifiable to subject a large number of patients to this procedure with a yield so small. It should be noted moreover that the yield of positive tests in sarcoidosis is essentially the same (Table 1) whether or not biopsy is restricted to macroscopic lesions. The question of specificity hinges not on too few reactions, but on too many!

Diagnostic Value of the Kveim Test

No hypothesis can explain away the flood of observations of positive reactions in diseases other than sarcoidosis (Tables 1, 2, and 3). To persist in claims of the diagnostic specificity of the Kveim reaction is to disregard the difficulties in preparation, standardization, and preservation of test materials that have recently come to light. The Chase-Siltzbach test material appears to evoke reactions much less often in other diseases,[36, 38] although prospective trials in glandular tuberculosis and other types of chronic lymphadenopathy have not been reported. The supply of this preparation is too limited to permit general investigative or clinical use, and whether preparations by these workers from other spleens will have similar characteristics or behave like those produced in England and Australia remains to be shown.

Until test materials that will not react frequently in other diseases can be regularly reproduced, the Food and Drug Administration is correct in discouraging clinical use of the Kveim test.

If the essential factors of Kveim test materials are identified, this may result in a test useful for the diagnosis of sarcoidosis. To establish its clinical value, the antigen should produce reactions that can be interpreted by competent general or dermatologic pathologists without special expertise in the niceties of granuloma differentiation. Commercial production and distribution of stable test materials should be feasible. The failure of these criteria to be met by any of the Kveim test materials thus far produced raises serious doubts about the future prospects of this reaction as a clinical test.

As Scadding[46] has pointed out, special pleading for its value as a "specific" test for sarcoidosis is likely to hinder more important studies of the Kveim reaction. It is noteworthy that our study of the relationship of the Kveim reaction to lymphadenopathy has led to endless argument regarding the "specificity" of the test, but little discussion of the observations regarding the mechanism of the reaction in the disease in which it most commonly occurs, i.e., sarcoidosis.

Hypothesis

Although lacking diagnostic and etiologic specificity, it need not be concluded that the Kveim reaction is nonspecific, reacting whimsically and erratically, without rhyme or reason. It is probable, rather, that Kveim test materials contain several antigens, which vary in kind and number according to the tissue source from which they are derived, as well as with subtle differences in preparation (Table 3).

Reactants to all or most of these antigens are commonly present in sarcoidosis, but reactants to some occur in many patients with tuberculosis, inflammatory gut disease, collagen disorders, and a variety of chronic lymphadenopathies. Genetic factors in responsiveness may be involved since Rees in a study of tuberculoid leprosy found positive Kveim tests only in Orientals,[47] and Izumi[35] has reported an astonishing frequency of positive reactions among normal Japanese.

I would suggest that the Kveim reaction *is* a specific immunologic response, resembling the Mitsuda reaction, which has not been given adequate attention in conventional immunologic classifications.

This reaction deserves far more intensive investigation than it has yet received. Further investigation of the Kveim reaction may or may not contribute to discovery of the cause of sarcoidosis, but other important benefits are to be anticipated from a thorough study of this largely neglected system of immunologic recognition.

Summary and Conclusions

The Kveim reaction is not a specific diagnostic test for sarcoidosis. The test materials in their present form evoke granulomatous responses in a variety of other diseases and fail to produce reactions in many patients with sarcoidosis. A reaction to the two generally available test materials does not establish the presence of active sarcoidosis, and a negative test does not exclude active sarcoidal granulomatosis.

Investigation of the Kveim reaction has in the past been preoccupied with a fruitless search for a single substance, the presumed cause of sarcoidosis. Future research should be directed toward elucidation of the factors common to sarcoidosis, tuberculosis, disseminated lupus, and inflammatory gut diseases that are responsible for the reactions elicited by many validated test materials.

References

1. Daniel, T. H., and Schneider, G. W.: Positive Kveim tests in patients without sarcoidosis. Amer. Rev. Resp. Dis. 86:98, 1962.
2. Kenney, M., and Stone, D. J.: Objective evaluation of the Kveim test in a double-blind study. Amer. Rev. Resp. Dis. 87:504, 1963.
3. Siltzbach, L. E.: Concepts of sarcoidosis in the light of Kveim reaction. In La Sarcoidose. Rapp. IVth International Conference, 1967. Paris, Masson et Cie, 1967, pp. 129–140.
4. McLean, R. L., Meltzer, H. D., and Lathan, S. R.: Kveim reaction in sarcoidosis. A comparison of two splenic suspensions applied simultaneously to the same patients. In La Sarcoidose. Rapp. IVth International Conference, 1967. Paris, Masson et Cie, 1967, pp. 182–188.
5. Israel, H. L., and Goldstein, R. A.: Relation of Kveim-antigen reaction to lymphadenopathy. New Eng. J. Med. 284:345, 1971.
6. Kooij, R.: The nature of the Kveim reaction. Acta Med. Scand. 176 (Suppl.) 425, 1964.
7. Scadding, J. G.: The Kveim controversy. Lancet 2:1372, 1971.
8. Siltzbach, L. E.: The Kveim test in sarcoidosis, a study of 750 patients. J.A.M.A. 178:476, 1961.
9. Hirsch, J. G., Cohn, Z. A., Morse, S. I., et al.: Evaluation of the Kveim reaction as a diagnostic test for sarcoidosis. New Eng. J. Med. 265:827, 1961.
10. Hurley, T. H., and Bartholomeusz, C.: The Kveim test. Results obtained in sarcoid and non-sarcoid patients with simultaneous use of Australian (C.S.L.) and American (Chase-Siltzbach Type I USA) Kveim suspensions. In La Sarcoidose. Rapp. IVth International Conference, 1967. Paris, Masson et Cie, 1967, pp. 194–200.
11. Siltzbach, L. E.: An international Kveim test study, 1960–1966. In La Sarcoidose. Rapp. IVth International Conference on Sarcoidosis. Paris, Masson et Cie, 1967, pp. 201–213.
12. Hurley, T. H., and Bartholomeusz, C. L.: An international Siltzbach-Kveim test study using an Australian (C.S.L.) test material (1966–69) Vth International Conference on Sarcoidosis, Prague, 1971, pp. 343–348.
13. Mitchell, D. N., Cannon, P., Dyer, N. H., et al.: The Kveim test in Crohn's disease. 2:571, 1969.
14. James D. G., and Sharma, O. P.: The Kveim-Siltzbach test. Report of a new British antigen. Lancet 2:1274, 1967.
15. Behrend, H., Rupec, M., and Deicher, H.: Zur Stellung des Kveim-tests in der Diagnostik der Boeck' schen sarkoidose. Med. Thor. 24:129, 1967.
16. Israel, H. L., and Sones, M.: Diagnosis of sarcoidosis with special reference to the Kveim reaction. Ann. Intern. Med. 43:1269, 1955.
17. Mitchell, D. N., Cannon, P., Dyer, N. H., et al.: Further observations on Kveim test in Crohn's disease. Lancet 2:496, 1970.
18. Karlish, A. J., Cox, E. V., Hampson, F., et al.: Kveim test in Crohn's disease. Lancet 2:977, 1970.
19. Mikhail, J., and Mitchell, D. N.: Mediastinoscopy: A diagnostic procedure in hilar and paratracheal lymphadenopathy. Postgrad. Med. J. 47:698, 1971.
20. Karlish, A. J.: The Kveim test in sarcoidosis. Oxford Med. Sch. Gaz. 23:26, 1971.
21. Bringel, C., and Lofgren, S.: Kveim reaction in collagen diseases. Presented at Symposium Européen sur la Sarcoidose, Geneva, September, 1971.
22. Willoughby, J. M. T., and Mitchell, D. N.: In vitro inhibition of leucocyte migration in Crohn's disease by a sarcoid spleen suspension. Brit. Med. J. 3:155, 1971.

23. Pagaltsos, A. S., Kumor, P. J., Willoughby, J. M. T., et al.: In-vitro inhibition of leucocyte migration by sarcoid spleen suspension in coeliac disease and dermatitis herpetiformis. Lancet 2:1179, 1971.
24. Topilsky, M., Williams, M. Siltzbach, L. E., et al.: Lymphocyte response in sarcoidosis. Lancet 1:117, 1972.
25. Becker, F. W., Deicher, H., Krull, P., et al.: Leucocyte-migration test in sarcoidosis. Lancet 1:120, 1971.
26. Hart, P. D., Mitchell, D. N., and Sutherland, L.: Association between Kveim test results, previous BCG vaccination, and tuberculin sensitivity in healthy young adults. Brit. Med. J. 1:795, 1964.
27. Israel, H. L., and Sones, M.: A study of BCG vaccination and the Kveim reaction. Ann. Intern. Med. 64:1, 1966.
28. Mikhail, J. R., Mitchell, D. N., Drury, R. A. B., et al.: A comparison of the value of mediastinal lymph node biopsy and the Kveim test. Vth International Conference on Sarcoidosis. Prague, 1971, p. 361.
29. Kooij, R.: "Kveim" test with a cow spleen suspension. Vth International Conference on Sarcoidosis, Prague, 1971, p. 384.
30. Hirako, T.: Kveim test on sarcoidosis and some other diseases. *La Sarcoidose.* Rapp. IVth International Conference on Sarcoidosis, Paris, 1967, p. 214.
31. Putkonen, T.: Uber die Kveim reaction bei Lymphogranulomatosis benigna. Acta Derm. Venereol. 25:393, 1945.
32. Gilroy, J.: Kveim test. Brit. Med. J. 3:369, 1971.
33. Nelson, C. T.: Observations on the Kveim reaction in sarcoidosis of the American Negro. J. Invest. Derm. 10:15, 1948.
34. Meyer, A., Nico, J. P., and Guize, L.: La Réaction de Kveim chez de jeunes adultes ou des enfants dont les réactions tuberculiniques sont restées négatives malgré deux vaccinations par le B.C.G. *In La Sarcoidose.* Rapp. IVth International Conference on Sarcoidosis, Paris, 1967, p. 162.
35. Kveim-Siltzbach test vindicated. (Editorial.) Lancet 1:88, 1972.
36. Hirsch, J. G., Nelson, C. T., and Siltzbach, L. E., The Kveim test. New Eng. J. Med. 284:1326, 1971.
37. Bartnik, W., and Zych, D.: The Kveim controversy. Lancet 1:154, 1972.
38. Siltzbach, L. E., Vieria, L. O. B. D., Topilsky, M., et al.: Is there Kveim responsiveness in Crohn's disease? Lancet 2:634, 1971.
39. Hannuksela, M., Alkio, H., and Selroos, O.: Kveim reaction in Crohn's disease. Lancet 2:974, 1971.
40. Chapman, J. A., Gleeson, M. H., and Taylor, G.: Kveim tests in Crohn's disease. Lancet 2:1097, 1971.
41. Israel, H. L., Sones, M., Beerman, H., et al.: A further study of the Kveim reaction in sarcoidosis and tuberculosis. New Eng. J. Med. 259:365, 1958.
42. Ringsted, J., and Ferebec, J. B.: On the standardization of the histopathologic reading of the Kveim test. Acta Med. Scand. 88 (Suppl.):425, 1964.
43. Drury, R. A. B.: Problems in histologic interpretation in sarcoidosis. Postgrad. Med. J. 46:478, 1970.
44. The Kveim controversy. (Editorial.) Lancet 2:750, 1971.
45. Karlish, A. J.: Measurements of Kveim specific nodules in sarcoidosis. *In La Sarcoidose.* Rapp. IVth International Conference on Sarcoidosis. Paris, Masson et Cie, 1967, p. 176.
46. Scadding, J. G.: The Kveim controversy. Lancet 1:260, 1972.
47. Rees, R. J. W.: The Kveim test in leprosy. Postgrad. Med. J. 46:486, 1970.
48. Hurley, T. H.: Personal communication.

The Kveim Test Is a Reliable Means of Diagnosing Sarcoidosis*

LOUIS E. SILTZBACH

Mount Sinai School of Medicine, New York

Since 1941, when Kveim[1] first described it, the phenomenon of Kveim reactivity has been accepted as being associated almost exclusively with sarcoidosis. The intracutaneous test, employing saline homogenates of selected human sarcoidal tissues, was quickly adopted in many centers as a mainstay in the diagnosis of sarcoidosis because of its simplicity and reliability. The test could be carried out on an ambulatory basis and often spared the patient one or more organ biopsies in a hospital. At the Mount Sinai Hospital, we have assessed more than 3500 biopsies of Kveim sites since 1946, and during the course of illness we have found microscopically positive reactions in about 80 per cent of patients with organ biopsy-confirmed sarcoidosis. False positive reactions have amounted to less than 1 per cent among nonsarcoid subjects in the same period. Equally favorable experiences with the Kveim test have been reported from many centers around the world,[2-4] and reliable test suspensions are currently being processed and are in diagnostic use in two other clinics in New York City, in Baltimore, and in European centers in Paris, Helsinki, Stockholm, Hanover, and Belgrade, among other cities. On the one hand, recent scattered reports of Kveim cross reactivity in patients with diverse disorders have raised questions about the test's specificity and have also stimulated speculation regarding possible etiologic and immunologic relationships between sarcoidosis and conditions which hitherto have been presumed to be completely unrelated to it. Data have now been coming to light which go far to explain many of the reported aberrant Kveim test results which, it turns out, were associated for the most part with the use of two batches of Kveim material from the same tissue source which had been distributed on an international scale.

---

* This work was supported by a research grant from the National Heart and Lung Institute, Public Health Service (HL 13853-15—Patho-Physiology Branch).

Two Unsatisfactory Batches of Kveim Test Suspensions

On December 18, 1971, Hurley and Lane[5] of the Commonwealth Serum Laboratory (CSL), Melbourne, Australia, announced through a letter in *The Lancet* of that date that the latest two batches of their Kveim test material—CSL batches #004 and #005—were being withdrawn from further issue because of their unreliability as test agents in the diagnosis of sarcoidosis. These faulty batches of test material prepared, respectively, in 1968 and 1970, had been dispensed from 1969 through 1971 to investigators in 40 countries, and a number of proformas being returned to the Commonwealth Serum Laboratories indicated that these materials were yielding aberrantly positive Kveim reactions in a high proportion of patients with diseases other than sarcoidosis and even among healthy control subjects.[6-10] These new results were quite unlike the highly satisfactory results of Kveim testing obtained with earlier products of the same human sarcoidal splenic tissue source (CSL batches #001, #002, #003).[11] Review of the techniques employed in processing the two erratic batches revealed that prewashed muslin had inadvertently been used to strain particles of the final product, and it was initially suspected at the laboratory that cotton fibers might have been introduced and could be causing confusing foreign body granulomas at the test sites. However, an additional preparation, CSL batch #006, made later from the same tissue source and processed without muslin filtration also behaved unpredictably as a test agent, an experience similar to one reported by Nelson with a human sarcoidal spleen he had used.[12] It had thus become obvious that the portions of the sarcoid spleen which remained had unaccountably become unsuitable as a source of diagnostic Kveim material. Before examining more closely the basis for doubts about Kveim specificity engendered by these adverse experiences with CSL #004 and #005 test suspensions, it may be helpful to recount briefly some previous challenges to the test's specificity and how these were met.

Sources of Error in Kveim Testing

It has been known for some time that not all human sarcoidal tissues make satisfactory sources of potent and specific Kveim test material. Since 1946 Kveim suspensions made from tissues of 52 patients with sarcoidosis have been assessed and calibrated in our laboratory and clinic at the Mount Sinai Hospital, New York for their specificity and sensitivity. Intracutaneous injections of Kveim preparations made from any new tissue sources are injected in parallel with our closely monitored Kveim suspension (Spleen J, Chase-Siltzbach, Type 1), which has been serving as an international reference standard since 1960. Only about half the test suspensions which have been evaluated have proved to be satisfactory for diagnostic purposes.

Until 1969 few reports appeared questioning the test's usefulness and, on closer scrutiny, the doubts raised by these earlier studies could be dissipated.

Thus, Israel and co-workers,[13] using a Kveim suspension they prepared from sarcoidal lymph nodes, reported in 1955 that 14 of 33 patients with tuberculosis exhibited positive Kveim reactions with their test material. But in 1958[14] these authors encountered not a single positive Kveim reaction among 29 patients with tuberculosis who were tested with material prepared from other sarcoidal lymph nodes obtained from the same patient source. As it turned out, the test suspensions these authors prepared were neither potent nor specific enough to be used in the diagnosis of sarcoidosis.

A similar resolution of doubts about the Kveim test respecting aberrant results encountered in nonsarcoid subjects with another Kveim suspension (Spleen A, Perlich's antigen) could be reached by parallel testing with our continuously validated Kveim reference material. Daniel and Schneider[15] found positive Kveim reactions among eight of 13 patients with histoplasmosis, coccidioidomycosis, and tuberculosis. But when, as a check on these unusual Kveim test results,[16] Lot 8, Type 1 (Spleen J) test material from our laboratory and the same Spleen A Kveim suspension Daniel and Schneider had used were injected intracutaneously in parallel in 16 nonsarcoid patients (11 with active pulmonary tuberculosis and five with various nonsarcoid neurologic disorders), the source of the confusing results with Spleen A became apparent (Table 1). The biopsy test site slides were read "double-blind" by three assessors, including the writer (Assessor III) and two of the original readers of Daniel and Schneider's slides. The 16 biopsy test sites of standard Lot 8 material were all read as negative Kveim reactions by the three assessors. In contrast, Spleen A (Perlich's antigen) had evoked substantial papules in nine of the 16 patients and the biopsy test papules often had a bizarre microscopic appearance, causing considerable disparity in the readings of the three assessors. Assessors I and II read five and eight test sites, respectively, as positive Kveim reactions while I placed eight sites in the equivocal category and only one site in the Kveim positive group. Spleen A test suspension had previously been shown by other investigators to have the capacity to elicit positive Kveim reactions in a high proportion of patients with biopsy-confirmed sarcoidosis. Yet Speen A suspension was decidedly unreliable as a test agent for the diagnosis of sarcoidosis because it also evoked granulomas haphazardly in nonsarcoid subjects who had been found Kveim-negative when tested with a standardized, closely monitored Kveim suspension, Lot 8, Spleen J.

Table 1. *Kveim Test Results with Two Different Sarcoidal Spleen Suspensions in 11 Patients with Active Tuberculosis and 5 Cases with Nonsarcoid Neurologic Disorders*

	Kveim nodule size at 4–6 weeks			Microscopic Kveim readings								
				Assessor I			Assessor II			Assessor III		
	>3 mm.	3 mm. or less	No. nodule	+	−	±	+	−	±	+	−	±
Spleen A	9	2	5	5	9	2	8	4	4	1	8	7
Lot 8, type I (Chase-Siltzbach)	0	1	15	0	16	0	0	16	0	0	16	0

Kveim Specificity in Two International Kveim Trials

In 1960, on recommendation of the conferees of the Second International Conference on Sarcoidosis, I employed a single sarcoidal splenic tissue source (Spleen J, Chase-Siltzbach, Type 1 test suspension) in an international Kveim test trial.[17] The test material was distributed to investigators in 37 countries around the world, and 3244 patients were Kveim tested. The international Kveim trial recorded a wide-scale specific responsiveness to the active fraction contained in the Kveim test suspension used, and the results strengthened the view that sarcoidosis was a distinct disease entity and was one and the same disorder around the world. The trial, moreover, confirmed the satisfactory level of specificity of the Kveim material used. False positive reactions were rarely encountered, occurring in only five (0.7 per cent) among 668 nonsarcoid subjects tested. Between 1966 and 1969 a second and similarily organized international Kveim trial encompassing 2038 subjects was undertaken by Hurley[11] of Mebourne, Australia. That investigator used a splenic sarcoidal tissue suspension prepared by the Commonwealth Serum Laboratories (CSL batches #0017 through #0032). This second Kveim trial confirmed the findings of the first trial with respect to the test's specificity and was characterized by a similarly low frequency of Kveim cross reactivity among nonsarcoid subjects; viz, false positive reactions occurred among six (0.8 per cent) of 722 subjects without sarcoidosis.

Faulty Batches of Kveim Test Material

But a vastly different story emerged with the international use of the next batches of CSL suspensions, series #004 and #005, prepared from the same splenic source in 1968 and 1970 and dispensed between 1969 and 1971 for eventual use in 2260 subjects.[18] CSL batches #004 and #005 yielded an inordinately high frequency of Kveim cross reactivity in nonsarcoid subjects including healthy volunteers and, as previously stated, these test materials had to be withdrawn from further issue.

It was the erratic behavior of these two batches of CSL test suspensions that was responsible for the appearance of a series of reports in which high frequencies of positive Kveim reactions were recorded in presumably unrelated disorders, such as nonsarcoid lymphadenopathy of diverse etiology, Crohn's disease and other diseases of the gut, collagen disorders, and isolated granulomatous hepatitis as well as in asthma, lung abscess, silicosis, chronic bronchitis, emphysema, idiopathic pulmonary fibrosis, lung carcinoma, and other malignancies, and in healthy volunteer subjects (Table 2). Because CSL batches #0017 through #0032 had previously been used with good effect in the second international Kveim trial,[11] it was assumed by most investigators using the new CSL batches #004 and #005 after 1969 that they could forgo a parallel series of Kveim tests in a control population and omit the parallel use of another validated Kveim suspension to ascertain whether the unusually high proportion of Kveim cross reactivity they

Table 2. *Kveim Test Results in Nonsarcoid Subjects with Two Different Lots of CSL Suspensions*

	CSL LOTS #001 TO 003			CSL LOTS #004 AND 005		
	Number Tested	Number Kv Positive	Per Cent Kv Positive	Number Tested	Number Kv Positive	Per Cent Kv Positive
Hurley and Bartholomeusz,[11]* 1966–1969	722	6	0.8	363	116	31
Hurley and Sullivan,[18]* 1969–1972						
Izumi et al.,[9] 1967–1971	36	2	5.5	164	84	51
Chretien,[10] 1967–1971				34	22	65

*International Kveim trial results which include data of Izumi et al.[14] and Chretien[10], among others.

were observing was bona fide or was to be ascribed to a lack of specificity in the CSL #004–#005 test material. These misleading results prompted the observers to postulate a series of hypotheses, including possible etiologic and immunologic relationships between sarcoidosis and these variegated disorders which now appeared to be associated with Kveim reactivity. Thus, Israel and Goldstein,[6] using CSL #004 test material soon after it was dispensed, observed six positive Kveim reactions among eight patients with four different diseases with lymphadenopathy not caused by sarcoidosis. They concluded that Kveim reactivity was a phenomenon common to lymphadenopathy regardless of cause.

Hirsch et al.,[19] in a combined series of personal observations and results from the first international Kveim test trial, found only two of 138 control patients with similar types of nonsarcoid lymphadenopathy who were Kveim positive with two validated Kveim suspensions (Spleen J and DM2). Israel and Goldstein had not performed concurrent Kveim tests with the same CSL #004 material in nonsarcoid subjects *without* lymphadenopathy. Likewise, Karlish et al.[7] were also unaware of the unreliability of the CSL #004 and #005 Kveim suspensions when they reported positive Kveim reactions in 33 of 78 (42 per cent) nonsarcoid patients with three gastrointestinal disorders: Crohn's disease, ulcerative colitis, and adult celiac disease. Kveim tests using the same CSL material in subjects without diseases of the gut were not performed for comparison. At about the same time, Bringel[8] also used the CSL #004 Kveim suspension to test 12 patients with various collagen disorders, mainly lupus erythematosus. Nine of the 12 patients showed microscopically positive Kveim reactions. Dissatisfied with these results, she reinjected her 12 patients with another closely monitored test suspension of satisfactory specificity, viz., Spleen J suspension. None of the 12 patients were Kveim positive with this material.

Chretien,[10] also unaware of the unpredictable behavior of the CSL #004 and #005 material, used these suspensions and found positive Kveim reactions just as frequently among patients without sarcoidosis as in those with sarcoidosis,

65 and 69 per cent, respectively. Chretien tested 110 patients with sarcoidosis and 34 patients with such varied conditions as tuberculosis, Hodgkin's disease, reticulum cell sarcoma, lung abscess, benign bronchial tumor, and asthma.

Comparison of Early and Later Batches of CSL Kveim Suspensions

The puzzling behavior of CSL series #004 and #005 Kveim suspensions remained unexplained until a study by Izumi and co-workers[9] from Kyoto became available. This was an analysis of the results of this study[20] which demonstrated conclusively the unreliability of those two Kveim suspensions as diagnostic agents in sarcoidosis and which led to their withdrawal from further issue by the Commonwealth Serum Laboratories in December, 1971. Between January, 1967, and June, 1971, Izumi and colleagues had made 583 Kveim tests in patients with sarcoidosis and other disorders as well as in healthy controls, using CSL test material exclusively. What endowed their study with its special importance was their use of two different bulk batches of CSL Kveim test material, one prepared in the Commonwealth Serum Laboratories in 1965 designated as CSL #002–#003 series and the other prepared in 1968, the CSL #004 series. As stated previously, the CSL #002–#003 series had been widely used in the second international Kveim trial and had been found to be highly specific in differentiating patients with nonsarcoid disorders from those with sarcoidosis. The CSL #002–#003 series of test suspensions were found to be equally reliable in the study of Izumi and co-workers (Table 2). Among nonsarcoid subjects tested with these two batches, and these included patients with tuberculosis, asthma, chronic obstructive lung disease, silicosis, lung carcinoma, as well as healthy controls, only two of 36 subjects were Kveim positive. But with the later batches of the CSL #004 series the nonsarcoid groups and the healthy controls exhibited positive Kveim reactions with extraordinary frequency, 84 of 164 individuals, or 51 per cent, responding. Even among the 29 healthy controls included in this group 13, or 45 per cent, were Kveim positive with the new material. Hurley and Sullivan[18] also recorded 116 instances (31 per cent) of Kveim cross reactivity among 363 nonsarcoid subjects tested with CSL #004–#005 in various clinics around the world.

Because the CSL #004 series of Kveim suspensions were eliciting granulomatous intracutaneous papules almost indiscriminately, one might have anticipated that among patients with sarcoidosis as well, a higher than usual frequency of positive Kveim reactions would be observed. This turned out to be so in the series of Izumi and co-workers, in which 26 of 46 (78 per cent) of patients with sarcoidosis of less than one year's duration were Kveim positive with the use of the early CSL #002–#003 series of suspensions, in contrast to 55 of 64 (88 per cent) being Kveim positive when tested with the CSL #004 series. But this difference in response to the two sets of CSL suspensions was even more dramatic when patients whose sarcoidosis was regressing were tested. Among them, seven of 26 (27 per cent) were Kveim positive with the CSL #002–#003 series as contrasted with 25 of 35 patients (71 per cent) in the regressed stage tested with the CSL

#004 material. Hurley and Sullivan[18] report similar findings with a larger series of CSL Kveim tests among 395 patients with sarcoidosis of less than two years' duration; for example, 63 per cent were Kveim positive with the CSL #001 through #003 suspensions as compared with 81 per cent among 344 patients tested with the later CSL #004–#005 material. Likewise, among 244 patients with sarcoidosis of longer than two years' duration or of indeterminate length, 51 per cent were Kveim positive with CSL #001 through #003 suspensions as compared with 74 per cent among 138 patients tested with the CSL #004–#005 suspensions. This increment in positive Kveim tests with the later test material no doubt resulted from the finding of positive Kveim reactions in patients with sarcoidosis who were really in the Kveim negative phase and would not have reacted when tested with satisfactory Kveim material.

These experiences emphasize that the crux of the matter is not whether a particular Kveim suspension can produce positive Kveim reactions in a high proportion of patients with active sarcoidosis, but whether the suspension can do so while at the same time it produces virtually no positive Kveim reactions in subjects without sarcoidosis. From the very outset, unlike its predecessors the CSL #001, #002 and #003 suspensions, the CSL #004 and #005 suspensions could not measure up to these criteria.

A continuing puzzle are the reports of Mitchell and colleagues[21, 22] from London of a high frequency of positive Kveim reactions in Crohn's disease as well as in ulcerative colitis and adult celiac disease when patients were tested with certain lots of the Colindale K 12 Kveim suspensions (Lots 5 and 14). In contrast to the findings of Mitchell et al., a combined report of Kveim test results among 135 patients with Crohn's disease observed in seven other clinics—Cardiff,[23] Manchester,[24] Reading,[25] Helsinki,[26] Hanover,[27] New Haven[28] and New York[29]—showed positive reactions in only four patients, or 3 per cent, a satisfactory level of Kveim cross reactivity (Table 3). Some of those observers used the same K 12 suspension but not the same lots Mitchell et al. used. (Tests made with the faulty CSL #004 series in patients with Crohn's disease have been excluded from these combined results.) Regrettably, supplies of the lots 5 and 14 of Colindale K 12 Kveim suspension are no longer available for continued study.

Table 3. *Kveim Reaction in 135 Patients with Crohn's Disease**

AUTHOR	Kv SUSP. BATCH/LOT	TOTAL TESTS	NO. Kv POSITIVE
J. Williams[23]	K 12-1,18,19	46	1
Chapman[24]	K 12-15	17	1
Karlish[25]	K 12-18,19	12	2
Hannukusela[26]	Fin LN	16	0
Behrend[27]	WG LN	6	0
Klatskin[28]	Spl J-10	6	0
Siltzbach[29]	Spl J-1,3,10	32	0
TOTAL		135	4 = 3%

*Excludes test made with CSL batches #004–005 and K-12 Lots 5 and 14. See text.

Criteria To Be Met by Satisfactory Kveim Suspensions

In Stockholm in 1963 at the Third International Conference on Sarcoidosis[30] the properties possessed by a satisfactory Kveim test suspension to be employed as a diagnostic agent in sarcoidosis were outlined.

First, with respect to potency, the test suspension should contain a high enough concentration of the granuloma-producing factor to evoke positive Kveim reactions in a majority of patients with active sarcoidosis—six or more of every 10 patients tested.

Second, a properly screened suspension elicits in responsive patients a histologically characteristic intracutaneous papule within four to six weeks. The Kveim papule grows slowly, and in about one third of responsive subjects measures 5 mm. or more in diameter after four to six weeks. Tissue particles in a satisfactory test suspension are fine and are evenly dispersed on shaking the vial. Simultaneous injection of an equal volume and concentration of a satisfactory test suspension yields, in a responsive subject, like-sized papules in four to six weeks. The papule is composed of compact and discrete masses of epithelioid cells and occasional giant cells with only a minor degree of fibrinoid necrosis and nonspecific inflammatory cellular reaction. Birefringent bodies may occasionally be present, but in small numbers.

Third, and most important, a diagnostically effective Kveim suspension is bland, producing in nonsarcoid subjects no sizeable papules and no true sarcoidal reaction histologically. Cross reactivity or false positive Kveim reactions should not exceed a level of 3 per cent. When such aberrant reactions are present at all, they should be characterized by small papules at six weeks which histologically exhibit few granulomas, poor in epithelioid cells more loosely arranged than the classically positive Kveim reaction elicited in patients with sarcoidosis.

It is to be stressed that no Kveim test suspension can qualify for diagnostic use in sarcoidosis unless its nonreactivity has been conclusively demonstrated in a sizeable group of a variety of nonsarcoid subjects. Should some particular nonsarcoid disorder be under investigation with regard to Kveim reactivity, it is of paramount importance that the same Kveim test material be *concurrently* studied in nonsarcoid disorders unrelated to the condition being focused upon. Obviously the level of sensitivity or potency of the test material when used in patients with active sarcoidosis must also be ascertained and monitored during such investigations. To repeat, it is not enough for a particular batch being used to provoke positive Kveim reactions with regularity in patients with active sarcoidosis; it is quite as important to know how the Kveim suspension behaves in nonsarcoid subjects.

Monitoring batches of Kveim suspensions need not be too onerous a task from a practical standpoint, provided a volume of Kveim batches is made up in quantities sufficient for several hundreds or thousands of test doses and preferably prepared from a sarcoidal spleen. As stated previously, satisfactory Kveim test material is currently being prepared for local use at several centers in this country and abroad. Efforts are continuing toward the establishment of a central source of specific test material so that general distribution of validated material can be resumed.

The intracutaneous Kveim test as currently used will be employed with profit in the diagnosis of sarcoidosis so long as recognized procedures for preparation of satisfactory Kveim suspensions are followed and accurate assessments of the microscopic responses at the injection site are made. Identification of the active fraction responsible for the formation of granulomas at Kveim sites in patients with active sarcoidosis will constitute a long step toward making reliable test material widely available and will, no doubt, cast much light on the enigma of the etiology and pathogenesis of sarcoidosis.

References

1. Kveim, A.: En ny og Spesifik kutan-reackjon ved Boeck's Sarcoid. Nord. Med. 9:169, 1941.
2. Putkonen, T.: Ueber die Intrakutanreaktion von Kveim (KvR) bie Lymphogranulomatosis benigna. Acta Dermat.-Venereol. 23 (Suppl. 10):1–194, 1943.
3. James, D. G., and Thomson, A. D.: The Kveim test in sarcoidosis. Quart. J. Med. 24:49, 1955.
4. Turiaf, J., and Battesti, J. P.: A propos de la spécificité du test de Kveim. Presse Méd. 79: 2211, 1971.
5. Hurley, T. H., and Lane, W. R.: The Kveim test. Lancet 2:1373, 1971.
6. Israel, H. L., and Goldstein, R. A.: Relation of Kveim antigen to lymphadenopathy. New Eng. J. Med. 284:345, 1971.
7. Karlish, A. J., et al.: Kveim test in Crohn's disease. Lancet 2:977, 1970.
8. Bringel, C.: Relationship Between Sarcoidosis and Collagen Disease. Preliminary Report, La Sarcoidose. Reports of European Symposium on Sarcoidosis, Geneva, 1972, p. 34.
9. Izumi, T., et al.: False positive reactions in the Kveim test using the CSL Kveim material. Proceedings of VIth International Conference on Sarcoidosis, Tokyo, Sept., 1972.
10. Chretien, J.: La sarcoidosis, est-elle une entité nosologique? La Sarcoidose. Reports of European Symposium on Sarcoidosis, Geneva, 1972, p. 9.
11. Hurley, T. H., and Bartholomeusz, C. L.: International Kveim trial. Proceedings Vth International Conference on Sarcoidosis, Universita, Karlova, Prague, 1971, p. 343.
12. Nelson, C. T.: The Kveim reaction in sarcoidosis. J. Chronic Dis. 6:158, 1957.
13. Israel, H. L., and Sones, M.: The diagnosis of sarcoidosis with special reference to the Kveim reaction. Ann. Intern. Med. 43:1269, 1955.
14. Israel, H. L., et al.: A further study of the Kveim reaction in sarcoidosis and tuberculosis. New Eng. J. Med. 259:365, 1958.
15. Daniel, T. M., and Schneider, G. W.: Positive Kveim tests in patients without sarcoidosis. Amer. Rev. Resp. Dis. 86:98, 1962.
16. Siltzbach, L. E.: The Kveim test in tuberculosis, beryllium disease, leprosy and sarcoidosis. Amer. Rev. Resp. Dis. 90:308, 1964.
17. Siltzbach, L. E.: An International Kveim Test Study, 1960–1966. In Rapp: *La Sarcoidose*. IVth International Conference on Sarcoidosis, 1966. Paris, Masson et Cie, 1967, p. 201.
18. Hurley, T. J., and Sullivan, J. R.: Results obtained with Australian Kveim test material 1966–1972. Proceedings VIth International Conference on Sarcoidosis, Tokyo, September 1972.
19. Hirsch, J. G., Nelson, C. T., and Siltzbach, L. E.: (Letter.) New Eng. J. Med. 284: 1326, 1971.
20. Kveim-Siltzbach test vindicated. (Editorial.) Lancet 1:88, 1972.
21. Mitchell, D. N., et al.: The Kveim test in Crohn's disease. Lancet 2:571, 1969.
22. Mitchell, D. N., et al.: Further observations on Kveim test in Crohn's disease. Lancet 2: 496, 1970.
23. Jones Williams, W.: The Kveim controversy. Lancet 2:926, 1971.

24. Chapman, J., et al.: The Kveim test in Crohn's disease. Lancet 2:1097, 1971.
25. Karlish, A. J., et al.: The Kveim test in Crohn's disease, ulcerative colitis and coeliac disease. Lancet 1:438, 1972.
26. Hannuksela, M., et al.: Kveim reaction in Crohn's disease. Lancet 2:974, 1971.
27. Behrend, H.: Kveim reaction in Crohn's disease. Quoted by Jones Williams, W.: Lancet 2:926, 1971.
28. Klatskin, G.: Personal communication, 1973.
29. Siltzbach, L. E., et al.: Is there Kveim responsiveness in Crohn's disease? Lancet 2:637, 1971.
30. Siltzbach, L. E.: Significance and specificity of the Kveim reaction. Acta Med. Scand. 176 (Suppl. 425):74, 1964.

Comment

The Kveim Test

Medical literature abounds with examples of similar or nearly identical clinical and anatomic syndromes that are caused by clearly different and distinct etiologic agents. Conversely there are numerous instances of different clinical and anatomic syndromes produced by the same well defined etiologic agent. It is not surprising, therefore, that in a disease of unknown etiology, with as nonspecific a structural abnormality as sarcoidosis is at present, the specificity of a diagnostic test involving a reaction to a biologic reagent should be brought into question.

One useful and important dividend of "controversies" such as this one on the diagnostic specificity of the Kveim test for sarcoidosis is that it helps to define the common ground for agreement and may offer useful hints or even reveal the basis for the disagreement. It is particularly true in the present instance, because both sides of the controversy are clearly stated and are based on different interpretations of essentially the same body of data.

Both essayists have quoted the same or overlapping data which show clearly that some lots of the Kveim reagent, prepared and tested in some laboratories, have given clearly positive diagnostic tests in the great majority of cases which clinically and histologically are diagnosed as sarcoidosis, and have not produced clearly positive reactions grossly and histologically in control groups of cases, including some cases of well defined granulomatous disease such as glandular (lymph node) tuberculosis. On the other hand, other lots of the reagent, presumably prepared according to the same criteria, produced positive reactions in similar or different proportions of cases of sarcoidosis but also gave positive reactions in patients with other disease entities, notably glandular tuberculosis and regional ileitis, or even in normal individuals.

From the practical point of view, based on the previous experience quoted by our essayists, the criteria for a suitable Kveim reagent established at Stockholm in 1963 and presented here by Siltzbach involve: (1) adequate potency of the reagent, arrived at by tests in known reactors, and, acknowledging the variable reactivity of patients with clinically and histologically "proved" sarcoidosis, the requirement permits acceptance if the reagent produces six positives among 10 cases; (2) a clearly defined histologic lesion produced by the reagent within a limited time (four to six weeks), during which the lesion goes through a predictable clinical course; added is the requirement that a known and previously tested reagent must produce the same predictable and definable lesion in the same individuals who are being tested; and (3) the requirement, equally important, that the reagent produce no similar lesion in nonsarcoid subjects or should only rarely do so (the figure 3 per cent is quoted as the maximum permissible).

Obviously certain other criteria could very well be included as corollaries: (1) there must be agreement on the diagnostic criteria of sarcoidosis (this may be the least controversial aspect but nonetheless still admits to certain errors because of the nonspecific nature of the lesions in this disease); (2) there must be agreement as to the stage of the disease and other criteria for selection of organs or tissues for preparation of the reagent; (3) a standardized method must be available for preparing and testing the reagent for activity and and specificity such as that given by Siltzbach; and (4) there should be a standard and reliable method of reading and interpreting the test to be acceptable for diagnosis of a positive reaction.

In reality Siltzbach has established a standard for the diagnostic specificity of the Kveim reaction based on his own reagents and on his group of patients who react with his reagent, or with those lots of his reagent that he deems acceptable. Theoretically this may really be a narrower specificity than is encompassed by the current clinical and anatomically confirmed cases of sarcoidosis. In other words, this essentially makes the diagnosis of the disease dependent on the positive Kveim test to a reagent he deems acceptable. It is a practical solution to the problems of diagnosis but not a final and absolute one.

The ultimate goal obviously must be the identification of the etiologic agent or the specific portion of that agent or its product within the Kveim skin test reagent that is responsible for the specific reaction. When that is clearly defined and its biologic specificity established, perhaps this controversy will be settled. Similar differences of opinion and uncertainties are to be expected in any situation in which the disease to be diagnosed is only a clinical and anatomically defined entity, the precise etiology of which is not yet determined.

Should the FDA approve the Kveim test reagent? In the present climate (as of early 1973), if I correctly judge the attitude of the agency and what is currently expected of it, it would not be justified in giving approval because of the difficulties in preparing, standardizing, preserving, and uniformly replicating and monitoring the specificity in the same manner that Siltzbach and some other workers seem to have succeeded in doing. Essentially it would require establishing centers where large numbers of "certified" patients are available and willing to cooperate in the repeated tests; this is quite a demand on patients for consent and cooperation in these days of consumerism. This becomes a particularly difficult problem with respect to the negative controls, which include adequate numbers of nonsarcoid patients who must also consent to the same type of procedure.

MAXWELL FINLAND

14

The Status of Smallpox Vaccination

Vaccination Should Be Abolished in the United States Except for Selected Populations
    by Alexander D. Langmuir

Routine Vaccination for All Is Still Indicated
    by Abraham Benenson

Comment
    by Maxwell Finland

Vaccination Should Be Abolished in the United States Except for Selected Populations

ALEXANDER D. LANGMUIR

Harvard Medical School

On October 1, 1971, the Surgeon General of the United States Public Health Service officially accepted the report of his Advisory Committee on Immunization Practices[1] that had recommended:

"... The practice of routine smallpox vaccination is no longer indicated in this country."

This decision culminated a period of intensive study and debate of the issue during the preceding decade. Thus, it was a deliberate action, although an abrupt reversal of one of the most traditional and presumably well founded epidemiologic doctrines in worldwide public health practice. As an active litigant in this issue and as a relatively recent but enthusiastic convert to the new policy, I welcome the opportunity to review the history of this controversy and to expound the epidemiologic evidence upon which the new policy was based. The epidemics in Yugoslavia and Bengal which developed subsequent to the new policy have provided a prompt and serious challenge to its validity, but not in my opinion a sufficient basis for changing it.

Smallpox was endemic in the United States until the early 1940's when it began to disappear, apparently spontaneously. By 1950 it had gone altogether. The reasons for its demise are presumably related to the advancing standard of living, the generally improved medical and preventive health services, and the steady waning of the antivaccination movement which had been so active, particularly in the mid-West. Certainly there had been no systematic program comparable to the present Global Eradication Program of the World Health Organization (WHO). But routine vaccination at or about one year of age and compulsory vaccination on entry into public school became increasingly widely accepted practices in most parts of the country. The basic "herd immunity" thus provided was considered by most of us in the medical and health professions to be the foundation upon which effective smallpox control must be based.

In 1962 Dick[2, 3] in Great Britain and in 1965 Kempe[4] in the United States challenged the doctrine that such routine vaccination of infants and children was essential. They argued that the "herd immunity" presumably achieved by this practice was of doubtful, if any, effect and that the continuing and cumulative human costs in the form of severe and fatal vaccine reactions greatly exceeded the risks of the disease. These views were considered rank heresy at the time as revealed in the public discussion of Dr. Kempe's paper at the American Pediatric Society meeting.[4] I personally was an articulate critic. Within less than a decade, however, the arguments so cogently marshaled by Dick[3] became accepted as national policy in both Britain and the United States.

During this decade, repeated studies were made to quantitate the extent and severity of vaccine reactions. Many American epidemiologists participated in field investigations and intensive control programs in collaboration with the WHO Global Eradication Program. A large body of data was accumulated for inclusion in the cost-benefit equation which determined the policy decision.

The Human Costs of Vaccination

Fifty or more years ago the human costs of vaccination were high, but the risk of the disease was much higher. With improved standards of vaccine manufacture and simplified techniques of vaccination, the incidence of severe reactions has declined. A finite residuum, however, persists. In a comprehensive study of vaccine complications in the United States in 1968, Lane and his colleagues[5] identified 16 cases of postvaccinial encephalitis with four deaths. All but one of these occurred in children under 10 years of age. There were 11 cases of vaccinia necrosum with four deaths distributed approximately equally among children and adults. Eczema vaccinatum was identified 126 times with one death, and generalized vaccinia 143 times with no deaths.

Summarizing the several studies made over the past decade, Neff[6] concludes, "there are probably 5 to 10 deaths, 200 hospitalized cases and several thousand minor complications a year caused directly by smallpox vaccination." Relating these estimates to the five to six million primary vaccinations and eight to nine million revaccinations performed annually, incidence rates for deaths range from one to two per million primary vaccinations and for severe reactions from 10 to 15 per million total vaccinations.

The risk of encephalitis has been found, both in this country and in Great Britain, to be higher under one year of age than at older ages. No substantiation could be found for the widely held belief that vaccine reactions increased in frequency and severity among adults.

This recent experience reveals that the residual human costs of routine smallpox vaccination are sufficiently important to receive serious consideration.

The Risks of the Disease

Quantification of the present risks of the disease in this country and projections of these risks into the future present difficult problems because no outbreaks of smallpox have occurred here since 1949. As long as smallpox exists anywhere in the world, however, a small but finite risk of importation persists. An estimate of this risk must be made by epidemiologic inference based on the status of smallpox in the world and the character of recent smallpox outbreaks that have occurred in nonendemic areas that are as reasonably comparable to the United States as can be identified.

THE WORLD INCIDENCE OF SMALLPOX

In 1945, as recently summarized by Foege, Foster, and Goldstein,[7] the majority of the world's population lived in smallpox endemic areas. The disease receded progressively, but in 1967, when the WHO embarked upon its Global Eradication Program, smallpox still appeared to be an entrenched endemic disease in Brazil, in sub-Sahara Africa, on the Indian Pakistan subcontinent and in Indonesia. Approximately 100,000 cases were annually recorded by the WHO, but reporting was known to be grossly deficient.

The initial strategy of eradication was to achieve effective mass vaccination of all age groups in the endemic countries.[8] The tactics were to improve and strengthen the existing health programs by insuring adequate supplies of potent heat stable, freeze-dried vaccine and to introduce simplified and far more acceptable methods of vaccination, namely, the jet injector and the bifurcated needle. The need for surveillance was recognized as an essential supporting feature to measure progress, to set priorities, and to provide a continuing audit.

It soon became apparent, however, as emphasized by Henderson,[9] that mass vaccination alone was an insufficient control measure. As high a proportion as 95 per cent of a population, as in Central Java, could be reached with vaccine and yet smallpox could continue to spread among the remaining 5 per cent. The employment of mobile surveillance teams to seek out individual cases, search for their sources, identify their contacts, and direct selective ring vaccination was found to be the most effective measure and essential to the elimination of foci of infection. Thus, a responsive and imaginative surveillance program became the key factor in achieving eradication of the disease.

The Eradication Program has been conspicuously successful. By October, 1971, the date of the Surgeon General's policy statement, smallpox had been eliminated from West and Central Africa and was rapidly disappearing in Brazil and in Indonesia, where well staffed programs were active and efficient in their pursuit of the last cases. Successful programs were also underway in East Pakistan, India, and Afghanistan. Ethiopia and Sudan remained problem areas, but plans to mount programs were progressing well. The trend of world incidence was sharply downward in spite of markedly improved reporting. The disease was clearly being confined to a few residual focal areas, and these seemed amenable to elimination.

Thus, the risk of importation of infection into the United States, which was low enough in the 1950's that no importations occurred, had declined further by the mid-1960's when the WHO Program was begun. The risk must have declined even further by 1971, and the trend seemed to be downward. This optimistic epidemiologic inference was an important factor influencing the policy decision.

THE CHARACTER OF OUTBREAKS

Mack[10] has identified and analyzed 49 importations of smallpox into Europe from 1950 to 1971. Of these, 45 were variola major and involved 640 indigenous cases with 109 deaths. Four outbreaks were variola minor with 256 cases and no deaths. Thirteen of the importations resulted in no transmission.

The epidemiologic pattern of the outbreaks was remarkably consistent and similar to the two outbreaks that had occurred in the United States in Seattle in 1946 and in New York City in 1947. The patients who imported the infection were recent arrivals from areas of high incidence (annual rates exceeding three per 100,000) in Asia, Africa, or South America. Fewer than half of these showed symptoms on arrival. Most had "valid" certificates of vaccination or revaccination. The patients were usually misdiagnosed, often for understandable reasons such as the existence of concurrent serious disease such as malaria, or the absence of a typical rash. Such patients were admitted to a general hospital, sometimes on an open ward. Only when the first generation of indigenous cases appeared among members of the hospital staff or patients would the true diagnosis become appreciated.

Subsequent cases occurred in very large measure among close and readily identifiable contacts. Of the 680 cases of variola major, 359 resulted from contact within a medical setting, 51 comprised members of other occupational groups such as laundry or mortuary workers, or members of a ship's crew. Of the remaining 270 cases, most were family or other direct face-to-face contacts. Only 44 were classified as unpredictable in that no specific history of contact was demonstrated. It was the general consensus that most of these unaccounted cases represented failure to conduct adequate contact histories, or the purposeful suppression of such a history in order to avoid quarantine, rather than long-range or airborne spread of infection.

Certain limited exceptions to this interpretation were recorded by Wehrle et al.[11] In Monschau, West Germany, in 1961 a hospitalized second generation case infected 19 other persons. Nine of these were face-to-face contacts, but 10 developed among seven patients, two members of the medical staff, and a carpenter in a neighboring ward at the end of a common corridor. In 1970 a single patient admitted to an isolation ward in Meschede, Germany, with a presumptive diagnosis of typhoid fever infected 17 other patients in the hospital who had no face-to-face contact with him. The implications are evident of airborne transmission of infection over considerable distances within an enclosed building. It should be noted, however, that in both instances the source case had a severe hacking cough and presumably was capable of producing highly infective aerosols. It should also be emphasized that both epidemics were promptly contained. Spread beyond the hospital setting was minimal.

Notable in the European experience was the concentration of cases among adults. Less than 15 per cent of cases of variola major were among children under 10 years of age. These were either acquired by exposure within hospitals or in the home from hospital-acquired cases. Spread through schools or nurseries or among childhood playmates was conspicuously infrequent. Three fourths of the adults gave a history of vaccination, usually 10 to 20 or more years previously, and 20 per cent of the children had also been vaccinated.

In many of the European outbreaks, public hysteria, either spontaneous or sometimes provoked, forced widespread mass vaccination programs, with all the inherent disadvantages known to be associated therewith. A similar officially sponsored mass campaign was launched following the New York City outbreak in 1947. Sober review fails to indicate that such heroic shotgun approaches were necessary.

It may be concluded from these critical evaluations of the European experience that imported smallpox is not usually a highly infectious disease but rather that it spreads slowly in localized areas. Once recognized, the 12-day incubation period provides a considerable amount of time for the alert health authority to contain the outbreak by case investigation, identification, and quarantine of contacts, and selective ring vaccination among those exposed. Even when the rare dangerous spreader causes cases by the airborne route, containment is still possible with these conservative measures.

The routine vaccination of infants and children does not contribute effectively to herd immunity. In developed countries the disease clearly does not spread among such groups, but rather among adults whose immunity has substantially, if not completely, waned.

The Revised Policy

The Advisory Committee's recommendations were based on the careful weighing of the continuing and cumulative human costs of routine vaccination against the evidently small and decreasing risk of the disease. The revised policy emphasizes the prevention of importation and the containment of any outbreak if an importation happens.

The specific recommendations are:[1]

    1. The effective vaccination of all travelers to or from countries where smallpox exists.

    2. The adequate immunization of all persons involved in health services.

    3. The maintenance of an alert surveillance program.

    4. The full support of the Global Smallpox Eradication Program.

This program is now in effect. The screening of travelers entering the country has been made much simpler and more selective because so few have been in endemic countries. The surveillance system in each state health department, backstopped by the epidemiologic and laboratory diagnostic services of the Center for Disease Control, has never been so alert nor staffed with so many experienced professional personnel. The Global Eradication Program is being pursued intensively.

The weakest link in the program is the vaccination of health personnel, specifically hospital workers of all types. The seriousness of this vulnerability is not so widely appreciated as it should be. It is perhaps inevitable that one or more importations of smallpox may have to occur before hospital administrators and medical staffs recognize their clear responsibility to maintain the immunity of all hospital personnel at a high level.

The possibility of such importations, while small, must be recognized. If one, or even several, occur, it would not negate the validity of the new policy. Only if importations lead to uncontrolled spread, primarily among infants and schoolchildren, should a return to routine vaccination of such groups be seriously considered. The Surgeon General's Advisory Committee did not believe that such an eventuality was sufficiently possible to justify the present high costs in complications of routine vaccination.

Subsequent Developments

These recommendations, formulated in consultation with representatives of the Ministries of Health of Canada and the United Kingdom, were promptly approved by the Committee on Infectious Diseases of the American Academy of Pediatrics (the Red Book Committee) and the Association of State and Territorial Health Officers during the fall of 1971. Since that time a number of anticipated as well as surprising events have taken place. These warrant careful review of the validity of the revised policy.

General acceptance of the new policy has been prompt and almost complete. All states but two have modified their laws, sanitary codes, or regulations or declared their intent to do so. The distribution of smallpox vaccine has been reduced by about two thirds. The requests for Vaccine Immune Globin for the treatment or prophylaxis of complications have fallen to less than 25 per cent of previous demand. Only a few voices of protest have been raised in the professional press.[12]

On the world scene, smallpox has disappeared from Brazil, with the last known case reported in April, 1971; and from Indonesia, where the last known case was in January, 1972. The reported world incidence, however, has increased. From a low of 30,812 cases in 1970, the total rose to 51,834 in 1971. This increase was due primarily to the successful expansion of major control programs in Ethiopia and Sudan with extensive vaccination, case finding, and reporting. More than 50 per cent of the total cases reported in 1971 emanated from these two countries. This increase, therefore, was an artifact of progress toward the goal of eradication of the disease from this last endemic focus on the African continent.[13]

The world incidence further increased in 1972 when an estimated total of

64,000 cases were reported. This resulted primarily from sharp increases in Bangladesh and in Central India following the repatriation of refugees of the Indo-Pakistan Conflict. Intensified control programs are in progress, but South Asia remains the largest focus of endemic smallpox in the world.[14]

The severest challenge of the new policy was the outbreak of variola major in Yugoslavia in March and April, 1972. It involved 176 cases with 36 deaths. The outbreak centered in the autonomous province of Kosovo which adjoins the Albanian border. The infection was most probably introduced by a Moslem pilgrim who, while returning from Mecca by bus, stopped in Baghdad, where an unreported break of smallpox was in progress.

The first indigenous generation comprised 11 cases, all spread by community contact in Kosovo and nearby communities. The second indigenous generation included 142 cases, mostly in Kosovo but also in two hospital-centered foci in Cacak and Belgrade where a patient with confluent smallpox was sent with the mistaken diagnosis of acute penicillin reaction.

The third, and last, generation of cases was limited to 23 cases, all but one of which developed among known contacts in quarantine. The outbreak led to an essentially nationwide mass vaccination program begun in the middle of the second generation when the extent of the outbreak was first appreciated. The resort to mass vaccination was understandable in view of the many ethnic, religious, political, and communication problems involved, but had more complete surveillance data been available more promptly, it seems reasonable that effective containment could have been achieved by more selective vaccination.[15, 16]

These developments subsequent to the adoption of the new policy warrant careful reconsideration of the wisdom of the change. The crucial question is whether the estimate of the risk of importation of the disease was in error. Certainly the increased incidence of smallpox in Ethiopia and Sudan cannot be a cause of worry. The increase in India and Bangladesh is a disappointment but an anticipated result of war. No exportations of smallpox from this traditionally highly endemic area have been reported. Prospects for renewed progress in the area are excellent.

The Yugoslavian outbreak was the first one to occur in that country since 1930 and the most severe outbreak in Europe since the end of World War II. In spite of its extent, only one exported case occurred in a worker returning to Hanover, Germany. No further spread resulted.

This outbreak vividly reinforces the fact that as long as smallpox exists anywhere in the world, no other spot is free of risk of the disease. This one extraordinary outbreak must not be weighed alone but rather, with the 49 other outbreaks in Europe during the past 20 years, it should be balanced with the 100 to 200 estimated vaccine deaths and 4000 hospitalized cases of vaccine complications that have occurred during the past 20 years in the United States.

In my judgment, only if repeated outbreaks of variola major occur in this country and turn out to be far more formidable to control than can be expected from the total European experience would there be a valid basis for reconsidering the policy of routine vaccination. In this remote eventuality, not only routine vaccination of children but routine revaccination of adults, as emphasized by Dick,[2] would be necessary.

References

1. Public Health Service Recommendation on Smallpox Vaccination. Morbidity and Mortality Weekly Report 20:339–345, 1971.
2. Dick, G.W.A.: Prevention of virus diseases in the community. Brit. Med. J. 2:1275–1280, 1962.
3. Dick, G.W.A.: Smallpox: A reconsideration of public health policies. Progr. Med. Virol. 8:1–29, 1966.
4. Kempe, C. H.: An evaluation of risks of smallpox vaccination in the United States. (Abstract and discussion.) J. Pediat. 67:1017–1022, Part 2, 1965.
5. Lane, J. M., Ruben, F. L., Neff, J. M., et al.: Complications of smallpox vaccination, 1968. National surveillance in the United States. New Eng. J. Med. 281:1201–1208, 1969.
6. Neff, J. M.: The case for abolishing routine childhood smallpox vaccination in the United States. Amer. J. Epidem. 93:245–247, 1971.
7. Foege, W. H., Foster, S. O., and Goldstein, J. A.: Current status of global smallpox eradication. Amer. J. Epidem. 93: 223–233, 1971.
8. Henderson, D. A.: Smallpox: The problem. Proceedings of the International Conference on the application of vaccines against viral, rickettsial, and bacterial diseases of man. Washington, D.C., Pan American Health Organization, Scientific Publication No. 226, 1971, pp. 139–143.
9. Henderson, D. A.: Epidemiology in the global eradication of smallpox. Int. J. Epidem. 1:25–30, 1972.
10. Mack, T. M.: Review: Smallpox in Europe 1950–1971. J. Infect. Dis. 125:161–169, 1972.
11. Wehrle, P. F., Posch, J., Richter, K. H., and Henderson, D. A.: An airborne outbreak of smallpox in a German hospital and its significance with respect to other recent outbreaks in Europe. Bull. WHO 43:669–679, 1970.
12. Piszczek, E. A., Lull, G. F., Stebbins, E. L., Adriani, J., and Niess, O.K.: Smallpox vaccination. (Letter to the Editor.) J.A.M.A. 222:1185, 1972.
13. Weekly Epidemiological Record, WHO, Geneva, 47:17–26, 1972, No. 2, January 14.
14. *Ibid*, 48:9–19, 1973, No. 2, January 12.
15. *Ibid*, 47:141–143, 1972, No. 14, April 7.
16. Lane, J. M. (Center for Disease Control, Atlanta): Personal communication.

Routine Vaccination for All Is Still Indicated

ABRAM S. BENENSON

University of Kentucky College of Medicine

Smallpox has been one of the most serious of the diseases afflicting mankind. With no respect for social class, it took its toll from the nobility and commoner alike. It was present in Europe, Asia, and Africa, and was brought by the early explorers to the Western Hemisphere where it greatly influenced the ultimate conquest and political boundaries. The pock-marked complexion was normal. The likelihood of acquiring and dying from smallpox was so great that variolation, the deliberate inoculation of smallpox material into the nose or skin of the healthy person, was considered a wise gamble, even though two to eight of each 100 persons would die from the resulting smallpox. These odds were clearly better than the 30 to 50 per cent who would die if they acquired the natural disease without protection. Until recently there have been societies among whom babies were not given a name until they had survived their inevitable attack of smallpox; it would seem that the baby supply exceeded the supply of names (or the cost involved in a naming ceremony)! Lord Macaulay[1] paints the picture of the times when he wrote that smallpox

"... was then the most terrible of all the ministers of death. The havoc of the plague had been far more rapid; but the plague had visited our shores only once or twice within living memory; and the smallpox was always present, filling the churchyards with corpses, tormenting with constant fears all whom it had not yet stricken, leaving on those whose lives it spared the hideous traces of its power, turning the babe into a changeling at which the mother shuddered, and making the eyes and cheeks of the betrothed maiden objects of horror to the lover. Towards the end of the year 1694, this pestilence was more than usually severe. At length the infection spread to the palace, and reached the young and blooming Queen."

The situation today presents a delightful contrast. To the bulk of the world's population, smallpox is an exotic disease. Pockmarks are seen rarely if at all, usually among older people. Except for a very small number of peripatetic individuals, United States physicians of today have never seen a case of smallpox. In their medical education, save for allusions to the disease, smallpox, its recognition and its management are not "relevant" to the needs of the physician and are left uncovered. The domain of smallpox has been steadily constricted. In the mid 1940's approximately 80 countries reported smallpox; in 1972 continuing transmission of disease is being reported from only seven countries on two continents (India, Pakistan, Bangladesh, and Nepal in Asia, and Ethiopia, Sudan, and Botswana in Africa). Smallpox was introduced and controlled in Yugoslavia, Germany, South Africa, Uganda, Iran, Iraq, Syria, Sri Lanka (Ceylon), and the African French Territory of Afars and the Issas. During 1972 endemic disease was controlled in Indonesia, with no new reported cases after January, and in Afghanistan with no new cases since October.[2]

How was this accomplished? The basic tool was presented to the professional community 175 years ago, but no dramatic decrease in the incidence of smallpox ensued. From the beginning, vaccination was resisted by an aggressive antivaccination movement; this was justified on theological grounds but was nurtured by fear of the illness associated with the vaccinial infection, necessary for immunity to develop. To complicate the case further, many of the early vaccines were low or lacking in vaccinia virus while replete with pyogenic bacteria, hepatitis virus, or other pathogens, so that vaccination could produce illness without conferring immunity to smallpox. To achieve a vaccinial infection when virus content was so low, vaccine was applied over large areas of skin using elaborate scarifiers, multiple insertion sites, cruciate incisions, and so forth. The subsequent severe reactions which not infrequently followed did the cause little good.

The use of the skin of the calf for propagating the virus eliminated the hazard of transmission of human disease. The establishment of laboratory controls, enforced by governmental authority, assured a product free of disease-producing contaminants and, at least at the time of production, a reasonable level of vaccinial infectivity as judged on the rabbit skin. Vaccine strains which produced larger and more consistent takes were selected, and "virulence" was fortified by man-rabbit-calf passages; this was to assure that each vaccination did in fact produce immunity.

In the United States smallpox vaccination was made compulsory for school admission in most states. The technique of vaccination in general use was modified by the introduction of the multiple pressure technique in the late 1920's. Smallpox can be considered to have become nonendemic in the United States by the mid 1930's, although isolated outbreaks did occur among nonvaccinated groups. However, the occurrence of smallpox among "vaccinated" military personnel and the introduction of the disease by them to the West Coast in 1946 drew attention to the need for a more potent vaccine for revaccination than for primary vaccination. This had been recognized by Leake,[3] who specified six to 10 pressures in the multiple pressure vaccination technique for primary vaccinations, but 30 pressures for revaccination. The question whether there should then be two smallpox vaccines, one for domestic use and one for revaccination of those who were to be at high risk of exposure, was resolved by the development of freeze-dried vaccine and greater attention to production and storage factors to assure high potency in stocks of liquid glycerinated vaccine.

The dramatic results of the WHO Smallpox Eradication Program are based on the availability of potent stable smallpox vaccine (freeze-dried), nontraumatic techniques for its administration (intradermal jet injection, and then the bifurcated needle in the multiple puncture technique), a surveillance program which detects cases early and breaks the chain of transmission to or from the contacts of the patient, and systematic vaccination.[4] When the program was initiated in 1967 smallpox was reported from 42 countries; in 12 of these the cases had been imported and the disease was not considered endemic. Today, as noted previously, in only seven or eight countries is smallpox still endemic, and WHO has set a goal for global eradication by April, 1974.

On September 25, 1971, the U.S. Public Health Service Recommendation on Smallpox Vaccination was published, accepting the recommendation formulated by its Advisory Committee on Immunization Practices,[5] which was:

"The Committee has reviewed the success achieved so far by the World Health Organization (WHO)-sponsored smallpox eradication effort and fully expects that it will continue. It now believes that the risk of smallpox in the United States is so small that the practice of routine smallpox vaccination is no longer indicated in this country.

"The Committee believes that public health efforts should be devoted to assuring adequate immunization of all personnel involved in health services and of all travelers to and from continents where smallpox has not been eradicated.

"Because of the rapidly declining incidence of smallpox in the world and the vastly reduced risk of its being imported into the United States, health officials in the United States should consider the discontinuation of compulsory measures as they relate to routine smallpox vaccination.

"The Public Health Service should regularly evaluate and distribute information on the progress toward worldwide smallpox eradication. This will provide a basis for future assessment of smallpox vaccination practices in the United States.

"Finally, physicians and public health agencies should intensify efforts to assure that all adverse vaccine reactions are reported and that the following contraindications to smallpox vaccination are scrupulously observed: (1) eczema and other forms of chronic dermatitis in the person to be vaccinated or in a household contact; (2) pregnancy; (3) altered immune states from disease or therapy."[6]

The Center for Disease Control states: "The decision of the Public Health Service to institute a policy of selective vaccination against smallpox in the United States was made only after the careful examination and quantification of many factors, including the risk of complications following smallpox vaccination, the probability of smallpox importation into the United States, and the anticipated extent of smallpox spread after importation."[6]

This decision has been welcomed by those who are worried by the risk of complications in their patients, and greatly disturbs those who are concerned with the continued health of the community. The factors on which the decision was made bear re-examination.

Risk of Complications Following Smallpox Vaccination

The strongest argument against continued routine smallpox vaccination lies in the risk of one death per million primary vaccinations based on the 1963[7] and 1968[8] national surveys in the United States. In contrast, there have been no deaths from smallpox in this country since 1949. Based on European experience with smallpox importations, it is estimated that there might be 20 smallpox deaths between 1969 and the end of the century if vaccination is discontinued, against the 210 deaths from smallpox vaccination itself which would occur with the continued routine vaccination program, based on the rate of seven deaths per year.[9] These data would be a serious contraindication to continued vaccination if valid, but their validity is subject to question.

There is no doubt that vaccinia virus can, under certain circumstances, become an invasive pathogen. The induced infection with vaccinia virus is terminated by the emergence of active immunity. Vaccination of those with immune deficiencies is hazardous, with the danger that the lesion will continue to progress to become progressive vaccinia (vaccinia necrosum). While this had previously carried a high case fatality rate, its prognosis has been greatly improved by the use of vaccinia immune globulin and thiosemicarbazone. In 1963 nine cases were reported with no deaths;[7] in 1968 11 cases with four deaths were reported.[8] Eight of the 1968 victims were over 15 years of age; seven (including one with "unknown vaccination status") followed revaccination. Of these, two had leukemia, three Hodgkin's disease, and one lymphoma. Among the four deaths, one was a 62 year old woman with chronic lymphatic leukemia, revaccinated as treatment for recurrent herpes simplex(!); another death followed primary vaccination of a microcephalic with cerebral palsy; and the third followed primary vaccination of a 16 year old girl "with previously undetected aplastic anemia." The fourth fatal case was a six year old boy with acute myelogenous leukemia which was in remission on vincristine and prednisone therapy; the vaccinial lesion cleared and was considered "cured" but he died approximately one month later of his leukemia. Whether this death is properly attributed to vaccination is a matter of judgment. It would seem that pre-existing disease was probably known in all these cases but possibly two—a 22 month old boy with Bruton's hypogammaglobulinemia and the girl with aplastic anemia (whose pallor should have been a warning). The patients with malignancy, one on antimetabolite therapy, and one on anticoagulants for ischemic heart disease, should not have been vaccinated unless exposed to smallpox. If vaccination is restricted to those who are well and thriving,[10] the problem of vaccinia necrosum will be greatly reduced.

Postvaccinal encephalitis (PVE) is a serious complication, which is noted to have an incidence of 2.9 per million primary vaccinations (and none after revaccination).[5] "'Postvaccinial central-nervous-system disease' includes a variety of disorders manifesting signs and symptoms of classic encephalitis, encephalopathy, demyelinization or neuropathy. *These entities are attributed to vaccinia because of their temporal relation to smallpox vaccination and because of the absence of any other etiology.* [Italics added.] The pathology of these diseases is similar to that seen with other viral central-nervous-system disorders."[8] Is it coincidental that 2.86 cases of encephalitis of unknown etiology were reported per 28-day period[11] in 1965 in New Jersey per million children one to nine years old? During that year cases of encephalitis of unknown etiology in the New England and the Middle Atlantic area showed no seasonal aggregation.[12] These cases were collected passively; i.e., they were reported by physicians usually seeking diagnostic help. A much higher rate would be expected to be reported following vaccination, since CNS involvement is looked for, and any aberrant behavior of the child is suspected to be the result of the procedure.

This is not to imply that postvaccinal encephalitis cannot be caused by vaccination, but it may well be overreported. The difference in incidence rates between the United States with one case per 345,000 primary vaccinations contrasts sharply with the Dutch experience of one in 4000. The rate of one per 152,000 primary vaccinations (6.5 per million) in the first year of life, and half that rate at higher ages,[5] contrasts with the German experience of one in 10,000 to 15,000 primary vaccinations of infants and one in 2000 to 3000 primary vaccinations among those two years or older.[13] Studies in Hamburg of the age incidence of postvaccinal convulsions among approximately 250,000 primary vaccinations reported an incidence of one convulsion per 1049 primary vaccinations (953 per million vaccinations) of children under three years old, with a peak incidence of one per 511 (1957 per million) among those 18 to 23 months old, and a minimal incidence of one per 15,405 (65 per million) in those under six months of age.[14] The facts on PVE are evidently unclear; it has not been the problem in the United States that it has in European countries. It is difficult to accept genetic differences; the more rigorous vaccination techniques and more virulent strains of vaccine which have been used in Europe are more likely explanations.

The morbidity caused by vaccination has been exaggerated by the emphasis placed on the minor side reactions. For example, generalized vaccinia is cited to occur in 242 per million primary vaccinations.[5] "The clinical spectrum of generalized vaccinia was broad. . . . In most cases the clinical descriptions obtained were insufficient to distinguish patients with vesicular or pustular rashes from those with maculopapular or erythema-multiforme-like rashes. There were no deaths, and no patients suffered serious sequelae."[8] And "the most common manifestation was satellite vesiculation around the vaccination site."[7] To minimize this technical error we had recommended that the vaccination site not be cleaned (and thereby superficially abraded).[10] Accidental infections have increased with the delay of vaccination to the second year of life and, at the worst, produce an aberrant scar. Erythematous urticarial lesions occur frequently without making the vaccinee sick. Lack of understanding of these interesting but unimportant phenomena have resulted in unnecessary concern and hospitalization. Stress is placed on exceedingly rare phenomena. There have been only about 20 cases of fetal vaccinia reported in all the medical literature and no apparent evidence that there is an increased risk of abortion, miscarriage, or fetal malformation, and virtually all after primary vaccination, but pregnancy is now accepted as a contraindication to vaccination or revaccination!

The important complications of smallpox vaccination then are largely the problems of an underlying disease, and deaths attributed to vaccination may properly be ascribed to the primary defect. Deaths were reduced by delaying vaccination to the second year of life. "As Conybeare has pointed out, in all countries delaying routine vaccination until the second year of life, the number of fatal cases due to some of the complications of vaccination will tend to diminish for by that time many of the susceptible individuals will have died from one or another infection of childhood."[13] Encephalitis of unknown origin had its highest incidence in the first year of life.[12]

Elimination of routine vaccination, while retaining it for members of the health professions and travelers to endemic countries, assumes that primary vaccination of the adult can be carried out without a significant increase in risk. The experience of U.S. military personnel is cited[9] as evidence of the safety of primary vaccination of adults; however, results obtained on a highly selected group of healthy individuals may not apply to the population at large. This United States experience is in sharp contrast to the European experience. In Austria the incidence of PVE was 55 times greater among those 11 to 14 years of age than among those one to three; deaths occurred 33 times more frequently.[15]

The mortality and morbidity from smallpox vaccination on which our policy for the future is based[5] are those associated with the vaccine strain, the concentration of virus (potency), and the vaccination method in use in the country today; as noted previously, these factors were selected for control of endemic disease and not designed for the needs of today. Studies carried out in several countries have shown that certain vaccine strains, used at reduced potency, and the use of other routes of administration result in lowered morbidity.[16] It has been argued that no new regimens can be validated without a field test involving millions of vaccinations, since PVE occurs approximately only three times in a million primary vaccinations. The data showing that encephalitis of unknown origin, unassociated with vaccination, occurs in the same frequency suggest that we can properly focus on the fever and vaccinial illness itself as the criteria for a safer vaccination regimen. The system designed for today's, rather than yesterday's, needs should be used in calculation of risks.

The Probability of Smallpox Importation into the United States

No one can argue with the declining probability of introduction as disease is eradicated from more and more endemic foci, even with increased mass travel in jumbo jets. However, while calculations may indicate the probability of only one importation every 12 years, Monte Carlo and Las Vegas are evidences that probabilities are only probabilities.

The Anticipated Extent of Smallpox Spread After Importation

Again, statistical analysis of the experience in 51 importations into Europe in the last two decades provides the comforting data that 15 importations per year would be required to produce the number of deaths now associated with vaccination. This assumes "vigilant surveillance and outbreak control." Early case detection and then selective (or ring) vaccination of contacts[17] is expected to contain any introduction. Reliance is placed on quarantine inspectors at international airports who will "observe travelers for signs of illness and check vaccination certificates of travelers from smallpox-infected countries."[5]

The predicted number of cases may be valid as an average over the long run. This low transmission rate is supported by observations in both Africa and Pakistan of several generations of smallpox within one family group; this is the basis for the statement that "smallpox is not the highly contagious disease it was once thought to be."[5] However, the microecology of smallpox is not fully understood. Transmission is clearly affected by climatic conditions; in East Bengal the disease bears the name of the season during which epidemics occur, springtime (Bashunto). While transmission usually occurs in a face-to-face contact, not only was the outbreak in Meschede, Germany, in 1970 spread by air currents within the hospital, but all the evidence suggests that infection actually left the patient's room through the window, rose on updrafts along the outside of the hospital and re-entered through windows to infect one patient in a second floor room and three in third floor rooms overhead.[18]

The outbreak in Yugoslavia in March, 1972, showed what can happen. After 42 smallpox-free years, a traveler with a valid vaccination certificate introduced the disease from Iraq. He had so mild an illness that he did not seek medical attention, but he infected 11 individuals; the contact with some of these was slight and his own illness was only uncovered in retrospect.[19] One of his contacts developed hemorrhagic disease, was hospitalized in his hometown, then was transferred to a larger hospital, thence to a dermatology clinic in Belgrade as a case of "unusual drug reaction secondary to penicillin." After 12 hours he was transferred to an intensive care unit at a surgical hospital, where he died 24 hours after admission. Only when his brother came down with smallpox a few days later did the correct diagnosis become apparent. This one man infected two patients and one visitor in the first hospital, caused eight secondary cases in the second hospital, eight in the third hospital, and 18 in the final hospital. The last group included all 13 patients in the intensive care unit, one doctor, one nurse, one hospital technician, and a wardrobe man in charge of patients' clothing. Including his brother, this one man infected 38 individuals, a new record.[20] This outbreak was controlled within a month, after 175 cases and 34 deaths. A mass vaccination campaign was carried out in which 95 per cent of the total population of Belgrade and 98 per cent of the Kosovo region (where the cases originated) were successfully vaccinated. Military personnel carried out the vaccination program; four hotels were taken over for isolation of all known contacts; in Belgrade, the Thousand Roses Motel was converted to a hospital.

Could this have happened in the United States? For anyone entering the United States after leaving Belgrade during this outbreak, no quarantine inspectors were in evidence. Vaccination certificates were checked by the immigration officer, and a single revaccination performed 48 hours earlier in Belgrade was properly accepted. Analysis of importations into Europe during the period 1950 to 1971 showed that at least 65 or probably 85 per cent of these importations were attributable to errors in revaccination.[21] Under these conditions a mild infection, such as that in the Yugoslav traveler, could easily have supervened during the next two weeks with little motivation to comply with the instructions on the card given by the immigration officer, if this had not by now been discarded or misplaced. The rest of the episode is as probable here as in Yugoslavia; the missed diagnoses, the public panic, even the inclusion of physicians and health workers among the diseased. Had some of these exposures occurred in the New York subway system during rush hour, a problem of greater magnitude would result. We have no isolation facilities in which we could house large numbers of smallpox patients, and in our social structure we are unlikely to requisition hotels, or to find large numbers of contacts willing to remain in quarantine facilities.

It is true that more people have died in the United States in association with (but not necessarily due to) vaccination than from smallpox. This has led to the argument that we are protecting our people from a disease which does not exist. It does not exist within our country, but it does exist and is still active among other populations. Although the immune status of our population, as measured by immunity to percutaneous vaccination, is lower than ideal, there have been no importations from India during the period 1950 to 1971 in contrast to seven importations into Germany; three times as many Americans as Germans have been temporary visitors to India.[20] Discontinuing vaccination because there have been no cases is analogous to discontinuing fire preventive measures because there has been no fire. Certainly the most intensive control measures are needed near known fire sources, but serious fires still occur in new buildings built of nonburning material.

The cost of smallpox vaccination has been padded by several factors. The incidence of postvaccinal encephalitis in the United States is no greater than that of encephalitis of unknown etiology among unvaccinated persons; PVE has no specific diagnostic criterion, other than its temporal association with vaccination. There does tend to be a clustering of central nervous system symptoms nine to ten days after vaccination;[8] this coincides with the fever after primary vaccination. Is this a real cost of vaccination? Generalized vaccinia connotes spread of vaccinia virus throughout the body with multiple foci of replicating vaccinia virus, a condition often a part of eczema vaccination; the rubric, however, as noted above, includes local lesions more properly classified as co-primary lesions and a variety of rashes which have no prognostic significance and could be considered "side reactions" rather than complications of vaccination. Finally, the "costs" are those which are produced by a methodology designed for the "attack phase" of smallpox control, rather than the "maintenance phase."

What are the prospects for global eradication? To date, we have no evidence of transmission of variola virus to man from any source other than man. The West African success gives every hope that smallpox can be eradicated. It calls for sincere determination at all governmental and health professional levels to detect and contain each possible case, and that there be no implication that the emergence of smallpox represents personal or national failure or dishonor. Concern of the effect of a case or outbreak of smallpox on the tourist trade is best answered by the successful season enjoyed by Yugoslavia in 1972. The global eradication program can succeed by April, 1974, but this should have been actually achieved before dropping our defenses.

George Dick, who is firmly against routine childhood vaccination, wrote:[13]

"Even with the apparent eradication of smallpox throughout the world, at which we must aim, and which is the ideal solution to the problem, there is always the possibility of smallpox virus emerging from the 'backwoods' or deep freezes when we thought it had gone and also the possible (perhaps remote) use of smallpox virus in 'bacteriological' warfare. We must have a sensible policy for the control of smallpox now and in the future."

Smallpox had been an effective biological warfare (BW) agent, but had lost its effectiveness when populations were relatively immune. The development of nonimmune populations will re-establish variola as an ideal lethal BW agent, with danger persisting as long as the virus lies in the deep freeze. That the "backwoods" may become important is shown by the isolation in Holland of virus strains from two different cynomolgus monkey kidney cell lines and in Moscow from the tissues of a chimpanzee caught in the Congo. These virus strains could not be distinguished from standard variola virus by any laboratory test. While the Dutch monkeys did come from Malaysia, which is not too far from Indonesia where smallpox was then occurring, the chimpanzee was caught in a search for monkeypox virus in an area where no smallpox had occurred for some time.

What is the sensible policy for now and the future? I disagree with the discontinuation of routine childhood vaccination, certainly for now. Until global eradication has been accomplished, we are assuming the race has been won and, like the hare, may be prematurely resting on our laurels. Our policy of no routine vaccination becomes a status symbol of progress and can be expected to motivate less prepared countries to conceal their smallpox cases and prematurely drop their defenses.

Discontinuance of childhood vaccination commits us to the possibility of mass adult vaccination, as well as selective vaccination of health workers and some travelers; in all tabulations vaccination of adults involves a greater incidence of PVE and vaccinia necrosum. It is argued by the British that childhood vaccination offers no great protection against complications when revaccination is carried out in the adult. This is clearly not confirmed by United States data,[5] which indicate virtual absence of significant complications on revaccination, except for vaccinia necrosum among those with disease of the hematopoietic system. Further, the fever and morbidity of the "normal" primary take, with our present technology, can have economic implications in the adult whose vaccination is unplanned, in contrast to the indisposition of the baby who is vaccinated in the prime of health.

Routine vaccination has been condemned because of the financial cost. These analyses include the cost of the physician's visit, coming to 69 per cent of the total costs. About 30 per cent is costed for lost earnings owing to time off work for vaccination and its complications. But vaccination and revaccination should be an integral part of comprehensive health care and should not be separated therefrom and charged for separately. There is a real cost in the vaccine, but vaccine production and competence in its production will have to continue for the foreseeable future. What would the comparable cost be if there were a bona fide introduction of smallpox, such as occurred in Yugoslavia?

We recommended[10] that vaccination be performed only on those in full health, using the very minimal trauma, and that all smallpox vaccinations be planned for a second procedure if a major reaction, indicative of multiplying virus, is not present seven days later; this policy I would continue. The immunizing strain, dose, and route which produce immunity with minimal side reactions should be used, based on comparisons of the morbidity they produce.[16] The use of sequential vaccines may prove best, but is not desirable. Contraindications to vaccination would be strictly respected. I favor vaccination of the thriving infant in the first three to six months of life, assuming the mother had been vaccinated and revaccinated; when this is done, it can be carried out with no systemic reaction. Revaccination at five- to 10-year intervals will maintain immunity with safety.

I would not argue for legal compulsion to assure that all members of our society be kept in a state of full smallpox immunity. Discontinuance of routine vaccination, on a compulsory basis, could be justified on the basis that it was no longer necessary; this then permits the physician and the patient to make the appropriate decision.[22] For those who are likely to go into the health services or are likely to enter the military forces or do extensive traveling, infantile vaccination of the healthy thriving infant seems safest. Even if revaccination is not performed every five to 10 years, the European experience was that of 52 per cent case fatality rates among those never vaccinated in contrast with 11 per cent of those whose last vaccination was over 20 years before; the contrast is even sharper among those over 50 years of age, where the comparable figures are 91 per cent (10 or 11) and 26 per cent, respectively;[20] and, as noted above, the United States data show that the primary vaccination protects against complications of adult revaccination. Since prediction of the future life pattern is difficult, infantile vaccination, in general, would continue.

It is unfortunate that, in justifying the discontinuance, principal emphasis was placed on the "risks" of vaccination, which were widely publicized in the news media so that there is now a public fear of vaccination. This seems to have extended even to those physicians who favor vaccination of their healthy patients but fear malpractice suits. However, truly informed consent, preferably in writing, avoids such suits and returns to the physician his obligation to give the patient the benefit of his best professional advice. This advice, and our recommendations for the future, will be subject to change when global eradication has been achieved and will be strongly influenced by the temper of the international climate at that time. While the proper action, in my judgment, has not been taken, change is permissible. Newer vaccines will justify a revision of emphasis with, I hope, a national trend toward a protected population.

I have previously used a quotation which has now become most appropriate. Written in 1802, very shortly indeed after Jenner reported the effectiveness of vaccination, it is even more pertinent 170 years later. James Bryce wrote:[23]

"Dr. Jenner has thus acted his part; it remains for the other members of society to act theirs; he has shown how important advantages may be obtained; it is theirs to carry this plan into execution by cooperating, both by example and by precept, to render general the practices of inoculation for cowpox; the reward being no less than exterminating one of the most loathsome and fatal diseases to which mankind are liable—the smallpox. I must here, however, observe that it is not the prevention of smallpox in a country, for a few years or perhaps a century, that ought to be regarded sufficient. . . . If it should then unfortunately so happen that the advantages resulting from cowpox are forgotten, or undervalued . . . then the smallpox may again be imported from some remote corner where the influence of cowpox was unknown. . . . Measures might be contrived not only for rendering vaccine inoculation general, but also for continuing it with unremitting diligence throughout future ages."

References

1. Macaulay, T. B.: *The History of England from the Accession of James the Second.* Volume 4. Philadelphia, E. H. Butler and Company, 1856, p. 369.
2. WHO Weekly Epidemiological Record 47:494–496, 1972.

3. Leake, J. P.: Questions and answers on smallpox and vaccination. Public Health Rep. 60: 221–238, 1927. (Revised 1946, reprint No. 1137.)
4. WHO Expert Committee on Smallpox Eradication: Second Report. WHO Techn. Rep. Ser. 493:9, 1972.
5. Center for Disease Control: Morbidity and Mortality Weekly Report 20:339–345, 1971.
6. Ibid., p. 342.
7. Neff, J. M., et al.: Complication of smallpox vaccination. I. National survey in the United States, 1963. New Eng. J. Med. 276:125–131, 1967.
8. Lane, J. M., et al.: Complications of smallpox vaccination, 1968. National surveillance in the United States. New Eng. J. Med. 281:1201–1208, 1969.
9. Lane, J. M., and Millar, J. D.: Routine childhood vaccination against smallpox reconsidered. New Eng. J. Med. 281:1220–1224, 1969.
10. Kempe, J. H., and Benenson, A. S.: Smallpox immunization in the United States. J.A.M.A. 194:161–166, 1965.
11. Landrigan, P. J.: Neurological disorder following measles-virus vaccination. Presented at Annual Meeting, American Public Health Association, November 15, 1972.
12. Communicable Disease Center: Encephalitis surveillance, 1965. Annual Summary, July 1, 1966, pp. 12–15.
13. Dick: G.: Smallpox: A reconsideration of public health policies. Progr. Med. Virol. 8:1–29, 1966.
14. Ehrengut, W., and Ehrengut-Lange, J.: Postvaccinal convulsions, age disposition and prognosis. Proceedings of the Symposium on Smallpox, Zagreb, Yugoslavia, 1969.
15. Berger, K., and Puntigam, F.: Die Altersdisposition bei postvakzinaler Enzephalitis. Dtsch. Med. Wschr. 85:1520–1524, 1960.
16. Benenson, A. S.: Possible alternatives to routine smallpox vaccination in the United States. Amer. J. Epidemiol. 93:248–252, 1971.
17. Foege, W. H., et al.: Selective epidemiologic control in smallpox eradication. Amer. J. Epidemiol. 94:311–315, 1971.
18. Gelfand, H. M., and Posch, J.: The recent outbreak of smallpox in Meschede, West Germany. Amer. J. Epidemiol. 93:234–237, 1971.
19. WHO Weekly Epidemiological Record 47:161–162, 1972.
20. Egli, D.: Yugoslavia. Conquest of an epidemic. World Health, October, 1972, pp. 28–30.
21. Mack, T. M.: Smallpox in Europe, 1950–1971. J. Infect. Dis. 125:161–169, 1972.
22. Katz, S.L.: The case for continuing "routine" childhood smallpox vaccination in the United States. Amer. J. Epidemiol. 93:241–244, 1971.
23. Bryce, J.: *Practical Observations on the Inoculation of Cowpox, Pointing Out a Test of a Constitutional Affection in Those Cases in Which the Local Inflammation Is Slight, and in Which No Fever Is Perceptible.* Edinburgh, Scotland, William Couch, 1802.

Comment

The Status of Smallpox Vaccination

We have become accustomed, in recent years, to accept with varying degrees of resignation, or even with equanimity, some radical and rather abrupt changes in attitudes toward social behavior, political actions, ingrained traditions and, in medicine, long accepted and practiced therapeutic and prophylactic measures. Yet there are always those, usually but not always a minority, who decry these changes and are deeply concerned about their possible immediate or long-term effects.

As with other similarly effective procedures that have come into use over the years, the acceptance of vaccination against smallpox, first introduced about 175 years ago, took a long time and, as pointed out by Benenson, this was complicated by many factors, not all of them related to the underlying principle of the effectiveness of cowpox vaccine in protecting humans against smallpox. It was only the serious nature of the full-blown disease when it achieved epidemic proportions, and the well demonstrated value of the available vaccines in limiting and preventing such epidemics, that finally led to full acceptance of routine vaccination and to making it compulsory in many nations throughout the world.

It is precisely this high degree of effectiveness that has brought increasingly into focus what Langmuir terms the "human cost" of vaccination, for some of the unwanted effects are indeed serious and sometimes fatal. In assessing the risk-to-benefit ratio for the justification of routine or compulsory vaccination, the fairly large number in the numerator, which includes the serious illnesses and deaths, has been considered fully acceptable in view of the very large size of the denominator, representing the millions of individuals subjected to vaccination and hence protected against this dreaded disease. This was true, and still is, wherever smallpox is endemic because of the marked susceptibility of exposed and unprotected individuals, the seriousness of the disease, and the high case-fatality ratio among those who become infected. By the same token, where cases are rare and occur only in small numbers and at long intervals, the value of vaccination has been questioned to the point that routine and compulsory vaccination has been discontinued recently in the United States and in several other countries.

In the preceding essays Langmuir and Benenson have corralled the arguments for and against the recommendation to discontinue routine vaccination. There are large areas of agreement between them, among which are the following:

1. There is or would be no need for vaccination if or when global eradication of smallpox is indeed achieved.

2. Global eradication of smallpox can be achieved within the next two or three years provided there is adequate cooperation of the populations and authorities within the endemic areas and barring unanticipated catastrophes, wars, or other militating circumstances. Recent progress to that goal is demonstrated in Figure 1.

Smallpox Cases per 100,000 Inhabitants—1967

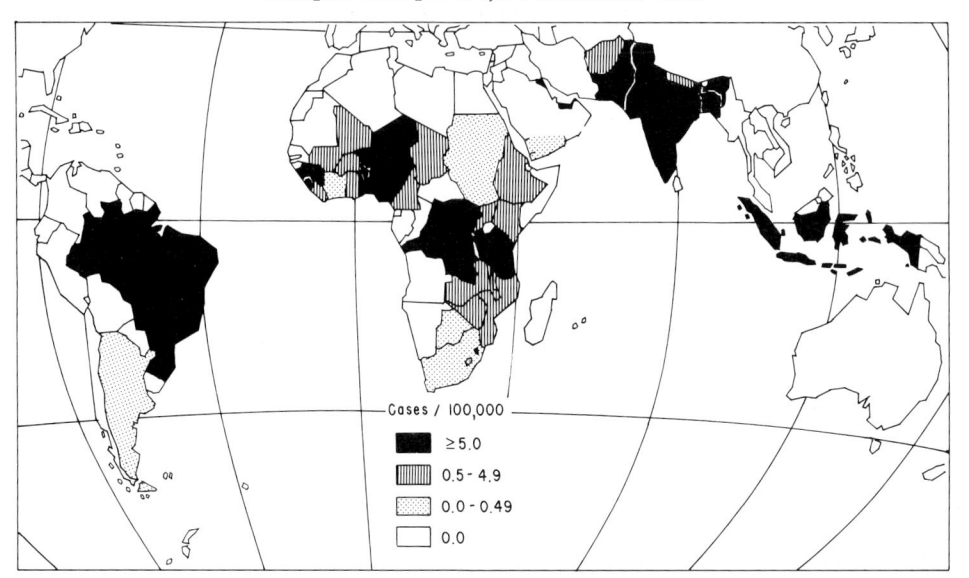

Smallpox Cases per 100,000 Inhabitants (Estimated)*—1972

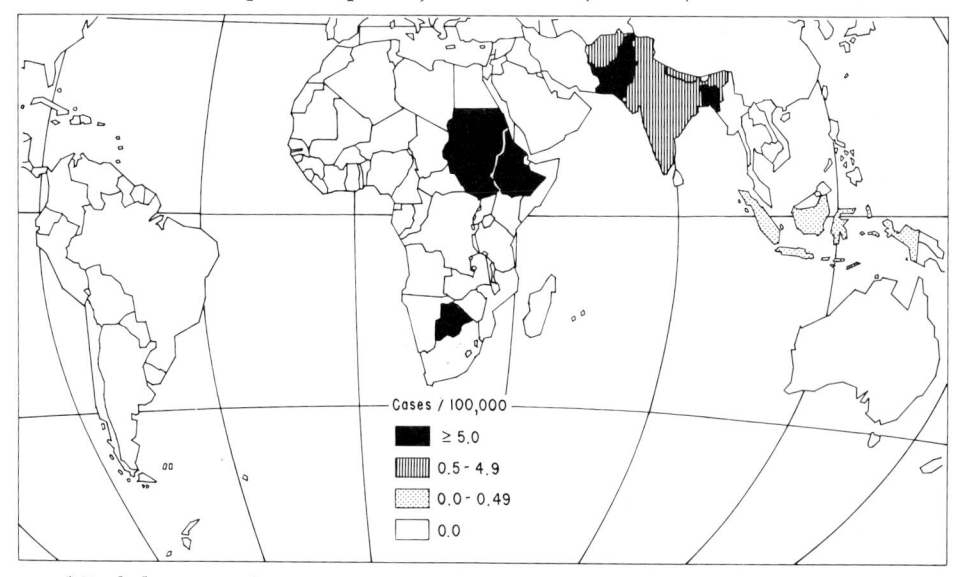

* Excludes imported cases.

Figure 1. Progress toward global eradication of smallpox from 1967 to 1972. (From Wkly. Epidem. Rec. 47:175, 1972.)

3. In the present situation, with some endemic foci reporting varying numbers of cases, it is still possible to reduce the number of importations of active cases and the spread of infection from such cases to susceptibles within clean areas to the point where the small risk of infection more than balances the human and economic costs of routine vaccination and thus can justify withdrawal of the procedure as a routine or compulsory measure. This would require: (a) restoration of orderly and fully cooperative governments in Bangladesh and other endemic countries, and return of conditions there to normal; (b) maintenance of effective surveillance in those countries and in all remaining endemic foci; (c) containment of outbreaks within the endemic foci by effective quarantine of cases and contacts and by "ring vaccination," that is, by intensive search for and effective immunizing of all possibly exposed individuals and their contacts within a reasonable radius; and (d) an effective reporting and alerting system to apprise authorities in all countries of the occurrence of any outbreaks in order to prevent exportation from those foci, and especially to prevent importation of such cases into the "clean areas."

4. Both essayists agree with the caveats that accompany the discontinuance of routine vaccination. These are: (a) vaccination and "adequate immunization" of all health-related personnel, especially in hospitals; (b) vaccination of all travelers to and from any area where active cases are occurring; (c) continuous vigilance and surveillance, including effective and worldwide reporting and alerting system; and (d) care to avoid vaccination of "high risk" individuals, that is, those most likely to suffer serious side effects; these include "allergic" individuals, particularly those with eczema or other diseases of the skin, immunodeficient individuals, and patients undergoing therapy with immunosuppressive or corticosteroid drugs. Also, such high risk individuals should not be exposed to vaccinated individuals during the infectious stage and, by the same token, those who are in contact with such individuals should not be vaccinated, or when vaccinated, should be removed from all such contacts until their vaccination scars are completely healed. Vaccination of the high risk individuals is justified only when the degree and nature of exposure to active disease is great enough to warrant the risk of vaccination. (e) Maintenance of a stock of good, active, effective and stable vaccine, and education of the health profession in its proper use. Currently available, properly prepared, and fully dried (lyophilized) vaccines satisfy the requirement for such a vaccine.

In view of these wide areas of agreement, what then is the basis of the controversy? First of all, Langmuir played an important role in the development and support of the global smallpox eradication program. He bases his conclusion on confidence that the eradication *will* be accomplished very soon. He seems to be the eternal optimist and activist who has vigorously pursued each program in which he has been concerned when he considered it to be well conceived, well planned, and justified by adequate supporting data. He also has great faith in the efficacy of surveillance programs designed to bring to light promptly any serious health problems that may arise, and to marshall the proper resources for their rapid and effective containment. This he did very successfully in establishing and maintaining the Epidemic Intelligence Program which he headed at the Communicable Diseases Center (now the Center for Disease Control) until his recent move to Harvard. Having himself established and demonstrated many times the effectiveness of such surveillance and developed a whole generation of young physicians and other health workers more or less in his image, he is naturally optimistic and supremely confident that it can and does work.

Benenson is also an experienced and scholarly "shoe-leather" epidemiologist and educator, well acquainted with the methodology and practices of surveillance and disease control. He places much less confidence in the infallibility of the human element involved in such activities. He appears to be less certain that complete eradication will indeed be accomplished in the very near future and considers the risk of importation of infection still a real one, believing that failure to recognize an imported case is still highly possible, and that serious smallpox may spread quite extensively from such cases before the spread is effectively halted. Examples of recent occurrence of this type are cited by both essayists. Moreover, having participated in the scientific, medical, and political decision making related to immunization programs, he realizes and points out in detail what he considers to be flaws in the successive arguments which led the Surgeon General to recommend discontinuance of routine and compulsory vaccination programs *at this time*, that is, before global eradication of smallpox has *in fact* been achieved. Item by item he exposes, on the one hand, the dark side of the picture with respect to the still present dangers of occurrence and spread of the disease. On the other hand, he calls attention to the possible fallacies in interpreting and possibly exaggerating the risks of vaccination against which those dangers must be balanced. The former are minimized and the latter he feels have been exaggerated by supporters of the new program.

Benenson feels, and there is some evidence to support him, that the arguments put forth to justify the Surgeon General's proposal have made it difficult to induce health workers and even travelers to be vaccinated because the risks of infection have been minimized and the risks of vaccination have been exaggerated.

The facts are the same, but their interpretation and the weight placed on them differ substantially. Is this not the basis of most controversies? Is this not the basis of the philosophy of the optimist-activist who looks only to the future, is confident of the decision he makes to achieve his goal, and acts on it, often knowing full well, but choosing to discount the risks? Or he feels confident that he can cope with the problems as they arise and is willing to accept those risks. This is in contrast to the more conservative individual who would rather live with what he knows to be the facts in the real world about him and with which he has learned to cope, until he is fully satisfied that the proposed alternative is indeed adequately justified.

MAXWELL FINLAND

15

Management of Adult-Onset Diabetes

ORAL ANTIDIABETIC AGENTS HAVE A LIMITED PLACE IN MANAGEMENT AND MAY BE HARMFUL
    by Albert I. Winegrad, Rex S. Clements, Jr., and Anthony D. Morrison

ORAL HYPOGLYCEMIC AGENTS ARE WORTHWHILE
    by Robert F. Bradley

COMMENT
    by Arnold S. Relman

Oral Antidiabetic Agents Have a Limited Place in Management and May Be Harmful*

ALBERT I. WINEGRAD, REX S. CLEMENTS, JR., and ANTHONY D. MORRISON

University of Pennsylvania School of Medicine

The manner in which most physicians now manage their patients with adult-onset diabetes might best be termed "benign neglect." In part, this is a consequence of the continuing controversy over the aims and the efficacy of presently available therapy. Just how benign current practice really is remains to be determined; however, it includes certain aspects that are difficult to justify, such as the common misuse of the sulfonylurea compounds and the biguanide derivatives.

The indications for continued medical intervention are not so obvious in adult-onset diabetics as in juvenile diabetics since, irrespective of their age at diagnosis, patients with the adult-onset form of the disease exhibit little tendency to ketoacidosis. There is general agreement that efforts to lower the blood glucose are indicated in patients who are symptomatic as the result of hyperglycemia, and that delay in the effective treatment of symptomatic hyperglycemia in adult-onset diabetics may be a major factor in the development of hyperglycemic nonketotic coma. At the time of diagnosis, patients with adult-onset diabetes are a heterogeneous group not only with regard to symptoms, but also with regard to the presence of the complications of diabetes and the coexistence of other conditions (e.g., hypertension and arteriosclerotic cardiovascular disease) that might be expected to alter their prognosis. There is little agreement as to benefit of therapy other than that designed to relieve symptoms directly related to hyperglycemia.

---

* This review was supported in part by Grant AM04722, National Institutes of Health, U.S.P.H.S., and a grant from the John A. Hartford Foundation. Dr. Winegrad is the recipient of Research Career Development Award GM06405 from the National Institute of General Medical Sciences.

What Is the Value of "Control"?

Physicians are divided on the value of attempts to achieve an approximation of normal glucose metabolism in the hope that this will influence the development or progression of the late complications. (It is symptomatic of the state of the field that measures to modify other demonstrable abnormalities, such as hyperlipoproteinemias, have received minimal consideration.) Much of the present controversy over the value of "control" is nonsense. The players in this philosophical sport are trapped by the definitions and unstated assumptions that constitute the rules of this game. In the treatment of adult-onset diabetics, convenience is the overriding consideration in the minds of most physicians, which may be understandable since the value of treatment in asymptomatic patients is disputed. The effort and expense required to achieve and to document an approximation of normal blood glucose concentrations throughout the day preclude this type of treatment for most patients. None of the reported clinical trials designed to evaluate the value of "control" has made a serious attempt to achieve normalization of blood glucose fluctuations. The frequency with which this goal can be achieved in a large population of adult-onset diabetics by presently available means has never been evaluated. In essence we have been subjected to a heated dispute over the value of a form of therapy that is only rarely attempted and even more rarely achieved.

Recent studies suggest that fluctuations in the blood glucose concentration in nondiabetic subjects on a normal diet are restricted to a relatively narrow range. However, when evaluating blood glucose concentrations in adult-onset diabetics, physicians almost invariably apply arbitrary standards that bear little relationship to the levels observed in nondiabetics. In addition, it is commonly assumed that if there were a relationship between the blood glucose level and the pathological processes responsible for complications, it should be apparent from comparisons of groups of patients who have had persistently differing degrees of *abnormal* blood glucose levels. Although the basis of this belief is difficult to perceive, it is rarely questioned. A blood glucose concentration that fluctuates between 110 mg. per cent and 180 mg. per cent in a 39 year old man throughout the day cannot be considered normal, even though most physicians would consider this good or excellent "control."

One of the undisputed aspects of the recent reports of the University Group Diabetes Program (UGDP)[1,2] is the record of the quality of "control" achieved in adult-onset diabetics treated in university medical centers by a variety of therapeutic regimens, most of which are similar to those now commonly employed. None of the treatment groups in the UDPG study had a normal fasting blood glucose at any time during the initial four plus years of the study. Diurnal fluctuations in blood glucose on the patients' usual diet and with their usual physical activity were not assessed. However, at regular intervals the patients were given a 50-gm. oral glucose load one half hour after their morning medication, and the blood glucose was determined one hour later. Although the *lowest* mean blood glucose level at one hour was observed in the patients treated with adjusted insulin dosages, even in this group the mean one-hour value was in excess of 200 mg. per cent in more than half the tests during the initial four plus years. It is difficult to assemble totally appropriate age and sex matched control data, but in a recent study of normal males with no family history of diabetes (ages 22 to 28), the mean blood glucose one hour after a 50 gm. glucose load was 90.6 ± 5.7 mg. per cent,[3] and in the studies of Neel et al.[4] the mean blood glucose one hour after a 100 gm. glucose load in patients with no family history of diabetes (ages 30 to 39) was 104.3 ± 7.1 mg. per cent in males and 93.7 ± 6.9 mg. per cent in females.* The data available would suggest that most of the patients in the UDPG study had persistently abnormal fluctuations in blood glucose concentration irrespective of the treatment prescribed. Although the UDPG study was a pioneer effort to improve the quality of clinical trials, it shares one of the common deficiencies of such studies in that it included no group of patients who had an essentially normal range of blood glucose fluctuation throughout the day.

Another frivolous aspect of the current controversy is the simplistic fashion in which the pathogenesis of the late complications of diabetes is viewed by most physicians. Each of the diverse clinical syndromes lumped into this unfortunate term has a very complex pathological basis, and in some instances a distinction must be made between processes responsible for acute symptoms and those which operate in the production of predisposing pathological lesions. There is little to support the widespread belief that each of the late complications is primarily a reflection of diabetic microangiopathy. There is no convincing evidence that alterations in capillary structure play a determining role in the pathogenesis of the common symmetrical peripheral neuropathic syndromes associated with diabetes mellitus,[5] nor is there convincing evidence that this process contributes to the increased frequency with which arterial occlusions occur in specific portions of the vascular system. In patients dying of diabetic nephropathy the pathological findings almost invariably include alterations other than those unique to diabetes mellitus; thus, arteriolosclerosis and intimal fibrosis of the renal arteries are often present.[6] Therefore, in any organ system, the pathological changes that are associated with diabetes mellitus may very well be subject to modification by independently determined genetic and environmental factors. However, this is rarely considered in efforts to evaluate the factors responsible for the clinical course in diabetics. As an example, although the recent studies of Hazzard et al.[7] would suggest that inherited abnormalities in lipoprotein metabolism are commonly associated with myocardial infarction, the distribution of patients with such abnormalities has not yet been assessed in clinical trials of diabetic therapy.

Another reason why caution must be exercised in the evaluation of clinical trials is the problem of asymptomatic but irreversible pathology in the patients studied. It is notoriously difficult to date the onset of an abnormality in glucose tolerance in adult-onset diabetics, and this problem is magnified by the recent realization that asymptomatic adult-onset diabetes may occur in children and young adults and does not appear to progress to the ketosis-prone type of the

---

* The effects of sex and increasing age on fasting blood glucose levels, and on the response to a 100-gm. oral glucose tolerance test in patients with no family history of diabetes have been well documented in patients up to age 39.

disease.[8] Thus, the presence of asymptomatic pathology in newly diagnosed adult-onset diabetics cannot be used as a telling argument against a relationship to the metabolic abnormalities associated with diabetes mellitus.

The failure to consistently observe improvement in specific diabetic complications following the institution of "stricter control" is frequently used as evidence that the pathogenesis of these conditions is unrelated to the consequences of an impaired insulin secretory mechanism. To cite but one example of the limitations of this reasoning, recent studies have demonstrated that the majority of a group of newly diagnosed adult-onset diabetics with normal standard neurologic examinations and without symptoms of neuropathy could be shown to have widespread functional abnormalities in their peripheral nervous system when suitably sensitive techniques were employed.[9] Biopsies of peripheral nerves from asymptomatic adult-onset diabetics without clinical evidence of neuropathy have also revealed pathological changes similar to those found in the nerves of patients with clinical neuropathy (although of a lesser degree).[10] Thus, the development of the clinical manifestations of diabetic neuropathy may represent a late stage in the pathological process and have irreversible elements. Whether or not patients with clinically apparent peripheral neuropathy respond to efforts to improve "control" can provide little information concerning its pathogenesis or its prevention. The host of invasive techniques which would be required to assemble suitably characterized subjects for study (e.g., coronary angiography, renal and peripheral nerve biopsies, fluoroscein retinography, and so forth) almost precludes meaningful large scale clinical trials.

Many physicians also believe that the controversy over the relationship between the metabolic derangements that result from an altered insulin secretory mechanism and alterations in the capillary basement membrane in diabetics has been resolved and that the two are clearly unrelated. This stems from the provocative studies of Siperstein and associates, who were the first to apply quantitative techniques to the assessment of capillary basement membrane thickness (CBMT).[11] They recognized the inherent technical problems in attempting to measure CBMT in many organs and demonstrated that skeletal muscle biopsies provide a means of obtaining suitable material for study from large numbers of patients. Their data indicated that muscle CBMT was significantly greater in diabetics and that the degree of thickening appeared to be unrelated to the duration of known disease or to its "severity." Moreover, their studies suggested that in patients genetically at high risk for the development of diabetes mellitus, increased muscle CBMT was present prior to the development of a detectable abnormality in glucose tolerance. Siperstein's work has been a major contribution and stimulus. However, some of his observations and interpretations have been seriously challenged by Kilo et al., who have concluded that muscle CBMT is usually within normal limits at the outset of clinical diabetes mellitus and increases with duration of disease.[12] There are differences in methodology and in patient selection in these studies, and the resulting controversy has not been resolved. The studies of Østerby suggest that in the kidney the alterations in glomerular capillary structure are not present at the outset of clinical diabetes in young adults but progress with increased duration of the disease.[13] Thus, it would be premature to conclude that the demonstrable metabolic abnormalities in diabetes mellitus are totally unrelated to the development or progression of alterations in capillary structure. A similar conclusion would have to be drawn with regard to data available from studies of experimental diabetes in animals, particularly in view of recent preliminary reports of the production of retinal capillary microaneurysms in rats with chronic streptozotocin diabetes.[14]

From this cursory review it would appear that at the present time the physician treating adult-onset diabetics has a clear responsibility to prevent symptomatic hyperglycemia; the advantages of maintaining a normal or nearly normal range of blood glucose fluctuations remain to be evaluated but cannot be excluded. The choice of therapeutic aims must be a conscious decision by the physician, and one in which an informed patient participates. The patient's age, the presence of other serious medical problems, the presence or absence of specific clinical complications, and the patient's motivation are practical considerations.

The Importance of Weight Control

Whether the physician believes that the prevention of symptomatic hyperglycemia is an adequate goal in a given patient, or whether a strenuous effort is undertaken to achieve a normalization of glucose metabolism, the relationship between increased body weight and hyperglycemia that so frequently exists in adult-onset diabetics must be considered. In the UGDP study the adult-onset diabetics averaged +33 per cent of ideal body weight at the outset.[15] It has been observed repeatedly that many adult-onset diabetics will exhibit improvement in their degree of hyperglycemia if a significant reduction in body weight can be achieved. (Whether this is due to weight reduction per se or to a decrease in carbohydrate intake remains to be determined.[16, 17]) The UGDP studies provide an indication of the effectiveness of present efforts to achieve weight reduction and the resultant improvement in diabetic "control." All the patient groups in the UGDP study exhibited a fall in mean body weight at the time of the first follow-up visit. However, the maximum decrease for any group was 4.2 lbs (less than 3 per cent of initial mean weight), which was observed in the patients treated with diet plus a placebo. In this group the early weight loss was not sustained, and the mean body weight remained close to 98 per cent of the initial weight throughout the subsequent four plus years. The initial weight loss was associated with a fall in both the mean fasting blood glucose level and in the glucose level observed one hour after the ingestion of 50 gm. of glucose. Subsequently both of these parameters of "control" rose progressively throughout the remainder of the study. Although the patients receiving tolbutamide or insulin (in fixed or varying dosages) also received dietary instruction, their initial weight loss was less than that observed in the placebo group, and no further reduction in mean body weight was observed during the subsequent four years. These data suggest that current efforts to achieve weight reduction in adult-onset diabetics are ineffective, at least as currently practiced in medical outpatient clinics.

The difficulties encountered in achieving weight reduction in chronically obese nondiabetic subjects have been well documented, and the psychiatric implications of food to some patients are recognized; however, it is not certain that the experience with these chronically obese patients provides a meaningful index of the results that could be obtained in patients with adult-onset diabetes. Weight reduction remains the safest and cheapest means of achieving "control" sufficient to prevent hyperglycemic symptoms in the majority of adult-onset diabetics. Moreover, in the absence of significant weight reduction, the efficacy of other agents employed to lower blood glucose appears to be considerably reduced. The manner in which weight reduction is usually undertaken ensures failure in a large percentage of patients. Diet instruction is confusing and reflects the pseudoscience that presently surrounds the question of an appropriate diet for adult-onset diabetics.

Dietary instructions should be as simple as possible. The justification for modifications in dietary composition remains to be established; however, in the face of evidence of persistent abnormalities in plasma lipoproteins, we suggest modifications similar to those recently outlined by Fredrickson and his co-workers.[18] One of the factors that may contribute to the failure of diet therapy is the long period between follow-up visits—three-month intervals being not uncommon. The commercial weight reduction groups have demonstrated the value of reinforcement provided by frequent weight checks, and brief visits in which weight is checked by an office nurse can be helpful in many patients. Increased physical activity is often dismissed as of little benefit; however, for most 40 year old Americans a 15-minute daily walk would represent a significant increase in physical activity. A conscientious effort to increase physical activity is, in our hands, a significant factor in those patients in whom a reduction in weight and improved glucose levels are achieved. (It is of interest that a recent study, thus far reported only in abstract, suggests that the abnormal pattern of insulin secretion observed in markedly obese nondiabetics can be normalized by physical training without a decrease in body fat.[19])

Although there are many adult-onset diabetics in whom lifelong patterns of overeating and limited physical activity are practically immutable, the fact remains that serious efforts to encourage reduced caloric intake and increased physical activity have been abandoned by many physicians. There is little justification for the use of any pharmacologic agent in asymptomatic adult-onset diabetics until the possibility of attaining improved "control" by weight reduction has been given an adequate trial. It is now common practice, however, to begin sulfonylurea or phenformin treatment from the outset in asymptomatic adult-onset diabetics. One of the results of this practice is that the necessity for weight reduction is minimized in the patient's mind. Moreover, the patient is instructed that the oral hypoglycemic agents may provoke hypoglycemic symptoms which can be relieved by the ingestion of free carbohydrate. For many patients, who are understandably anxious about their newly diagnosed disease, this becomes a sanctioned invitation to unrestricted caloric intake. It is not surprising that significant weight reduction and maintenance of normal body weight are rarely achieved under these conditions, for both physicians and patients have come to view the nature and amount of the drug ingested as the major consideration in "controlling" adult onset diabetes.

Limited Effectiveness of Oral Hypoglycemic Agents

If the physician resorts to pharmacologic agents to prevent symptomatic hyperglycemia in adult-onset diabetics before demonstrating the necessity for their use, then one might hope that he would at least document the effectiveness of the agent employed. Since a fixed dosage of 1.5 gm. per day of tolbutamide was employed, the data derived from the UGDP study are not completely applicable. However, all the sulfonylureas have a relatively narrow effective dosage range, and the experience of this study is probably not too unrepresentative of the long-term efficacy of sulfonylureas in adult-onset diabetics in whom significant weight reduction is not achieved. In the UDGP study there was an initial improvement in fasting blood sugar and also in the blood glucose level observed one hour after a glucose load. This improved "control" paralleled the initial and transient weight loss which had occurred in these patients. Subsequently there was a progressive rise in mean fasting blood glucose and over the remaining four plus years it rarely differed from that of the group receiving a placebo by more than 15 mg. per cent (the mean values in both groups being persistently abnormal). The blood glucose level after a glucose load also tended to increase progressively in the patients treated with tolbutamide, and the mean value was rarely more than 20 mg. per cent different from that of the placebo group. At the end of four plus years the mean value in the group treated with tolbutamide was 244 mg. per cent, whereas the value for the placebo group was 251 mg. per cent. Thus, one may question whether the use of tolbutamide under these conditions significantly reduced the frequency with which *abnormal* blood glucose levels were present in these patients, or with which symptomatic hyperglycemia developed.

The mechanisms responsible for the development of refractoriness to sulfonylurea therapy in patients in whom an initial response is observed are still uncertain, and the data on its incidence are difficult to interpret.[20] Values ranging from 0.3 to 30 per cent have been reported, and there is a suggestion that the incidence increases with known duration of diabetes. The uncertainty results, in part, from differences in patient selection, in criteria for failure, and in the extent to which other factors such as weight gain and dosage were considered. Unfortunately physicians exercise little selectivity in administering sulfonylurea or biguanides to adult-onset diabetics, ignore the limitations imposed by obesity, and are slow to raise the question of efficacy. One can only guess at the number of patients presently receiving these drugs in whom their withdrawal would not significantly alter the daily fluctuations in blood glucose levels. Our own experience would suggest that it represents a significant fraction of the patients who have received the drug for a prolonged period and in whom obesity persists.

In general, both physicians and patients are reluctant to stop oral hypoglycemic therapy once it has been instituted. In many instances random blood glucose values of 200 to 300 mg. per cent are observed over a period of months to years before the physician reluctantly concludes that the drug has become ineffective. The usual course under these circumstances is to resort to another sulfonylurea in the hope of finding one that is "effective," and often to combine this with a biguanide. The pernicious aspect of the current misuse of the sulfonylureas and the biguanides is that many patients are subjected to the expense and potential hazard of long-term treatment to attain a relatively limited goal—freedom from hyperglycemic symptoms—while the agents are used under conditions in which their efficacy is restricted and is only rarely adequately assessed.

The foregoing comments should not be misinterpreted. There are a number of adult-onset diabetics in whom the use of the sulfonylureas can produce further improvement in the range of fluctuations of blood glucose over that resulting from the correction of obesity. These agents may also be effective in some non-obese adult-onset diabetics. We do not eschew the use of sulfonylureas in efforts to prevent symptomatic hyperglycemia, or to achieve an approximation of normal fluctuations in blood glucose. In both instances, however, the consequences of effective weight reduction should first be demonstrated if obesity is present. If the addition of a pharmacologic agent is required, the relative merits either of insulin or of a sulfonylurea must be considered. We do not believe that the biguanides have an established place in the treatment of diabetics.

Many physicians are reluctant to accept the fact that the sulfonylureas and the biguanides are not appropriate agents in circumstances in which rapid correction of the metabolic abnormalities is required. An obvious instance is when ketonemia develops either in association with an acute infection or following the institution of therapy for an unrelated disease that requires the use of agents that can impair endogenous insulin secretion and/or decrease its apparent effectiveness. In these circumstances insulin is indicated, since neither the sulfonylureas nor the biguanides provide significant protection against the development of ketoacidosis. Even in the more common situation in which the previously untreated patient presents with marked polydipsia, polyuria, and weight loss without ketonemia, one cannot predict with any certainty whether the patient will respond to sulfonylurea or biguanide therapy. Under these circumstances, and particularly if there is an associated illness that predisposes to dehydration, it is wiser to use insulin for the acute correction of hyperglycemia and the relief of symptoms. Nonetheless, many physicians attempt trials at treatment with the sulfonylureas or the biguanides with a resulting delay in effective therapy that in some instances may contribute to the development of hyperglycemic nonketotic coma.

The use of insulin to achieve acute improvement does not imply that the patients will necessarily require exogenous insulin once they have been stabilized for a significant period. When there is a demonstrated requirement for the addition of a pharmacologic agent to correct symptomatic hyperglycemia, there is a curious reluctance to employ insulin in the management of adult-onset diabetics. This stems, in part, from the misconception that these patients are invariably insulin hypersecretors and that insulin resistance is a major factor in the pathogenesis of this syndrome. The bulk of the present evidence (which Kipnis has admirably reviewed[21]) clearly indicates that most adult-onset diabetics exhibit an impaired insulin secretory mechanism when compared with appropriately matched age, sex, and weight groups. Moreover, although obesity in both the normal and diabetic individual is associated with an apparent decrease in the biologic effectiveness of insulin, the diabetic state per se does not appear to be associated with any significant degree of insulin antagonism (if one excludes specific circumstances such as ketoacidosis). Insulin remains the preferred pharmacologic agent because of its assured and continued efficacy and its protective value in circumstances in which acute impairment of endogenous insulin secretion and/or effectiveness may arise. Since 1972 there have been improvements in the purity of the commercial insulin preparations available, as the result of the application of methods developed to separate insulin, pro-insulin, and related peptides. Preliminary data suggest that these newer preparations *may* significantly reduce the immunologic responses to the administration of porcine and bovine insulin and the associated clinical problems.[22, 23] However, the present methods for the administration of insulin to adult-onset diabetics are far from ideal. We have no practical method of reproducing the timed relationship between food ingestion and insulin secretion that occurs in normals nor of selectively exposing the liver to the pulses of insulin that normally occur in portal venous blood after eating. Therefore, there is little reason to believe that present forms of insulin treatment reproduce normal physiology.

The primary advantage of the sulfonylureas is that they can be administered orally. The resulting convenience is a real but not necessarily compelling consideration when there is a manifest requirement for a pharmacologic hypoglycemic agent. The specific circumstances in a given patient should determine the choice, and while our own preference is to employ insulin, there is no good reason why a carefully controlled trial—preferably with one of the shorter acting sulfonylureas—should not be undertaken. The physician should, however, consider the possibility that contraindications to the use of sulfonylureas may exist (e.g., renal impairment or liver disease) and that sulfonylurea therapy may influence the metabolism of other pharmacologic agents (e.g., bishydroxycumarin and sulfonamides). The limitations of our knowledge concerning the role of insulin deficiency in certain situations lead us to prefer the use of insulin in patients with manifest symmetrical peripheral neuropathy with or without associated chronic foot ulcers, and in individuals in whom repeated skin infections or poorly healing surgical wounds are present. However, it must be admitted that this is clearly a prejudice on our part.

Hazards of Treatment with Sulfonylureas

Insulin or sulfonylurea therapies are not without hazard. With insulin the major concerns are hypoglycemia and problems resulting from the administration of foreign protein(s). The safety of treatment with the sulfonylureas is, however, the point most fiercely disputed at the moment. It should be apparent from the initial section of this discussion that we have serious reservations about the conclusions that can be drawn from any of the published clinical studies, irrespective of the elegance of the statistical methods employed to deal with their inherent deficiencies. A causal relationship between the treatment prescribed in the UDPG study and the subsequent clinical course of these patients would be difficult to establish on the basis of the information available. The excess cardiovascular mortality observed in the groups treated with tolbutamide and phenformin cannot be dismissed, since the manner in which these agents were employed mirrors the misuse of these agents in common practice. If subsequent data provided by the UDPG group provide evidence of an unusual form of coronary artery disease in the patients treated with tolbutamide and phenformin, or of an unusual propensity to cardiac arrhythmias, to pulmonary emboli, or to shock in the patients who died of cardiovascular disease, the case may be strengthened. However, although we feel that the sulfonylureas have a limited role in the treatment of adult-onset diabetes, we would not abandon their use on the basis of the findings of the UDPG study. Nevertheless, this study has served the useful purpose of reminding physicians that the use of sulfonylureas and biguanides is not without hazard, and that as with any pharmacologic agent, the possibility of unanticipated effects must be considered.

Hypoglycemia and hypersensitivity reactions have been the major problems encountered in the use of the sulfonylureas. Hypoglycemia resulting from these drugs can be prolonged and may be fatal; this is particularly true of long acting compounds such as chlorpropamide. Many of the reported instances have resulted from the unwarranted administration of this agent to patients with impaired renal function.[24] In addition, it has been recognized that chlorpropamide can induce a syndrome characterized by hyponatremia, impaired mental function, and evidence of inappropriate antidiuretic hormone activity.[25] The pernicious aspect of this syndrome is that in elderly patients (in whom it has been most frequently observed) the impaired mental function could easily be attributed to other causes. There is little reason to believe that the effects of the sulfonylureas are restricted to the pancreatic β-cells. Specific compounds have been shown to alter thyroid function,[26] to modify adenyl cyclase activity in cardiac muscle,[27] to augment antidiuresis,[25] and to alter lipolytic activity in isolated adipose tissue.[28] However, with the exception of the UGDP study, the reported incidence of serious problems resulting from the use of the shorter acting sulfonylureas has been remarkably low. Nonetheless, the prolonged administration of sulfonylureas to adult-onset diabetics does entail an obvious risk. As with any pharmacologic agent, this risk must be justified in terms of the indications for its use, and is not acceptable unless the agent is demonstrated to be effective.

Why Do We Use the Biguanides?

As we have previously mentioned, we find it difficult to justify a role for the biguanides in the treatment of diabetics and would discourage their use. It is doubtful that these agents would be employed at all if it were not for the fact that they can be administered orally. While there are gaps in our knowledge of the manner in which insulin and the sulfonylureas lower blood glucose levels in diabetics, there is some reassurance that these effects are mediated, in part, by the correction of metabolic abnormalities resulting from an altered insulin secretory mechanism. Whether the long-term effects of the sulfonylureas result primarily from an action on the pancreatic β-cells is a point that is difficult to document, but the ability of these agents to stimulate insulin secretion in adult-onset diabetics in whom they are effective is undisputed. In contrast, the manner in which phenformin lowers blood glucose in human diabetics, or in animals with alloxan diabetes, remains an enigma, but the fragmentary data available are not reassuring. An effect on insulin secretion has been excluded, although some residual endogenous insulin secretion is necessary for phenformin to be effective in lowering blood glucose. Kruger et al. have reported that phenformin impairs intestinal glucose absorption in man;[29] this compound also increases peripheral glucose utilization, albeit with an increased rate of lactate production.[30] The applicability of data derived from other species must be questioned because of the marked species variation in susceptibility to the hypoglycemic effects of phenformin. Thus, Kreisberg and associates dispute any effect of phenformin on decreasing hepatic glucose production or release in man.[30] However, at high concentrations phenformin does inhibit gluconeogenesis in isolated perfused rat liver.[30] In none of the isolated tissues in which the effects of phenformin have been examined is there clear evidence that phenformin restores a pattern of metabolism resembling that observed in the animal with a normal insulin secretory mechanism.

More to the point, biguanides are ineffective in the prevention of ketoacidosis, and there is no evidence that they have the assured efficacy of insulin in the management of acute symptomatic hyperglycemia. It is obviously not a suitable agent to use in those patients in whom a serious effort to achieve a normal range of blood glucose fluctuation is undertaken with the aim of correcting the underlying derangements in tissue metabolism that may contribute to the pathogenesis of the late complications. In patients in whom efforts at weight reduction have failed to remove the threat of symptomatic hyperglycemia, biguanides have no obvious advantage over insulin or the sulfonylureas (unless one wishes to view its effects on glucose absorption as an advantage). There is thus no obvious requirement for biguanides in the treatment of adult-onset diabetes, unless one will accept its use as an adjuvant to ineffective treatment with sulfonylureas. Since suitable alternatives are available, the justification for the additional risk entailed in this practice escapes us. The UDPG study reported a significant excess cardiovascular mortality in the groups treated with phenformin, but again the causal nature of this relationship is difficult to establish. However, there remains the distinct possibility that phenformin may represent a pharmacologic hazard in a group of patients who tend to develop general or local circulatory insufficiency. We believe this may contribute to the association between phenformin administration and the development of clinical lactic acidosis.[31]

Lactic Acidosis

The pathogenesis of lactic acidosis in those instances in which there is no obvious evidence of local tissue hypoxia is poorly understood. However, it is clear that in many tissues the rate of lactate production under normal conditions is in a range that represents only a small fraction of the tissues' total capacity. In many tissues the rates of conversion of glucose to pyruvate and lactate are kept at a small fraction of total capacity by chemical signals generated as a consequence of the operation of the Krebs cycle and the electron transport system in which oxygen is the final acceptor. The effect of anoxia on the rate of lactate production in a tissue such as muscle results from a decrease in the signals which are usually generated as a consequence of respiration and an increase in glycolysis. Under these conditions the end product of glycolysis appears primarily as lactate, since a secondary consequence of impaired respiration is an increase in the cytoplasmic free NADH/NAD ratio, which is one of the factors determining the ratio of lactate/pyruvate in the cytoplasm. There is no doubt that in lactic acidosis, as in diabetic ketoacidosis, the rate of production of a normal product can be increased to levels that threaten the organism's existence. Lactate released into the circulation by other tissus is removed in large part by the liver, where it is utilized to a considerable degree for the resynthesis of glucose. The only value of this simplistic outline is to stress the point that factors that permit the expression of the tremendous latent capacity for lactate production in many tissues, or which impair the capacity of the liver to dispose of lactate, may eventuate in lactic acidosis. It is well established in adult-onset diabetics that chronic phenformin administration results in significant elevation of blood lactate concentrations. While in most patients the levels observed give little cause for concern, the effect does appear to be dose related.[32] There is, therefore, the possibility that at sufficiently high concentrations phenformin might induce lactic acidosis in humans either by increasing peripheral lactate production or by decreasing hepatic utilization, or both. This would appear to be the case since there are well documented instances in which phenformin was taken for suicidal purposes, with the subsequent development of lactic acidosis.[33]

The biguanides are unlikely to be the sole cause of the increased frequency of lactic acidosis in diabetics, since this syndrome has been observed in patients who are not receiving these drugs. Adult-onset diabetics are, as a group, individuals at increased risk to the development of a number of acute conditions which may produce local circulatory changes conducive to the development of either increased lactate production or impaired disposition. It seems difficult to exclude the possibility that, under these circumstances, the presence of biguanides may potentiate the development of lactic acidosis. The efforts to exclude this possibility are not totally convincing; thus, the failure of biguanides to potentiate markedly the rise in blood lactate in rats exposed to low oxygen tensions ignores the relative insensitivity of this animal to the effects of these compounds. We find ourselves in agreement with Oliva, who concluded: "It remains possible that the association of phenformin and lactic acidosis is coincidental since lactic acidosis may occur in diabetic subjects not taking phenformin, as well as in non-diabetic subjects. The weight of the indirect evidence, however, strongly suggests that phenformin plays a causal or contributory role in the production of lactic acidosis."[31] It is interesting that the only death specifically ascribed to lactic acidosis in the UDPG study occurred in a patient in the group receiving phenformin.[2] In sum, since phenformin fills no unique requirement in the treatment of adult-onset diabetes, since its mode of action is uncertain but unlikely to be corrective of derangements resulting from an impaired insulin secretory mechanism, and since its relationship to lactic acidosis is unsettled, there is no valid reason to employ it in these patients.

Summary

The present state of treatment for adult-onset diabetes is admittedly inadequate, except for the prevention of symptomatic hyperglycemia. The data derived from clinical studies and from experimental work provide no basis for excluding the possibility that normalization of blood glucose fluctuations may significantly modify the development and progression of diabetic complications. However, the value of this form of therapy has never been adequately tested, and its immediate aims are difficult to achieve with present methods. It is an approach that should be considered primarily in younger diabetics without evidence of irreversible pathology who are capable of making an informed commitment to this form of treatment.

In the majority of adult-onset diabetics the aim of therapy is of necessity restricted to the prevention of symptomatic hyperglycemia, and irrespective of the arbitrary assessments of "control" employed, most of these patients will have blood glucose levels which persistently fluctuate in the abnormal range. The use of any pharmacologic agent in this group of patients should be justified by excluding the possibility that reduced caloric intake and increased exercise will not remove the threat of symptomatic hyperglycemia.

In present practice the sulfonylureas and the biguanides are often used without adequate indication and under circumstances in which they are unlikely to be of any benefit. In addition, patients are exposed to the expense and potential hazard of prolonged treatment with these agents without adequate concern for their efficacy.

Insulin is the drug of choice when ketoacidosis threatens, or when an acute improvement in symptomatic hyperglycemia is required. In asymptomatic patients with a demonstrated requirement for a pharmacologic hypoglycemic agent, we believe insulin to be preferred, but a well controlled trial of a sulfonylurea is not necessarily contraindicated. Biguanides have no role in the treatment of diabetes mellitus.

References

1. The University Group Diabetes Program: A study of the effects of hypoglycemic agents on vascular complications in patients with adult-onset diabetes. I: Design, methods and baseline results. II: Mortality results. Diabetes 19 (Suppl. 2):747–830, 1970.
2. Knatterud, G. L., Meinert, C. L., Klimt, C. R., et al.: The University Group Diabetes Program: A study of the effects of hypoglycemic agents on vascular complications in patients with adult-onset diabetes. IV. A preliminary report on phenformin results. J.A.M.A. 217:777–784, 1971.
3. Förster, H., Haslbeck, M., and Mehnert, H.: Metabolic studies following the oral ingestion of different doses of glucose. Diabetes 21:1102–1108, 1972.

4. United States Department of Health, Education, and Welfare, Public Health Service, Division of Chronic Diseases: *Genetics and the Epidemiology of Chronic Diseases.* Washington, D.C., Government Printing Office, PHS Publication No. 1163, 1965, p. 113.
5. Winegrad, A. I.: Diabetic neuropathy. (Editorial.) New Eng. J. Med. 286:1261–1262, 1972.
6. Warren, S., Le Compte, P. M., and Legg, M. A.: *The Pathology of Diabetes Mellitus.* Philadelphia, Lea & Febiger, 1966, pp. 200–201.
7. Hazzard, W. R., Goldstein, J. L., Schrott, H. G., et al.: Hyperlipidemia in coronary heart disease: Lipoprotein characteristics of a classification based on genetic analysis. J. Clin. Invest. 51:43a–44a, 1972.
8. Fajans, S. S.: What is diabetes? Definition, diagnosis, and course. Med. Clin. N. Amer. 55:793–805, 1971.
9. Chochinov, R. H., Ullyot, G. L. E., and Moorhouse, J. A.: Sensory perception thresholds in patients with juvenile diabetes and their close relatives. New Eng. J. Med. 286: 1233–1237, 1972.
10. Chopra, J. S., Hurwitz, L. J., and Montgomery, D. A. D.: The pathogenesis of sural nerve changes in diabetes mellitus. Brain 92:391–418, 1969.
11. Siperstein, M. D., Unger, R. H., and Madison, L. L.: Studies of muscle capillary basement membranes in normal subjects, diabetic and prediabetic subjects. J. Clin. Invest. 47:1973–1999, 1968.
12. Kilo, C., Vogler, N., and Williamson, J. R.: Muscle capillary basement membrane changes related to aging and to diabetes mellitus. Diabetes 21:881–905, 1972.
13. Østerby, R.: Diabetic glomerulopathy. A quantitative electron microscopic study of the initial phases, Diabetes: Proceedings of the Seventh Congress of the International Diabetes Federation, Buenos Aires, August 23–28, 1970 (International Congress Series No. 231). Edited by R. R. Rodriguez and J. Vallance-Owen. Amsterdam, Excerpta Medica, 1971, pp. 793–803.
14. Leuenberger, L., Cameron, D., Stauffacher, W., et al.: Ocular lesions in rats rendered chronically diabetic with streptozotocin. Ophthal. Res. 2:189–204, 1971.
15. Goldner, M. G., Knatterud, G. L., and Prout, T. E.: The University Group Diabetes Program: Effects of hypoglycemic agents on vascular complications in patients with adult-onset diabetes. III. Clinical implications of the UGDP results. J.A.M.A. 218: 1400–1410, 1971.
16. Grey, N., and Kipnis, D. M.: Effect of diet composition on the hyperinsulinemia of obesity. New Eng. J. Med. 285:827–831, 1971.
17. Brunzell, J. D., Lerner, R. L., Hazzard, W. R., et al.: Improved glucose tolerance with high carbohydrate feeding in mild diabetes. New Eng. J. Med. 284:521–524, 1971.
18. Levy, R. I., Fredrickson, D. S., Shulman, R., et al.: Dietary and drug treatment of primary hyperlipoproteinemia. Ann. Intern. Med. 77:267–294, 1972.
19. Björntorp, P., Fahlén, M., Grimby, G., et al.: The effects of physical training and acute physical work on plasma insulin in obesity. Europ. J. Clin. Invest. 2:274, 1972.
20. Krall, L. P.: The oral hypoglycemic agents. *In* Marble, A., White, P., Bradley, R. F., and Krall, L. P. (eds.): *Joslin's Diabetes Mellitus.* Philadelphia, Lea & Febiger, 1971, p. 315.
21. Kipnis, D. M.: Insulin secretion in normal and diabetic individuals. Advances Intern. Med. 16:103–134, 1970.
22. Schlichtkrull, J., Brange, J., Christiansen, A. H., et al.: Clinical aspects of insulin-antigenicity. Diabetes 21(Suppl. 2):649–656, 1972.
23. Root, M. A., Chance, R. E., and Galloway, J. A.: Immunogenicity of insulin. Diabetes 21 (Suppl. 2):657–660, 1972.
24. Seltzer, H. S.: Drug-induced hypoglycemia: A review based on 473 cases. Diabetes 21:955–966, 1972.
25. Weissman, P. N., Shenkman, L., and Gregerman, R. I.: Chlorpropamide hyponatremia: Drug-induced inappropriate antidiuretic-hormone activity. New Eng. J. Med. 284: 65–71, 1971.
26. Brown, J., and Solomon, D. H.: Effects of tolbutamide and carbutamide on thyroid function. Metabolism 5:813–819, 1956.
27. Lasseter, K. C., Levey, G. S., Palmer, R. F., et al.: The effect of sulfonylurea drugs on rabbit myocardial contractility, canine purkinje fiber automaticity, and adenyl cyclase activity from rabbit and human hearts. J. Clin. Invest. 51:2429–2434, 1972.
28. Stone, D. B., Brown, J. D., and Cox, C. P.: Effect of tolbutamide and phenformin on lipolysis in adipose tissue in vitro. Amer. J. Physiol. 210:26–30, 1966.

29. Kruger, F. A., Altschuld, R. A., Hallobough, S. L., et al.: Studies on the site and mechanism of action on phenformin. II. Phenformin inhibition of glucose transport by the rat intestine. Diabetes 19:50–52, 1970.
30. Kreisberg, R. A., Owen, W. C., and Siegal, A. M.: Hyperlacticacidemia in man: Ethanol-phenformin synergism. J. Clin. Endocrinol. 34:29–35, 1972.
31. Oliva, P. B.: Lactic acidosis. Amer. J. Med. 48:209–225, 1970.
32. Craig, J. W., Miller, M., Woodward, H., et al.: Influence of phenethylbiguanide on lactic, pyruvic, and citric acids in diabetic patients. Diabetes 9:186–193, 1960.
33. Davidson, M. B., Bogarth, W. R., Challoner, D. R., et al.: Phenformin hypoglycemia and lactic acidosis. New Eng. J. Med. 275:886–888, 1966.

Oral Hypoglycemic Agents Are Worthwhile

ROBERT F. BRADLEY

Joslin Clinic, Boston, Massachusetts

The controversy evoked by the University Group Diabetes Program (UGDP) results reported in December, 1970,[1] and a few months later,[2] has quite properly rekindled the interest of clinicians in the need for intensive dietary therapy of the adult maturity-onset diabetic and has provided another example of *possible* insidious effects of foreign compounds administered to humans. It has also exhumed the more basic controversy, namely, that relating to the benefits, if any, which can be gained from the rigid metabolic control of diabetes mellitus, as reviewed previously in the first edition of this text.[3]

The UGDP study by all odds had the best designed and the most laudable objectives of any yet undertaken. Unfortunately as they "eyeballed" the data week by week and month by month and saw first a cluster of deaths in patients treated with variable doses of insulin and then a somewhat larger cluster in those treated with tolbutamide, the biostatisticians held sway. Clinicians, shaken by their lack of expertise in biostatistics and forgetting that the study was not intended to evaluate mortality results,[4] bowed graciously to the intonations of those who extrapolated the data to the maturity-onset diabetic population at large. The tragedy of this issue rests both in the possibility that the implications of the UGDP study are entirely correct, and the equal possibility that they are completely invalid, i.e., that the observed cardiovascular events resulted from a repository of individuals treated with tolbutamide or phenformin who were greater cardiovascular risks at baseline.[5]

Regardless of the many arguments that have been presented pro and con, one must keep in mind the preliminary nature of the results, namely, that the total cardiovascular deaths occurring in the UGDP study represented only 8 per cent of those diabetic patients comprising the entire study population.

The sulfonylureas (carbutamide, tolbutamide, chlorpropamide, acetohexamide, tolazamide, glybenzcyclamide) and biguanides (phenformin, metformin, and buformin) lower blood glucose levels by differing mechanisms. Such an effect of these oral hypoglycemic agents used singly or in combination has been well documented in appropriately selected hyperglycemic individuals and accounts for their widespread usage in the United States and other countries during the past 17 years. In many of the more responsive patients with maturity-onset diabetes, normal blood glucose levels are more readily attainable than with diet or insulin.

Despite numerous reports during the early years of their clinical use that these compounds would effectively lower blood glucose levels in 50 to 75 per cent of maturity-onset diabetics who were not insulin dependent or ketoacidosis-prone and whose diabetes began at age 40 or older, physicians familiar with insidious long-term problems of the diabetic have from the beginning been concerned that patients so treated might be less well controlled and more prone to premature development of these complications than individuals treated with insulin. Experience has provided ample evidence that for one reason or another oral hypoglycemic agents lose their effectiveness at varying but relatively short intervals of time after initiation of treatment. The rate of such "secondary failure" depends upon many factors, including patient selection and dietary cooperation, therapeutic objectives, and the manner in which the oral hypoglycemic agents are used. A lucid presentation of "primary" vs. "secondary failure" and the effect their definition has upon long-term "failure" has recently been published.[6] The element of convenience for middle-aged and elderly people is obvious, but always has had to be balanced against the increased cost for those who took more than minimal doses and the possibility that physicians and patients alike would rely too heavily upon their effectiveness, so that diet would be either ignored or less carefully followed.

If benefit is to be anticipated from lowering blood glucose levels as well as reversing lipid, protein, and other metabolic abnormalities associated with insulin deficit, what should be the blood glucose levels attained? From the early days of their use, many sets of criteria have been utilized by those involved in the study of diabetic patients. In general, these have fallen into two categories: (1) those who consider the oral hypoglycemic agents effective despite blood glucose levels in excess of normal, provided the symptoms of diabetes have been relieved and remain so, and (2) others, such as Marble and his associates,[7] including this author, whose objective has been normoglycemia and aglycosuria, in accordance with the criteria originally published by Camerini-Davalos et al. in 1957[8] (Table 1). In defense of the former is the fact that in many maturity-onset diabetic patients whose blood glucose levels remain elevated despite dietary adherence, the addition of oral hypoglycemic agents lowers blood glucose levels to a degree comparable to that readily obtained with insulin and relieves symptoms, so that little would be gained by insisting upon a more rigid standard of metabolic control. Recognizing that evidence for the benefits of tight metabolic control remains controversial, the adoption of such standards would seem to be reasonable. On the other hand, if it is true that protection from long-term complications is attainable only through the more rigid control of blood glucose levels, the latter criteria should be applied, and if the standards are not attained, more relentless application of diet and insulin if necessary is required. At present the fundamental controversy continues to be that related to the possible benefits of such control. Considerable new evidence is available today, unfortunately no

Table 1. *Joslin Clinic Standard for Blood Glucose Control in Diabetic Patients Treated with Oral Hypoglycemic Compounds: Standards of Control* and Degree of Control†*

RELATION TO FOOD	GOOD Blood Sugar‡ (mg./100 ml.)	GOOD Urine Sugar (per cent)	FAIR Blood Sugar‡ (mg./100 ml.)	FAIR Urine Sugar (per cent)	POOR
Fasting	110	Trace	130	0.1	All other cases
1 hr. p.c.	150	0.3	180	0.5	
2 hr. p.c.	130	0.1	150	0.3	
3 hr. p.c.	110	Trace	130	0.1	

*For purpose of classification as to degree of control 70 per cent or more of values must conform with standards listed in the table.
†These standard values are the highest acceptable.
‡Glucose as determined by the Somogyi-Nelson procedure.

more conclusive than the data of 20 years ago. Meanwhile the practicing physician is busily and assuredly attempting to lower blood cholesterol levels, but is not certain how assiduously to work toward lowering blood glucose levels, and if so, how much.

A major concern has been the possibility that these oral agents might produce or allow the earlier development of the following: (1) islet cell failure with consequent decompensation of endogenous insulin function and greater activity of the diabetes; (2) infections; (3) neuropathy; (4) cataracts; (5) onset or more rapid progression of microangiopathy; and (6) greater morbidity and/or mortality from accelerated macroangiopathy, particularly that involving the coronary, cerebral, and peripheral vasculature. Because no good evidence had ever been presented to suggest that oral hypoglycemic agents were "antidiabetic," which would mean that they were inherently capable of delaying or preventing these more serious problems, the only reasonable benefit to be expected would be consequent to a net increase in the effectiveness of endogenous insulin, as indicated by lowering of the blood glucose level over and above that obtainable with diet. Thus, if significant lowering of blood glucose levels could not be attained and then maintained, there would be no basis for using any of the currently available oral hypoglycemic agents. The extent to which oral hypoglycemic agents have succeeded or failed with regard to these potential problems will be briefly reviewed.

ISLET CELL FUNCTION

That sulfonylureas lower blood glucose levels primarily by increasing insulin secretion from the pancreas has been definitely proved.[6] However, it has long been contended by some investigators that extrapancreatic effects of sulfonylureas, particularly those related to hepatic glucose release, contribute to the effects upon glucose.[6] Recently considerable data have confirmed extrapancreatic actions, which are demonstrable in the absence of insulin at cellular sites and with concentration of drug compatible with the clinical setting.[9] In addition, a portion of the effects of sulfonylureas may relate to inhibition of cyclic AMP phosphodiesterase, with a consequent net increase in cyclic AMP.[10]

One must also keep in mind the significant, and sometimes serious, hypoglycemia induced by sulfonylurea drugs. None of those currently available is an exception. Some of these enhanced hypoglycemic effects of the sulfonylureas have been related to the coincident use of other drugs such as salicylates, monamine oxidase inhibitors, phenylbutazone, sulfonamides, sulfisoxazole, sulfaphenazole, coumarin anticoagulants, and phenyramidol.

Occasional patients on sulfonylurea drugs are suspected of having a rapid loss of endogenous insulin function because it appeared necessary after a short period of treatment to give insulin to control the diabetes. Such observations obviously have suggested that the sulfonylurea might have accelerated the depletion of pancreatic insulin. However, studies in animals chronically treated with sulfonylureas have not supported this concept. Rather, there has been consistent histologic evidence of an increase in the number of beta cell mitoses, hypertrophy of the islets, and an increase in mass of islet tissue.[6, 9]

No data have been presented to suggest that biguanides "wear out" the insulin mechanism. The means by which biguanides lower blood glucose levels in diabetics, but not in normal humans, remains uncertain. By whatever means they act, these substances lower blood glucose levels in diabetic individuals having some available endogenous or exogenous insulin, albeit more gradually than is noted in responsive diabetic individuals following sulfonylureas. Available endogenous or administered insulin simply appears to be more effective when phenformin or other biguanides are administered. In the absence of any demonstrable effect of these compounds upon the pancreatic islet cell, it is not surprising there is no evidence thus far that diabetes is worsened metabolically by their administration.

A number of studies have suggested that sulfonylureas or biguanides may ameliorate "chemical" or "latent" diabetes[6] (as defined by the American Diabetes Association[11]). Although inconclusive, observations of no adverse effects have now accumulated for a sufficient number of years to allow one to assume that at least no worsening of the diabetes is likely to be produced.

INFECTION

At one time the increased susceptibility of the diabetic to invasive local and systemic infection accounted for an important portion of the morbidity and mortality among diabetics. With improved control of diabetes following the availability of insulin and the proper use of antibiotic treatment, infections in the diabetic now pose much less of a problem.

Recent studies have helped to clarify the issue as to whether the diabetic is indeed more susceptible to infection. Defects in host defense can be related to the degrees of hyperglycemia and/or ketoacidosis.[12, 13] Uncontrolled diabetes of short duration may not be associated with a great likelihood of infection, but when present over a period of weeks and months the patient becomes more susceptible. Thus far no studies have clearly defined the critical degree or duration of uncontrolled diabetes, but metabolic control is well accepted as a fundamental part of the preventive program in avoiding fungal infection and active tuberculosis, as well as bacterial infection. Perhaps the most common and easily demonstrable example clinically is the persistence of Candida infections producing vulvovaginitis in the female and balanitis in the male, responding poorly to specific therapy such as nystatin or gentian violet but dramatically improving with the cessation of or marked improvement in excessive glycosuria and hyperglycemia. Such improvement is readily shown to occur in the diabetic patient responsive to oral hypoglycemic therapy, with rapidity of improvement comparable to that obtained with insulin. Similar responses can be obtained in certain patients with nearly normal endogenous insulin reserve upon application of diet and, of course, with the administration of insulin.

To date there has been no indication in patients responsive to oral hypoglycemic agents, when properly combined with reasonable dietary adherence, that new infection or aggravation of existing infection has occurred as a result of the use of oral rather than insulin therapy.

NEUROPATHY

No controlled studies have proved that metabolic control prevents the development of neuropathy. However, neuropathy, particularly the more severe types such as amyotrophy, anesthetic feet, Charcot joints, and so forth, classically develops in the adult who seems to have had a short duration of diabetes, but who was unknowingly hyperglycemic for a period of time, or in the patient with known diabetes of longer duration in whom therapy was inappropriate or inadequate. Although diabetic patients may at times have an exacerbation of symptoms due to neuropathy following treatment of any kind, and although on occasion hypoglycemia may itself induce neuropathy, the *usual* clinical observation is that following improved metabolic control by whatever means, many manifestations of neuropathy improve sooner or later.

Recent biochemical data demonstrating the presence of the polyol pathway in nerve suggest a mechanism by which increased ambient glucose concentrations in the Schwann cell activate the formation of sorbitol,[14] so that nerve function may be compromised. To date the critical circulating blood glucose levels for activation of this pathway have not been clearly demonstrated, but its possible major metabolic role in the production of neuropathy provides further evidence for the desirability of keeping blood glucose levels as close to normal as is readily obtainable.

CATARACTS

At least two morphologic types of cataract occur in diabetes. These are: (1) the snowflake, flocculent, or metabolic cataract, occurring mainly in juveniles with grossly uncontrolled diabetes; and (2) the senile cataract due to sclerosis of the lens nucleus, indistinguishable from that seen in the nondiabetic and the commonest type observed in adult diabetic patients. The more rapid maturation of senile cataract in the diabetic than in the nondiabetic has recently been re-emphasized by studies showing grossly poorer diabetic control in patients having cataract extraction than among the average patients attending a diabetic clinic.[15] These observations, and demonstrations of the appropriate enzymes in the lens of man for activation of the polyol pathway by existing hyperglycemia,[16, 17] lend considerable support to the long-held opinion that poorly controlled diabetes is a factor in the rate of maturation in senile cataract as well as in the development of metabolic or snowflake cataract.[15, 18]

Although of lesser importance, the well known relation of refractive changes in the eye of the diabetic to changing blood glucose levels would be still another basis for adequate blood glucose control, at least in terms of the quality of daily living.

Microangiopathy

The microangiopathy of diabetes involves small blood vessels, particularly capillaries supplying many tissues. The possible value of careful metabolic control in protecting the individual from clinically important retinal and/or renal vascular disease has been the subject of major controversy for 25 years. The UGDP study was directed in major part toward seeking an answer to this question. Thus far, neither the prospective UGDP study nor other studies, all wholly or in part retrospective in nature, have proved conclusively that significant benefit is to be gained from any tighter control of the metabolic components of diabetes than is necessary to avoid the symptoms of diabetes, ketoacidosis, and so forth. Detailed reviews of this subject have either supported no relationship between careful metabolic control and the prevention of microangiopathy,[19] or indicated that such control improves the chances of preventing severer grades of clinical microangiopathy, such as retinitis proliferans and/or nephropathy with renal failure.[20]

Despite the lack of unanimity concerning this controversy, recent biochemical data tend to shift the weight of evidence in the direction of favoring tight metabolic control. In particular, the observations of Spiro regarding the role of hyperglycemia as a stimulus to the biosynthesis of basement membrane material of the renal glomerulus,[21, 22] and observations of basement membrane thickening showing an apparent correlation with duration of insulin deficit,[23] appear to bolster the practice of those physicians who strive for normoglycemia.

Meanwhile, although not specifically related to effects upon microangiopathy, sufficient data have accumulated to support the role of striving for normoglycemia as assiduously as possible in assuring survival of the fetus of the diabetic mother.[24, 25]

Macroangiopathy

Although neuropathy, increased susceptibility to infection, and microangiopathy are the most specific manifestations of diabetes mellitus and are of particular concern because of their adverse effects upon many younger patients, the overall greatest problem in terms of morbidity and mortality is that related to involvement of medium and larger vessels, especially the coronary, cerebral and lower extremity arteries. The prevalence of such vascular lesions is high in the

Table 2. *Causes of Death in 912 Diabetics
(Per Cent of Total Deaths)
1966–1969**

Vascular disease, total	74.3
Cardiac	54.6
Renal	8.0
Cerebrovascular	10.0
Gangrene, "circulatory"	1.7
Cancer	12.8
Infectious, Non-TBC	5.9
All others	6.0

*Experience of the Joslin Clinic.

general population, but cardiovascular disease as a cause of death is nearly doubled in the diabetic. Table 2 shows that cardiovascular causes account for at least two thirds of the mortality in the diabetic population as a whole. With such a high frequency and with so many factors other than diabetes playing a potential role, any attempts to assess the possible benefits of diabetes treatment are extremely difficult to evaluate. An additional problem in trying to judge the effects of therapy directed toward improved diabetes control is that in the adult maturity-onset diabetic the duration of hyperglycemia is extremely difficult to ascertain, except in those individuals who have been subjected to blood glucose measurements from early in life either because of a family history or as part of routine examinations.

Many observations relate vascular disease of medium-sized arteries to the presence of hyperglycemia.[26] Perhaps the earliest, and certainly one of the most striking, has been derived from the huge autopsy series of Bell at the University of Minnesota[27] (Table 3), which points out the extraordinary prevalence of peripheral vascular disease and gangrene in the hyperglycemic individual. Such associations appear to justify efforts of physicians within reason to provide "metabolic control" of diabetes.

In the clinical use of oral hypoglycemic agents, the assumption has been that lowering blood glucose would reverse the metabolic abnormalities related to insulin deficits, such as those in protein and lipid metabolism, much as such defects are reversible with comparable degrees of blood glucose lowering following insulin. As has been summarized elsewhere,[28] various types of circulating lipid abnormalities are reversible with sulfonylureas in those patients who have sufficient endogenous insulin, such that blood glucose levels fall to normal following the administration of one of these oral agents. On the other hand, a number of

Table 3. *Results of Autopsies Following Atherosclerotic Gangrene**

	NONDIABETIC (59,733) (PER CENT)		DIABETIC (2130) (PER CENT)		RATIO OF FREQUENCY
Age	M	F	M	F	Diabetic/Nondiabetic
20–40	0	0	3.4	0	All Ages > 40
40–60	0.1	0.08	14.7	14.0	M 53:1
60–80	0.45	0.46	24.3	24.6	F 71:1

*From Bell, E. T.: Amer. J. Clin. Path. 28:27, 1957.

reports have demonstrated persisting abnormalities in cholesterol, free fatty acids, and triglycerides in individuals who were receiving a sulfonylurea, but on close inspection of the data, "control" was determined only by measurements of fasting blood glucose levels, and even these were persistently elevated. However, abnormalities in circulating lipids associated with imperfect management of diabetes using oral hypoglycemic agents have been shown to be reversible by the addition of sufficient insulin to improve blood glucose levels.[28] This observation has been one of the factors which have supported the use of more rigid blood glucose criteria as an objective in treatment with oral hypoglycemic agents, be they sulfonylureas or biguanides. Thus far there is no clear-cut evidence that blood lipid abnormalities due to relative insulin deficit are more or less likely to be preventable or reversible at comparable blood glucose levels whether insulin or oral hypoglycemic agents are used.

A real problem has been the tendency for physicians to use oral hypoglycemic agents not in an ideal manner, but rather for the sake of convenience, with too little emphasis upon diet, adequate choice or dosage of the agent used, or proper selection of the patient. In such situations, obviously, the performance of oral hypoglycemic agents should be less effective than that of insulin, assuming that control of blood glucose and lipid abnormalities are indeed important in slowing down progression of macroangiopathy.

The above observations are critical in evaluating studies such as the University Group Diabetes Program (UGDP), which recorded more cardiovascular deaths in patients receiving tolbutamide or phenformin than in those treated with diet and placebo, diet and standard dose of insulin, or diet and a variable dose of insulin. The results may be interpreted as follows: (1) If it is true that tolbutamide, as a result of an inotropic effect upon the myocardium[29] or via some other mechanism, and an unrelated compound such as phenformin, through some unidentified mechanism, actually contribute to cardiovascular death, the seriousness of this particular end point would weigh so heavily that the use of these oral hypoglycemic agents should be summarily discontinued. (2) On the other hand, if these oral agents were seemingly less effective because of their improper use, the question is whether the results would be improved by correct usage and what the criteria should be for such usage. (3) The third possibility is that inadvertent significant differences in baseline cardiovascular risk factors accounted for the less favorable cardiovascular mortality experience in those treated with tolbutamide or phenformin and that the study does not prove or disprove lack of effectiveness for tolbutamide up to the time it was discontinued from the study (October, 1969) or for phenformin (discontinued January, 1971). The latter is more than a mere possibility, for the interpretations of UGDP results by the investigators, the American Diabetes Association,[30] the Council on Drugs of the American Medical Association,[31] and the U.S. Food and Drug Administration[32] are based upon statistical grounds that do not take into account the clinical background of knowledge concerning coronary heart disease in the diabetic. The many flaws in the UGDP study make any extrapolation of the results to the diabetic population at large extremely hazardous, and a number of objections remain apparent to the clinician:

1. In placebo treated patients not a single myocardial infarction was recorded among the cardiovascular deaths.

2. A characteristic feature of cardiovascular mortality in the diabetic is the female predisposition to dying, equaling or exceeding that observed among males.[26] UGDP findings of fewer than one half as many cardiovascular deaths in females as compared to males in placebo treated diabetics indicated a lack of full expression of the effects of diabetes upon cardiovascular mortality in this group; i.e., the diabetes was milder and/or of shorter duration, or the numbers were too small.

3. Cardiovascular risk factors at baseline were present wtih greater frequency in patients on tolbutamide than in those treated with placebo or with small fixed doses of insulin ("insulin standard"). Although only one factor, blood cholesterol levels equal to or greater than 300 mg./100 ml., reached statistical significance in its greater frequency in tolbutamide treated patients, out of a total of 10 baseline risk factors, nine occurred more often in the tolbutamide treated than in the placebo group. On comparison with "insulin standard" treated patients, seven cardiovascular risk factors were present at baseline with greater frequency in tolbutamide treated patients as compared to three affecting more patients in the "insulin standard" group.

4. The prevalence of coronary heart disease as evidenced by "significant ECG abnormality" at baseline was extremely low in all treatment groups (Table 4), especially in view of the higher frequencies of digitalis usage, of angina pectoris, and of ECG abnormalities in diabetics of comparable age reported in the literature.[26, 33] When the original baseline findings were reported by the UGDP investigators in 1967, different criteria for ECG abnormality were used, so that on the basis of the electrocardiogram, a distinctly greater prevalence of coronary heart disease was reported in the tolbutamide as compared to placebo, insulin standard, or insulin variable groups of patients.[34]

5. The duration of diabetes among patients entering the UGDP study were indeterminate. However, elevated fasting blood glucose and greater increments of post glucose blood levels were found in more tolbutamide treated patients at baseline than in any other treatment group. Therefore, more tolbutamide treated patients had severer and/or longer durations of diabetes mellitus.

6. For an end point (cardiovascular mortality) having an extremely high prevalence in the diabetic population in which a number of risk factors, both

Table 4. *UGDP Study—1967* vs. 1970†*
Selected Baseline Cardiovascular Risk Factors

	PLACEBO		TOLBUTAMIDE		INSULIN STAND.		INSULIN VARIABLE		TOTAL	
	No.	Per Cent	No.	Per Cent	No.	Per Cent	No.	Per Cent	No.	Per Cent
Significant ECG abnormality 1967	30	(15.2)	48	(24.0)	40	(19.3)	39	(19.3)	157	(19.4)
Significant ECG abnormality 1970	6	(3.0)	8	(4.0)	11	(5.3)	8	(4.0)	33	(4.1)
History of digitalis use	9	(4.5)	15	(7.6)	12	(5.8)	10	(5.0)	46	(5.7)
History of angina pectoris	10	(5.0)	14	(7.0)	16	(7.7)	7	(3.5)	47	(5.8)

*Reference 34.
†Reference 1.

known and unknown, were present, the number of individuals reaching that end point was too small to permit a definitive conclusion.

Summary

The benefits of oral hypoglycemic agents are limited to those diabetic patients who are responsive, in that symptoms of diabetes are absent and blood glucose levels are significantly and consistently lowered (20 per cent or more) below pretreatment values. Under these conditions, benefits may be summarized as *definite* or *qualified*.

DEFINITE

1. Convenience.
2. In those with diminished vision, arthritis, or other problems, who find injection of insulin difficult or impossible.
3. For individuals whose diabetes is not controllable by diet and whose employment and/or economic status might be jeopardized by the taking of insulin.
4. In certain patients with allergy to insulin, in whom desensitization is difficult or cannot readily be maintained.
5. In truly responsive diabetics in whom normoglycemia is more readily attained than with insulin.

QUALIFIED

If lowering of lipid and other metabolic abnormalities related to insulin deficit are important in protecting the diabetic from earlier progression of vascular lesions and neuropathy, as well as from infection, the use of oral hypoglycemic agents is of benefit in patients who attain "significantly" lower blood glucose values than are attainable by use of diet alone. My criteria for such blood glucose values are that on two out of three occasions the blood glucose, whenever drawn, is normal.

Data from the UGDP study have thus far contributed nothing to the controversy regarding the effectiveness of blood glucose control and are sufficiently in doubt as to the apparent lesser benefits of tolbutamide and phenformin as compared to diet alone or diet and insulin, so that the results cannot at present be extrapolated to the diabetic population at large. They do not warrant discontinuation of the appropriate routine clinical use of oral hypoglycemic agents.

References

1. The University Group Diabetes Program: A study of the effects of hypoglycemic agents on vascular complications in patients with adult onset diabetes. II. Mortality results: Diabetes 19(Suppl. 2):789, 1970.

2. Knatterud, G. L., Meinert, C. L., Klimt, C. R., Osborne, R. K., and Martin, D. B.: Effects of hypoglycemic agents on vascular complications in patients with adult-onset diabetes. IV. A preliminary report on phenformin results. J.A.M.A. 217:777, 1971.
3. Marble, A.: Control of diabetes lessens or postpones vascular complications. In Ingelfinger, F. J., Relman, A. S., and Finland, M. (eds.): Controversy in Internal Medicine. Philadelphia, W. B. Saunders Company, 1966, p. 491.
4. Feinstein, A. R.: An analytic appraisal of the University Group Diabetes Program (UGDP) Study. Clin. Pharmacol. Ther. 12:167, 1971.
5. Keen, H., and Jarrett, R. J.: Effects of oral hypoglycemic agents on cardiovascular disease. In Fajans, S. S., and Sussman, K. E. (eds.): Diabetes Mellitus: Diagnosis and Treatment. Vol. III. New York, American Diabetes Association, Inc., 1971, p. 167.
6. Krall, L. P.: The oral hypoglycemic agents. In Marble, A., White, P., Bradley, R. F., and Krall, L. P. (eds.): Joslin's Diabetes Mellitus. 11th ed. Philadelphia, Lea & Febiger, 1971, p. 302.
7. Balodimos, M. C., Gleason, R. E., Bradley, R. F., and Marble, A.: Long-term tolbutamide therapy in diabetes. A controlled study of the frequency of cardiovascular disease and other findings. In Butterfield, W. J. H., and Van Westering, W. (eds.): Tolbutamide . . . after Ten Years. Proceedings of the Brook Lodge Symposium, Augusta, Michigan, March 6–7, 1967. Amsterdam, Excerpta Medica Foundation, 1967, p. 270.
8. Camerini-Davalos, R., Root, H. F., and Marble, A.: Clinical experiences with carbutamide (BZ-55). Diabetes 6:74, 1957.
9. Lebovitz, H. E., and Feldman, J. M.: Oral hypoglycemic agents: Mechanisms of action. In Fajans, S. S., and Sussman, K. E., (eds.): Diabetes Mellitus: Diagnosis and Treatment. Vol. III. New York, American Diabetes Association, Inc., 1971, p. 147.
10. Roth, J., Prout, T. E., Goldfine, I. D., Wolfe, S. M., Muenzer, J., Grauer, L. E., and Marcus, M. L.: Sulfonylureas: Effects in vivo and in vitro. (NIH Conferences.) Ann. Intern. Med. 75:607, 1971.
11. Fajans, S. S.: Classification and natural history of genetic diabetes mellitus. In Fajans, S. S., and Sussman, K. E. (eds.): Diabetes Mellitus: Diagnosis and Treatment. Vol. III. New York, American Diabetes Association, Inc., 1971, p. 89.
12. Bagdade, J. D.: Infections. In Fajans, S. S., and Sussman, K. E. (eds.): Diabetes Mellitus: Diagnosis and Treatment. Vol. III. New York, American Diabetes Association, Inc., 1971, p. 211.
13. Younger, D., and Hadley, W. B.: Infection and diabetes. In Marble, A., White, P., Bradley, R. F. and Krall, L. P. (eds.): Joslin's Diabetes Mellitus. 11th ed. Philadelphia, Lea & Febiger, 1971, p. 621.
14. Prockop, L. D.: Diabetic neuropathy. In Fajans, S. S., and Sussman, K. E. (eds.): Diabetes Mellitus: Diagnosis and Treatment. Vol. III. New York, American Diabetes Association, Inc., 1971, p. 347.
15. Clinical aspects of cataract in diabetes. In Caird, F. I., Pirie, A., and Ramsell, T. G. (eds.): Diabetes and the Eye. Oxford, Blackwell Scientific Publications, 1969, p. 127.
16. Winegrad, A. I., Clements, R. S., and Morrison, A. D.: In Fajans, S. S., and Sussman, K. E. (eds.): Diabetes Mellitus: Diagnosis and Treatment. Vol. III, New York, American Diabetes Association, Inc., 1971, p. 269.
17. The metabolism of the lens in relation to lens opacities in diabetes. In Caird, F. I., Pirie, A., and Ramsell, T. G. (eds.): Diabetes and the Eye. Oxford, Blackwell Scientific Publications, 1969, p. 140.
18. Bradley, R. F., and Ramos, E.: The eyes and diabetes. In Marble, A., White, P., Bradley, R. F., and Krall, L. P. (eds.): Joslin's Diabetes Mellitus. 11th ed. Philadelphia, Lea & Febiger, 1971, p. 478.
19. Knowles, H. C., Jr., Guest, G. M., Lampe, J. Kessler, M., and Skillman. T. G.: The course of juvenile diabetes treated with unmeasured diet. Diabetes 14:239, 1965.
20. Marble, A.: Angiopathy in diabetes: An unsolved problem. (The Banting Memorial Lecture.) Diabetes 16:825, 1967.
21. Spiro, R. G.: Pathophysiology. B. Biochemical basis of the diabetic microangiopathy. In Fajans, S. S., and Sussman, K. E. (eds.): Diabetes Mellitus: Diagnosis and Treatment. Vol. III, New York, American Diabetes Association, Inc., 1971, p. 275.
22. Spiro, R. G., and Spiro, M. J.: Effect of diabetes on the biosynthesis of the renal glomerular basement membrane. Diabetes 20:641, 1971.
23. Kilo, C., Vogler, N. J. and Williamson, J. R.: Basement membrane thickening in diabetes. In Fajans, S. S., and Sussman, K. E. (eds.): Diabetes Mellitus: Diagnosis and Treatment. Vol. III. New York, American Diabetes Association, Inc., 1971, p. 289.

24. White, P.: Pregnancy and diabetes. *In* Marble, A., White, P., Bradley, R. F., and Krall, L. P. (eds.): *Joslin's Diabetes Mellitus.* 11th ed. Philadelphia, Lea & Febiger, 1971, p. 581.
25. Pedersen, J.: Management of the pregnant diabetic. *In* Fajans, S. S., and Sussman, K. E. (eds.): *Diabetes Mellitus: Diagnosis and Treatment.* Vol. III, New York, American Diabetes Association, Inc., 1971, p. 235.
26. Bradley, R. F.: Cardiovascular disease. *In* Marble, A., White, P., Bradley, R. F., and Krall, L. P. (eds.): *Joslin's Diabetes Mellitus.* 11th ed. Philadelphia, Lea & Febiger, 1971, p. 417.
27. Bell, E. T.: Atherosclerotic gangrene of the lower extremities in diabetic and non-diabetic persons. Amer. J. Clin. Path. 28:27, 1957.
28. Bradley, R. F.: Cardiovascular disease. In Marble, A., White, P., Bradley, R. F., and Krall, L. P. (eds.): *Joslin's Diabetes Mellitus.* 11th ed. Philadelphia, Lea & Febiger, 1971, p. 429–430.
29. Levey, G. S., Palmer, R. G., Lasseter, K. C., and McCarthy, J.: Effect of tolbutamide on adenyl cyclase in rabbit and human heart and contractility of isolated rabbit atria. J. Clin. Endocr. 33:371, 1971.
30. Ricketts, H. T.: Editorial Statement. October 7, 1970. Diabetes 19(Suppl. 2):iii–v, 1970.
31. A.M.A. Council on Drugs: Statement regarding the University Group Diabetes Program (UGDP) Study. November 2, 1970. Diabetes 19(Suppl. 2):vi–vii, 1970.
32. *Food and Drug Administration Current Drug Information Bulletin,* October 30, 1970.
33. Bryfogle, J. W., and Bradley, R. F.: The vascular complications of diabetes mellitus. A clinical study. Diabetes 6:159, 1957.
34. Klimt, C. R., Meinert, C. L., Miller, M., and Knowles, H. C.: University Group Diabetes Program (UGDP): A study of the relationships of therapy to vascular and other complications of diabetes. *In* Butterfield, W. J. H., and Van Westering, W. (eds.): *Tolbutamide . . . After Ten Years.* Amsterdam, Excerpta Medica Foundation, 1967, p. 261.

Comment

Management of Adult-Onset Diabetes

The central issue here is the status of oral hypoglycemic agents. There is no doubt that these drugs can lower the blood sugar in the majority of patients with adult-onset diabetes who are not insulin dependent. But what are the indications for the use of these agents? How frequently, and for how long, can one expect to maintain effective diabetic control in those patients who respond initially? Most important of all, does the long-term use of oral agents produce any complications beyond those to be expected in comparable groups of patients treated with diet alone or with diet and insulin? These questions, the present controversy makes clear, are not much closer to resolution now than they were 10 or 15 years ago, when oral agents first came into widespread use.

Concerning the indications for the use of these agents, the two papers in this section seem to differ more in emphasis than substance. Bradley, reflecting the current philosophy of the Joslin Clinic, stresses the usefulness and convenience of hypoglycemic pills in a wide variety of adult-onset patients and seems to suggest that pills ought to be used in all diabetic patients whose blood glucose levels can be adequately controlled by this means. Winegrad and his colleagues, on the other hand, while conceding the convenience and apparent effectiveness of pills in many patients, emphasize that these agents are often used unnecessarily and unwisely. They urge that oral agents should not be used without an adequate prior trial of weight reduction.

Elimination of obesity by diet and exercise is an admirable goal, certainly worth trying if achievable, but it seems to me that we must recognize how seldom even the most conscientious physician succeeds in getting his middle aged overweight patients to change permanently their eating and exercise habits. It is far easier for the patient to take a pill than it is to change ingrained patterns of behavior. If he believes that a pill will lower his blood sugar and control his diabetic symptoms, the average diabetic is not likely to accept his physician's advice to try diet and exercise instead, unless perhaps there is clear-cut evidence that he will be much better off in the long run.

Both essays refer to the phenomenon of "secondary failure" and agree that the incidence is variable because acquired resistance to pills depends upon many factors. Nevertheless, Bradley implies that the proper use of oral agents will keep the blood sugar and serum lipids under satisfactory control in a large percentage of those who respond initially, while Winegrad and his colleagues say that there is very little information to support this view.

As for the much discussed UGDP study of cardiovascular complications in patients treated with oral agents, both contributors agree that the data are not convincing. This, in fact, appears to be the prevailing view of most practicing physicians, for at present there seems to be no inclination to avoid the use of tolbutamide, or any of the other sulfonylurea drugs, in the long-term management of responsive diabetics. For reasons that are not necessarily related to the UGDP study, the status of phenformin is more uncertain. Winegrad and colleagues argue that this agent should not be employed because it meets no special need, its mechanism of action is not likely to correct the underlying metabolic defects of insulin deficiency, and it probably causes severe lactic acidosis in some patients. Bradley, in defending the thesis that "oral hypoglycemic agents are worthwhile," does not distinguish between the sulfonylureas and phenformin. In my view, however, the weight of evidence clearly supports Winegrad's position on phenformin. Although there may well be good reason for continuing the prudent use of the sulfonylureas, it is hard to avoid real concern about the biguanides.

The whole question of vascular disease in diabetes remains, of course, the primary concern of all those who treat this disease. Both essayists here agree that the relation of control to vascular complications remains unsettled but, as might be expected, Bradley believes that the avilable evidence justifies efforts to maintain strict control of blood sugar, whereas Winegrad and his colleagues are more skeptical. This perennial issue was the subject of one of the controversies in the first edition of this series, and it is reviewed again briefly in the chapter "Controversy I Revisited."

ARNOLD S. RELMAN

16

Thyroid Nodules

Most Solitary Thyroid Nodules Should Be Removed
    by Leslie J. DeGroot

Thyroid Nodules: Surgery Is Usually Not Necessary
    by Monte A. Greer

Comment
    by Robert D. Utiger

Most Solitary Thyroid Nodules Should Be Removed*

LESLIE J. DEGROOT

University of Chicago

Physicians unimpressed with the malignant potential of thyroid nodules defend their position with statements that these nodules rarely prove to be lethal neoplasms, that growth of those which are histologically differentiated cancers can be suppressed by thyroxine, and that, in any event, surgery would not help patients who have an aggressive or invasive tumor. The position we have taken is certainly diametrically opposed to the foregoing in spirit, if not always in practice. We recognize that to prove without doubt the merits of a particular point of view is as difficult in this area of medicine as in many others. Faced with the uncertainty of the data base as discussed later, we usually advise our patients to have what appear to be discrete thyroid nodules resected, as soon as convenient, by a knowledgeable surgeon.

It may be important to note that the problem herein considered is in regard to nodules that come to the attention of an examining physician, not necessarily the entire incidence of nodules in the population. The prevalence in the general population of thyroid nodules, at least half of which appear to be single, may be in the order of 4 per cent, judging from the data of the Framingham study.[1] It can be assumed that the prevalence of microscopically or macroscopically detectable nodularity that could be observed by a pathologist would be considerably greater, if we extrapolate from data obtained on autopsies prior to 1955.[2] (Of course, the influence of increased iodide intake in the past five to 10 years on the histologic picture of the thyroid is unknown and may have reduced the incidence from figures obtained two decades ago.) Again, estimating from the Framingham study, nodules develop or at least become recognizable with an incidence of approximately 0.1 per cent per year.[3] We are, however, not discussing in this article the problem of what to do with every thyroid nodule in the population. Rather, we are discussing the appropriate therapy for those that come to the

---

* Supported in part by United States Public Health Service Grant AM-13,377.

attention of the physician, which may represent a distinct subpopulation. Probably less than one quarter of the nodules in the population eventually do come to surgery.[3] Of those that filter through the selection process, including "cocktail party" observation, family physician screening, palpation by the gynecologist, referral to an internist, endocrinologist, or surgeon, and finally reach the microscope of the pathologist, a significant proportion turn out not to be discrete nodules, but rather to be multinodular goiters in which one portion of the gland is especially prominent. This may account for half of all the alleged single thyroid nodules.[4] The final incidence of pathologically diagnosed thyroid carcinoma in specimens resected because of the presence of a "clinical solitary nodule" is variable, but typical figures are 8 to 20 per cent.[4-6] Over the past three and a half years in our own institution, 104 patients have been operated on for a suspicion of thyroid carcinoma, and of these 36 per cent had the diagnosis established at surgery. Of 64 patients presenting with what clinically appeared to be a single nodule, 33 per cent had cancer. Less than 10 per cent of the total number had multinodular goiter. A reminder that this experience may not be typical comes again from the Framingham study, in which, of nearly 60 nodules resected over a period of 15 years, none was declared malignant by the pathologist. Perhaps this indicates a peculiarity of this series, which selected a population group, rather than those who came to the physician for care.

What is the prognosis, with or without treatment, of these malignancies found in specimens of thyroid nodules? Obviously one cannot tell for certain. The tumors are similar in type to all thyroid tumors; therefore, the majority are papillary or mixed papillary-follicular tumors with fewer pure follicular and rare solid or anaplastic carcinomas. In general, the death rate for thyroid carcinoma represents approximately one quarter the diagnosed incidence rate, approximately 24 per million people per year.[7] While it would be comforting to believe that the difference between the incidence and death rates represents the effectiveness of surgical and medical therapy, it may represent as well the remarkable benignity of this tumor, which many patients carry with them throughout their lives and to their death from other causes. About all that can be stated with certainty is that some patients do die annually of thyroid carcinoma. If the surgeon removes a nodule which is really an invasive tumor, prior to the time it has metastasized, or while it is still subject to the defense mechanisms of the body, presumably a cure is effected. Quantitating this result of resection of thyroid nodules is impossible. While no controlled series is available, it seems obvious that some carcinomas, presenting first as nodules, will cause death. Of 38 thyroid cancer patients personally cared for in the past three and a half years, six have succumbed to their lesions. Three of these patients presented with single nodules, which had been present for one to six years before initial surgery and which might have been cured by appropriate early treatment. Two of the deaths were in patients with differentiated mixed tumors, indicating the lethal nature of this process. And, on the converse side, surgery does apparently cure 5 to 15 per cent of patients with anaplastic tumors,[8,9] patients whose outlook is otherwise most ominous.

Studies are available which suggest that thyroid nodules can be made to disappear by administration of desiccated thyroid.[10-12] Unfortunately, histologic diagnosis is lacking in the best known series.[10,12] My observation, coinciding with that of many other authors,[13, 14] is that nodules very rarely "go away" with such therapy. Does this treatment prevent the spread of malignancy? Again, data are unsatisfactory. We do know that "incidentally observed" thyroid tumors, even those metastatic to the neck, are very slow growing and infrequently fatal.[15] However, proof that thyroid hormone alone controls their growth is not available.

The essential reason for operation on a thyroid nodule is the hope and expectation that prompt surgery can eradicate a potentially lethal neoplastic process before uncontrollable metastatic spread or local invasion has occurred. But, one might ask, since the majority of thyroid nodules are pathologically benign, why not select those that are probably malignant and leave the others in place? This is a desirable goal, and much thought has been given to it. A direct approach to this differentiation might be to do needle or aspiration biopsy. Two objections may be cited to this idea: First, there is reluctance on the part of most surgeons to needle a possible malignancy, on the grounds that tumor cells could be spread.[16] More important is the difficulty in interpretation of limited biopsy material. It is hard enough to predict malignancy from permanent sections—the accuracy of biopsy or aspiration diagnosis would be questionable.

Patient age, duration of lesion, biologic function, presence of local symptoms, evidence of physiological suppressibility, lymph nodes, heredity, and prior x-ray treatment have been suggested as important determinants acting for or against need for surgery, and may be individually considered. Benign thyroid adenomas are predominantly a lesion of adults and, in fact, as stated previously, subclinical micro- or macroscopic adenomas become common with advancing age.[2] A palpable nodule in an individual under age 21 is highly suspicious of malignancy. In older individuals, perhaps above the age of 40 or 50, the frequency of benign nodules increases. But it is not established among older patients recognized as having single nodules that a significantly lower proportion are, in fact, malignant.

Recently discovered lesions might be assumed to be of greater danger than those known to have existed in the neck for several years. Yet our experience and that of others[17] is replete with the occurrence of malignancies in nodules known to have been present in the patient's neck for up to 40 years. In one recent review, a thyroid nodule had been detected on an average of six years prior to the diagnosis at surgery of thyroid malignancy.[13]

The presence of a diffusely multinodular gland, this differentiation being based either on physical evidence of palpation or on scanning, is usually interpreted as a sign of safety.[18] Multinodular goiters coming to surgery have a significant incidence of carcinoma (1 to 17 per cent), but this is believed to represent a process of selection and not to be typical of the process in the general population.[5, 6] The same sanguine approach does not hold if there is one area within a multinodular goiter which seems different from the entire remainder of the gland on the basis of its palpation characteristics or functional characteristics, or if there are perhaps two discrete nodules in a gland that is otherwise normal.

Isotope scanning of the thyroid is suggested as a way of differentiating lesions of significance, "cold" lesions being more dangerous than "warm" or "hot" lesions. It is obvious that most cold (inactive in accumulation of isotope) nodules are, in fact, benign, and frequently cystic. Nodules that are clearly hyperfunctional (or "hot"), and especially those that produce overt hyperthyroidism, are rare and are probably less frequently malignant than cold nodules, although exact statistics on such a comparison are not available.[19, 20] A sufficient number of hot nodules, due to or associated with carcinoma, have been reported (see review of Miller and Hamburger[21]) to establish with certainty the principle that presence of a hot nodule does not exclude the possibility of malignancy in the gland.[22, 23]

Several new techniques have been introduced for scanning, all holding promise for selection of dangerous lesions. It is reported that lesions "cold" on conventional radioiodine scan, but "active" on selenomethionine scan, are typically malignant.[24] Experience is not yet available to allow definition of the percentage of false negatives in this procedure, which is certainly an innovative approach. Fluorescent thyroid scanning[25] offers the possibility of quantitating the distribution of stable I^{127} in thyroid nodules, but preliminary experience does not prove it to be a more discriminating diagnostic tool than radioisotope scanning. Use of echo imaging has recently been reported; it can delineate cysts from solid structures, but this information will not allow certain prediction of histologic pattern.[26] Thyroid thermography also has been done and might hold promise, although it obviously is not a definitive procedure.[27]

Suppressibility of a nodule by desiccated thyroid surely suggests a physiologic derangement rather than the presence of an autonomously growing tumor. In my experience desiccated thyroid usually causes regression of the normal tissue surrounding a nodule and sometimes, therefore, makes the nodules appear to be smaller, and with greatest rarity leads to its gradual disappearance. In such instances I am usually led to the bigoted position of believing that my original diagnosis was erroneous and that the lesion probably represented another process, such as thyroiditis. Thyroid carcinomas may also appear to or actually become smaller on thyroid hormone replacement therapy.[13] The problem with this approach is simply that the vast majority of nodules do not disappear on suppression, and some shrinkage is not diagnostic.

What about local phenomena in relation to the lump? Fixation of the nodule to strap muscles or trachea is alarming, although characteristically a benign thyroid adenoma is fixed to the thyroid and moves with deglutition. It is, however, separable from overlying muscles and sometimes can be moved rather freely within the substance of the thyroid itself. Pain or tenderness in the nodule could indicate local invasion, but most commonly represents hemorrhage into a benign or neoplastic lesion which has outgrown its blood supply; it is often associated with sudden swelling. Regression may follow over a period of days or weeks. It is alleged by some experienced observers that benign tumors tend to be more flat and almond-shaped in profile, whereas malignancies tend to be more firm and more discretely bulging. Hoarseness may occur from pressure, or by infiltration of a recurrent laryngeal nerve by a neoplasm. Obviously the presence of a fixed lesion associated with pain, having a hard, bulging characteristic, and causing hoarseness, or any one of these features, should signal some degree of alarm. Absence of these findings is inconsequential.

The presence of lymph nodes must definitely be taken as a signal of danger. Epithyroid nodes are frequently found in patients with Hashimoto's thyroiditis and Graves' disease, but they are infrequent in patients with benign adenomas, and their presence in these lesions leads to the suspicion of a mitotic process or an immunologic reaction to a mitotic process.

Heredity may play a role in selection. There are rare patients who combine some portion of the "multiple endocrine adenoma syndrome, Type II," characterized by pheochromocytomas, medullary thyroid carcinomas, hyperparathyroidism, and mucosal neuromas.[28-30] Further, some patients have evidence of multiple thyroid malignancies in their family.

The most important bit of information regarding a nodule is a history of prior neck radiation. Any significant prior dose of radiation should be viewed with alarm. Exposure to 100 to 700 rads during the first three or four years of life is associated with a 1 to 3 per cent incidence of thyroid malignancy occurring from 10 to 30 years later.[31-33] Radiation during adolescence or early adulthood for acne or for other reasons has also been incriminated in the causation of this disease. Although knowledge of this association was available in 1952, patients are currently being seen with presumed radiation-related tumors who received x-ray treatments through 1958.

Thus, from my point of view, it is obvious that most rules available for selection of dangerous lesions are of minimal assistance. Some clear indicators for operation are obvious. Recent growth of a nodule, the presence of disturbing local symptoms, a history of radiation, young age, presence in a male, or a family history of thyroid malignancy are all signs pressing for operation. On the other extreme, the chance discovery of a minimal-sized adenoma, perhaps less than 1 cm., in an elderly woman, especially in the presence of some other medical process altering life expectancy, speaks for medical management.

In addition to the major indications for surgery just outlined, there are several other situations that might be classified as "minor" indications for operative intervention. Occasionally nodules develop into masses of significant size that are clearly a continuous distraction because of their appearance and merit removal for that reason alone. Some nodules produce pain, hoarseness, a sense of choking, or neck fullness—symptoms that are sufficient to disturb the patient and warrant removal. Rarely a functioning lump produces thyrotoxicosis, which then must be controlled by one of the available modalities of treatment, either radioactive iodide or surgery.

The most important requirement for operation is the selection of an experienced surgeon in an institution with an adequate pathology department. The patient should be pretreated for several weeks with some form of thyroid hormone to suppress normal thyroid tissue, and thus make the operation easier and delineate the abnormal tissue. The surgeon should be prepared to do a lobectomy, if the lesion is benign, or "near total" thyroidectomy and appropriate lymph node or neck dissection if the lesion is malignant. The first operation is the time to do definitive surgery. Although a surgeon with minimal experience in the area can perform a nodulectomy, an adequate near-total thyroidectomy and modified radical neck dissection require experience if damage to the recurrent laryngeal nerves or induction of hypoparathyroidism is to be avoided. In this day of specialization, patients deserve operation by a surgeon who has more than a casual interest in the field. In fact, in the absence of such surgical skill, medical therapy may offer fewer problems for certain patients with nodules than those associated with the performance of inadequate surgery.

The operative complications of lobectomy for a benign adenoma should be almost nil, and hospitalization is usually for three to five days. Obviously the incidence of risks and complications goes up if a malignancy is discovered and total thyroidectomy plus node dissection is required. This risk is more than balanced by the benefits,[34-36] since long-term survival of intrathyroidal or locally metastatic thyroid carcinoma is nearly equal to that of the rest of the population, after adequate surgery. Histologic examination must be done at the time of the procedure by a pathologist having competence in this area, where differential diagnosis is by no means easy. Occasionally the difficulty of interpreting frozen sections will lead to resection of a tumor which is ultimately classified as benign on permanent section. In my view the performance of an occasional unnecessary total thyroidectomy is not a serious problem in the hands of a surgeon who has few operative complications. On the other hand, the necessity of reoperation at a later date for erroneously undiagnosed malignancies is an all too common phenomenon and does not offer the patient the best chance of operative cure without complications. After operation all patients should be on long-term replacement therapy with thyroid hormone. This rule also applies to those few patients in whom medical management is elected. While the recurrence of "solitary" nodules is infrequent, this therapy is convenient and inexpensive and presumably provides some protection against the occurrence of another lesion.

References

1. Vander, J. B., Gaston, E. A., and Dawber, T. R.: Significance of solitary nontoxic thyroid nodules. Preliminary report. New Eng. J. Med. *251:*970, 1954.
2. Mortensen, J. D., Woolner, L. B., and Bennett, W. A.: Gross and microscopic findings in clinically normal thyroid glands. J. Clin. Endocr. *15:*1270, 1955.
3. Vander, J. B., Gaston, E. A., and Dawber, T. R.: The significance of nontoxic thyroid nodules. Ann. Intern. Med. *69:*537, 1968.
4. Cole, W. H., Majarahis, J. D., and Slaughter, D. P.: Incidence of carcinoma of the thyroid in nodular goiter. J. Clin. Endocr. *9:*1007, 1949.
5. Sokal, J. E.: The problem of malignancy in nodular goiter—Recapitulation and a challenge. J.A.M.A. *170:*61, 1959.
6. Veith, F. J., Brooks, J. R., Grigsby, W. P., and Selenkow, H. A.: The nodular thyroid gland and cancer. New Eng. J. Med. *270:*431, 1964.
7. Hakama, M.: Different world thyroid cancer rates. *In* Hedinger, C. E. (ed.): *Thyroid Cancer.* International Union Against Cancer Monograph Series, Vol. 12. Berlin, Springer-Verlag, 1969, page 66.
8. McDermott, W. V., Morgan, W. S., Hamlin, E., and Cope, O.: Cancer of the thyroid. J. Clin. Endocr. *14:*1336, 1954.
9. Rafla, S.: Anaplastic tumors of the thyroid. Cancer *23:*668, 1969.
10. Greer, M. A., and Astwood, E. B.: Treatment of simple goiter with thyroid. J. Clin. Endocr. *13:*1312, 1953.
11. Schneeberg, N. G., Stahl, T. J., Maldia, G., and Menduke, H.: Regression of goiter by whole thyroid or triiodothyronine. Metabolism *11:*1054, 1962.
12. Astwood, E. B., Cassidy, C. E., and Auerbach, G. D.: Treatment of goiter and thyroid nodules with thyroid. J.A.M.A. *174:*459, 1960.

13. Glassford, G. H., Fowler, E. F., and Cole, W. H.: The treatment of nontoxic nodular goiter with desiccated thyroid: Results and evaluation. Surgery 58:621, 1965.
14. Taylor, S.: Limitations of thyrotropin suppression in the treatment of nodular goiter and thyroid carcinoma. In Werner, S. C. (ed.): Thyrotropin Proc. Conf. Thyrotropin. Springfield, Illinois, Charles C Thomas, 1963, p. 353.
15. Hazard, J. B.: Small papillary carcinoma of the thyroid. Lab. Invest. 9:86, 1060.
16. Hamlin, E., and Vickery, A. L.: Needle biopsy of the thyroid gland. New Eng. J. Med. 254:742, 1956.
17. Glass, H. G., Waldron, G. W., Allen, H. C., and Brown, W. G.: A rational approach to the thyroid malignancy problem. Amer. Surg. 26:81, 1960.
18. Means, J. H., DeGroot, L. J., and Stanbury, J. B.: Multinodular goiter. In *The Thyroid and Its Diseases*. New York, McGraw-Hill Book Co., 1963, Chapter 15.
19. Kendall, L. W., and Condon, R. E.: Prediction of malignancy in solitary thyroid nodules. Lancet 1:1071, 1969.
20. Horst, W., Rosler, H., Schneider, C., and Labhart, A.: 306 Cases of toxic adenoma: Clinical aspects, findings in radioiodine diagnostics, radiochromatography and histology: Results of ^{131}I and surgical treatment. J. Nucl. Med. 8:515, 1967.
21. Miller, J. M., and Hamburger, J. I.: The thyroid scintigram. I. The hot nodule. Radiology 84:66, 1965.
22. Attie, J. N.: The use of radioactive iodine in the evaluation of thyroid nodules. Surgery 47:611, 1960.
23. Dische, S.: The radioisotope scan applied to the detection of carcinoma in thyroid swellings. Cancer 17:473, 1964.
24. Thomas, C. G., Pepper, F. D., and Owen, J.: Differentiation of malignant from benign lesions of the thyroid gland using complementary scanning with selenomethionine and radioiodide. Ann. Surg. 170:396, 1969.
25. Hoffer, P. B., Gottschalk, A., and Refetoff, S.: Thyroid scanning techniques: The old and the new. Current Prob. Radiol. 2:5, 1972.
26. Thijs, L. J.: Diagnostic ultrasound in clinical thyroid investigation. J. Clin. Endocr. 32:709, 1971.
27. Samuels, B. I.: Thermography: A valuable tool in the detection of thyroid disease. Radiology 102:59, 1972.
28. Sipple, J. H.: Association of pheochromocytoma with carcinoma of thyroid gland. Amer. J. Med. 31:163, 1961.
29. Schimke, R. N., Hartmann, W. H., Prout, T. E., and Rimoin, D. L.: Syndrome of bilateral pheochromocytoma, medullary thyroid carcinoma, and multiple neuromas. New Eng. J. Med. 279:1, 1968.
30. Sapira, J. D., Altman, M., Vandyk, K., and Shapiro, A. P.: Bilateral adrenal pheochromocytoma and medullary thyroid carcinoma. New Eng. J. Med. 273:140, 1965.
31. Duffy, B. J., Jr., and Fitzgerald, P. J.: Cancer of the thyroid in children: A report of twenty-eight cases. J. Clin. Endocr. 10:1296, 1950.
32. Clark, D. E.: Association of irradiation with cancer of the thyroid in children and adolescents. J.A.M.A., 159:1007, 1955.
33. Hempelmann, L. H.: Risk of thyroid neoplasms after irradiation in childhood. Science 160:159, 1968.
34. Wilson, S. M., and Bock, G. E.: Carcinoma of the thyroid metastatic to lymph nodes of the neck. Arch. Surg. 102:285, 1971.
35. Buckwalter, J.: Surgical treatment of thyroid carcinoma. Arch. Surg. 98:579, 1969.
36. Woolner, L. B., Beahrs, O. H., Black, B. M., McConahey, W. M., and Keating, F. R., Jr.: Long term survival rates. In Hedinger, E. (ed.): *Thyroid Cancer*. International Union Against Cancer Monograph Series, Vol. 12. Berlin, Springer-Verlag, 1969, pp. 326–331.

Thyroid Nodules:
Surgery Is Usually Not Necessary

MONTE A. GREER

University of Oregon Medical School

The problem of the single thyroid nodule has been hotly debated for the past quarter century. The controversy relates to whether such nodules are likely to be malignant and best treated by immediate excision or whether the probability of malignancy is very low and the patient may run a greater risk from the knife than from the nodule. In general, surgeons tend to favor an operative approach and internists a less physical attack. However, as with our major political parties, there are defectors to the opposite view in both camps. A rational decision on what to do with the nodule should be individualized for each patient. In order to proceed on a scientific rather than emotional basis, some valid information relating to the various risks and underlying physiological processes must be available to the responsible physician.

The Prevalence of Thyroid Nodules

Thyroid nodules are very common. Enlargement of the thyroid gland is probably the most frequent endocrine abnormality, more prevalent even than diabetes mellitus. In some large population groups living in endemic goiter areas, over 50 per cent of the individuals are afflicted. Although endemic goiter has largely disappeared from North America, careful examination of large unselected populations in areas which have never been considered "goiter belts" indicates that approximately 2 to 4 per cent of the population have clinically detectable single thyroid nodules.[1,2] In actual fact, the prevalence of thyroid nodules must be considerably higher than this. Additional thyroid nodules are often found during surgery for single nodules, and thyroid nodules are commonly found in postmortem examination of individuals in whom thyroid abnormalities had not been detected in life. It is therefore reasonable to accept that approximately 2 per cent of the population will have clinically detectable single thyroid nodules. It is these patients about whom the controversy in management exists.

Prevalence of Thyroid Cancer

Death from thyroid cancer is uncommon. The annual death rate from thyroid cancer is estimated at 0.5/100,000 population in the United States.[3, 4] This compares with the death rate from breast carcinoma of approximately 15/100,000, a thirty-fold difference.

Criteria for histologic diagnosis of thyroid cancer are not universally agreed upon.[5] Typical histologic characteristics of thyroid cancers which will cause the death of an individual, such as capsular invasion, frequent mitoses, and cellular irregularity, are also frequently seen in thyroids which are hyperplastic as a normal response to increased TSH secretion induced by physiologic or pharmacologic challenges such as iodine deficiency or administration of antithyroid drugs. Even in the absence of these last two factors, the histologic appearance of thyroid tissue on which a diagnosis of malignancy is based does not permit definite conclusions about the subsequent morbidity or mortality unless it is of a rapidly growing type such as anaplastic carcinoma, which almost invariably causes the demise of the patient.

The diagnosis of thyroid cancer is much more frequently made by the surgical pathologist than the death rate from the disease would seem to warrant. This is undoubtedly, at least in part, due to the difficulty in selecting adequate diagnostic criteria. Some authors have reported microscopic evidence of malignancy as high as 20 per cent in nodules removed solely because they were clinically detectable.[6] Although it is usually stressed that single nodules are more likely to be malignant than multinodular glands, some have found malignancy in over 10 per cent of the multinodular goiters removed surgically.[6] This should be considered in relation to the report by Mortensen et al.[7] that careful postmortem examination of the thyroid glands from 821 patients with clinically normal thyroids revealed that "occult" primary thyroid carcinoma occurred as often in patients without clinical evidence of thyroid disease as in patients with clinically recognized thyroid nodules who were surgically treated. The frequency was 4 per cent in both groups, although all the patients with clinically normal thyroids had died of other causes and had never had any therapy directed to their thyroid.

There is also an obvious discrepancy in the incidence of malignancy in nodules at surgery and the mortality figures for thyroid cancer. If one takes the 20 per cent incidence of malignancy in single thyroid nodules and accepts that 2 per cent of the general population has a single thyroid nodule, one obtains a prevalence of thyroid cancer, limited to those patients with clinically detectable single thyroid nodules and excluding all other patients who might have thyroid malignancy, of 400/100,000 population. Yet the death rate from thyroid cancer is only 0.5/100,000. This is almost a 1000 to 1 ratio and suggests that, if the histologic diagnosis was accurate, thyroid malignancy is usually very benign. If one accepts the 4 per cent incidence of malignancy of Mortensen et al.,[7] the ratio of patients with malignant thyroid nodules to death from thyroid cancer is reduced to 160:1. However, the same ratio would also exist for patients with clinically normal thyroids. A large percentage of thyroid cancers which are responsible for the death of the patient are not first detected in a single thyroid nodule. Thus, the true ratios would probably be skewed even further.

Pathogenesis of Thyroid Nodules

Current evidence indicates that thyroid nodules often develop as the result of stimulation of the gland by thyrotropin. In the rat, iodine deficiency produces an increase in TSH secretion as a compensatory mechanism for the decreased circulating thyroid hormone level resulting from inadequate iodine substrate.[8] This continuous supranormal TSH secretion initially results in diffuse enlargement of the thyroid gland. However, after several months nodules develop in the thyroid.[9] These frequently have different morphologic characteristics from the surrounding thyroid tissue and may differ considerably from the paranodular portion of the gland in their ability to metabolize radioiodine. Eventually some of these nodules become malignant and may cause the death of the animal.

Thyroid hyperplasia and nodularity do not occur in previously hypophysectomized iodine-deficient animals or in those given adequate physiologic replacement doses of thyroid hormone. If the thyroid enlargement has been present a relatively short time, hypophysectomy or administration of thyroid hormone will produce a decrease in thyroid size to the normal level. However, if the goiter has been present for several weeks or months, the thyroid always remains larger than normal, although considerably reduced in size compared to iodine-deficient animals in which TSH secretion has not been reduced.[10]

The above observations indicate that a complete reduction of thyroid size to normal is unlikely to occur in patients who have had goiters or nodules for a long period and is consistent with clinical observations that thyroid hormone is less efficacious in shrinking longstanding goiters than those which have recently developed.[11]

It is not understood why some patients may develop a localized enlargement of their gland (nodule) as a compensatory mechanism rather than a diffuse thyroid enlargement, even in the early phases of compensatory adjustment. Certain clones of thyroid cells may be more sensitive to TSH and respond with hypertrophy and hyperplasia more readily than others. In the rat, the rate of iodine metabolism can increase in response to iodine deficiency to a profound degree before there is any appreciable thyroid enlargement.[8] Thus, there may be stimulation of function in the paranodular thyroid tissue without any clinically detectable growth of such tissue. There is considerable variation in the uniformity of thyroid enlargement in patients with goiter. Most commonly one lobe is enlarged more than the other and the isthmus is affected to variable degrees. Often one sees appreciable enlargement of only one lobe. Such diversity is probably an expression of local heterogeneity in response to TSH. This is seen in a more extreme form in the development of a thyroid nodule. Any thyroid enlargement which results from a compensatory reaction to an inability of the gland to secrete adequate thyroid hormone without increased TSH stimulation should decrease in size, or at least not grow further, when TSH secretion is inhibited by administration of exogenous thyroid hormone.

Hot, Warm, and Cold Nodules

Thyroid nodules are usually classified as hot, warm, or cold on the basis of thyroid scans following administration of radioiodine or radioactive pertechnetate. A hot nodule will have much greater avidity for the radioisotope than the paranodular tissue, a warm nodule will have approximately the same concentration, and a cold nodule will have much less avidity. Hot nodules presumably represent the main functional portion of the thyroid and are either autonomous of TSH, thus producing sufficient thyroid hormone to suppress TSH secretion and secondarily the paranodular tissue, or they are more sensitive to TSH than the paranodular tissue. The autonomous nodules can be distinguished by the fact that they do not decrease in function or size when thyroid hormone is administered.

Cold nodules have relatively little affinity for radioiodine and therefore have been assumed to also be nonresponsive to TSH and autonomous. However, although hot nodules rarely decrease in size following administration of thyroid hormone, cold nodules may do so, indicating that they are not always autonomous. Recent studies have shown that slices from cold human thyroid nodules will respond to TSH stimulation in vitro with increases in ^{32}P incorporation and adenyl cyclase activity although they will not respond with an increase in radioiodine metabolism.[12] Such cold nodules probably have developed from clones of thyroid cells in which there is a defective cellular mechanism for iodide concentration or organic binding of iodine similar to the known inherited biosynthetic defects which usually affect the whole gland.[13]

A higher incidence of histologic malignancy has been recorded in cold than in warm or hot nodules.[14] On this basis, some authors feel that cold nodules, in particular, should be removed surgically. However, approximately half of all thyroid nodules are "cold" on scanning. The great discrepancy between death rates from thyroid cancer and the incidence of thyroid nodules documented above would thus be reduced only by half. This still leaves a very low risk from morbidity or mortality from thyroid cancer in patients with cold nodules.

Treatment

The choice of therapy for any condition is preferably based on statistical evaluation of the risks and benefits to be derived from the various alternatives. Although removal of a thyroid nodule, with or without lobectomy, by a first-rate thyroid surgeon carries little risk, it is nevertheless not an innocuous procedure. There is a probably unavoidable death rate from anesthetic accidents, cardiac arrhythmias, and so forth, of approximately 0.1 per cent. With less experienced surgeons the degree of technical skill also becomes an important factor. In my opinion, a further major consideration is the medicolegal responsibility of the surgeon. Many reports recommend total thyroidectomy for thyroid malignancy, often with additional radical neck dissection to prevent metastatic spread, because multicentric occult thyroid carcinomas are often found. Once the surgeon is told by the pathologist that there is malignant tissue in the thyroid, he may feel obliged to do a total thyroidectomy and a radical neck dissection even though he may not be philosophically committed to this principle himself. The risks and mutilation consequent upon such radical procedures are, of course, much greater than simple removal of the thyroid nodule. Since a large proportion of single thyroid nodules occur in young women, the potential cosmetic defects alone are enough to give one pause. Additional factors to be considered are the economic losses from the expense of the surgery, hospitalization, and the time lost from work.

There also is the uncertainty whether "prophylactic" removal of thyroid nodules, even in those cases with histologic malignancy, provides any real safeguard against future morbidity or mortality from thyroid cancer. I know of no adequately controlled study which permits an answer. Certainly some patients will die from thyroid cancer; most of these have had previous thyroid surgery. Reports from some clinics in which it is the policy to operate on all patients with nodular thyroids, whether single or multiple, indicate that there is a high incidence of malignancy in the surgically removed glands and that a certain portion of these patients subsequently die from thyroid cancer. In one study approximately half the patients refused surgery in spite of vigorous urging. In a follow-up of these nonoperated patients up to seven years, no clinical evidence of malignancy was known to have developed.[6]

In a nonselected population of over 5000 persons, 218 were found to have nontoxic thyroid nodules (4.2 per cent). These lesions were followed for approximately 15 years and none showed evidence of malignancy at the end of that time.[1] Our own experience is similar. We have not seen any development of thyroid malignancy in unoperated patients with single thyroid nodules in a 25-year experience. It is possible that some of our patients may have developed thyroid cancer and been treated elsewhere. However, because our philosophy in the treatment of thyroid nodules is well known in the community, it is unlikely that any such patients would not be forcefully brought to our attention.

It is obvious to the reader by now that I do not believe in routine surgical removal of thyroid nodules. Hot nodules, usually representing hyperfunctional autonomous tissue, can be treated by surgical excision if they are active enough to produce hyperthyroidism. On the other hand, since the paranodular tissue is essentially nonfunctional, they can be treated more cheaply, safely, and just as effectively with radioiodine. The nonfunctional normal portion of the gland will regain activity as soon as the abnormal nodule has been destroyed.

Warm or cold nodules are treated by administering thyroid hormone in amounts adequate to suppress TSH secretion (which can be evaluated by following the radioiodine uptake or, if T_3 is given, depression of the plasma thyroxine concentration). Our usual plan is to give 0.3 mg. sodium-L-thyroxine daily, but it is sometimes necessary to adjust the dose up or down. After the initial examination and evaluation, with careful measurement of the size of the nodule, thyroid hormone therapy is instituted. The patient is followed biweekly for the first month, monthly for six months, every three months for six months, semi-annually for two years, then annually indefinitely. Since the thyroid hormone is given to compensate for an assumed biosynthetic defect in producing thyroid hormone, the expected response is a decrease in the size of the nodule, or at least no increase in its size. In my experience approximately half the nodules decrease in size and some become clinically undetectable. The length of time required for a nodule to disappear completely has varied from two weeks to more than two years. However, if no appreciable decrease in size has occurred by the end of the first year, the chances for regression at a later date are small. The fact that some nodules fail to decrease completely in size may be related to the observations in the rat,[10] mentioned previously, in which it was found that longstanding thyroid enlargement did not return completely to normal even when TSH secretion was abolished.

If the nodule enlarges during administration of adequate amounts of thyroid hormone to suppress thyroid function, the basic assumption on which thyroid therapy was instituted would seem incorrect for such a patient. In these individuals surgery seems warranted since an autonomous expanding lesion is certainly much more suspicious of malignancy. We have had four patients in whom surgery was undertaken for this reason. Surprisingly, in none of these was there histologic evidence of malignancy. We have a 10-year follow-up on two of these patients. Neither has developed any clinical evidence of malignancy nor any further thyroid enlargement, but both have been maintained on continuous thyroid hormone therapy.

In the rare patient who shows evidence of malignancy on the first examination, e.g., a hard irregular infiltrating mass, cord paralysis, or lymph node involvement, we recommend immediate surgery. I have seen several such individuals, but they present quite a different clinical picture from the usual patient with a single firm, rubbery, well circumscribed, smooth, nontender nodule.

Our approach to the therapy of the thyroid nodule is the same regardless of the age or sex of the patient. Nodules in children or males are considered by some to be much more likely to be malignant than those in adult females. However, childhood death from thyroid cancer is very rare, and the mortality from this disease is twice as high in women as in men[3,4] compared to a fourfold higher incidence of single nodules in the female.[1] The danger of death from thyroid cancer in the two "high risk" groups therefore is not appreciably different from that in adult women. The important points to keep in mind are: (1) There is no valid evidence that surgery reduces the morbidity or mortality from thyroid cancer compared to a nonoperated control group. (2) Surgery may accelerate the malignant development of thyroid tumors if increased TSH secretion is necessary to counteract a reduction in functioning thyroid tissue. (3) Nodules showing autonomous growth will be recognized early with the plan of therapy described here.

Since nodules may arise as a compensatory adjustment to an inefficient biosynthetic mechanism for producing thyroid hormone, withdrawing thyroid medication should lead to the recurrence of a nodule which has disappeared or decreased with replacement therapy. This phenomenon has often been observed.[15] We therefore recommend that patients continue with thyroid hormone for the duration of their life. This is especially important in individuals who have had a reduction in their functional thyroid mass as a result of surgery, radioiodine therapy, or other destructive processes.

References

1. Vander, J. B., Gaston, E. A., and Dawber, T. R.: The significance of nontoxic thyroid nodules. Ann. Intern. Med. 69:537, 1968.
2. Slater, S.: The occurrence of thyroid nodules in the general population. Arch. Intern. Med. 98:175–180, 1956.
3. *Facts on the Major Crippling and Killing Diseases in the United States Today.* New York, National Health Education Committee, 1964.
4. Silverberg, E., and Holleb, A. I.: Cancer Statistics 1971. Cancer 21:13, 1971.
5. Perloff, W. H., and Schneeberg, N. G.: The problem of thyroid carcinoma. Surgery 29:572, 1951.
6. Cerise, E. J., Randall, S., and Ochsner, A.: Carcinoma of the thyroid and nontoxic nodular goiter. Surgery 31:552, 1952.
7. Mortensen, J. D., Woolner, L. B., and Bennett, W. A.: Gross and microscopic findings in clinically normal thyroid glands. J. Clin. Endocr. 15:1270, 1955.
8. Studer, H., and Greer, M. A.: *The Regulation of Thyroid Function in Iodine Deficiency.* Stuttgart, Hans Huber, 1968.
9. Matovinovic, J., Hilbert, R. D., Armstrong, W. F., et al.: Thyroid tumor and thyroid transplant tumor in iodine-deficient rat. *In* Cassano, C., and Andreoli, M. (eds.): *Current Topics in Thyroid Research.* New York, Academic Press Inc., 1965.
10. Greer, M. A., Studer, H., and Kendall, J. W.: Studies on the pathogenesis of colloid goiter. Endocrinology 81:623, 1967.
11. Bruns, P.: Beobachtungen und Untersuchungen über die Schilddrüsenbehandlung des Kropfes. Beitr. Klin. Chirurg. 16:521, 1896.
12. DeRubertis, F., Yamashita, K., Dekker, A., et al.: Effects of thyroid-stimulating hormone on adenyl cyclase activity and intermediary metabolism of "cold" thyroid nodules and normal human thyroid tissue. J. Clin. Invest. 51:1109, 1972.
13. Stanbury, J. B.: Familial goiter. *In* Stanbury, J. B., Wyngaarden, J. B., and Frederickson, D. S. (eds.): *The Metabolic Basis of Inherited Disease.* New York, McGraw-Hill Book Co., Inc., 1966, p. 215.
14. Perlmutter, M., and Slater, S. L.: Which nodular goiters should be removed? A physiologic plan for the diagnosis and treatment of nodular goiter. New Eng. J. Med. 255:65, 1956.
15. Greer, M. A., and Astwood, E. B.: Treatment of simple goiter with thyroid. J. Clin. Endocr. 13:1312, 1953.

Comment

Thyroid Nodules

Controversy concerning the management of patients who have a solitary nodule of the thyroid gland has occurred for two reasons: The first is that a precise diagnosis cannot be made nonoperatively with any certainty. Secondly, it has not been clearly established that early surgical excision of the types of thyroid carcinoma which present as a solitary nodule is beneficial. A solitary nodule of the thyroid gland is a localized palpable abnormality of the gland. It represents not one disease entity, but many diseases. Anatomically such nodules may be localized thyroiditis, a thyroid cyst, an adenomatous nodule (in a thyroid gland that often turns out to have multiple nodules on pathological examination), thyroid adenoma, or thyroid carcinoma, and pathological distinction among them may be very difficult. Little is known about the pathogenesis or natural history of any of these lesions. (Greer's statement implicating chronic TSH stimulation as a cause of solitary nodules is not supported by any direct evidence in humans.)

Patients who have a solitary nodule may require some kind of therapy for several reasons. These include the possibility that the nodule is a thyroid carcinoma, that it is responsible for hyperthyroidism, or that it is producing significant compression or cosmetic symptoms. These latter findings generally raise no controversy concerning management. It is the fear that a solitary nodule may be a thyroid carcinoma that has led to recommendations that most such patients be treated surgically. Even though thyroid carcinoma may be a rare cause of death, patients do have significant disability or die from it, and their survival may be prolonged by surgical treatment. The real question is, "Can patients whose nodule is likely to be a thyroid carcinoma be identified clinically?"

The preceding two papers appear to argue that such selection is not possible and furthermore appear to argue for dramatically different courses of action for the management of patients with solitary thyroid nodules. However, I do not believe the views of Greer and DeGroot are so divergent as appears at first glance. Greer believes most patients with a solitary thyroid nodule should receive thyroid hormone therapy, but then goes on to admit that he recommends surgery for patients whose nodules appear clinically to have some "evidence of malignancy" or in whom further enlargement of the nodule occurs despite thyroid therapy. Greer also states that no evidence of thyroid cancer has become apparent in any unoperated patients whom he has followed over a period of many years. This suggests either that all the patients whose nodules contain thyroid carcinoma are selected (or even preselected) for surgery initially by the aforementioned (but unfortunately unclearly stated) criteria or that he is dealing with a very different group of patients than is DeGroot and the rest of us.

On the other hand, DeGroot outlines a series of clinical findings which he considers to constitute "pressing" indications for surgery. Since some (?many) patients do not have these findings, presumably surgery is not recommended. Furthermore, his statement that 33 per cent of 64 patients who had a solitary thyroid nodule were found to have thyroid carcinoma suggests that selection is being exercised, since this figure is the highest incidence figure for the presence of thyroid carcinoma in solitary nodules of which I am aware. Thus, I would submit that both Greer and DeGroot do, in fact, make decisions concerning whether or not patients with a solitary nodule should have the nodule surgically excised and pathologically examined; i.e., both individualize therapy. Further, while the data given in the two papers are not comparable, both would appear to be "missing" few thyroid carcinomas.

When the decision is to not operate, a further though less momentous controversy arises—whether or not to administer thyroid hormone. (There are no serious objections to treatment with thyroid hormone, though I agree with DeGroot that it is not usually effective in producing significant reduction in nodule size.) Despite our present inability to make a precise nonoperative diagnosis of the solitary nodule with great certainty, it seems clear that judicious application of historical, physical, and laboratory findings can and should be used to avoid indiscriminate use of any form of therapy in the patient who has a solitary nodule of the thyroid gland. Let us hope that new tools allowing more precise nonoperative diagnosis will become available in the future.

ROBERT D. UTIGER

17

The Prolonged Therapeutic Use of Adrenocortical Steroids

GLUCOCORTICOID THERAPY: AN OVERMALIGNED REPUTATION WITH UNTAPPED POTENTIAL BENEFIT
 by William McK. Jefferies

HAZARDS OF PROLONGED CORTICOSTEROID THERAPY
 by Philip K. Bondy

COMMENT
 by Arnold S. Relman

Glucocorticoid Therapy: An Overmaligned Reputation with Untapped Potential Benefit

WILLIAM McK. JEFFERIES

Case-Western Reserve University School of Medicine

The status of glucocorticoid therapy in clinical medicine today is confused, to say the least. By many it has been denounced as a dangerous drug whose use is not justified except in critical illnesses or emergencies; by a few it has been defended as a useful therapeutic tool whose hazards have been exaggerated. A brief consideration will reveal that an odd and rather unique situation has developed in which a therapeutic agent of great promise has achieved such a bad reputation that its potential benefit has been stifled. How soon the medical profession and the public will awaken to the truth that the hazards of glucocorticoid therapy have been misinterpreted to a great extent, that some dosages are as safe as or safer than aspirin, and that the therapeutic potential of the safe dosages has been barely touched, remains to be seen.

In 1949 after Hench and his associates first reported the effects of cortisone upon rheumatoid arthritis,[1] it rapidly became known as "the wonder drug." In addition to antirheumatic, anti-allergic and anti-inflammatory effects, it had the fantastic property of counteracting malaise, fatigue, and anorexia, the nonspecific clinical symptoms that cause a person to feel ill when his or her body is fighting the results of damage inflicted by infection or injury. Unfortunately, in the dosages that were given, cortisone also produced undesirable and even hazardous side effects. Patients' faces became round and florid, their skin became thin, ecchymoses appeared, their bones became porotic and spontaneous fractures occurred, peptic ulcers developed, and resistance to infection or other stresses became impaired. Not every patient treated developed these complications, but some did, and this was sufficiently alarming to cause many physicians who had been extolling the virtues of this therapeutic agent to reverse their position and say that it was too dangerous to use.

Meanwhile new, more potent derivatives such as prednisone, prednisolone, triamcinolone, methyl prednisolone, dexamethasone, and betamethasone were introduced with the expectation that they would produce clinical benefit with fewer undesirable side effects. After an initial resurgence of hope, it soon became evident that, except for less tendency to cause sodium retention, an effect that was hazardous chiefly for patients with cardiac, renal, or hepatic disease, the derivatives could produce all the other undesirable side effects of cortisone, plus perhaps a few additional ones. Medical literature abounded with reports of grim complications of glucocorticoid therapy, optimism gave way to pessimism, and soon a situation developed in which alarm became so great that perspective was lost.

The dangers of glucocorticoid therapy came to be taken for granted. It was assumed that any dosage of any glucocorticoid was potentially hazardous. Often reports of undesirable effects would fail to state the dosage and duration of administration, implying that all dosages were capable of producing similar effects. The term "cortisone therapy" came to be applied indiscriminately to all types of glucocorticoid treatment, making it difficult to evaluate differences between glucocorticoid preparations or even to determine what steroid a patient had received. Many statements appeared to the effect that all glucocorticoid therapy was dangerous; hence, it should not be started except as a last resort and should be discontinued as soon as possible. For almost 20 years physicians have been indoctrinated with this concept.

Statements that glucocorticoid therapy might not be all bad were considered heresy by many. Occasional reports implying that its dangers might have been exaggerated were overlooked or ignored. For example, Bowen and his associates reported from the Mayo Clinic in 1960[2] that a review of the records of 2114 patients with rheumatoid arthritis revealed no difference in incidence of peptic ulcer in those treated systemically with glucocorticoids compared with those who had not received glucocorticoids! Yet patients with rheumatoid arthritis had a three to four times greater incidence of peptic ulcer than the general patient population. This was probably the result of salicylate therapy, but how many physicians today are aware that glucocorticoid therapy is apparently less apt to produce peptic ulcer than salicylates?

Robbins[3] in 1968 stated that experience with several thousand patients treated with prednisolone (dosages not indicated) resulted in the appearance of active peptic ulcers de novo in only four, whereas 41 active ulcers, already present, healed with an ulcer regimen while glucocorticoid therapy was continued.

Savage[4] in 1965 reported that metyrapone tests indicated that, in short courses of up to two months' duration, doses up to 80 mg. prednisolone daily did not impair pituitary response to stress. He further stated that "long courses with small doses such as 5 mg. prednisolone per diem also leave the pituitary intact and, in addition, do not result in side effects." He went on to say, "In rheumatoid arthritics on relatively low dosage (of prednisolone) . . . a number of our most severe rheumatoids have gone through many winters in England without getting more chest or other infections than the rest of the population."

An editorial[5] in the New England Journal of Medicine in 1965 included the statement, "It should be pointed out, however, for reassurance of those with adrenal insufficiency, that corticosteroid therapy in replacement dosage (that is, 37.5 mg. of cortisone per day) is not only life-saving but essentially devoid of undesirable side effects except, of course, in patients with coexisting diabetes mellitus, hypertension or peptic ulcer diathesis." Actually, these exceptions are not justified, because there is no evidence that daily dosages of cortisone totaling less than 37.5 mg., at least when divided into three or four doses, will increase insulin requirements or in any way aggravate diabetes mellitus or hypertension. On the contrary, there is suggestive evidence that such dosages may help to stabilize labile diabetics and provide some protection against hypoglycemic reactions. The relative safety of glucocorticoids, especially in small doses, in patients with peptic ulcer has been cited previously.[2,3] If suitable precautions are employed, such as antacid therapy in patients with peptic ulcer and antibiotic therapy in patients with bacterial infections, especially tuberculosis, there are no specific contraindications to low dosage glucocorticoid therapy.

In 1967[6] a report was published documenting the safety of low dosage glucocorticoid therapy in 371 patients treated for six months to nine years, with no development of peptic ulcer or any other side effect encountered with larger doses. The low dosages referred to in this report were cortisone or hydrocortisone, 5 mg. 4 times daily, or less. A comparable dosage of prednisone would be 1 mg. 4 times daily, but with small doses there seems to be no advantage in using the more potent derivatives instead of the natural steroids. The optimum duration of therapy with low dosages varies with individual patients and with the nature of the disorder being treated, but there is ample evidence that they may be continued indefinitely without harm, and in disorders such as rheumatoid arthritis and chronic asthma it may prove advisable for some patients to take such dosages the rest of their lives.

These statements and reports have apparently gone relatively unnoticed. The general attitude of apprehension regarding glucocorticoid therapy has persisted. The fact that cortisone and hydrocortisone are natural hormones produced by the adrenal cortex has largely been forgotten. The fact that patients with adrenal insufficiency are treated with doses of cortisone acetate or hydrocortisone up to 40 mg. daily for years without ill effects has made little impression. The fact that practically every arthritis clinic has patients who are maintained on dosages equivalent to 30 mg. or less daily of hydrocortisone for years without evidence of hypercorticism or impairment of resistance to stress has been virtually overlooked.

How could this occur? Why should there be an apparent failure to believe evidence that glucocorticoids in small doses are remarkably safe? The answer probably lies in a peculiar combination of factors.

The dosages of cortisone and hydrocortisone given for arthritis in the first years after their introduction usually started at 100 to 300 mg. daily, later decreasing to 50 to 75 mg. daily for maintenance. It came to be assumed that large doses were necessary for antirheumatic, anti-allergic and anti-inflammatory effects. When it was found that adrenalectomized patients could be maintained on 40 mg. daily, it became evident that doses greater than this were excessive and could produce hypercorticism, but by this time the harmful effects of hypercorticism were so deeply impressed upon the medical profession and the public that it was assumed that even maintenance dosages would be potentially harmful. Only those physicians who were treating patients with adrenal insufficiency realized that such dosages were not producing the undesirable effects seen with larger doses. Even when arthritics were found to benefit from dosages less than 40 mg. hydrocortisone daily or its equivalent, it was assumed that such dosages were potentially hazardous.

Meanwhile, interesting therapeutic effects were being found with small doses. They were initially used in women with fertility problems associated with irregular menses, hirsutism, and high urinary 17-ketosteroids.[7] The results were so encouraging that they were given to women with ovarian dysfunction regardless of whether they had associated hirsutism, acne, elevated 17-ketosteroids, or infertility.[8] Eighty per cent of these women benefited from this therapy.[9] The small dosages were also found to be helpful in treating acne, hirsutism, and chronic cystic mastitis. Perhaps the most dramatic effects occurred in women with functional uterine bleeding, a condition that has been notoriously disturbing to gynecologists, as manifested by the numbers of D and C's and hysterectomies performed for this disorder. A hysterectomy certainly is not a satisfactory solution to a problem of this nature in a young woman who is anxious to have children. With 5 mg. of hydrocortisone 4 times daily, practically every patient with this disorder has developed regular ovulatory menstrual cycles.[9]

These small dosages have also been found to have antirheumatic and antiallergic effects.[6] This should not be surprising, since almost every arthritis clinic has some patients who are maintained in a reasonably good clinical state with dosages equivalent to 30 mg. hydrocortisone daily or less, but who develop an exacerbation of symptoms when the steroid is withdrawn. It has been assumed that such beneficial effects must result from a summation action, because it was generally acknowledged that antirheumatic and anti-allergic effects depended upon large "pharmacologic" doses of steroid. Studies, however, clearly demonstrated that the small dosages do not cause a summation effect.[6] A dosage of 10 mg. daily of cortisone acetate (2.5 mg. 4 times a day) depresses normal endogenous adrenal production by about 25 per cent and a dosage of 20 mg. daily (5 mg. 4 times a day) depresses it about 50 per cent. The remaining function is adequate for normal responses to stress; patients have undergone major surgical procedures while on these dosages without difficulty, even though the administration of the steroid is stopped before the operation and not resumed until the patient is able to take oral medication. Patients receiving these dosages also respond normally to standard injections of ACTH. During treatment, levels of plasma 11-oxycorticosteroids and 17-hydroxycorticosteroids remain normal, as do levels of urinary 17-hydroxycorticosteroids. It is, therefore, evident that dosages of cortisone acetate or hydrocortisone totaling less than 40 mg. daily cause a decrease in endogenous production of hydrocortisone just sufficient to maintain a normal circulating level of this hormone. Therefore, they would not be expected to cause signs and symptoms of hypercorticism.

The beneficial effects in patients with ovarian dysfunction, acne, and hirsutism apparently result from a demonstrated ability of these small dosages to decrease adrenal production of androgen and estrogen. Such actions also appear to explain the beneficial effects of this therapy in some cases of oligospermia. The mechanisms of the antirheumatic and anti-allergic effects at any dosage remain to be clarified. Experience in our clinic with over 1000 patient years of low dosage therapy with cortisone acetate or hydrocortisone (5 mg. or less 4 times daily) has confirmed its safety, with no incidence of hypercorticism or impairment of resistance to stress or infection.

With such an impressive array of clinical benefits, such a therapeutic agent should be welcomed and achieve wide usage. But not cortisone. The value and safety of small doses is not even mentioned in advertisements or package inserts by the pharmaceutical companies that distribute it. This seems odd, but is apparently due to a peculiar quirk in drug regulations whereby a different therapeutic use for an old drug, even though the dosage might be smaller, must receive essentially the same investigative treatment as a new drug. Hence, for a pharmaceutical company to be able to state that an old drug has additional therapeutic effects, investment must be made in studies similar to those necessary for a new drug in order to receive authorization for the statement. Such studies are obviously desirable, but they are expensive. Because the patents on cortisone and hydrocortisone have expired, pharmaceutical companies have little incentive to undertake the expense necessary to satisfy the regulations when any other company would be able to manufacture and sell the product once an authorization was granted. Until drug regulations provide protection for the investment of a pharmaceutical company under such circumstances, low dosage glucocorticoid therapy will not receive the promotion that the medical profession has come to expect for an effective therapeutic agent.

Other factors have contributed to the failure of the value and safety of this therapy to be recognized. One has been a tendency to confuse cortisone and hydrocortisone with their more potent derivatives. Because of the lumping of all glucocorticoid therapy under the term, "cortisone therapy," many physicians seem to have forgotten that cortisone and hydrocortisone are much less potent, milligram for milligram, than prednisone, prednisolone, or the other derivatives. A dosage of 5 mg. 4 times daily of cortisone acetate or hydrocortisone is quite safe, but 5 mg. of prednisone 4 times daily can produce all the hazardous side effects of hypercorticism.

Also, because cortisone and hydrocortisone are more effective in divided dosage,[6] this therapy has the inconvenience of requiring that patients take four doses daily for optimum effects. This entails more time in the physician's office for explanation of the schedule and more difficulty on the part of the patient in following it. Most patients are willing to accept this inconvenience if the reason is explained and after they realize its beneficial effect. It would be interesting to determine whether timed-release preparations would work as well when given every 12 hours, but as yet no such preparations of these agents have been made available. It should be noted that a study of the effectiveness of prednisolone in controlling the symptoms of rheumatoid arthritis when administered as a single dose versus four divided doses revealed a definite tendency for greater effectiveness of divided doses.[10] No similar studies with cortisone acetate or with hydrocortisone have been reported, but it would be anticipated that with the shorter half-life of these less potent agents in the circulation, the advantage of four divided doses over a single dose would be even greater.

The use of several doses per day should be contrasted with the alternate day program that was recommended by Harter and the Thorn group.[11, 12] The latter schedule was suggested as a method to lessen the occurrence of side effects with large "pharmacologic" doses of glucocorticoids. Its chief advantage was stated to be less likelihood of persistent complete adrenal suppression. Because small dosages do not produce side effects or complete adrenal suppression, and because they require divided daily doses for optimum effects, there is no reason to administer them on an alternate day schedule. In fact, Harter et al.[11] report that two patients who had been maintained on only physiologic doses of steroids (5 to 10 mg. prednisone or the equivalent per day) could not be maintained on every other day therapy.

The investigation of low dosage glucocorticoid therapy has been handicapped by an attitude on the part of some authorities that everything is known about the clinical effects of cortisone and hydrocortisone, so there is no reason to spend more time and effort studying them further. Such an attitude is not valid because, although much is known about the harmful effects of large doses of glucocorticoids, virtually nothing is known about the mechanism of any of their beneficial clinical actions!

The result of this combination of factors is a unique situation in which a therapeutic agent with promising potential in several broad clinical areas has been practically ignored. In addition to its antirheumatic and anti-allergic effects, as well as its beneficial effects upon ovarian and testicular dysfunction, acne, and hirsutism, low dosage glucocorticoid therapy appears to have antimalaise and antifatigue effects that warrant careful study. This aspect of the clinical effects of glucocorticoids has apparently been completely neglected. The observation by Kass and Finland[13] that cortisone could make a patient with lobar pneumonia feel well produced such alarm, because of the possible masking of signs and symptoms of disease, that the feasibility of its being used safely in the treatment of at least some types of illness or injury in a nonspecific manner has apparently not been considered.

It is time that the unfortunate predicament of glucocorticoid therapy be corrected. Unreasonable fear must be put aside. The potential benefits and hazards of these agents must be put in proper perspective. Promising leads should be investigated without being handicapped by unjustified timidity. An attitude that all glucocorticoid therapy is dangerous is as absurd as one that all thyroid or all estrogen therapy is dangerous. Drug regulations must be changed to encourage, rather than stifle, the development of new uses for old medications. Physicians must realize that the occurrence of undesirable side effects with large doses does not necessarily imply that they will occur with smaller doses. If this were the case, no drug could be used safely! Some rather serious side effects can occur as a result of the prolonged ingestion of too much food, but that does not justify the stopping of eating any food at all!

References

1. Hench, P. S., Kendall, E. C., Slocumb, C. H., and Polley, H. F.: Effect of hormone of adrenal cortex (17-hydroxy- 11-dehydro-corticosterone; compound E) and of pituitary adrenocorticotropic hormone on rheumatoid arthritis. Proc. Staff Meet. Mayo Clin. 24:181, 1949.

2. Bowen, R., Jr., Mayne, J. G., Cain, J. C., and Bartholomew, L. G.: Peptic ulcer in rheumatoid arthritis and relationship to steroid treatment. Proc. Mayo Clin. 35:537, 1960.
3. Robbins, J. J.: Steroid effects, a credibility gap between fact and opinion. (Correspondence). New Eng. J. Med. 279:328, 1968.
4. Savage, O.: The place and problems of corticosteroid therapy. Brit. J. Clin. Pract. 19:657, 1965.
5. Editorial: Pharmacologic effects of adrenal corticosteroids. New Eng. J. Med. 273:875, 1965.
6. Jefferies, W. McK.: Low dosage glucocorticoid therapy. Arch. Intern. Med. 119:265, 1967.
7. Jefferies, W. McK., Weir, W. C., Weir, D. R., and Prouty, R. L.: The use of cortisone and related steroids in infertility. Fertil. Steril. 9:145, 1958.
8. Jefferies, W. McK.: Further experience with small doses of cortisone and related steroids in infertility associated with ovarian dysfunction. Fertil. Steril. 11:100, 1960.
9. Jefferies, W. McK.: Glucocorticoids and ovulation. In Greenblatt, R. B. (ed.): Ovulation. Philadelphia, J. B. Lippincott Company, 1966, p. 63.
10. Nugent, C. A., Ward, J., MacDiarmid, W. D., McCall, J. C., Baukol, J., and Tyler, F. H.: Glucocorticoid toxicity. Single contrasted with divided daily doses of prednisolone. J. Chron. Dis. 18:323, 1965.
11. Harter, J. G., Reddy, W. J., and Thorn, G. W.: Studies of intermittent corticosteroid dosage regimen. New Eng. J. Med. 269:591, 1963.
12. Thorn, G. W.: Clinical considerations in the use of corticosteroids. New Eng. J. Med. 274:775, 1966.
13. Kass, E. H., and Finland, M.: Role of adrenal steroids in infection and immunity. New Eng. J. Med. 244:464, 1951.

Hazards of Prolonged Corticosteroid Therapy

PHILIP K. BONDY

Chester Beatty Research Institute, London

In order to explore areas of controversy in the therapeutic use of corticosteroids, it may be well first to dispose briefly of the noncontroversial aspects of such treatment. It is obvious that steroids should be given to patients who are unable to produce what they need, as a result of destruction or surgical ablation of the adrenal glands, or because of pituitary insufficiency. In addition, patients with congenital adrenal hyperplasia resulting from a deficiency of one of the enzymes essential for the biosynthesis of cortisol also require treatment with corticosteroids. In these patients the proper dose of steroid is one which replaces the missing hormone. For cortisol, this is about 20 mg. twice a day. Patients without a functioning adrenal cortex, and some patients with the adrenogenital syndrome resulting from congenital adrenal hyperplasia may also need a salt-retaining steroid such as 9α-fluorocortisol (Fludrocortisone).

The most important point about this type of treatment is that it supplies hormones which are missing in the patient and which are essential to survival, so the treatment must be continued for the remainder of the patient's life. It is indefensible to attempt to reduce, taper, or discontinue treatment in such patients. Moreover, since there is need for the mineralocorticoid effect, it is not advisable to use a steroid derivative such as triamcinolone or dexamethasone which has been modified to eliminate this effect.

The remainder of this chapter, therefore, does not apply to this type of patient, but concerns those individuals receiving corticosteroids to suppress inflammation or immune reactions.

There are certain dangers in giving corticosteroids, and these should be recognized and carefully weighed against the potential advantages of using the medications. The damaging effects of the steroids are not a result of idiosyncrasy or sensitivity, as is the case with many medications. Rather, they reflect the excessive exhibition of normal actions of the compounds as a result of administration of doses which are larger than physiological or which are administered for prolonged periods. Thus, the necessary ability to promote gluconeogenesis is exaggerated into pathological destruction of protein and resulting osteoporosis, peptic ulcer, dermal striae, and even cerebral atrophy, while the normally protective anti-insulin effect results in unmasking diabetes. Adrenocortical secretion is normally controlled by a series of feedback mechanisms of which the corticosteroids are the major suppressing limb. Prolonged suppression, leading to adrenal cortical atrophy and inhibited ability of the hypothalamic-pituitary-adrenal system to respond to stress, interferes with the patient's ability to survive trauma, infection, or surgery and may threaten his life.

With these considerations in mind, it is essential that the use of steroids be restricted to those situations in which they are known to be effective; that the dose be adjusted to the minimum resulting in adequate therapeutic response; and that the duration of treatment be as brief as is consistent with adequate control of the patient's disorder. It must constantly be kept in mind that the steroids do not, in themselves, cure any disease. The most they can do is to suppress the inflammatory or immune reaction while the disorder takes its course under the influence of more specific forms of treatment.

Errors in the use of corticosteroids can be considered under several headings, although in any given instance it is common to see more than one type of error at work.

The most serious mistake is to give these substances to patients who cannot benefit from them. For example, hypertrophic osteoarthritis cannot be improved by steroids, since inflammation plays only a trivial part in its pathogenesis. Even in inflammatory joint disease such as rheumatoid arthritis, the steroids are useless after the process has burned out and the joints are ankylosed. In these circumstances there is no reason to expect improvement of symptoms (aside from the nonspecific effects of mild euphoria often produced by steroids), and the bone and muscle atrophy produced by the treatment aggravates the total disability of the arthritic at this stage of the disease. Moreover, parallel treatment with salicylates exaggerates the danger of peptic ulceration. Thus, there is no advantage to treatment with steroids in these circumstances, and there are excellent arguments against their use.

A second type of error, and one almost as serious, is to give the steroid for longer than necessary. Even very large doses of corticoids are usually well tolerated if they are given for only a few days. During this period only trivial amounts of protein destruction can occur; the feedback inhibition does not continue long enough to produce lasting derangement of hypothalamic-pituitary controls; and peptic erosions do not have time to develop. But if the dose is continued for more than a week or so, appreciable muscle and bone atrophy may occur, emotional disturbances are quite common, and the risk of gastrointestinal complications becomes appreciable. After about a month of treatment these problems are further complicated by deranged pituitary feedback function, skin atrophy with striae, muscular weakness, Cushingoid changes of face and body contours, osteoporosis, and often carbohydrate intolerance. Thus, the patient is at minimal risk if the objectives of treatment can be achieved within a few days and at maximal risk when treatment is prolonged beyond a month. This does not mean that prolonged treatment is always inadvisable; indeed, in proper circumstances it may be lifesaving. But it does mean that the physician should reconsider carefully as the duration of treatment lengthens to be certain that continuation of treatment is justified.

A third error is to prescribe too large a dose of steroid. As has already been mentioned, this is usually a trivial matter when treatment will continue for only a day or two, but when prolonged treatment is required the dose should be adjusted to the minimum which will achieve the desired effect. This requires an assessment both of the patient's response and of the ultimate objective which it is reasonable to expect. For example, if a patient with chronic rheumatoid arthritis has good control of pain but continues to suffer from limitation of motion in the affected joints, it is important to know how much of the stiffness is due to irreversible fibrosis and how much to continuing inflammation. If steroids in a small dose raise the platelet count of a thrombocytopenic patient from 5000 to 50,000 per cu. mm., is it justifiable to give a larger dose in order to bring the count to a normal 200,000? Clearly, if adequate function has been restored, so that the arthritic has achieved maximal motion compatible with the degree of fibrosis, and the thrombopenic patient is no longer in danger of hemorrhage, increasing the dose is not justified. Indeed, in these circumstances the dose should be titrated downward to find the minimum capable of providing adequate control. Even continuing a constant dose without periodic re-evaluation is an error.

What is the minimum effective dose of steroid which can reduce symptoms or control inflammation? This minimal effective dose is different for each patient and varies from one disease to another. In some instances it may be extremely low. I have seen patients with chronic hepatitis whose liver enzyme profile deteriorated when the dose of prednisone was reduced to 2.5 mg. per day, whereas it remained normal at 5.0 mg. per day. A few asthmatics may have substantial relief with as little as 5 mg. of prednisone twice a week. Is this a placebo effect? I doubt it, since other medications have failed to help, but I cannot be certain.

A fourth error is to give steroids for relief of a derangement attributed to one problem when it is a result of another for which steroids are useless or even dangerous. If increasing doses of steroids are given to control fever in an arthritic patient when the fever is a result of an unrecognized infection, the patient's ability to handle his complication will be reduced and his survival threatened because of an incorrect diagnosis. On the other hand, certain diseases such as disseminated lupus erythematosus may produce symptoms resembling those associated with steroid overdose. A patient with lupus who becomes psychotic almost always needs more, not less steroid.

A fifth error is to give steroids systemically when appropriate results could be achieved by local application. The use of steroids as enemas, skin creams, and eye drops may reduce the systemic effect considerably, while permitting good local control. It should not be assumed, however, that such local applications will not have any systemic effect. The inflamed or abraded skin and the ulcerated colon can absorb considerable amounts even of insoluble steroids, especially if the area of application is large. Even the intact normal colon will absorb enough dexamethasone to cause measurable suppression of ACTH secretion. Thus, local application is helpful, where possible, but it is not foolproof.

Special schedules of steroid administration may also be helpful in minimizing the undesirable effects of prolonged treatment. The most successful is to give the total amount needed in 48 hours as a single dose every alternate morning. This schedule works well with steroids of intermediate or short duration of action, such as prednisone or cortisone, since the pituitary-suppressing and gluconeogenic effects are largely dissipated during the second 24-hour period. On the other hand, such alternate day treatment does not work with long-acting compounds whose action persists beyond 40 hours. Moreover, although many patients are well controlled with alternate day treatment some fail to respond. Other schedules such as treating for three or four sequential days of each week have no advantages over continuous treatment.

What are the dangers or problems in concluding prolonged steroid therapy? After only a short period of treatment the medication can be stopped abruptly and completely without risk or symptoms. When therapy has been prolonged beyond about a month, however, such sudden discontinuation usually causes a period of reduced adrenal function associated with weakness, anorexia, myalgia, and low blood pressure. At this time the plasma steroid concentration is low and response to ACTH is minimal. These symptoms can be alleviated by slow withdrawal of the steroids; but even under these circumstances some patients develop a withdrawal syndrome during which plasma cortisol is normal and the response to ACTH is adequate. The symptoms mimic those of adrenal insufficiency and include myalgia, arthralgia, desquamation of the skin, nausea, and irritability.

Although these symptoms can be alleviated by retreatment with steroids for short periods, an additional disability may persist for nine months or more after treatment is stopped and the patient is no longer receiving any medication. It is during this period that the hypothalamic-pituitary-adrenal system gradually recovers its normal ability to respond to stresses. The period cannot be shortened by treating with ACTH—indeed, it may be prolonged by this treatment—and during this time there is a substantial though small risk that trauma or infection could precipitate acute adrenal insufficiency with collapse, shock, and death. This danger must be kept in mind and appropriate brief periods of supporting steroid treatment prescribed for the patient during the danger period if he is stressed. Alternatively, if the stress is predictable and controllable (for example, a surgical operation) steroid coverage may be omitted as long as generous amounts of intravenous glucocorticoid medication are kept close at hand during the operation and immediately thereafter while the patient is kept under close supervision.

Steroids are powerful medications. Used properly they can relieve distress, preserve function, and prolong life. But used carelessly, for situations in which they are ineffective, or in doses which are larger than necessary, or for longer than necessary, they can increase disability, prolong illness, and kill. Knowing this, the physician is obligated to evaluate the potential gains in light of the dangers. It would be folly to take large hazards for small gains; but when much might be accomplished, much could justifiably be risked.

Comment

The Prolonged Therapeutic Use of Adrenocortical Steroids

Dr. Jefferies contends that long-term low dosage therapy with adrenal steroids (less than 40 mg. per day of cortisol equivalent) is essentially free of side effects and in support cites his wide personal experience with low doses of steroids in the management of ovarian dysfunction. He suggests that similar doses would be safe and effective as "antirheumatic" and "anti-allergic" therapy. Dr. Bondy, on the other hand, stresses the risks of using steroids in any dose as nonspecific anti-inflammatory agents. He urges that physicians be cautious in their use, employing these agents only when necessary, only in the lowest effective dosage, and only in the therapy of serious illness that will respond to such therapy.

Setting aside the controversial question of the use of adrenal steroids in the treatment of ovarian disorders, the issue between our two essayists may boil down simply to a matter of emphasis. Both seem to agree that too much adrenal steroid medication is bad and, although he does not explicitly say so, I think it is fair to assume that Dr. Jefferies would concur with Dr. Bondy's opinion that one should not use steroids as anti-inflammatory or anti-allergic agents if less dangerous modalities of therapy will suffice.

Is this difference in emphasis of much practical importance? I think it is. Those physicians who are not sufficiently impressed with the harmful potential of steroids tend to be more easily persuaded that this type of therapy is "necessary" in a given patient, and they also tend to be less aggressive in attempting to lower the dosage or wean the patient entirely off medication once an initial response has occurred.

For practical purposes the issue concerns the use of steroids in rheumatoid arthritis and asthma, since these are the two common disabling diseases that are symptomatically improved by steroids.

A comparison of therapeutic practices in different parts of the country would, I am sure, reveal wide variations in the frequency with which patients with rheumatoid arthritis or chronic asthma are treated with adrenal steroids. Such differences probably reflect the attitudes of physicians, and not the underlying nature of these diseases as they occur in different clinics. The dilemma, then, is a real one: Do the undoubted symptomatic benefits of long-term adrenal steroids as anti-allergic and anti-inflammatory agents in these two diseases justify the risk of side effects? Can one, in fact, maintain symptomatic improvement without incurring the side effects of therapy?

Unfortunately there are no published data to provide clear quantitative answers. I suspect that the issue may never be definitively settled because of the subjective nature of many of the phenomena involved. We must remember that adrenal steroids produce an elevation of mood as well as a modification of the inflammatory reaction. Reduction of dosage after sustained administration often causes depression and fatigue and renders chronically ill patients far more susceptible to the discomforts of their underlying disease. Furthermore, a given dose that initially is adequate to suppress symptoms often becomes less effective with time; at least such seems to be the case in rheumatoid arthritis.

In this sense, adrenal steroids may be considered addictive, because the chronic administration of these agents tends to be a self-perpetuating process, which often leads the patient to demand more than the minimum maintenance dosage that might have been expected to be safe and effective. Under these difficult circumstances it takes all the skill a good physician can muster to prevent his patient from becoming habituated to a chronic dose of steroid that may ultimately do more harm than the disease which the steroid is intended to alleviate.

ARNOLD S. RELMAN

18

Treatment of Crohn's Disease

The Usefulness of Adrenocortical Steroids
 by Joseph B. Kirsner

The Usefulness of Azathioprine
 by Bryan N. Brooke

The Case for Surgical Treatment
 by Donald J. Glotzer

A Conservative Approach
 by Thomas A. Warthin

Comment
 by Franz J. Ingelfinger

The Usefulness of Adrenocortical Steroids

JOSEPH B. KIRSNER

Department of Medicine, The University of Chicago

The cause of regional enteritis is not known; hence, no specific or curative treatment is available. Therapy, as for inflammatory bowel disease in general, is symptomatic, comprehensive, and empirical, including physical rest, restoration of general health, elimination of infection, and control of associated emotional problems. Surgical intervention is required frequently for various complications, including stenosis of the bowel with obstruction, abscess formation, uncontrollable bleeding, and fistula formation.

Adrenal corticosteroids do not cure regional enteritis or completely prevent recurrences. However, although controlled studies are yet lacking, steroids in many instances appear to be useful symptom-controlling agents when administered in sufficient quantities under careful supervision. Their capacity to diminish the vascular and tissue responses to inflammation of whatever etiology is helpful in controlling the inflammatory reaction of Crohn's disease. They also are immunosuppressive agents, but conclusive evidence of this action and, indeed, of the role of immunology in regional enteritis is lacking. Steroids serve as "facilitating" agents; they restrain progression of the disease, they reduce thereby the likelihood of complications, and they promote the patient's favorable response to the total therapeutic program.

Adrenal steroids are prescribed as adjuncts, never as the sole treatment. The indications are moderate to severe Crohn's disease, uncomplicated but unresponsive to, or recurrent despite, conventional therapy; diffuse ileojejunitis, too extensive for surgery; progressive recurrent inflammation after previous resections, when further surgery is to be avoided; Crohn's disease of the colon not requiring surgical intervention; and the presence of systemic complications, notably acute iritis, erythema nodosum, and hemolytic anemia, problems known to respond to steroid medication.

The beneficial effects in regional enteritis are characterized clinically by the subsidence of fever, toxemia, abdominal discomfort, and diarrhea, by increased appetite, by weight gain as nutritional deficits are corrected under steroid influence, and by a general sense of well-being. Obstructive symptoms resulting from inflammation and edema of the bowel also respond promptly. Laboratory indications of improvement include the return of an elevated sedimentation rate to normal, improvement in the plasma proteins and blood counts, and disappearance of occult blood from the feces. Occasionally an associated inflammatory abdominal mass may decrease in size or may disappear. Fistulas usually are unchanged, although shrinkage has been reported. The roentgen changes of Crohn's disease do not disappear completely, but in nonstenosing disease the coarsened mucosal pattern and the degree of narrowing may improve.

The preferred preparations are hydrocortisone and prednisone; but other steroids, e.g., methyl prednisone, may also be helpful. The necessary quantities of steroids, as in ulcerative colitis, tend to be large. The initial oral doses are for hydrocortisone, 200 to 300 mg., and for prednisone, 40 to 60 mg., given in one or several doses daily. Alternate day steroid therapy in which the two-day dose is given every other day, to lower the incidence of side effects while maintaining therapeutic benefit, has not been consistently effective in patients with inflammatory bowel disease. As in other disorders, the response to steroids varies among individuals, and in the same person at different times, requiring identification of the appropriate preparation and the effective dosage for a given patient. Since a favorable clinical response depends upon adequate nutrition, treatment must include restoration of the bodily stores of protein, either before steroids are prescribed or concurrently.

Once improvement has been established, the quantity of steroids is decreased gradually toward an effective maintenance level, negotiated over a period of months. As illustrated for prednisone, "early" dose reductions may be from 40 to 30, then 25 and 20 mg. daily, each decrease undertaken only after the favorable clinical course has been maintained despite the lower steroid intake. Subsequent decreases are to 17.5, 15.0, 12.5, and 10.0 mg. daily, each decrement taking at least two to four weeks, occasionally longer. After 10 mg., the decreases are to 7.5, 5.0, and 2.5 mg., each reduction being made over periods of one or two months. Steroids can then be discontinued completely. Continued control then depends upon the general measures noted earlier. Some patients with Crohn's disease not requiring surgery seem to remain under better control with small quantities of steroids, ranging from 5 to 15 mg. prednisone or 20 to 60 mg. hydrocortisone daily for long periods. At this dosage the incidence and the severity of side effects have been minimal.

Steroids are usually continued for months and, in some instances, for years, although efforts are made repeatedly to eliminate the medication. The complete removal of steroids is not easy, requiring patience and time. Clinically premature and excessively rapid decreases in the quantity of steroids often precipitate flareups and also a relative adrenal insufficiency. Steroid dependency is encountered occasionally, but this problem can be negotiated with continued control of disease. The intramuscular injection of ACTH, 40 to 80 units once or twice each week, is advocated by some physicians, but I am not enthusiastic about this therapy and have not used it.

The initial course of steroids probably is the most effective in patients with inflammatory bowel disease, and this experience reinforces the need for the careful initial use of this medication, avoiding inadequate doses, premature and excessive reductions in quantity, and indifference to the overall therapeutic requirements. Occasionally, during prolonged steroid medication and especially after interrupted therapy, the beneficial response tends to diminish and may disappear, including not only the effect upon the bowel disease but also the side effects; e.g., the cushingoid facies may decrease. The mechanism of this waning response is not known but it often is associated with undernutrition and it may be reversed with improvement in nutrition. The response to steroids may also be restored by increasing the quantity or by changing from hydrocortisone to prednisone and vice versa.

Steroids are contraindicated in regional enteritis in the presence of perforation of the bowel and peritonitis; in the presence of pyogenic complications (e.g., perirectal or ischiorectal abscess or liver abscess); when the clinical situation is dominated by mechanical obstruction caused by cicatricial narrowing of the intestine; and perhaps in patients with severe psychiatric difficulties. Steroids are not necessarily contraindicated in the presence of fistula formation provided the comprehensive program is maintained. Steroids are not necessarily contraindicated in bleeding from the bowel, for the underlying inflammation and ulceration may respond to the anti-inflammatory program. A history of pulmonary tuberculosis does not exclude steroids, providing the indications otherwise are acceptable and isoniazid is administered concurrently. Severe hypertension and osteoporosis usually are contraindications to prolonged steroid medication.

Adrenal steroids may induce various complications, especially during prolonged used in large amounts. Constant vigilance, the maintenance of adequate nutrition, and frequent monitoring of the serum electrolytes are necessary to reduce their frequency and severity. The early side effects, especially cushingoid appearance and growth of hair, may be disagreeable, especially to young female patients, but they are reversible changes. Indeed, the development of a cushingoid facies is a clinical indication of an adequate steroid dosage. If it does not develop, the patient's gastrointestinal symptoms probably will not respond to the steroid prescribed. The most commonly encountered biochemical side effect, hypokalemia, is corrected easily. The long-term hazards include aggravation or development of diabetes mellitus, especially in patients wih a family history of diabetes; osteoporosis with concomitant bony problems, including fractures, aseptic necrosis of the hip, and collapse of vertebrae; increased susceptibility to infection, bruising, growth retardation in children, steroid myopathy, posterior subcapsular cataracts, and steroid psychosis.

Since steroids do not cure regional enteritis or even guarantee against recurrences, and since they may cause significant side effects, can their long-term use be justified in terms of the "risk-benefit" balance? In my experience the answer to this important question is yes. The initial consideration here is the experienced use of steroids by physicians thoroughly familiar both with the pharmacology of the drugs and with the nature of inflammatory bowel disease. The physician also must be aware of the "facilitating" influence of steroids rather than curative effects and must adjust therapy accordingly. Inexperienced, casual administration of steroids accounts for many of the steroid-related problems encountered in the management of inflammatory bowel disease and for therapeutic failures. Proper awareness of the advantages and limitations of steroids and continuing supervision of the patient have greatly reduced the number and severity of complications. Diabetes mellitus, should it occur, can be managed with dietary restrictions and oral hypoglycemic agents. Peptic ulcer has been very infrequent, in my experience; and psychotic reactions have been rare. On the other hand, the growth retardation observed in some young patients presents a difficult therapeutic challenge, especially since the growth retardation may be as attributable to active Crohn's disease as to steroids. The inexpert administration of steroids, therefore, does not seem to be a sufficient reason for not utilizing this helpful medication in the management of a disorder for which no curative medication is yet available; and wherein even the most skillful and well prepared resective surgery does not guarantee against recurrences, progression of the disease, and the development of problems such as short bowel syndrome, bile salt deficiency, steatorrhea, B_{12} deficiency, and malnutrition.

Can the long-term administration of relatively large amounts of steroids be justified as a means of providing long-term control of a chronic recurrent disease such as regional enteritis? The answer to this question, in my judgment, is no, except unavoidably perhaps in those patients with recurrent disease of the remaining small bowel and/or colon after one or several operaions. Administration of large quantities of steroids for years without unmistakable and sustained clinical benefit at the risk of precarious general health of the patient cannot be justified. For purposes of long-term management, the bowel disease, when it is not extensive (to the degree of nonresectability), probably is best removed surgically, with the hope that the enteritis does not recur or that recurrences will be relatively mild. Long-term steroid therapy may be virtually unavoidable in the presence of extensive small bowel disease, recurrent despite one or more surgical attempts to remove diseased bowel. In this desperate situation, long-term steroids may be administered together with intensive nutritional support in an effort to reduce the hazard of complications. The apparent steroid-sparing effects of azathioprine (Imuran) may offer another approach to this problem, although azathioprine also is a potentially dangerous drug and its long-term effects in inflammatory bowel disease as yet are unknown. This aspect of the therapeutic dilemma should be clarified within the next few years as ongoing double-blind controlled studies with azathioprine are completed. The possibility that both steroids and azathioprine may eventually contribute to the increased development of neoplasia by inhibition or alteration of our normal immunologic surveillance mechanisms is an important consideration which cannot be evaluated in our present knowledge.

Since surgery is so often necessary in patients with regional enteritis, why complicate the operative problem with steroids? In this situation the anti-inflammatory benefits of steroids, by reducing the tissue reaction, may, in fact, facilitate definitive surgery, provided the general support of the patient also is accomplished. In our experience steroids, given properly and with adequate supportive measures, do not jeopardize the success of necessary surgical intervention or increase the hazard of postoperative recurrence. Wound healing may be delayed slightly, but healing proceeds satisfactorily with adequate protein levels and blood counts.

Do not steroids increase the risk of penetration through the bowel wall to produce more enteric fistulas and also perforations of the bowel? Our experience indicates a negative response to this question. Fistula formation is as common among nonsteroid- as in steroid-treated patients. Frank perforation of the bowel in regional enteritis is not common; but when it occurs, the perforation usually is proximal to an area of intestinal obstruction. Stenosis of the bowel (a characteristic of the regional enteritis process), and mechanical obstruction of an inflamed bowel, in addition to the inflammatory process per se, are important contributory factors. The assumption that steroids increase the tendency to perianal fistula formation and anal ulceration has not been documented conclusively.

Does the use of steroids promote the progression of regional enteritis? Not in our experience. The progression of regional enteritis is related to its continuing activity and to the severity of the tissue reaction and to undernutrition; it occurs more often following surgical intervention than following the use of steroids.

Do steroids promote the occurrence of systemic complications, presumably by diminishing host resistance? There is no evidence for this assumption. In the presence of severe inflammatory bowel disease, the use of steroids may not prevent the development of systemic complications; but, more often, steroids are dramatically helpful in quickly controlling various systemic complications, e.g., acute iritis which, if not controlled fully and promptly, may lead to blindness.

Thus, in conclusion, steroids are useful "facilitating" adjuncts in the management of Crohn's disease. With proper awareness of their potential advantages and limitations, experience in their administration, and knowledge of inflammatory bowel disease, use of steroids is capable of contributing to the control of a chronic, recurrent, often progressive intestinal disease for which there are no curative measures and which rarely spontaneously heals completely.

The Usefulness of Azathioprine

BRYAN N. BROOKE

University of London at St. George's Hospital Medical School

We are perplexed and thwarted by an inflammatory disease which displays an almost malignant potential for recurrence, though not a similar mortality. It is now abundantly clear that the longer a series of cases is reviewed, the higher the recurrence rate. This was revealed in early reports. In 1955 Cooke[1] revealed 45 per cent recurrence at two years, 68 per cent at five years, and 78 per cent at 10 years in 90 patients treated medically and surgically; in 1954 the Mayo Clinic[2] reported 80 per cent recurrence at 15 years in a surgical series of 270 patients. More recently, using actuarial methods, Lennard-Jones,[3] together with Stadler,[4] ascertained that one third of all patients with an ileal resection have relapsed symptomatically after five years, and this proportion has risen to one half after 10 years. After resection and ileorectal anastomosis for Crohn's colitis a 50 to 60 per cent recurrence rate was observed in two series.[5,6] Recently Cooke[7] has reviewed his cases 17 years later in a group now containing more than 300 patients, indicating slight improvement over his previous figures but no substantial change —32 per cent at two years, 50 per cent at five years, and 69.5 per cent at 10 years.

Thus, a patient with Crohn's disease once under care is, like the poor, always with us. Once treated, the patient will remain under observation for life. The disease, therefore, calls for therapeutic ingenuity from a wide choice of treatments. To date the choice has been limited to corticosteroids and extirpation of the gross lesions by surgery, together with supportive therapy for secondary phenomena such as malabsorption and anemia. Insoluble sulfonamides, in particular salicylazosulfapyridine, have been tried and have proved ineffective.

Though there can be no doubt that corticosteroids are capable of inducing a remission in individual cases, the long-term effects are now in question, all the more so in that no prospective controlled studies have yet been reported. Steroids are sometimes effective in inducing a remission in acute disease; they are more so in young patients who have a short history and have had no previous surgery,[8] and in widespread disease in the small bowel,[9] though improvement is not always sustained.[10] They are ineffective in the presence of fistula, stricture, or abscess; their use has been disappointing when the colon is involved,[11] in recurrence following surgery, and when used prophylactically as maintenance therapy to prevent such recurrences.[12] Apart from the usual disadvantages inherent in steroid treatment, Cooke and Fielding[13] have drawn attention to the following specific points: the probability of operation per annum was double in those patients treated with steroids compared with the rest of their group of 300 cases; mortality for those thus treated was significantly higher—24 out of 124 in the steroid-treated group, that is, four and a half times greater than the expected death rate in a matched normal population and two and a half times greater than in those patients with Crohn's disease not treated with steroids.

The most that can be said for steroid therapy is that it restores a sense of well-being and brings about a beneficial effect as regards symptoms while sometimes correcting hematological abnormalities or maintaining any gain after their correction by other means. While it cannot be denied that this represents a substantial advance in the absence of other effective remedies, there is no evidence that this form of therapy has any long-term effect upon the disease. Moreover, interference with growth and development places limitations upon the use of steroids in young patients. Finally, more than a suspicion is arising that a cancer hazard exists in longstanding disease, as it does in ulcerative colitis. Wyatt,[14] when reporting a case of carcinoma of the small intestine in Crohn's disease, collected 16 further cases from the literature and demonstrated, in all but two cases, a mean duration of the disease of 15.7 years before the clinical demonstration of cancer, and a mean age of onset of cancer of 42.7 years, in contrast with 60.8 years for cancer in the small bowel without antecedent inflammation[15]—statistics singularly similar to those for ulcerative colitis.

It is natural, therefore that a search should be made elsewhere for a new line of treatment. Faute de mieux the direction has turned toward immunosuppressive drugs, in particular azathioprine. It cannot be said, however, that this trend is soundly based in scientific proof of immunologic disturbance. Since the evidence of immunologic disorder is conflicting in the extreme, the use of immunosuppressives is empirical, for Crohn's disease may represent a state of anergy on the one hand, or delayed hypersensitivity on the other.

The idea initially gained ground from the histologic appearances of the granuloma which is present in 60 per cent of specimens and resembles those seen in sarcoidosis, leprosy, tuberculosis, and beryllium poisoning. In all these conditions the granuloma is accepted as evidence of delayed hypersensitivity induced by an infective or toxic agent. Slaney,[16] who was able to reproduce the granuloma in the intestine of rabbits, used horse serum injections after sensitization to the same serum; it has not, however, proved possible to reproduce this model by means of bovine serum albumin in my laboratories, though Freund's complete adjuvant alone when injected subserosally has met with intermittent success[17]—a point which may be of significance, as will be seen later, since Freund's adjuvant contains killed *Mycobacterium tuberculosis*.

The granuloma is not the sole histologic straw in the wind. The epithelioid cell, which may be an outward and visible sign of delayed hypersensitivity, is an integral part of the granuloma, but lymphocytes are also undoubtedly increased in number generally throughout tissue involved in the disease. The lymphocyte has a prominent nucleolus when about to transform into a plasma cell. Aluwihare[18, 19] has found this phenomenon to be more prominent in Crohn's disease than in ulcerative colitis. But this raises the question whether it is an indication of hyperactivity or a sign of arrest. Aluwihare has also noted the proximity of lymphocytes to epithelioid cells and macrophages, an advantageous position if lymphocytes are needed to pass on antibody to these cells.

These are straws in the wind which have led to numerous attempts to prove an immunologic basis for Crohn's disease. It appears certain that there is no circulating humoral antibody. A fecal antigen may be a cause, since diversion of the fecal stream by short circuit is followed by improvement, and the reintroduction of fecal contents into defunctioned colon is followed by exacerbation,[20] but it is unlikely that this is a humoral antibody. Eggert et al.[21] reported a case of Crohn's disease in a patient with agammaglobulinemia; moreover, humoral antibodies to casein are low in Crohn's disease[22]—in contrast to ulcerative colitis— indicating a reduced immunity to a naturally occurring ingested antigen. Dykes[23] demonstrated the inhibition of macrophage migration by fecal extracts from patients with Crohn's disease, the first real indication of a possible fecal antigen invoking a cellular immune reaction. In this respect the notable feature of the site of recurrence after resection has been constantly overlooked; that this is at the former anastomotic site would lend credence to the idea that a fecal antigen might induce a local hypersensitivity reaction wherever it could gain access through the mucosa. The discovery of a transmissible substance from extracts of Crohn's tissue creating lesions indistinguishable from the granulomata of Crohn's disease after injection into the footpads of mice[24] in no way runs counter to this proposition, though another explanation is possible, albeit on a basis of cellular hypersensitivity.

Mycobacteria may be partially destroyed by mycobacteriophage, as occurs in tuberculoid leprosy,[25] tuberculosis, and sarcoidosis;[26,27] some cellular degradation products of the bacteria remain and are antigenic. This is the so-called lysogenous state. Before Crohn's disease was described, cases were thought to represent a form of ileocecal tuberculosis. Possibly particles of dead or partially destroyed tubercle bacilli persist in Crohn's disease to invoke the lysogenous state. Though whole tubercle bacilli have not hitherto been demonstrated in Crohn's disease, Aluwihare[18,19] has identified intramural bacteria in six of 11 specimens examined by electron microscopy. Kane's[17] ability to obtain Crohn's type granulomata in rabbits using Freund's adjuvant alone may be explicable in the light of the lysogenous theory. But a report from Minnesota indicates that mycobacteriophage can be cultured from the sera of Crohn's patients with no greater frequency than in normal patients.[28]

The pursuit of the lymphocyte for evidence of delayed hypersensitivity has provided equivocal results and must, to date, be regarded as unfruitful. Leukocytes from patients with Crohn's disease, like those from ulcerative colitis, are toxic to colonic epithelium.[29-31] However, lymphocyte transformation was impaired in patients with Crohn's disease studied by Walker and Greaves[32] and Brown and his colleagues.[33] Bendixen[34] alone and with Weeke[35] found no inhibition of leukocyte migration by mucosal homogenates in cases of Crohn's disease, whereas migration was inhibited in ulcerative colitis.

The failure to obtain positive evidence from leukocyte studies may indicate a state of anergy. Indeed, the toxic effect of lymphocytes on colonic epithelium is not to be found in Crohn's disease when these cells are applied to the mucosa of ileum.[25] Verrier Jones and his colleagues[36] demonstrated an inability in Crohn's patients to develop delayed hypersensitivity to the dinitrochlorobenzene skin test. Williams[37] found the Mantoux reaction to be negative more frequently in Crohn's disease than ulcerative colitis, but this could not be confirmed by Fletcher and Hinton.[38] Similarly the Kveim test has proved equivocal, and the explanation for this only serves to indicate the pitfalls for investigators in the immunologic field.[39]

Despite the equivocal experimental evidence, we decided to try the effects of immunosuppression in advanced and complicated cases no longer responding to the usual forms of treatment. Azathioprine was chosen because of its proved success in transplant cases and its lymphocyte specificity. Encouraged by early results,[46] we have now extended its use to include the primary treatment for ileal disease and colitis and as maintenance therapy following surgery to ascertain whether recurrence can be avoided or delayed.

At the time of writing 39 patients have received or are continuing to receive the drug and have been under surveillance for nine to 36 months. It is always difficult to record in a reproducible way clinical improvement, or the reverse, in a disease with such protean manifestations as Crohn's disease. A system has therefore been evolved allocating a numerical score to certain clinical parameters (Table 1); the better the result, the lower the score. In Figure 1 is shown the clinical status of 22 patients before and after receiving azathioprine as the only form of treatment. All but two have improved, one remaining in status quo, the other deteriorating. The parameters have improved sufficiently in seven patients to place them in the range of normal health (at or below the level of 1). Submitting the differences in each sample to analysis of variance (Anova Class 1),[41] the changes seen in the whole group before and after treatment indicate a highly significant improvement ($P>0.001$). In Figure 2 are considered seven patients in whom surgery was a necessary adjunct during the course of azathioprine; four deteriorated while on the drug before operation, two improved at this stage, and one showed no change. Analysis of variance here gives no clue as to whether the drug or the intervention of surgery improved the situation ($P=0.005$). Eight of the 10 patients submitted initially to surgery and then given azathioprine (Fig.

Table 1. *Score System for Progress Assessment of Crohn's Disease*

	0	1	2
Abdominal pain	None	Present but able to work and/or sleep	Unable to work or sleep
Diarrhea (stool frequency)	0–3	4–6	>6
Weight	Gained >5 kg.	Presentation weight	Loss of >5 kg.
Anal lesions	Nil	Fissures or superficial ulcers	Fistulas, abscesses, or deep ulcers
Mass	None	Induration	Mass
Fistulas Abdominal or viscerovisceral	None	Present with purulent or no discharge	Gut contents discharging
Hemoglobin	♂ >13.5 gm. ♀ >11.5 gm.	13.5–10.5 gm. 11.5– 8.5 gm.	<10.5 gm. < 8.5 gm.
Albumin	Normal >3.0 gm.	3 – 2 gm.	< 2 gm.

3) improved, one remaining unchanged and another showing deterioration. Though there is significant change (P=0.005→0.001), again no deduction can be made as to the part played by surgery or azathioprine. Taking Figures 2 and 3 in conjunction, it can be seen that when certain indications for surgery already

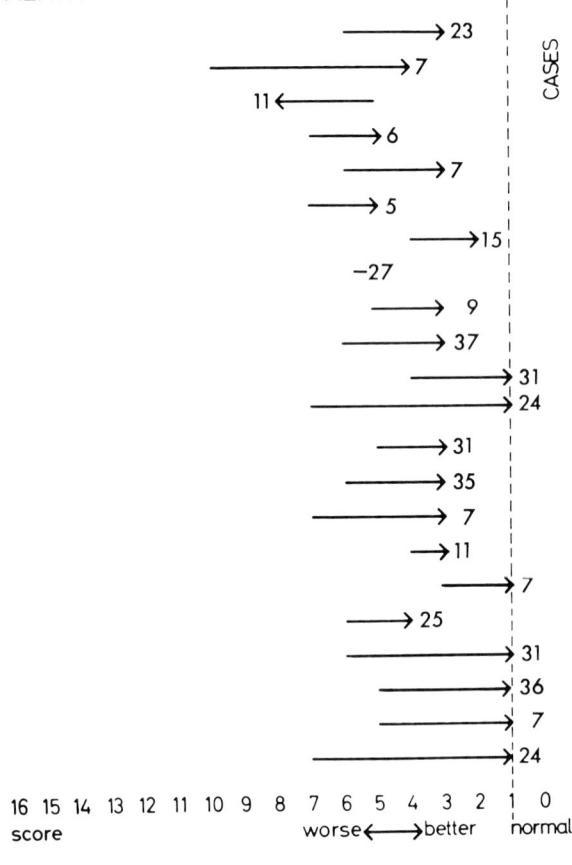

Figure 1. The figure related to each arrow indicates the duration in months of follow-up since the institution of azathioprine therapy.

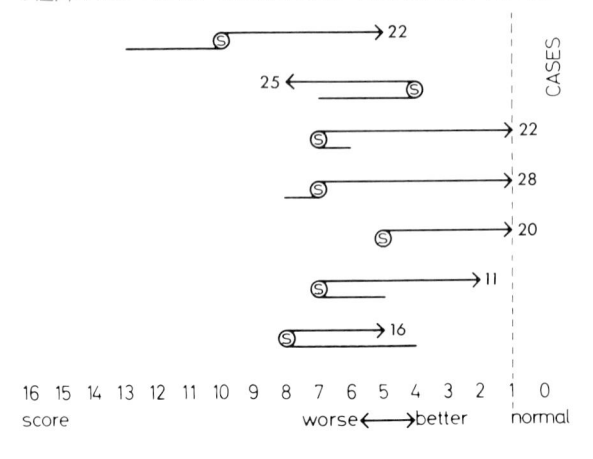

Figure 2. The figure related to each arrow indicates the duration in months of treatment with azathioprine.

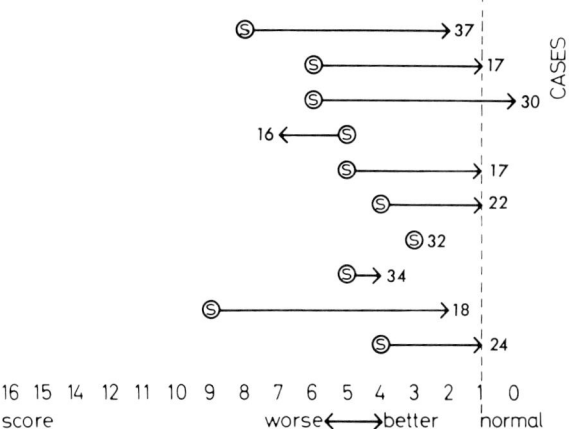

Figure 3. The figure related to each arrow indicates the duration in months of treatment with azathioprine.

exist (obstruction, abscess, or a palpable mass), azathioprine will not remove the need for surgery.

The drug has proved effective in inducing a remission in acute ileitis, generalized small intestinal disease, and colitis, and in the presence of abdominal and multiple anal fistulas.[42]

Initially the dosage of azathioprine used was the same as for organ transplantation—4 mg./kg. for 10 days followed by 2 mg./kg.[40, 43] Leukopenia not infrequently occurred during the loading period; it was therefore decided to abandon the higher dosage since in transplantation this was required chiefly for rapid immunosuppression, which is unnecessary in Crohn's disease. A clinical response in Crohn's disease, when it is forthcoming, is noticeable within one to three weeks. The white cell count is monitored on alternate days during the initial period of three to four weeks. Should the count fall to 3000, the drug is withheld. The white count returns to normal within five to seven days; when immunosuppressive therapy is restored leukopenia does not recur.

A far greater problem arises as to cessation of treatment. Improvement is usually noticeable within a week, but restoration to normal health may require as long as six months to a year. What may happen when the drug is stopped is entirely unpredictable. In some of our cases improvement has been maintained, particularly those successfully treated for acute Crohn's colitis. But by contrast four of our patients with a good response and in normal health have relapsed on withdrawal or reduction of the drug, in one patient after continuous therapy for nearly three years. In every case restoration to full dosage of 2 mg./kg. has reversed the situation and induced remission again. There appears to be no measurement, such as sedimentation rate, by which the appropriate moment for withdrawal may be chosen.

The problem is a serious one because of the fears of carcinogenicity. This fear arises from certain animal experiments; while it is not possible to induce malignancy in rats with azathioprine, it has been achieved in New Zealand black mice. Six of eight mice given azathioprine from two months of age developed lymphoma.[44] However, this strain of mice has been found to carry a latent virus, and it is possible that azathioprine depresses resistance to potential oncogenetic properties of the virus. To turn to man, alarming reports have come from Starzl and his colleagues.[45] But it must be borne in mind that the vast majority of cases of malignancy have occurred in transplant cases, many of them with incipient episodes of rejection and variously treated with steroids, thymectomy, antilymphocyte globulins, and irradiation. It is therefore difficult to assess the effect of azathioprine alone in this respect. At the time of writing 52 out of a total of over 5000 transplant patients have developed malignancies, most of these arising in one center in the United States. Out of over 4000 treated with azathioprine for disorders as various as chronic active hepatitis, rheumatoid disease, systemic lupus, autoimmune hemolytic anemia, idiopathic thrombocytopenic purpura, psoriasis, and fibrosing pulmonary alveolitis, only three cases of malignancy have been reported. One patient had had ulcerative colitis for 14 years and was found to have carcinoma of the colon. The other two were more sinister in the light of the animal experiments, for lymphoma was found in one and retroperitoneal sarcoma in the other. However, as a further twist to this story, in a recent controlled trial of azathioprine for rheumatoid arthritis 27 patients received the drug for 30 months. None of the treated patients developed malignancies, but three of the control group died of cancer.[46] If Crohn's disease is proved to be premalignant,[14] and azathioprine to be an effective drug in controlling the disease and yet to be occasionally oncogenic, a situation will prevail presenting difficult therapeutic decisions.

The potential for superinfection arising from immunosuppression is another disadvantage too well known to be discussed here. It calls for therapeutic vigilance. Though septicemia has been encountered in our series, no deaths have occurred. Azathioprine has been administered to the time of operation and has been instituted within 48 hours of surgery without ill effect.

Finally, there is the objection of teratogenicity. This has arisen because of experiments with mice.[47] Fortunately in this regard the experience in humans is clear-cut and encouraging, for no malformation has been seen in numerous pregnancies reported in renal transplant patients receiving immunosuppression.[48-50] Our own experience endorses this. One woman delivered a normal baby after receiving the drug not only throughout pregnancy but for two years preceding it. We also had the opportunity of studying a four month fetus in a woman who needed hysterotomy for unrelated reasons while under treatment for Crohn's disease. No abnormalities could be detected. Moreover the opportunity was taken to administer radioactive azathioprine (labeled with ^{35}S) before operation. Urine collections from the mother taken during the operative period contained radioactive material, but no significant activity was observed in thin tissue slices of the fetus placed in a spark chamber. This can only be regarded as an indication that azathioprine does not enter the fetus, for the metabolism and degradation of the drug is uncertain. All that may be said is that that portion which carries the sulfur molecule does not cross the placenta; this may not be the active and potentially teratogenic moiety.

In conclusion, despite uncertainty as to whether Crohn's disease is an expression of immunologic disorder, therapy based somewhat empirically on this assumption has been shown to yield beneficial results in the short term.[40, 43, 51-54]

Controversy is now properly engaged upon the propriety of using a drug which may have oncogenic properties. At the same time—and for the first time in the management of this disease—prospective controlled trials are being undertaken to test azathioprine, an attempt never yet made for corticosteroid therapy. The results are as yet equivocal, for one report[55] is favorable; the other, not.[58] A new line of treatment has been put in train which will require testing not only against other drugs but over a long term in order to assess its ability to reduce the recurrence rate. It is uncertain whether azathioprine acts as an anti-inflammatory or immunosuppressive agent in this disease. Its metabolic pathways and breakdown products in man are as yet unknown. Nor is it known whether the therapeutic effects are related specifically to azathioprine and less to immunosuppression; one of our patients responded well to azathioprine after cyclophosphamide had failed.[40]

References

1. Cooke, W. T.: Nutritional and metabolic factors in the aetiology and treatment of regional iletis. Ann. Roy. Coll. Surg. Eng. 17:137, 1955.
2. Van Patter, W. N., Bargen, J. A., Dockerty, M. B., Feldman, W. H., Mayo, C. W., and Waugh, J. M.: Regional enteritis. Gastroenterology 26:347, 1954.
3. Lennard-Jones, J. E.: Crohn's disease: Natural history and treatment. Postgrad. Med. J. 44:674, 1968.
4. Lennard-Jones, J. E., and Stadler, G. A.: Prognosis after resection of chronic regional ileitis. Gut 8:332, 1967.
5. Baker, W. N. W.: Ileorectal anastomosis for Crohn's disease of the colon. Gut 12:427, 1971.
6. Burman, J. H., Cooke, W. T., and Williams, J. A.: The fate of ileorectal anastomosis in Crohn's disease. Gut 12:432, 1971.
7. Cooke, W. T.: The results of treatment in Crohn's disease. In Brooke, B. N. (ed.): Clinics in Gastroenterology. 1:521, 1972.
8. Schofield, P. F.: Natural history and treatment of Crohn's disease. Ann. Roy. Coll. Surg. Eng. 36:258, 1965.
9. Howel Jones, J., and Lennard-Jones, J. E.: Corticosteroids and corticotrophin in the treatment of Crohn's disease. Gut 7:181, 1966.
10. Swan, C. H. J., and Cooke, W. T.: Treatment and prognosis in diffuse jejuno-ileitis. Reported to the British Society of Gastroenterology, September, 1971.
11. Howel Jones, J., Lennard-Jones, J. E., and Lockhart-Mummery, H. E.: Experience in the treatment of Crohn's disease of the large intestine. Gut 7:448, 1966.
12. Sparberg, M., and Kirsner, J.: Long term corticosteroid therapy for regional enteritis. Amer. J. Dig. Dis. 11:652, 1966.
13. Cooke, W. T., and Fielding, J. F.: Corticosteroid or corticotrophin therapy in Crohn's disease (regional enteritis). Gut 11:921, 1970.
14. Wyatt, A. P.: Regional enteritis leading to carcinoma of the small bowel. Gut 10:924, 1969.
15. Brookes, V. S., Waterhouse, J. A. H., and Powell, D. J.: Malignant lesions of the small intestine; a ten year survey. Brit. J. Surg. 55:405, 1968.
16. Slaney, G.: Hypersensitivity granulomata and the alimentary tract. Ann. Roy. Coll. Surg. Eng. 31:249, 1962.
17. Kane, S.: Experimental pathology of Crohn's disease. In Brooke, B. N. (ed.): Clinics in Gastroenterology 1:295, 1972.
18. Aluwihare, A. P. R.: Electron microscopy in Crohn's disease. Gut 12:509, 1971.
19. Aluwihare, A. P. R.: Electron microscopy in Crohn's disease. In Brooke, B. N. (ed.): Clinics in Gastroenterology 1:279: 1972.
20. Oberhelman, H. A., Kohatsu, S., Taylor, K. B., and Kivel, R. M.: Diverting ileostomy in the surgical management of Crohn's disease of the colon. Amer. J. Surg. 115:231, 1968.

21. Eggert, R. C., Wilson, I. D., and Good, R. A.: Agamma-globulinemia and regional enteritis. Ann. Intern. Med. 71:581, 1969.
22. Taylor, K. B.: Immune mechanisms in gastroenterology. In Badenoch, J., and Brooke, B. N. (eds.): Recent Advances in Gastroenterology. London, J. & A. Churchill, 1965, p. 24.
23. Dykes, P. W.: Delayed hypersensitivity in Crohn's disease. Proc. Roy. Soc. Med. 63:906, 1970.
24. Mitchell, D. N., and Rees, R. J. W.: Agent transmissible from Crohn's disease tissue. Lancet 2:168, 1970.
25. Watson, D. W.: Immune responses and the gut. Gastroenterology 56:944, 1969.
26. Mankiewicz, E., and Van Walbeek, M.: Mycobacteriophages: their role in tuberculosis and sarcoidosis. Arch. Environ. Health (Chicago) 5:122, 1962.
27. Mankiewicz, E., and Liivak, M.: Mycobacteriophages isolated from human sources. Nature (London) 216:485, 1967.
28. Parent, K., and Dodd Wilson, I.: Mycobacteriophage in Crohn's disease. Gut 12:1019, 1971.
29. Perlmann, P., and Broberger, O.: In vitro studies in ulcerative colitis. Cytotoxic action of white blood cells from patients on human fetal colon cells. J. Exp. Med. 117:717, 1963.
30. Watson, D. W., Quigley, A., and Bolt, R. J.: Effect of lymphocytes from patients with ulcerative colitis on human adult colon epithelial cells. Gastroenterology 51:985, 1966.
31. Shorter, R. G., Spencer, R. J., Huizenga, K. A., and Hallenbeck, G. A.: Inhibition of in vitro cytotoxicity of lymphocytes from patients with ulcerative colitis and granulomatous colitis for allogenic colonic epithelial cells using horse antihuman thymus serum. Gastroenterology 54:227, 1968.
32. Walker, J. G., and Greaves, M. F.: Delayed hypersensitivity and lymphocyte transformation in Crohn's disease and proctocolitis. Gut 10:414, 1969.
33. Brown, S. M., Taub, R. N., Present, D. H., and Janowitz, H. D.: Short-term lymphocyte cultures in regional enteritis. Lancet 1:1112, 1970.
34. Bendixen, G.: Specific inhibition of in vitro migration of leucocytes in ulcerative colitis and Crohn's disease. Scand. J. Gastroent. 2:214, 1967.
35. Weeke, B., and Bendixen, G.: Serum immunoglobulins and organ-specific cellular hypersensitivity in ulcerative colitis and Crohn's disease. Acta Med. Scand. 186:87, 1969.
36. Verrier Jones, J., Housley, J., Ashurst, P. M., and Hawkins, C. F.: Development of delayed hypersensitivity to dinitrochlorobenzene in patients with Crohn's disease. Gut 10:52, 1969.
37. Williams, W. J.: A study of Crohn's syndrome using tissue extracts and the Kveim and Mantoux tests. Gut 6:503, 1965.
38. Fletcher, J., and Hinton, J. M.: Tuberculin sensitivity in Crohn's disease. Lancet 2:753, 1967.
39. Lancet: Kveim-Siltzbach test vindicated. 1:188, 1972.
40. Brooke, B. N., Hoffmann, D. C., and Swarbrick, E. T.: Azathioprine for Crohn's disease. Lancet 2:612, 1969.
41. Dowsett, D. J., and Priest, R.: Short programmes for statistical analysis using FOCAL. Decus Catalogue, 1970.
42. Brooke, B. N.: The treatment of Crohn's disease with azathioprine. In Badenoch, J., and Brooke, B. N. (eds.): Recent Advances in Gastroenterology. 2nd ed. London, Churchill Livingstone, 1972.
43. Brooke, B. N., Javett, S. L., and Davison, O. W.: Further experience with azathioprine for Crohn's disease. Lancet 2:1050, 1970.
44. Casey, T. P.: Azathioprine (Imuran) administration and the development of malignant lymphomas in mice. Clin. Exp. Immunol. 3:305, 1968.
45. Starzl, T. E., Porter, K. A., Andres, G., and Halgrimson, C. G.: Long term survival after renal transplantation in humans: (with special reference to histocompatibility matching, thymectomy, homograft glomerulonephritis, heterologous ALG, and recipient malignancy). Ann. Surg. 172:437, 1970.
46. Harris, J., Jessop, J. D., and Chaput de Saintouge, D. M.: Further experience with azathioprine in rheumatoid arthritis. Brit. Med. J. 4:463, 1971.
47. Rosenkrantz, J. G., Githens, J. H., Cox, S. M., and Kellum, D. L.: Azathioprine (Imuran) and pregnancy. Amer. J. Obstet. Gynec. 97:387, 1967.
48. Gillibrand, P. N.: Systemic lupus erythematosus in pregnancy treated with azathioprine. Proc. Roy. Soc. Med. 59:834, 1966.
49. Board, J. A., Lee, H. M., Draper, D. A., and Hume, D. M.: Pregnancy following kidney

homotransplantation from a non-twin: Report of a case with concurrent administration of azathioprine and prednisone. Obstet. Gynec. 29:318, 1967.
50. Kaufman, J. J., Goodwin, W. E., and Goldman, R.: Successful normal childbirth after kidney homotransplantation. J. A. M. A. 200:338, 1967.
51. Drucker, W. R., and Jeejeebhoy, K. N.: Azathioprine: an adjunct to surgical therapy of granulomatous enteritis. Ann. Surg. 172:618, 1970.
52. Kasper, H., Zimmermann, H. D., and Nägele, E.: Treatment of regional ileitis (Crohn's disease) with azathioprine. German Med. Monthly 15:521, 1970.
53. Kyle, J.: The management of chronic Crohn's disease. Ulster Med. J. 40:59, 1971.
54. Patterson, J. F., Norton, R. A., and Schwartz, R. S.: Azathioprine treatment of ulcerative colitis, granulomatous colitis and regional enteritis. Digest. Dis. 16:327, 1971.
55. Willoughby, J. M. T., Kumar, P. J., Beckett, J., and Dawson, A. M.: Controlled trial of azathioprine in Crohn's disease. Lancet. 2:944, 1971.
56. Rhodes, J., Bainton, D., Beck, P., and Campbell, H.: Controlled trial of azathioprine in Crohn's disease. Lancet. 2:1273, 1971.

The Case for Surgical Treatment

DONALD J. GLOTZER

Harvard Medical School

In assessing a role for any treatment in nonspecific inflammation of the intestine, including Crohn's disease, the empiric state of the art must be acknowledged at the outset. Currently two major categories of disease are recognized: (1) ulcerative colitis, and (2) Crohn's disease involving the small intestine, the large intestine, or both. In the absence of known etiology this is a tentative classification which is based upon certain shared clinical, distributional, radiologic, and pathologic features, not all of which are necessarily present in a given instance and none necessarily specific. Empiricism certainly also characterizes the medical treatment of Crohn's disease, for which there is no specific treatment, or even conclusive data substantiating the effectiveness of any of the agents used, whether corticosteroids, salicylazosulfapyridine, or azathioprine.

Because surgical treatment is also empiric, the results of operation must be judged, not on a preconception of how a disease should behave, but by how the treatment works in a given clinical situation. Crohn's disease of the colon may or may not be the same disease process as the classic one involving only the small intestine. If it is the same disease process, the response to surgical treatment may be different just as the location of the lesion is different. Additional considerations in the surgery of colonic Crohn's disease are the necessity for differential diagnosis with ulcerative colitis and the fact that operative treatment may necessitate ileostomy with its attendant physical and psychologic handicaps. These considerations militate against lumping the classic disease of the small intestine described by Crohn with granulomatous colitis and ileocolitis as is usually done.

Small Intestinal Crohn's Disease

ACUTE ILEITIS

Relatively little controversy exists concerning the management of acute enteritis. The diagnosis is usually made at laparotomy for suspected acute appendicitis. Most authorities agree that if symptoms are truly of recent onset, the disease is usually self-limited and therefore no treatment, medical or surgical, is necessary.[1-4] Because of the self-limited course of the disease some have questioned any relationship of this entity to chronic Crohn's disease.[3, 5] In some studies, mostly emanating from Europe, a high percentage of patients with acute enteritis either have transient high hemagglutination titers for Yersinia species, or these organisms have been isolated from the feces or the appendix.[6-8] There has been some confirmation of this finding from American studies as well.[9]

After acute ileitis is found, the only real decision to be made is the advisability of appendectomy—the pitfall being the possibility of a postoperative fecal fistula, especially should the pathologic process prove to be chronic Crohn's disease. If the cecum is soft, pliable, and uninflamed, the incidence of postoperative fistula is low. When or if a fistula occurs, diseased ileum rather than the appendiceal stump is the most common site of origin.[10] If the appendix is removed, further confusion in the diagnosis of possible right lower quadrant inflammatory disease is minimized.

Chronic Enteritis

Recurrences after excision of all apparently diseased intestine became evident shortly after Crohn described this entity in 1932, and this tendency has considerably dampened enthusiasm for operation as the primary or definitive treatment of this disease. Characteristically the neoterminal ileum is the site of such recurrent inflammation, which as a rule stops abruptly at the anastomosis with the colon. The reason for the propensity toward postoperative recurrence is not known. Possibilities include development or retention of skip disease, unknown factors related to juxtaposition of ileum to the colon, or the existence of subliminal inflammation in the retained intestine in which the pathologic process proceeds slowly and inexorably.

The optimal length of the proximal resection margin is not known. Although it is reasonable to assume that a wider resection margin would provide greater protection against recurrence than a more conservative resection, such evidence as is available does not verify this.[11]

The view that operation "causes" recurrence or spread of disease is widely held. I have observed two recurrences of disease in the neoterminal ileum in the immediate, in-hospital postoperative period, making it difficult to escape the feeling that operation hastened the development of disease in this segment in these two patients. Furthermore, spontaneous longitudinal spread of regional enteritis is not common, insofar as can be determined by x-ray studies, although spontaneous spread to the large intestine has been observed.[12, 13] However, the exact extent of disease may not always be obvious on x-ray examination. Moreover, since an increase in the extent of severity of the disease leads to operation, it is difficult to be certain that the disease would not have spread longitudinally if operation had not been necessary.

It is often said that if patients operated upon for Crohn's disease are followed long and closely enough, particularly with careful roentgenographic study, the recurrence rate will approach 100 per cent. I have found no published report of such a high recurrence rate, although the methods of evaluating recurrence rates have been variable and not always optimal. At times determination of recurrent disease has been based solely upon symptoms, reoperation, or hospital readmission, leading to overestimation or underestimation of the true recurrence rate. Perhaps the most accurate assessment of the recurrence rate would be based upon serial x-ray study regardless of the clinical status of the patients, with pathologic verification where reoperation becomes necessary. Furthermore, the length of follow-up is obviously important and varies from report to report. Recognizing these shortcomings, Table 1 lists the recurrence rates after resection and anastomosis from a number of major reports and presents the criteria upon which the diagnosis of recurrence was based as well as the length of follow-up. Resection is the operation preferred by most surgeons now, although it is by no means certain that exclusion bypass would not be as effective in comparable patients. Nonexclusion bypass seems to give considerably poorer results[1] and is not recommended. On the average about a 50 per cent recurrence rate is reported for resection and anastomosis.

More sophisticated statistical methods are used in more recent reports.

Table 1. *Recurrence After Resection in Small Intestinal Crohn's Disease*

AUTHORS	DATE OF REPORT	NO. OF PATIENTS	FOLLOW-UP PERIOD	METHOD OF DETERMINATION OF RECURRENCE	RECURRENCE RATE (%)
Hawthorne and Frobese[14]	1949	15	1-14 yrs.	Radiologic and/or pathologic	73
Van Patter et al.[11]	1954	203	2 yrs.	Clinical	62
Brown and Daffner[15]	1958	28	1 yr.	Not stated	54
Jackson[16]	1958	86	2 yrs.	Hospital readmissions	55
Stahlgren and Ferguson[17]	1961	43	1 yr.	Radiologic and/or pathologic	49
Barber et al.[18]	1962	75	5 yrs.	Reoperation	16
Atwell, Duthie and Goligher[1]	1965	146	3 yrs.	Radiologic and/or pathologic	50
Schofield[4]	1965	49	5 yrs.	? Reoperation	18
Lennard-Jones and Stalder[19]	1967	71	5 yrs. 10 yrs.	Radiologic and/or pathologic	23 51
Colcock[20]	1967	312	5-15 yrs.	Reoperation	25
Goligher, DeDombal, and Burton[21]	1971	79	5 yrs. 10 yrs. 15 yrs.	Radiologic and/or pathologic	40 62 70

Lennard-Jones and Stalder,[19] using the life table method, reported a probability of recurrence based on x-ray and pathologic criteria, of 23 per cent within five years and 51 per cent at 10 years. The graphs of cumulative recurrence of Goligher, DeDombal and Burton[21] show a recurrence rate for small bowel disease of about 40 per cent at five years, 62 per cent at 10 years and 70 per cent at 15 years. In these and most other studies, second resections have about the same or a slightly higher risk of recurrence.

Despite the data on the high recurrence rate after operation for Crohn's disease there are still advocates of early "radical" operation who argue that early resection keeps the disease from spreading and forestalls complications, particularly anorectal fistulas.[5] It seems to me that the good results reported by Wenckert and associates[5] can be explained by a comparatively short follow-up period rather than by extirpation of all disease. I therefore accept a fireman's role for the surgeon in regional enteritis—the treatment of complications of the disease—most often obstruction, abscess, and fistula.

Certainly if a patient requires minimal or no therapy to control symptoms, no operation or "specific" medical treatment should be considered. In more severe disease, salicylazosulfapyridine, corticosteroids, or even azathioprine should be used, although their efficacy has not been proved for aborting acute attacks, preventing recurrent attacks, or forestalling operation. An objective evaluation of these therapies should be forthcoming from a nationwide cooperative study now in its infancy. Cooke and Fielding[22] have suggested that corticosteroids are harmful in regional enteritis. If the chronic administration of corticosteroids is necessary to control symptoms, the side effects of this therapy may produce more morbidity than the treatment is worth. Acute obstruction unresponsive to gastrointestinal suction and perhaps to a brief period of corticosteroids or severe obstructive symptoms obviously necessitate operation. Patients with intra-abdominal abscess or those in whom the question of abscess is raised are candidates for operation if the only alternative is the use of corticosteroids. I have seen patients with suspected or unsuspected abscess who have been given these agents who then have developed perforation of the intestine, with disastrous consequences. Since the accompanying abscess is often incompletely drained by the fistula, patients with enteroenteric or enterocutaneous fistulas in general, should be operated upon, especially if corticosteroids are necessary to control symptoms. I treated one unusual patient with total involvement of the small intestine with very severe disease in the terminal ileum who responded to resection of the worst portion of the disease combined with continued postoperative corticosteroid therapy when all else failed. Finally, the patient with chronic disability, weight loss, and inability to function is a candidate for surgical treatment.

Despite this list of situations in which operation should be strongly considered, I do not wish to convey an attitude other than one of reasonable conservatism. It is quite clear that operation does not have a stellar track record in Crohn's disease of the small intestine. My quarrel is with the degrees of chronic invalidism sometimes tolerated to avoid operation, in which cases surgical treatment offers a reasonable chance for long periods of freedom from symptoms, or occasionally even "cure." It is my current practice to administer prophylactic salicylazosulfapyridine postoperatively in an attempt to forestall recurrences, based on an impression that x-ray evident and/or symptomatic recurrences have responded to this agent. No matter how reluctant one is to advise operation for chronic regional enteritis, an estimated 70 per cent of patients will require at least one intestinal operation in the course of their disease.[2]

Colonic Crohn's Disease

Although involvement of the colon by Crohn's disease had previously been described, it remained for Lockhart-Mummery and Morson,[23] and subsequently Lindner and associates,[24] to differentiate this entity clearly from ulcerative colitis and to emphasize its frequency. Now that the features of the disease are so well known, in most instances the diagnosis can be made on clinical and radiologic grounds. The concept of Crohn's disease involving the colon seems to explain heretofore confusing diagnostic problems in inflammatory bowel disease such as the nature of segmental ulcerative colitis, right-sided colitis, and regional enteritis with simultaneous or metachronous "ulcerative colitis." However, perhaps the most important implication of this diagnosis concerns the expected results of operation, if and when that becomes necessary.

Brooke has said of ileocolitis that "the disease is incurable medically or surgically."[25] Similarly a group at the Mt. Sinai Hospital, New York, has cautioned, "Because the tendency to recurrence is always present, we believe that patients with granulomatous colitis, like those with regional ileitis, should be managed medically as long as possible and surgery performed only for complications"[24] These views represent the prevailing posture taken regarding the surgical treatment of Crohn's disease involving the colon.

It has become evident that as many as 60 per cent of patients previously treated as though they had ulcerative colitis in fact had what is now considered granulomatous or Crohn's colitis or ileocolitis.[26] Has treatment in the past been incorrect based on mistaken diagnosis, and if so why was this not evident for so many years? Moreover, what is entailed in "managing medically as long as possible"? Because of the necessity for ileostomy, operation has never been the primary treatment for ulcerative colitis, even though colectomy has been assumed to be curative. In absolute terms, when medical management fails in both ulcerative and granulomatous colitis, it has failed, and in theory there should be no difference in the therapeutic approach save for caution about the expected results of operative treatment. However, differences do enter into the management and timing of operation, perhaps best illustrated by a case report.

Case report

A 19 year old boy entered the hospital in July, 1965, with abdominal cramps, weight loss, and non-bloody diarrhea of a few weeks' duration. Roentgenographic study of the colon demonstrated a segmental area of mucosal spiking and narrowing just distal to the hepatic flexure as well as patchy, asymmetric lesions proximal and distal to the splenic flexure. The terminal ileum appeared normal by x-ray study, as did the rectum by proctoscopic examination. Treatment with salicylazosulfapyridine was of no avail. Prednisone 60 mg. per day for three and a half weeks also failed to prevent continued fever, weight loss, and diarrhea. If this patient had ulcerative colitis, a colectomy would have been recommended at this point. However, we had learned to recognize granulomatous colitis, and at that time were inclined to accept the recommendations about deferring operation as long as possible. Consequently the patient was treated with prednisone 120 mg. daily and salicylazosulfapyridine 4 gm. every 24 hours. Although he became quite cushingoid, the patient's appetite improved and for the first time he gained weight and became afebrile. Unexplained twinges of right lower quadrant pain represented the only disquieting aspect of this patient's course prior to the sudden onset of generalized peritonitis resulting from a perforation of a totally masked right lower quadrant abscess. After a double-barreled ileostomy and drainage of the abscess, the patient made a surprisingly uneventful recovery. Two years later, cramps, purulent discharge from the colon, and spread of the inflammatory process in the colon demonstrated by x-ray examination led to a total abdominoperineal colectomy in June, 1967. Typical microscopic features of Crohn's colitis, including granulomas with giant cells and sinus tracts, were found on microscopic examination of the specimen. The patient has remained well since.

This disaster could have been avoided with a slightly more aggressive view of the role of operation in Crohn's disease of the colon. Stimulated by this case and our failure to observe the bleak outlook after operation predicted for patients with granulomatous disease simulating ulcerative colitis, a review was undertaken of our experience with Crohn's disease at the Tufts-New England Medical Center in Boston.[27] It soon became obvious that a number of patients with obvious clinical features of Crohn's colitis (segmental disease, internal or perirectal fistulas, or rectal sparing) did not have on histologic examination the noncaseating granulomas diagnostic of Crohn's disease. Furthermore, some patients with Crohn's colitis have more subtle features of the disease that could be missed by such a retrospective review. Hence, in an effort to detect all patients in whom proximal extension of disease or frank regional enteritis might have developed after colonic resection, we decided to determine the course of *all* patients with any kind of inflammatory disease involving the colon. The results are summarized in Table 2. The comparatively few patients who had anastomotic procedures had a greater than 50 per cent recurrence rate, results comparable to those previously reported. On the other hand, the course was considerably more favorable in those patients in whom a total colectomy and ileostomy was the operative procedure. Although a few patients, both with ulcerative colitis and granulomatous colitis, required ileostomy revisions, including the resection of ileum, none developed a progressively more proximal enteritis, leading to nutritional impairment and chronic illness. The closest approximation to this course of events was seen in a patient who died of a perforated duodenal ulcer postoperatively after the last of several ileostomy revisions. The "recurrent" ileal disease seen in this patient consisted of punched-out ulcerations more typical of nonspecific prestomal ileitis than of regional enteritis.[28] It thus appeared that the majority of patients, irrespective of whether they were believed to have ulcerative colitis or granulomatous colitis, were well in the long run after total colectomy, and that the postoperative courses of the two diseases were for the most part quite similar. Although most prior reports did not detail the type of operation done, recurrence after proctocolectomy appeared to be uncommon when this operation was specified.

To determine whether we could document any case of typical regional enteritis after ileostomy, and to assess the relative value of anastomotic procedures, a similar study was carried out at the Beth Israel Hospital in Boston.[29] I have already alluded to the fact that there is no absolute criterion upon which to

Table 2. Results of Operation in Inflammatory Bowel Disease*

CLASSI-FICATION	NO. OF PATIENTS	NO. WITH ILEAL INVOLVEMENT	NO. SURVIVING OPERATION	TYPE OF PROCEDURE	MEAN FOLLOW-UP IN YEARS	NO. TOTALLY WELL PATIENTS	COMMENT
Proved and clinical Crohn's colitis	7	4	7	Anastomotic	7.0	?1†	7 recurrences in 4 pts., 2 with and 2 without ileal disease
Ulcerative colitis	48	11	43	Ileostomy and colectomy	7.0	43	2 pts. required late ileostomy revisions
Proved Crohn's colitis	15	8	14	Ileostomy and colectomy	7.5	11	4 pts. required late ileostomy revisions
Clinical Crohn's colitis	9	7	9	Ileostomy and colectomy	6.8	7	3 pts. required late ileostomy revisions, 1 resulting in death (see text)

*Modified from Glotzer, D. J., et al.: New Eng. J. Med. 277:273–279, 1967.
†Lost to follow-up at 6 months.

Table 3. *Correlation of Clinical and Microscopic Classifications**

CLINICAL CLASSIFI-CATION	NO. OF PATIENTS	A MUCOSAL AND SUBMUCOSAL DISEASE	B TRANSMURAL DISEASE WITHOUT FISSURES OR GRANULOMAS	C SINUS TRACTS (FISSURES) PRESENT	D NON-CASEATING GRANULOMAS PRESENT
Ulcerative colitis	53	27(51%)	18(34%)	3(6%)	5(9%)
Crohn's colitis	42	10(24%)	6(14%)	8(19%)	18(43%)

*Modified from Glotzer, D. J., et al.: New Eng. J. Med. 282:582–587, 1970.

base a diagnosis of Crohn's disease of the colon, whether clinical, radiologic, or pathologic. The spectrum of histologic changes found in both "ulcerative" and "granulomatous" colitis is documented in Table 3, which confirms earlier findings of Valdes-Dapena and Vilardell for "ileocolitis."[30] Moreover, the pathologic features affecting the colon in granulomatous colitis, although sharing certain characteristics with regional enteritis, showed important differences. Typically granulomatous colitis was not the thick-walled stenosing disease with muscle hypertrophy, submucosal edema, lymphatic dilatation, and huge lymphoid aggregates seen classically in small intestinal Crohn's disease. This fact alone may account for the belated recognition of granulomatous colitis.

In this series the mortality was essentially the same in each disease whether based on patient mortality from all causes or that related to bowel disease or operation. There were 19 patients requiring surgical treatment in whom the distribution of disease allowed a resection of a portion of the colon or colon and small bowel with subsequent anastomosis. Nine of the 19 patients in this group subsequently required an ileostomy and colectomy; the seven who survived this reoperation remained well. Of 10 patients with intestinal continuity still maintained, seven were doing well, including five who were free of disease nine to 28 years after operation (all with extensive ileal disease); two had recurrence and one had died of intercurrent disease. In toto, then, 14 of 19 patients in this group were doing well after a resection and anastomoses as the initial operative procedure.

The course after operation in patients having a colectomy and ileostomy as the initial or as a secondary operative procedure is shown in Table 4. Although the patients with features of granulomatous colitis required an ileostomy revision

Table 4. *Ileostomy Revisions After Colectomy for Inflammatory Bowel Disease**

CRITERIA USED	ULCERATIVE COLITIS	CROHN'S COLITIS	STATISTICAL SIGNIFICANCE
Clinical	8/45(18%)	9/27(33%)	NS
Microscopic	7/45(15%)	10/24(42%)	$P<0.05$
Combined	5/28(13%)	12/34(35%)	NS

*Modified from Glotzer, D. J., et al.: New Eng. J. Med. 282:582–587, 1970.

more often than those with features of ulcerative colitis, the differences in the frequency of ileostomy revisions were not statistically significant except when the diagnosis of granulomatous disease was based solely upon microscopic criteria. It may emerge in the future that the microscopic features will offer an important prognostic index. Involvement of the ileum did not seem to affect the outcome.

Is the need for an ileostomy revision after operation for granulomatous colitis itself indicative of recurrence? The problem of differentiating inflammation associated with ileostomy dysfunction (which may occur even after ileostomy for familial polyposis) and that resulting from recurrence of the underlying inflammatory disease is considerable. The ileal inflammation which may occur after resection for ulcerative colitis is usually termed "ileostomy dysfunction," "postcolectomy ileitis," or "prestomal ileitis." If it is assumed that *any* ileal inflammation after ileostomy for Crohn's disease is recurrent Crohn's disease, it would be as logical to deem the comparable happenstance in ulcerative colitis "recurrent ulcerative colitis." In our studies, therefore, we have compared the incidence of the complication in each disease without attempting to assign an etiology to the process. To be sure, at one extreme the inflammatory process in the ileum after ileostomy for granulomatous colitis may contain microscopic granulomas and sinus tracts, and in further instances be completely indistinguishable from regional enteritis and thus incontrovertibly represent recurrence. Whatever the pathology, however, the problem can usually be solved by revision of the ileostomy and resection. Thus, in the four cases in our own series in which the resected ileal specimen contained noncaseating granulomas, all were well five to 19 years after ileostomy revision.

Even granting the dubious assumption that the necessity for an ileostomy revision is prima facie evidence of recurrence of granulomatous disease, our data indicate a more favorable outlook for Crohn's disease of the colon than is usually cited for small intestinal Crohn's disease. The recent data of Goligher and his associates[21] seem to corroborate this contention. Their curves of cumulative postoperative recurrences for large and small intestinal Crohn's disease are shown in Figure 1. The curve for colonic disease is strikingly below and to the right of that for small intestinal Crohn's disease. This trend is also well shown by their data for recurrences after specific operations (Fig. 2), in which the lowest recurrence rate of any operation for Crohn's disease was after proctocolectomy. Jones, Lennard-Jones and Lockhart-Mummery[31] also reported a favorable response to operation in that only one of 29 patients surviving total or subtotal colectomy and ileostomy for granulomatous colitis had recurrent ileitis.

Those who warn of the dire consequences of colectomy for colonic Crohn's disease should study their entire population of patients with inflammatory disease, place them in one or the other category blindly or prospectively, and then assess the results so obtained for both ulcerative and granulomatous colitis. Retrospective classification of the original colonic disease as granulomatous because ileal inflammation occurs after ileostomy is another logical error which I suspect has been committed in some instances. With a scheme of analysis that allows us to examine the courses of the most ulcerative-colitis-like patients and the most granulomatous-colitis-like patients we are unable to identify a group of patients

Figure 1. Curves comparing cumulative recurrences after operation for small and large intestinal Crohn's disease. (Modified from Goligher, DeDombal, and Burton.)

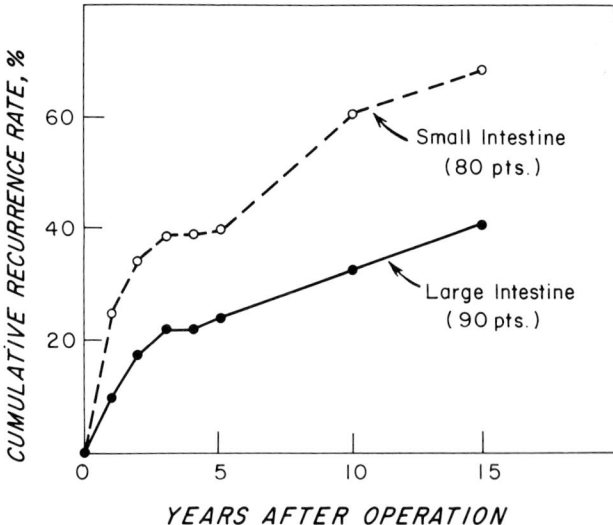

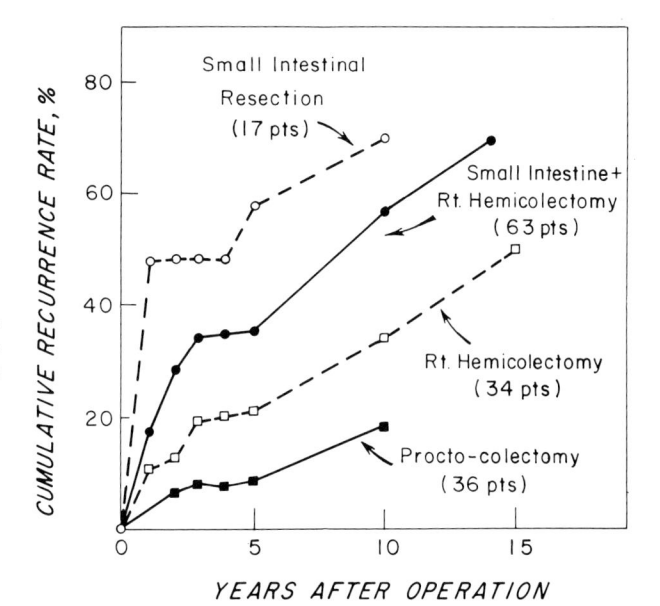

Figure 2. Cumulative recurrences after various operative procedures for Crohn's disease. (Modified from Goligher, DeDombal, and Burton.)

who have been immune from all further difficulty after operation or a group who uniformly or even usually have been doomed to multiple operations or chronic invalidism. Some of the worst results of operation in inflammatory colon disease were found in those patients who had ulcerative colitis as indicated by all possible criteria. Although we have encountered no patient in the two series of cases we studied in whom a short bowel syndrome developed, such patients do exist, and I have treated a few whose primary operations were performed elsewhere. Some patients also have extensive small intestinal and even duodenal inflammation in conjunction with their colonic disease as their initial extent of involvement, or may subsequently develop disease in these areas. The existence of patients with such extensive disease would seem to have little bearing upon the advisability of operation for the majority of patients with Crohn's disease of the colon whose disease fortunately is more limited.

My position is that in Crohn's disease of the colon there is little more reason to recommend an ultraconservative policy regarding surgical treatment than in ulcerative colitis, based on an objective comparison of the actual results of this therapy in these diseases. In the patient with segmental colonic disease allowing resection and anastomosis this should be done when medical management fails since there is a reasonable expectation of long-term palliation or cure. Recurrences certainly occur, but the ultimate outcome is usually not nearly so gloomy as advertised, even if a later ileostomy is the ultimate price for restoration of health. In such patients, and in those in whom ileostomy and colectomy is the primary operative procedure, the outcome is substantially the same in both ulcerative and granulomatous colitis. In both diseases the necessity for an ileostomy is the most cogent reason for a conservative approach and applies equally to both diseases. The chances are good for ultimate rehabilitation by operation of the patient with Crohn's disease involving the colon.

References

1. Atwell, J. D. Duthie, H. L., and Goligher, J. C.: The outcome of Crohn's disease. Brit. J. Surg. 52:966–972, 1965.
2. Banks, B. M., Zetzel, L., and Richter, H. S.: Morbidity and mortality in regional enteritis. Report of 168 cases. Amer. J. Dig. Dis. 14:369–379, 1969.
3. Gump, F. E., Lepore, M., and Barker, H. G.: A revised concept of acute regional enteritis. Ann. Surg. 166:942–946, 1967.
4. Schofield, P. F.: The natural history and treatment of Crohn's disease. Ann. Roy. Coll. Surg. Eng. 36:258–279, 1965.
5. Wenckert, A., Brahme, F., and Nilsson, R.: Operations indikationer vid Crohn's sjukdom. Nord. Med. 83:334–339, 1970.
6. Daniels, J. J. H. M.: Enteral infection with Pasteurella pseudotuberculosis. Isolation of the organism from human faeces. Brit. Med. J. 2:997, 1961.
7. Winblad, S., Nilehn, B., and Sternby, N. H.: Yersinia enterocolitica (Pasteurella X) in human enteric infections. Brit. Med. J. 2:1363–1366, 1966.
8. Sjostrom, B.: Acute terminal ileitis and its relation to Crohn's disease. In Engel, A., and Laurson, T. (eds): Regional Enteritis (Crohn's disease). Stockholm, Nordiska Bokhandelns Forlag, 1971, pp. 73–77.
9. Weber, J., Finlayson, N. B., and Mark, J. B.: Mesenteric lymphadenitis and terminal ileitis due to Yersinia pseudotuberculosis. New Eng. J. Med. 283:172–174, 1970.
10. Marx, F. W.: Incidental appendectomy with regional enteritis (advisability). Arch. Surg. 88:546–551, 1964.
11. Van Patter, W. N., Bargen, J. A., Dockerty, M. B., et al.: Regional enteritis. Gastroenterology 26:347–450, 1954.
12. Brahme, F.: Granulomatous colitis: Roentgenologic appearance and course of the lesions. Amer. J. Roentgenol. 99:35–44, 1967.
13. Ettinger, A.: Focal granulomatous colitis. Observation of its course. Gastroenterology 58:189–196, 1970.
14. Hawthorne, H. R., and Frobese, A. S.: Chronic stenosing regional enteritis. Surgical pathology and experience in surgical treatment. Ann. Surg. 103:233–241, 1949.
15. Brown, C. H., and Daffner, J. E.: Regional enteritis. II. Results of medical and surgical treatment in 100 patients. Ann. Intern. Med. 49:595–606, 1958.

16. Jackson, B. B.: Chronic regional enteritis. A survey of one hundred twenty-six cases treated at the Massachusetts General Hospital from 1937 to 1954. Ann. Surg. *148*:81–87, 1958.
17. Stahlgren, L. H., and Ferguson, L. K.: The results of surgical treatment of chronic regional enteritis. J.A.M.A. *175*:986–989, 1961.
18. Barber, K. W., Waugh, J. M., Beahrs, O. H., et al.: Indications for and the results of surgical treatment for regional enteritis. Ann. Surg. *156*:472, 1962.
19. Lennard-Jones, J. E., and Stalder, G. A.: Prognosis after resection of chronic regional ileitis. Gut *8*:332–336, 1967.
20. Colcock, B. P.: Surgical treatment of regional enteritis. Amer. J. Surg. *114*:398–401, 1967.
21. Goligher, J. C., DeDombal, F. T., and Burton, I.: Surgical treatment and its results. In Engel, A., and Larrson, T. (eds.): *Regional Enteritis* (Crohn's disease). Stockholm, Nordiska Bokhandelns Forlag, 1971, pp. 166–176.
22. Cooke, W. T., and Fielding, J. F.: Corticosteroid or corticotrophin therapy in Crohn's disease (regional enteritis). Gut *11*:921–927, 1970.
23. Lockhart-Mummery, H. E., and Morson, B. C.: Crohn's disease (regional enteritis) of the large intestine and its distinction from ulcerative colitis. Gut *1*:87–105, 1960.
24. Lindner, A. E., Marshak, R. J., Wolf, B. S., et al.: Granulomatous colitis: A clinical study. New Eng. J. Med. *269*:379–385, 1963.
25. Bockus, H. L., et al.: Regional enterocolitis. (Symposium.) Dis. Colon Rectum *8*:1–10, 1965.
26. Bacon, H. E., and Pezzutti, J. E.: Granulomatous ileocolitis: Report of 61 cases. J.A.M.A. *198*:1330–1334, 1966.
27. Glotzer, D. J., Stone, P. A., and Patterson, J. F.: Prognosis after surgical treatment of granulomatous colitis. New Eng. J. Med. *277*:273–279, 1967.
28. Knill-Jones, R. P., Morson, B., and Williams, R.: Prestomal ileitis: Clinical and pathologic findings in five cases. Quart. J. Med. *154*:287–297, 1970.
29. Glotzer, D. J., Gardner, R. C., Goldman, H., et al.: Comparative features and course of ulcerative and granulomatous colitis. New Eng. J. Med. *282*:582–587, 1970.
30. Valdes-Dapena, A., and Vilardell, F.: Granulomatous lesions in ileocolitis. Gastroenterologia *97*:191–204, 1962.
31. Jones, J. H., Lennard-Jones, J. E., and Lockhart-Mummery, H. E.: Experience in treatment of Crohn's disease of large intestine. Gut *7*:448–452, 1966.

A Conservative Approach

THOMAS A. WARTHIN

Harvard Medical School

Rational therapy should be designed to interfere with the abnormal processes that produce Crohn's disease. When one looks at the dozen or so unproved theories of the cause of the disorder and seriously reviews the natural history and epidemiology of the illness, the logical conclusion must be conservatism in therapy. There are, of course, specific exceptions such as surgery for obstruction and fistula formation, but these actions are basically conservative. This philosophic approach has been the result of an opportunity to follow carefully and personally 50 patients with Crohn's disease for periods of 10 to 25 years, a largely male population of veterans of World War II and the Korean Conflict. That significant observations can be made in a meticulous and continued follow-up experience with such a small group of patients was demonstrated by the fact that in 1956 I found involvement of the colon in Crohn's disease in 10 of 24 patients.

The current enthusiasms in etiology include infection, disorder of immunity, granulomatous hypersensitivity, and genetic factors. New bits of evidence seem to have overlapping results. Thus, the increased occurrence of the disease in certain families gives strength to both the genetic and infective theories. More recent careful electron microscopic information suggests that a disordered immune state exists and that following innocuous fecal bacterial entry a hyperactive but ineffective response develops in the wall of the intestines.[1]

Recent symposia in England and Sweden have reviewed the unproved similarities to sarcoid and the primacy of the submucosal response of the lymphocyte and plasma cells to whatever agents(s) is involved in the lymphatics and vessels of this layer.[2,3] It is believed that the granulomatous changes are a secondary manifestation, perhaps to foreign material entering the submucosa as a result of the primary inflammatory changes. The designation granulomatous ileocolitis should therefore be discarded and the use of the eponym continued until the etiology is finally discovered.

The observations that diversion of the intestinal stream from affected bowel loops is usually followed by a slow disappearance of the pathologic process suggest that there is a specific sensitivity reaction either to an ingested substance or to an organism. With rare exceptions, it is hazardous to draw diagnostic or etiologic conclusions from a response, or lack of reaction, to a specific therapy.

Thus, the occasional brilliant performance of an immunosuppressive agent or corticosteroids offers little of scientific value in relation to the etiology of the treated disorder.

In recent years British and Norwegian studies of the incidence and epidemiology of this disorder[4] have provided contrasting statistics to investigations in Baltimore.[5] These figures are helpful, but they are not static. Of equal import, and too often neglected, has been the basic evidence furnished by Burrill Crohn and the large surgical clinics such as the Cleveland, Lahey, and Mayo Clinics that this disease, while recognized for over 150 years, struck the United States and then Northern Europe in almost epidemic fashion in the second quarter of the 20th Century. Was this the result of the acute introduction of an infective or sensitizing agent into the intestinal tracts of a susceptible population, or was it more purely "a disturbed ecology of the human race" as suggested by Crohn at the Eighth International Congress of Gastroenterology? It will be most interesting to watch the incidence among blacks in the United States. Recently in Baltimore the first hospitalization rates per 100,000 population for Crohn's disease in whites was 1.35 and 0.04 for nonwhites. If more young blacks give up "soul foods" for hamburgers, milk shakes, and the other staples of the diet of United States and North European white young, will increases occur? Will the almost nonexistent recognition of the disease among the rice eating Orientals and the Hindus of India remain the same after exposure to young Americans and Europeans possibly carrying an infective agent? In modern Japan the disorder is now no longer uncommon. It is likely that the next decade will bring helpful answers in epidemiology related directly to the etiology.

Probably the most difficult aspect of Crohn's disease is the delineation of its natural history. Prognostic projections in relation to medical or surgical therapy are almost impossible to make because the disease is so varied in course and activity. There are several points worth noting. The disorder is uncommon under the age of 10 years, yet has its peak incidence between the ages of 15 and 30 years. One half of the patients have symptoms for one to four years prior to a diagnosis being established. Somewhere between 10 and 20 per cent of cases are acute, with lesions that will either disappear or fail to progress after the diagnosis is established at exploratory laparotomy. After 30 years of involvement, the disorder seems to become relatively inactive. Patients who were diagnosed prior to World War II are all essentially well. They also fared very well on the canned combat type diets in overseas areas, while others were doing poorly in the United States military camps.[6] In spite of a current prevalence of three to four per 100,000, the disorder has never been reported to my knowledge as an incidental finding at postmortem examination. Patients with active Crohn's disease who develop chronic congestive heart failure appear to go into a remission of their intestinal disorder.

Various clinics have reported "cures" after primary resection in 30 to 60 per cent of their patients. The remainder will be subjected to an average of 2.8 more surgical procedures per patient.[8] Obstruction, fistula formation, and sepsis are the main indications for operation. Death as the result of an operation or from the disease itself is unlikely. Less than 10 per cent of patients followed for many years die from either of these two causes. Finally, periods of significant rest and tranquility seem to ameliorate symptoms not related to the type of complications that warrant surgery.

Treatment

Conservative therapy is based on an intensive program of rest and supportive measures, diet, antibacterial therapy, and the early recognition of complications requiring surgical intervention. It is a vivid example of treating the patient "as a whole."

Rest

Rest and tranquility as preached by Trudeau were used in the treatment of tuberculosis until 1945, but disappeared as a therapeutic regimen because more specific antibacterial therapy became available. Until that time it was reasonably successsful. Crohn's disease is not intestinal tuberculosis, but there are so many similarities in their early pathophysiology, altered immune state, and clinical picture as to warrant the analogy. A program of rest, to be effective, must be applied before the complications of fistulas, sepsis, or obstruction develop. This is why patients get along for years with the disease, and it is only the complication that provokes enough attention to establish the diagnosis. Early diagnosis and meticulous conditioning are required. The current demand for "instant cure" must be met head on and the patient and his family persuaded that for many years a new life style will be necessary. The alternative is to risk a life of repeated surgery. Seven of 24 patients, who were persuaded 20 years ago to be shoe clerks, are still happily selling shoes today, with the same length of intestine (guts) as they started. The more aggressive 17 have required one or more operations.

Patients with Crohn's disease are competitors. Whether the high incidence of the disorder in North Europeans and Jews is based on genetics or is related to life styles and goals is unknown. But the similarities to the personality and behavior of patients with ulcerative colitis has long been recognized; in fact, it confused the recognition of the colonic involvement in Crohn's disease for 25 years. The point here is not that the emotions cause the disease, but that emotional reactions may control a patient's willingness to follow a long range program of rest and reduced competitiveness. If the individual doctor has little skill in relating to adolescents and young adults and parents he had best seek help.

Immediately upon establishing a clinical and radiologic diagnosis of Crohn's disease, a decision must be made whether a confirmatory exploratory laparotomy is the next step. In special instances this is desirable, and if the cecum is not involved, appendectomy can be safely performed. Since life styles are to be altered, one goes to the extreme needed to convince the individual appropriately. The patient remains in the hospital for several weeks while the physician or his delegate gets to know the problems, the day dreams, and the goals of the patient. The latter, meantime, is being diverted with satisfying bedside occupational therapy, not television programs which may be disturbing. One strives for

Utopia. Eighteen hours' bed rest a day for a month plus a proper complacence will usually see a disappearance of most intestinal complaints. Perhaps the alleged benefit of short-term corticosteroid therapy is the artificial contentment the drug provides as much as its anti-inflammatory effect.

The physician must individualize treatment for each patient, who then embarks on a long range program of 12 hours' bed rest a day, abstinence from competitive programs, and strict adherence to the minimal stress—i.e., basic school attendance without extracurricular activities, one 40 hour per week job, avoidance of irritating situations, and so forth. Follow-up diagnostic x-rays and other studies are made at six months and one year, and yearly thereafter. Any recurrence of symptoms requires a very careful review of potential transgressions. The appearance of erythema nodosum indicates renewal of activity and the necessity for a change in that patient's program. At least 25 per cent of patients with Crohn's disease will have a radiologic diagnosis of duodenal ulcer made during the early course of their illness.

It is most important to initiate a good rest program following resectional or diverting surgery, as the risk of recurrence is clearly highest during the first year after operation.[8,9] The patient must not be led to believe, "You've been operated on and are now cured." Is this the explanation for the variable cure rates seen after initial resectional surgery, which run from 30 to 60 per cent in different clinics?[7] Are not the patients without recurrence those whose life styles were significantly altered? Among my intelligent professional patients the relationship between recurrence of symptoms and overdoing their allocated work program is most precise.

DIET

Any disorder in which diversion of the intestinal stream is followed by a slow disappearance of the inflammatory process should include some concern about what we introduce into that intestinal stream. Until we know the etiologic substance, it seems wise to consider two actions: First, in acute states, temporary parenteral feeding or the use of nonresidue diets for two weeks combined with bodily rest will often bring about subsidence of inflammation and obstruction. This may be followed by a prolonged remission. Physicians who simultaneously administer corticosteroids with such a program are apt to attach excessive relevance to the drug. My experience of the past 14 years has convinced me that steroid therapy plays little part in the improvement.

Longer range diet therapy should begin with a detailed review of the dietary habits of the patient. As a group they drink twice as much milk as the average person of their age. They eat almost three times as much bread and butter.[6] They have an inordinate intake of sandwiches and prepared foods. The omission of milk certainly reduces intestinal gas and cramps, even in those who are not lactase deficient, and most are not. These are foods known to alter or increase intestinal bacterial growth. Does the lactase deficiency of blacks keep them from drinking milk excessively and, hence, acquiring Crohn's disease? Historically, effective pasteurization of milk, and the consequent great increase in the consumption of it, immediately preceded the appearance of the disorder here and abroad. Intake of wheat should be drastically reduced and potato or rice substituted. Many borderline problems of steatorrhea are improved by such a program. Consumption of low residue vegetables and desserts is encouraged. The usual vitamins are supplemented by nicotinic acid and B_{12} if prior surgery or anemia suggests their deficiency. Kidney stones, usually calcium in composition, may be prevented by an acid ash diet if of phosphate type or by reducing the hyperoxaluria associated with calcium oxalate stone formation.

Antibacterial Therapy

The evidence that bacterial agents are buried somewhere in the etiologic background is stronger today than it was a decade ago. Recent investigations using the electron microscope are suggestive but not so convincing as in the case of Whipple's disease.[1] There is evidence that large amounts of *Escherichia coli* type 0:14 antigen in the intestine might be the response modifying agent in certain hosts, permitting the establishment of inflammation.[3] Finally, does antibacterial therapy reduce the granulomatous reaction at the base of the lymphoid follicles, the "aphthoid" fissures and ulcers in the bowel wall which are the source of the serious fistulas and fibrotic complications requiring surgery? No answer is possible, but antibacterial therapy is probably helpful.

Many physicians in the United States prescribe Azulfidine (salicylazosulfapyridine), which we now know is broken down into its two major components in the lower small intestine and colon. Thus, it exerts both an anti-inflammatory and an antibacterial action. Doses up to 4.0 gm. per day are probably as effective as larger ones. There is abundant anecdotal evidence of concurrent healing of fistulas following administration of the drug, but no proof that there was a factual cause and effect relationship. The British seem to prefer tetracycline 1 gm. daily or ampicillin 1 to 2 gm. per day.[7] Toxic megacolon can occur in Crohn's disease, as well as ulcerative colitis. This may keep some physicians from using broad spectrum antibiotics, particularly when there is significant involvement of the colon.

Surgical treatment

Twenty-five years after Crohn's original description and recommendation of extirpative surgical resection of diseased intestine, it had become evident that conservatism in surgery was vastly better than a radical approach. Extensive involvement of the small intestine as demonstrated by x-ray is compatible with an active life. Surgery should be reserved for those structural complications such as stenosis, internal and external fistulas, and perforation with abscess formation. When surgery is performed it should be carried out with the intent of conserving normal small intestine, avoiding diversion operations, and performing resection whenever possible.[8] Anastomoses to the colon should be made as proximal as surgically feasible. The length of grossly normal intestine between the proximal line of resection and the diseased area does not seem to affect the possibility of recurrence. If recurrence appears it is often just proximal to the anastomosis or in the colon beyond.

Where greater controversy exists is in the management of colonic and rectal disease. This is not surprising since less than 15 years have passed since the recognition of this feature. Prior to that time patients were treated as having ulcerative or segmental colitis by ileostomy and colectomy. Surprisingly few later developed disease above the stoma. Possibly there is a lesson to be learned in that, of the entire gastrointestinal tract, we can live most comfortably without the colon. The following would seem therefore to represent conservative principles for an approach to colonic-rectal disease:

1. Do not seriously damage or cut the anal sphincter in treatment of perianal fistulas or abscess.

2. If colonic stricture develops, try resection and distal anastomosis once. A subsequent recurrence had best be treated by colectomy and ileostomy.[9] Strictures in the rectum and colon are apt to produce more complications than an equivalent stenosis in the small intestine.

3. Colostomy may seem successful for a few years, but in the long run fistulous disease of more serious character than ileostomy is apt to develop.

It appears that the physician caring for patients with Crohn's disease with significant colonic involvement must watch them with particular anxiety and be conservative in their medical management, otherwise he will need to subject them to more radical colonic surgery. This, it seems, carries a higher morbidity than small intestinal operations.

Corticosteroid Treatment

In 1960 I reviewed the results of 10 years of repeated short-term or chronic corticosteroid therapy in 25 patients. They were all alive, but had required a total of 48 operations. While this figure is fully in accord with those reported by Banks,[8] and many others, it seemed an excessive number. Operations denote complications which indicate a medical failure. It appeared to us that the anti-inflammatory benefits were being overturned by a high incidence of complications. Over the next 10 years 25 new patients were followed, and they and the original group were all treated without steroid, on a rest, diet, and Azulfidine program. Only 23 operations were required for the entire series of 50 during the second decade, and all are living and working, with two exceptions. One has died of opium addiction without active Crohn's disease, and the other is seriously ill with colonic disease treated too conservatively. Both were in the original steroid-treated group. Patients who were on the steroid programs required at least a year for safe, slow withdrawal from the drug, then returned to work and an active life.

At least 15 per cent of Crohn's disease patients receiving steroid therapy will at some time have significant genitourinary tract complications. One half of these will be infections often related to fistulous tracts into the bladder or prostate gland; the rest will have kidney stones. The stones are most often on the right in ileal disease and on the left in colonic involvement. Abnormalities in ureteric peristalsis are readily visible and seem related to extension of inflammation from the mesentery. The stones are of calcium composition. It is possible that steroid medication may increase this complication by its effects on calcium absorption and excretion. Intravenous pyelography should be part of a case review shortly after diagnosis and again within five years. In our series twice as many patients who received steroid medication developed duodenal ulcer as compared to the untreated group. In only one instance was this a serious complication.

After such an experience it is difficult not to believe that we have deluded ourselves in respect to significant benefit from this therapy in Crohn's disease. Until a factually controlled prospective study is made, the conservative approach to the management of Crohn's disease will not include the use of corticosteroids. Similarly, administration of more potentially dangerous immunosuppressive agents should be restrained until the evidence is clear and precise. Crohn's disease is a long, chronic, basically nonfatal condition, warranting a conservative approach that avoids therapy with hidden hazards.

References

1. Aluwihare, A. P. R.: Electron microscopy in Crohn's disease. Gut *12*:509, 1971.
2. Symposium on Crohn's Disease (Abridged). Proc. Roy. Soc. Med. *64*:157, 1971.
3. Mendeloff, A. I.: Crohn's Disease: Progress confounded. Ann. Intern. Med. 76:137, 1972.
4. Evans, J. G., and Acheson, E. D.: An epidemiological study of ulcerative colitis and regional enteritis in the Oxford area. Gut *6*:311, 1965.
5. Monk, M., Mendeloff, A. I., Siegel, C. I., and Lilienfeld, A.: An epidemiological study of ulcerative colitis and regional enteritis among adults in Baltimore. Gastroenterology 53:198, 1967.
6. Warthin, T. A.: Some epidemiological observations on the etiology of regional enteritis. Tran. Amer. Clin. Climat. Ass. *80*:116, 1968.
7. Lennard-Jones, J. E., and Morson, B. C.: Changing concepts in Crohn's disease. Disease-a-Month. Chicago, Year Book Publishers, Inc., 1969.
8. Banks, B. M., Zetzel, L., and Richter, H. S.: Morbidity and mortality in regional enteritis. Amer. J. Dig. Dis. *14*:369, 1969.
9. De Dombal, F. T., Burton, I., and Goligher, J. C.: Recurrence of Crohn's disease after primary excisional surgery. Gut *12*:519, 1971.

Comment

Treatment of Crohn's Disease

Any physican attempting to manage Crohn's disease of the bowels, small or large, deals with a disease (or perhaps several diseases) that is discouragingly real in its manifestations but quite intangible with respect to its nature. Some of the disagreements Dr. Glotzer has with others[1] concerning the efficacy of colectomy in treating granulomatous colitis may be attributed to the lack of agreement as to the criteria—clinical, radiologic, or pathologic—that permit the diagnosis of Crohn's disease. Several of the essayists appear convinced that immunologic mechanisms must be at work, but are also emphatic in pointing out the limited, fragmentary, and also contradictory evidence currently available to support their beliefs. Recurrence is an ever-present threat, no matter what the type of treatment and the degree of its initial success. It is thus not surprising that many a doctor will shun the either/or approach and will find himself forced to pursue a sequential plan of attack: first, a conservative regimen perhaps embellished with salicylazosulfapyridine, then corticosteroids, then bowel rest, then azathioprine, and finally surgical resection. Such floundering attempts to arrest the disease are discouraging to physician as well as patient, and it is even doubtful that the controlled therapeutic trials now being initiated on a multicenter basis will provide a clear-cut answer. Perhaps the money available to support research in this field should be concentrated on studies of pathogenetic mechanisms. But since the funds available are pitifully inadequate, the first order of business for patients with Crohn's disease and their doctors would appear to be the creation of the political organization that now unfortunately seems necessary in the U.S.A. if research in a given area is to obtain adequate support.

Reference

1. Korelitz, B. I., Present, D. H., Alpert, L. I., Marshak, R. H., and Janowitz, H. D.: Recurrent ileitis after ileostomy and colectomy for granulomatous colitis. New Eng. J. Med. 287:110–115, 1972.

FRANZ J. INGELFINGER

19

Aspirin and the Stomach

Aspirin Is Not a Major Cause of Acute Gastrointestinal Bleeding
 by M. J. S. Langman

Aspirin Is Dangerous for the Peptic Ulcer Patient
 by Howard M. Spiro

Comment
 by Franz J. Ingelfinger

Aspirin Is Not a Major Cause of Acute Gastrointestinal Bleeding

M. J. S. LANGMAN

Hurst[1] claimed that aspirin consumption was a likely cause of major gastrointestinal bleeding in half of all patients remaining when known causes, such as chronic ulceration, had been excluded from consideration, while Muir and Cossar[2] have suggested that recent aspirin ingestion could account for one eighth of all episodes of hematemesis and melena.

Experimental work in animals and clinical physiological studies in man have been used extensively to analyze the degree and cause of occult micro bleeding inducible by aspirin. It has demonstrated conclusively that lesions similar to acute gastric erosions can be induced in the stomach of animals given aspirin. It has also shown that occult bleeding (but not major bleeding) is a common concomitant and that aspirin can interfere with normal homeostatic mechanisms, for instance, facilitating acid back diffusion into the gastric mucosa.

However, the critical evidence in establishing a major role for aspirin in inducing hematemesis and melena in man must come from epidemiologic studies. Since no method has yet been devised which would allow prospective investigation of this problem, retrospective analyses remain the only available techniques. This is not necessarily a disadvantage, for in virtually all situations in which a specific factor is an important cause of disease, for instance, smoking and lung cancer or oral contraceptive agents and thromboembolism, retrospective case-control comparisons have pointed to that cause.

Epidemiologic Evidence Obtained from Controlled Investigations

The available evidence can be divided into three categories:
1. Uncontrolled studies showing the frequency of recent aspirin consumption in patients with acute gastrointestinal bleeding.
2. Controlled comparisons of the aspirin intake of individuals with hematemesis and melena.
3. Attempts to show that aspirin damage is the result of a specific type of bleeding lesion or occurs in identifiable "aspirin damage prone" individuals.

The first of these does no more than suggest an apparent association needing investigation, and any useful evidence must be obtained from the latter two types of investigation.

Case-control comparisons depend upon careful comparisons between the bleeding and nonbleeding group, but such analyses pose difficulties:

1. Bias, conscious or unconscious, during questioning is hard to avoid but cannot be mitigated by "blind" interrogation, for it is virtually impossible in this situation to question the patients and the control individuals without learning whether they belong to the test or control groups.

2. Aspirin and aspirin-containing compounds are common household remedies for minor ailments, and the initial symptoms of gastrointestinal bleeding could be mistaken for the onset of a flu-like illness. Investigators could well interpret this drug consumption as a factor precipitating bleeding.

3. The aspirin content of many preparations (Banks and Baron[3] were able to list over 300) is not obvious from their trade names; consequently, individuals in the patient or control groups may be unaware that they have taken aspirin. It is also probably very easy for an individual admitted to a hospital to forget the, to him, insignificant event of having taken an aspirin-containing tablet.

Such difficulties emphasize the need for good controls, but it is doubtful if these have always been obtained.[4-6]

Table 1 lists the controls used in eight major and commonly quoted investigations.[7-14] The variety selected probably reflects the difficulties of investigators in choosing well, and all those cited are open to criticism. The individual in the next bed could, for instance, have been admitted with a stroke and have a poor memory for antecedent events, or else could have been admitted some considerable time before and might not remember his previous salicylate intake. By con-

Table 1. *Control Groups Used in Investigations of the Role of Aspirin in Inducing Gastrointestinal Hemorrhage*

AUTHORS	% ASPIRIN TAKERS	TYPE OF CONTROL USED
Muir and Cossar, 1955	Approx. 5	Occupant of the bed on the right-hand side of the patient with bleeding
Brown and Mitchell, 1956	40	Hospital admissions to medical, surgical and gynecological wards
Kelley, 1956	4	Patients with myocardial infection
Lange, 1957	18	Ulcer patients without evidence of bleeding
Allibone and Flint, 1958	44	Nonthoracic surgical emergency or accident cases
Alvarez and Summerskill, 1958	17	Dyspeptic patients referred to an outpatient clinic
Muir and Cossar, 1959	16	Occupant of the bed on the right-hand side of the patient with bleeding
Parry and Wood, 1967	32	All other patients admitted to medical wards during the survey period

trast, a patient with arthritis would be expected to have taken aspirin recently and is scarcely a reasonable control.

Unselected control groups containing individuals with a variety of diseases contain subgroups with differing salicylate intakes. Thus Parry and Wood[13] found only a quarter of their control patients admitted with gastrointestinal, cardiovascular, hematologic and neurologic disorders had taken aspirin recently compared with half the remaining controls.

The selection of dyspeptic individuals or patients with proven ulcers but no bleeding could also be unwise, for salicylates are commonly considered to exacerbate ulcer symptoms. Such controls might therefore have limited their salicylate intake voluntarily or in response to their physician's advice.

When these points are taken into account it is not unexpected to find that the proportions of recent aspirin takers found in the eight control series varied from 4 to 44 per cent. A threefold difference from 25 to 72 per cent was also found in the test groups, though it should be noted that the test groups contained uniformly higher proportions of aspirin takers than the controls.

Some of the variability can be accounted for by the differing time periods for recent aspirin intake (from six hours to two weeks before admission) which were chosen for study. Standardization to a common base of 48 hours can be done for four of these studies,[8, 12-14] and the results are given in Table 2. The bleeding groups contain 51 to 58 per cent of recent aspirin takers, while the controls vary from 11 to 26 per cent. Marked differences between test and control groups remain, but for the reasons stated earlier these do not necessarily reflect directly the true likelihood of aspirin inducing acute bleeding. Clear evidence of a strong causal relationship must be sought elsewhere.

Aspirin as a Cause of Acute Hemorrhage from a Specific Gastrointestinal Lesion

The situation could be clarified if a specific lesion causing hemorrhage could be identified. In all investigations it has been found that the patients with non-

Table 2. *Proportions of Individuals Taking Aspirin Within 48 Hours of Admission*

SOURCE	HEMORRHAGE GROUP			CONTROL GROUP		
	Total No.	No. Taking Aspirin Within 48 Hours	% Taking Aspirin Within 48 Hours	Total No.	No. Taking Aspirin Within 48 Hours	% Taking Aspirin Within 48 Hours
Brown and Mitchell, 1956	50	20	58*	72	19	26
Alvarez and Summerskill, 1958	103	53	51	103	11	11†
Muir and Cossar, 1959	106	57	54	106	17	16
Parry and Wood, 1967	95	48	55	542	122	23

*Aspirin taken within 48 hours of admission or onset of symptoms.
†Aspirin taken within 48 hours of visit to the outpatient department.

chronic ulcer bleeding, the acute erosion or radiologically negative group, contain the highest proportion of aspirin takers. Such evidence cannot exculpate aspirin as a cause of chronic ulcer bleeding, though it does suggest that the radiologically negative subgroup could be profitably studied to try and define more closely a specific aspirin lesion.

Typical acute gastric erosions can be found in animals given salicylates and in the resected stomachs of patients given aspirin shortly before partial gastrectomy. However, these lesions differ from those found clinically in one critical respect; hematemesis and melena do not occur.

Clear separation of the group with gastroscopically visible acute erosions from the remainder of the x-ray negative acute bleeding group has been carried out by two groups of investigators. One found a higher aspirin intake in the patients with erosions,[15] while the other found the reverse to be true.[12] The differences may reflect only chance small number variation, but they cannot be said to confirm that acute erosion is the specific aspirin lesion.

Histologic examination of mucosal biopsy specimens and assessment of gastric acid output have likewise failed to show any clear difference between patients with radiologically negative bleeding who had and who had not taken aspirin recently beforehand.[16]

A consistent relationship between radiologically negative bleeding and hemorrhage therefore remains, but a specific aspirin lesion has yet to be demonstrated. Furthermore, when aspirin was deliberately readministered to individuals who had suffered from "aspirin-induced" bleeding, none suffered from acute hemorrhage, and occult bleeding did not differ in degree from that occurring in control individuals.[13]

Interaction Between Aspirin and Other Factors Causing Bleeding

It has been suggested that the coincidence of aspirin intake with other factors leads to overt hemorrhage. "The gun must be loaded in order for an explosion to occur when salicylates pull the trigger."[17]

ALCOHOL

Allibone and Flint[11] found no obvious association between aspirin intake and alcohol consumption in inducing upper gastrointestinal ulcer complications, though Astley,[18] Brown and Mitchell,[8] Jennings,[19] and Needham and his colleagues[20] all claimed that alcohol was a significant cofactor in inducing aspirin bleeding. However, closer examination of the data of Astley[18] and Brown and Mitchell[8] shows that the frequency with which aspirin and alcohol were taken together by their bleeding patients was no greater than would be expected by chance in the groups which they studied. Thus 23 of 31 male patients with bleeding studied by Astley had taken aspirin shortly beforehand, and 16 had taken alcohol. The observed figure of 10 who had taken both together was in fact slightly less than the expected chance value of 12.

The data of Jennings[19] likewise show that 17 per cent of the aspirin takers with bleeding had a simultaneous history of recent alcohol intake compared with 21 per cent of those with no aspirin intake—the reverse of expectation if aspirin and alcohol were cofactors.

Though Needham and his colleagues[20] found a significant association between recent alcohol and aspirin consumption in the histories of patients with acute bleeding, closer analysis of their data shows that the relationship holds virtually only for chronic duodenal ulcer and is nonexistent in the gastritis group; this latter presumably including the "aspirin erosion" group and having the strongest simple relationship with aspirin consumption.

There is, thus, no good evidence that alcohol is an important cofactor in inducing acute hemorrhage from the stomach, though it may well increase the severity of occult bleeding by a few milliliters per day.

OTHER FACTORS

Jennings[19] considered that a variety of influences, including physical strain, mental strain, smoking, hypertension, and acute and chronic infections, were important cofactors in inducing bleeding. Examination of his data shows, in fact, fewer patients with strain, physical or mental, or who were smokers in his aspirin takers than in the remainder. There was a slight (and probably insignificant trend) for a positive association between recent aspirin intake and chronic infections and hypertension, but the only substantial positive association was for acute respiratory infections. Such a relationship might reasonably be expected, for aspirin is the drug of choice for many upper respiratory tract infections and does not necessarily imply an interrelationship causing bleeding.

A single well conducted study[21] suggests that aspirin consumption and subclinical vitamin C deficiency are important cofactors and, if confirmed, would give strong support to the suggestion that aspirin can cause acute hemorrhage under certain limited conditions.

Other Epidemiologic Evidence

Since case-control studies cannot be interpreted unequivocally, it is reasonable to examine other epidemiologic evidence to see if this can allow a definite conclusion to be attained about the importance of aspirin as a major cause of bleeding. Schiller, Truelove, and Gwyn Williams,[22] in analyzing hematemesis and melena statistics for the Radcliffe Infirmary, Oxford, a hospital serving a population of about 300,000, found no evidence that the frequency of admission for acute upper gastrointestinal bleeding was increasing despite the fact that the apparent recent aspirin intake of the patients rose steadily during the 15 years of the study. These figures probably do no more than reflect the frequency of questioning about aspirin intake as the drug became established, at least in the inquirers' minds, as a possible major cause of bleeding.

National statistics comparing total aspirin consumption or sales with total admission rates for bleeding would be of more interest. Such figures have, for instance, been used in comparing the mortality from asthma with the sales of bronchodilator aerosols whereby a reasonable correlation was established.

The British public consumes approximately 6000 million tablets containing aspirin each year, or about 100 tablets per head of population per year.[23] The actual distribution of the total drug intake is hard to establish, but the figures must imply that the random chances of having recently taken aspirin at hospital admission are extremely high. There is no reason to believe United States habits differ materially for aspirin has been detected in 37 per cent of blood donations in Connecticut.[24] Yearly consumption of aspirin and aspirin-containing products has changed little or has perhaps fallen slightly in the United Kingdom in the last 10 years (though paracetamol consumption has risen). By contrast, admission rates for hematemesis and melena from undiagnosed sources (i.e., substantially if not totally the x-ray negative bleeding group) have risen (Table 3). The lack of parallelism with aspirin consumption is obvious.

Table 3. *Estimated Total Admission Rate of Patients with Hematemesis and Melena (Cause Unknown) in England and Wales, 1958–1969**

YEAR	NO. OF PATIENTS
1958	4460
1959	4941
1960	5557
1961	5438
1962	5559
1963	5660
1964	5900
1965	6466
1966	6181
1967	5960
1968	8757
1969	7351

*Calculated from unpublished data from Hospital Inpatient Enquiry 10 per cent sample.

Conclusion

Patients with hematemesis and melena, particularly those who are found to have no evidence of a chronic gastroduodenal ulcer have been repeatedly shown to contain a higher proportion of recent aspirin consumers than control populations. The weaknesses inherent in these controlled retrospective studies, allied to the problems as yet unsolved in defining specific circumstances under which aspirin, a universally and frequently consumed drug, causes bleeding, make it impossible to state that aspirin plays a major role in inducing gastroduodenal bleeding.

References

1. Hurst, A.: Aspirin and gastric haemorrhage. Brit. Med. J. 1:768.
2. Muir, A., and Cossar, I. A.: Aspirin and gastric bleeding: Further studies of calcium aspirin. Amer. J. Dig. Dis. 6:1115, 1961.
3. Banks, C. N., and Baron, J. H.: Drugs containing aspirin. Lancet 1:1165, 1964.
4. Davis, J. S.: Gastrointestinal haemorrhage and salicylates. Lancet 2:1121, 1958.
5. Allibone, A., and Flint, F. J.: Gastrointestinal haemorrhage and salicylates. Lancet 2:1121, 1958.
6. Salter, R. H.: Aspirin and gastrointestinal bleeding. Amer. J. Dig. Dis. 13:38, 1968.
7. Muir, A., and Cossar, I. A.: Aspirin and ulcer. Brit. Med. J. 2:7, 1955.
8. Brown, R. K., and Mitchell, N.: The influence of some of the salicyl compounds (and alcoholic beverages) on the natural history of peptic ulcer. Gastroenterology 31:198, 1956.
9. Kelly, J. J.: Salicylate ingestion: A frequent cause of gastric hemorrhage. Amer. J. Med. Sci. 232:119, 1956.
10. Lange, H. F.: Salicylates and gastric haemorrhage 2. Manifest bleeding. Gastroenterology 33:770, 1957.
11. Allibone, A., and Flint, F. J.: Bronchitis, aspirin, smoking, and other factors in the aetiology of peptic ulcer. Lancet 2:179, 1958.
12. Alvarez, A. S., and Summerskill, W. H. J.: Gastrointestinal haemorrhage and salicylates. Lancet 2:920, 1958.
13. Parry, D. J., and Wood, P. H. N.: Relationship between aspirin taking and gastroduodenal haemorrhage. Gut 8:301, 1967.
14. Muir, A., and Cossar, I. A.: Aspirin and gastric haemorrhage. Lancet 1:539, 1959.
15. Valman, H. B., Parry, D. J., and Coghill, N. F.: Lesions associated with gastroduodenal haemorrhage in relation to aspirin intake. Brit. Med. J. 4:661. 1968.
16. Langman, M. J. S., Hansky, J. H., Drury, R. A. B., and Jones, F. A.: The gastric mucosa in radiologically negative acute gastrointestinal bleeding. Gut 5:550, 1964.
17. Grossman, M. I., Matsumoto, K. K., and Lichter, R. J.: Fecal blood loss produced by oral and intravenous administration of various salicylates. Gastroenterology 40:383, 1961.
18. Astley, C. E.: Gastritis, aspirin and alcohol. Brit. Med. J. 4:484, 1967.
19. Jennings, G. H.: Causal influences in haematemesis and melaena. Gut 6:1, 1967.
20. Needham, C. D., Kyle, J., Jones, P. F., Johnston, S. J., and Kerridge, D. F.: Aspirin and alcohol in gastrointestinal haemorrhage. Gut 12:819, 1971.
21. Russell, R. I., Williamson, J. M., Goldberg, A., and Wares, E.: Ascorbic acid levels in leucocytes of patients with gastrointestinal haemorrhage. Lancet 2:603, 1968.
22. Schiller, K. F. R., Truelove, S. C., and Gwyn Williams, D.: Haematemesis and melaena with special reference to factors influencing the outcome. Brit. Med. J. 2:7, 1970.
23. Aspirin and blood donors. Lancet 1:477, 1972.
24. Schwartz, A. D.: Blood 38:815, 1971.

Aspirin Is Dangerous for the Peptic Ulcer Patient

HOWARD M. SPIRO

Yale University School of Medicine

I believe that the person who has had a peptic ulcer should not take aspirin in any circumstances. I am persuaded that the evidence for this conviction is clear for the patient with the gastric ulcer and that, while statistical proof that aspirin may also harm the duodenal ulcer patient is harder to come by, circumstantial witness suggests a link between aspirin damage and these two "peptic" cousins. If no other analgesic agent were available, such caution would not be possible, but as there are many reasonable if more costly substitutes for aspirin, prudence requires that patients with duodenal or gastric ulcer avoid all aspirin-containing compounds. Let me confess that I take aspirin if necessary, that I believe it is an excellent drug with a long history of widespread and apparently innocent use, that there can be few drugs with as profound effects (only just now beginning to be recognized) or with as excellent a safety record, but this panegyric should not obscure the fact that aspirin is not good for the patient with a peptic ulcer.

In my comments the reader should recognize that, regardless of the studies adduced, I see the potential for aspirin harm as predictable only in ulcer patients and I believe that it would be wrong to draw wider conclusions. In the discussion which follows I shall use the term "peptic ulcer" to refer to all patients with either duodenal or gastric ulcer. I consider the person who has had a bona fide ulcer in the past to have a predilection for ulcer forever and I use the term "ulcer patient" in that sense. "Once an ulcer always an ulcer." It might be just as well at this point to express another prejudice: I know of no way in which the peptic ulcer patient can prevent the onset of major complications or difficulties by dietary control, I am not a believer in "prophylaxis," I do not accept as proved the countless myths of drugs which prevent recurrences (and sometimes I envy the very real castles built on those clouds); but I do believe, as will become clear, that if the patient with peptic ulcer avoids aspirin, he avoids positive harm.

Clinical Evidence

Aspirin Dyspepsia

Let us begin with anecdotal evidence, since this kind is easiest for the clinician to come by and in the only just now waning "basic science" mood usually least believed. Aspirin dyspepsia occurs, it has been estimated, in about one quarter of all users, but this is an unpredictable event. In some unpublished observations on symptomatic aspirin intolerance some years ago, I noted that almost all college students could take two tablets of aspirin four times a day for three days without noting heartburn or indigestion and that it was only with increasing age that persons without a history of duodenal ulcer began to have "heartburn" on taking customary doses of aspirin. Therefore, I think that age has something to do with symptomatic aspirin intolerance, even if it probably does not play a role in aspirin-induced major bleeding.

Aspirin dyspepsia is even commoner in patients with peptic ulcer, and my general impression is that about two thirds of ulcer patients will note some heartburn on taking just a few aspirin tablets. Most often this pain is exactly the same as "ulcer pain." Indeed, many a person with a duodenal ulcer will have noted that the taking of aspirin usually reproduces his ulcer pain, but the clinician may have to inquire specifically about this sequence.

On the very simplest level, therefore, it makes as much sense to avoid medications which give pain as it does to avoid foods which bring on distress, even if any general prohibition now seems a little old fashioned. "Eat anything which does not hurt you and avoid anything which gives pain" is a good kind of hedonism for the ulcer patient in remission. Orange juice also often gives the peptic ulcer patient heartburn, and the cynic (presumably my adversary in this volume) could inquire whether I forbid my patients orange juice! Many an ulcer patient does tell his physician that he cannot take orange juice on an empty stomach, and if the evidence ever comes in as strongly that orange juice is associated with gastrointestinal bleeding as is aspirin, I will make enemies of the orange growers. But not yet!

Duodenal Ulcer Intractability

Sometimes aspirin dyspepsia is a cause of persistent refractory duodenal ulcer symptoms, and the clinician may find that all that is needed to cure "intractability" is the interdiction of all aspirin-containing compounds; it is remarkable how otherwise well informed persons with a duodenal ulcer may refrain from labeled aspirin quite dutifully and yet take a proprietary compound which combines an alkalizer with a little citric acid and aspirin. The alkalizer gives relief, the citric acid tastes good, and the aspirin (regardless of what form it may take in solution) may lead to more heartburn, which then makes the patient take more of the fizzy stuff, and so it goes on and on. Such products may be excellent for the general public, but they have not been proved innocent for the patient with an ulcer in his duodenum or stomach.

Some patients may not even take aspirin for pain or headache, but only for sleep, and may not consider this aspirin "for headache," so the physician must make his inquiries specific. Many practitioners must have had the experience of worrying over a patient with persistent night pain from a duodenal ulcer, suddenly discovering that he has been taking several aspirin tablets as a sedative at bedtime, and then relaxing as the ulcer pain disappears when the patient gives up his nocturnal aspirin tablets.

Aspirin Injury to the Gastric Mucosa

Let us look at more objective evidence, even as we re-emphasize that anecdotes are not so bad as some editors think, since the categorical imperative in medicine runs along the line that if something happens once, it will happen again. Evidence that aspirin injures the gastric mucosa lies in more than just the fiery witness of heartburn.[1] Aspirin produces gastric erosions,[2] it leads to an increased fecal blood loss,[3] it has been associated (in retrospective studies only, alas) with overt gastrointestinal bleeding, and[4] in retrospective but statistically responsible studies it has been associated, at least in Australia, with the now well known increased incidence of gastric ulcer among women.[2]

ULCERATIONS AND EROSIONS—THE BARRIER BREAKERS

Every study that I have reviewed shows that aspirin compounds lead to erosive lesions in the human and animal stomach, regardless of whether these studies have involved gastroscopy, the administration of aspirin just before gastrectomy and subsequent examination of the resected specimen, or some arcane experimental procedure which measures the leakage of electrolytes into the gastric lumen and the shedding of epithelial cells.

The mechanism of aspirin-induced injury to the stomach is now well known, the currently popular "back diffusion" concept providing the requisite scientific basis for clinical prejudice.[3] There is no evidence that aspirin injures the stomach by increasing gastric secretion,[4] and although gastroscopists once used to describe undissolved aspirin tablets lying in their own erosions in the stomach, today there is considerably less interest in strictly local irritative effects of undissolved aspirin tablets.[5,6] Instead a more generalized injury to the stomach seems likely to account for the events.[7] The normal stomach secretes hydrochloric acid, but does not reabsorb it, and in effect maintains a "barrier" against the reabsorption of gastric acid. This barrier is raised by the "tight junction" which each epithelial cell maintains with its neighbors. Junction to junction, the epithelial cells guard against acid injury until various noxious physiological events or substances, among them aspirin, loosen the tight junctions at the borders of the epithelial cells and so render the mucosa "leaky." Then hydrochloric acid seeps back through the mucosa to set up a chain of events which result in vasodilatation and pepsinogen stimulation[8] and ultimately in erosions and, depending upon the amount of gastric acid present, in bleeding. In a sense, then, aspirin permits acid to bore a hole in the stomach.

These events have been studied with the electron microscope and with the scanning electron microscope, which provide dramatic details of the rupture of intercellular bonds and intracellular damage, especially condensation and aggregation of chromatin with cytoplasmic edema, that attest to cellular injury.[9] At least in the experimental animal these subcellular studies so underline the inevitability and invariability of gastric damage from aspirin that the observer wonders how some of us get away with taking aspirin at all! Electron microscopic studies suggest that the cell is injured from inside by aspirin, within a minute or so of aspirin exposure; this immediate injury is diffuse and stands in contrast to the relatively localized erosions and ulcerations which may be seen grossly some hours later. That the electron microscope shows changes inside the cell so soon after exposure is an important consideration; the scanning electron microscopic views of cells dropping out of the epithelium and shrinking away from their neighbors provide dramatic evidence of the loosening of the tight junctures.[10] The differences between these studies reflect, I believe, differences in the times of observations. They both agree in recording the remarkable cellular injury from small amounts of aspirin in the stomach.

ACID LEVELS AND GASTRIC INJURY

Injury depends upon the presence of acid, and experimental studies make me conclude that acid itself accounts for erosions and bleeding. Aspirin in the anacid stomach is nowhere near so bad an actor: the patient with achlorhydria is less susceptible to the induction of erosions or to bleeding. To be sure, even the patient with pernicious anemia, and therefore with complete anacidity, may display some gastric erosions on exposure to small amounts of aspirin, and even such patients have a somewhat increased incidence of gastric bleeding after aspirin;[11] but these events are rarely as dramatic in the quantities of blood generated or in the number of erosions as in the normal subject with his normal gastric acid. We may note that not only is there less acid present to produce damage, but the patient with atrophic gastritis absorbs aspirin more slowly and to a lesser degree than normal.

Lesser injury and less absorption of aspirin also characterize the stomach bathed with aspirin buffered to pH 7;[12, 13] this, of course, is to be expected. Giving alkali along with aspirin should reduce aspirin injury to the stomach because it reduces the absorption of aspirin as well as the amount of noxious acid available for injury. This is indeed the case, and confirmatory studies have included gastroscopic evidence of erosions and measurement of fecal blood loss.[14] For example, the taking of 0.6 gm. of aspirin with 100 ml. of soda bicarbonate prevented the gross bleeding, ecchymoses, and petechiae observed in normal college students when the same amount of aspirin was taken with 100 ml. of 0.1 N hydrochloric acid. This is the basis used for the claims of several popular effervescent aspirin combinations, and it does seem likely that such effervescent alkaline buffered preparations do not increase fecal blood loss.[12]

Acid is bad in the presence of barrier breakers regardless of their nature; several observers have claimed that the frequency of stress ulceration is reduced by continuous adequate neutralization in the stomach. Again, acid apparently is the culprit. Since I know that most duodenal ulcer patients have lots of acid in their stomach, since they are subject to all kinds of stress, since aspirin is a "barrier breaker" that can be avoided, I advise them to avoid the dangers of aspirin along with its benefits, even though they cannot yet prevent bile reflux, psychic or physical distress, along with several other more physiological attacks against their gastric mucosal integrity. I do not believe that this is alarmism, but only simple good sense.

How about alcohol, that other popular barrier breaker? Because I recognize how many tensions dissolve in alcohol taken in social amounts (at least as defined in New Haven) and because there is no good evidence overall that alcohol in moderation is harmful to the peptic ulcer patient when not taken along with aspirin, I do not caution against its moderate use. Alcohol comes off better than aspirin when it comes to mood elevation; any pleasures induced by aspirin must surely be autistic.

Minor Bleeding

Aspirin has been shown time and again to induce minor gastrointestinal bleeding and even iron deficiency anemia in patients who take it chronically even without symptomatic evidence of aspirin intolerance. This probably occurs in about two thirds of normal persons, or even more. Its magnitude in patients with erosions or ulcerations in the stomach and duodenum has not, so far as I can tell, been studied. It seems clear that this bleeding must arise from the erosions which are so often demonstrated, but no clear relationship has been established between this micro bleeding which seems to occur in normals and in ulcer-bearing patients alike and the massive hematemesis or melena which appears to be "idiosyncratic" and unpredictable in nature. Indeed, some observers even deny any relationship between the gastroscopically visible erosions and fecal blood loss.[15] Recent observations that aspirin increases mucosal blood flow may provide further evidence of why aspirin is so consistently associated with bleeding of some degree.[16]

Massive Bleeding

Studies of overt bleeding following the use of aspirin are usually retrospective, it has been pointed out,[1] and consist of recording the amount of aspirin taken during the interval just preceding hospitalization, the bleeders being put in one group, the controls in another, and their aspirin intake compared. In one study[17] of 1634 admissions for acute gastrointestinal bleeding, about two thirds of the patients with an ulcer and two thirds of those with "acute lesions" (that is, with negative x-rays) had taken aspirin. These observers emphasized the regularity of aspirin intake in their patients; nearly half had taken more than two doses of aspirin each week for a long period; in them aspirin intake was not an isolated event. Gastric ulcer patients who had bled were even more likely to have taken aspirin just preceding the bleeding.

Presumably such a comparison defines the role of aspirin in precipitating clinically significant gastrointestinal bleeding, but admittedly the accuracy of such a study depends entirely upon the memory and reliability of the patients questioned.[12] If aspirin intake for about a week before hospitalization is taken as the measure, the control population may be found to take aspirin in percentages ranging from 4 to 44 per cent, while in those patients who have bled, the percentage taking aspirin during the week before hospitalization ranges from 25 to 72 per cent. This is suggestive, but such large variations detract from confidence. If the aspirin intake in the 48-hour period before admission is the criterion, then the bleeders have taken aspirin 51 to 58 per cent of the time, while control patients have taken it only 11 to 25 per cent, a much more impressive distinction. There are many such studies, and they all suggest that aspirin has something to do with massive gastrointestinal bleeding despite their retrospective nature and even though we can never be certain whether the patient takes aspirin for symptoms of bleeding which is already under way or whether the aspirin has been its immediate cause. Nevertheless, the data seem to be all in one direction; smoke usually means fire, and I would believe that the evidence links aspirin with massive bleeding from the gastrointestinal tract.

Now of course the burden of such studies is to show that aspirin causes bleeding in a significant proportion of patients who do not have a chronic gastric or duodenal ulcer; but if such patients can be made to bleed, there is nothing to suggest that the patient with a duodenal ulcer is at a lesser risk. Although the evidence is strong that patients in whom the cause of bleeding has not been demonstrated radiologically are especially likely to have taken aspirin, the possible association of aspirin intake with bleeding from a chronic duodenal ulcer cannot be dismissed. Aspirin intake seemed to be a factor in 80 per cent of bleeders with an acute gastric erosion, 52 per cent of those with bleeding from a duodenal ulcer, and 49 per cent of those bleeding from a gastric ulcer, while only 32 per cent of controls had been taking aspirin.[18] This is representative of many studies which condemn aspirin as the cause of massive bleeding in nonulcer patients and studies which suggest that aspirin may be linked with bleeding from a duodenal ulcer. As gastroscopy has not been used routinely, even the judgment that a duodenal ulcer-bearing patient is bleeding from his duodenal ulcer and not from aspirin-induced gastritis is inferential. It has always seemed possible that even patients thought to have bled from a duodenal ulcer have, in fact, bled from aspirin-induced gastritis. The predictable wider use of panendoscopy in the next few years should help with this distinction. The decision is after all an important one, because bleeding from erosive gastritis carries with it no necessary assurance of another hemorrhage, while bleeding from a duodenal ulcer has a statistically respectable likelihood of recurrence.

I do not know why massive bleeding is unpredictable and "idiosyncratic," I cannot predict who will bleed from peptic ulcer and who will not, and I recognize that major hemorrhages and acute erosive gastritis may have nothing at all to do with peptic ulcer. Yet, these are some more reasons why I request my patients with peptic ulcer to avoid aspirin.

EFFECT ON BLEEDING FACTORS

Aspirin even in doses as small as three or four tablets has many effects upon blood coagulation, as is increasingly being recognized,[19] and these changes persist for three to seven days. I suspect that in most patients with massive gastrointestinal bleeding these phenomena may have little to do with the clinical situation, yet since aspirin alters platelet physiology so profoundly it cannot be ignored. Aspirin prevents the aggregation of platelets, causes a slight prolongation of bleeding time in normal subjects and in those with von Willebrand's disease, while in hemophiliacs even one aspirin tablet severely interferes with clotting. This witness is impressive and it all points in the same direction, that aspirin cannot be good for the duodenal ulcer patient.

It has been suggested that clinically inapparent vitamin C deficiency may also underline aspirin-induced bleeding in the duodenal ulcer patient. Ulcer patients tend to be vitamin C deficient, and such a comment only confirms my prejudices!

Gastric Ulcer

I see no question at all as regards the harmful nature of aspirin in the patient with gastric ulcer, and it seems hardly believable that there could be any "controversy" about this, so strong is the evidence. In one study 60 per cent of patients with gastric ulcer, 23 per cent with duodenal ulcer, and only 10 per cent of controls had taken aspirin each day.[20] Evidence for bile reflux as a cause of back diffusion and barrier breaking in the gastric ulcer patient, evidence of back diffusion in the lower acid levels in the gastric ulcer stomach, clinical evidence that women who have gastric ulcer take aspirin in larger quantities for longer periods and more regularly than other persons all strongly testify to the fact that aspirin is bad for the gastric ulcer patient. Are gastric ulcer and duodenal ulcer the same disorder? That they look alike is not guarantee enough, but the reasons already adduced and their general association lead me to act as if they were, at least as far as aspirin is concerned. There seems to me no argument about aspirin and gastric ulcer, at least in 1973.

Other Forms of Aspirin

What about aspirin in its many disguises or forms? I am confused by the conflicting evidence which arrives at many different conclusions. Enteric-coated aspirin may protect against gastrointestinal bleeding or it may not; there is evidence in both directions. Buffered aspirin in the usual over-the-counter tablet probably does not provide a safe alternative, since the amount of buffer in most buffered aspirins would hardly seem capable of preventing erosions, as it certainly does not neutralize acid in the stomach. While it may have a lesser malign effect upon gastrointestinal bleeding, this has not been proved, and the relationship between micro bleeding and massive bleeding has yet to be established. Again evidence goes both ways, some stating that buffering in the usual amounts does not decrease micro bleeding,[21] others claiming it does. Aspirin given along with soda bicarbonate certainly seems in Davenport's studies to have been less harmful;[22] what it does to the duodenal ulcer patient and how the claim that sodium acetyl salicylate is less harmful in its general effects on the duodenal ulcer patient I do not know.

Aspirin of small particle size is apparently less likely to produce bleeding than that of coarser size, yet from the electron microscopic studies already noted which suggest that aspirin injury occurs within a few moments of exposure, I doubt that attempts at reducing the length of contact of aspirin particles with the stomach will make much difference. From the evidence that intravenous aspirin may be harmful I conclude that buffering may reduce the incidence of micro bleeding, but that major hemorrhages will prove as difficult to prevent and to predict as ever. If taking aspirin with food does not lessen the degree of microscopic blood loss,[23, 24] it seems doubtful that any degree of buffering will eliminate microscopic bleeding.

I do not recommend buffered aspirin to duodenal ulcer patients, therefore, and as for aspirin in some other form, whether by rectum or by enteric coating or intravenously, I likewise have very little confidence in recommending it to my patients. Studies of the effect of these different modes of aspirin administration upon the stomach are confusing. There is evidence that intravenous aspirin can increase fecal blood loss,[25, 26] and that it may not.[27] Since the evidence goes both ways, I suspect the positive and avoid aspirin in duodenal ulcer patients. I'm inclined to agree with Grossman's 1961 belief that "there is at present no route of administration or dosage form of salicylates of proven safety in these patients."[25]

Conclusions

There are alternatives to aspirin. I do not know why aspirin produces erosions only sporadically, I am uncertain whether aspirin "pulls the loaded trigger" to induce erosions in patients who are under other stress, but if that is indeed the case, aspirin can be eliminated when other stresses remain. I recognize the usefulness of aspirin even though, submitted as a new drug to the FDA tomorrow, I suspect it would have to undergo several years of testing. The point in what I have stated here is not that aspirin is a bad drug generally, but simply that it is a bad drug for ulcer patients.

References

1. Langman, M. J.: Epidemiological evidence for the association of aspirin and acute gastrointestinal bleeding. Gut *11*:627–634, 1970.
2. Duggan, J. M., and Chapman, B. L.: The incidence of aspirin ingestion in patients with peptic ulcer. Med. J. Aust. *1*:797–800, 1970.
3. Ivey, K. J.: Acute hemorrhagic gastritis: Modern concepts based on pathogenesis. Gut *12*:750–757, 1971.
4. Jabbari, M., and Valberg, L. S.: The role of acid secretion in aspirin induced gastric mucosal injury. Canad. Med. J. *102*:178–181, 1970.
5. Menguy, R.: Gastric mucus and the gastric mucous barrier. Amer. J. Surg. *117*:806–812, 1969.
6. Menguy, R.: Gastric mucosal injury by aspirin. Gastroenterology *51*:430–432, 1966.
7. Lev, R., Siegel, H. I., and Jerzy-Glass, G. B.: Effects of salicylates on the canine stomach: A morphological and histochemical study. Gastroenterology *62*:970–980, 1972.

8. Johnson, L. R.: Pepsin secretion during damage by ethanol and salicylic acid. Gastroenterology 62:412–416, 1972.
9. Hingson, D. J., and Ito, S.: Effect of aspirin and related compounds on the fine structure of most gastric mucosa. Gastroenterology 61:156–177, 1971.
10. Frenning, B., and Obrink, K. J.: The effect of acetyl and acetylsalicylic acids on the appearance of the gastric mucosal surface epithelium in the scanning electron microscope. Scand. J. Gastroent. 6:605–612, 1972.
11. St. John, D. J., and McDermott, F. T.: Influence of achlorhydria in aspirin induced occult gastrointestinal blood loss: Studies in Addisonian pernicious anemia. Brit. Med. J. 1:450–452, 1970.
12. Cooke, A. R.: Aspirin and gastrointestinal bleeding. Aust. Ann. Med. 2:171–2, 1970.
13. Cooke, A. R., and Hunt, J. N.: Absorption of acetylsalicylic acid from unbuffered and buffered gastric contents. Amer. J. Dig. Dis. 15:95–102, 1970.
14. Thorsen, W. B., Western, D., Tanaka, Y., and Morrissey, J. F.: Aspirin injury to the gastric mucosa. Arch. Intern. Med. 121:499–506, 1968.
15. Kuiper, D. H., Overholt, B. F., Fall, D. J., and Pollard, H. M.: Gastroscopic findings and fecal blood loss following aspirin administration. Amer. J. Dig. Dis. 14:761–769, 1969.
16. Augur, N. A., Jr.: Gastric mucosal blood flow following damage by ethanol, acetic acid, or aspirin. Gastroenterology 58:311–320, 1970.
17. Duggan, J. M.: Gastrointestinal hemorrhage, gastric ulcer, and aspirin. Aust. Ann. Med. 2: 135–138, 1970.
18. Valman, H. B., Parry, D. J., and Coghill, N. F.: Lesions associated with gastric and duodenal hemorrhage in relation to aspirin intake. Brit. Med. J. 2:661–665, 1968.
19. Kaneshiro, M. M., Mielke, C. H., Kasper, C. K., and Rapoport, S. I.: Bleeding time after aspirin in disorders of intrinsic clotting. New Eng. J. Med. 281:1039–1042, 1969.
20. Gillies, M. A., and Skyring, A.: Gastric and duodenal ulcer. The association between aspirin ingestion, smoking, and family history of ulcer. Med. J. Aust. 2:280–285, 1969.
21. Beeken, W. L.: Effect of five salicylic containing compounds upon loss of 51 chromium labelled erythrocytes from the GI tract of normal man. Gut 9:475–479, 1968.
22. Davenport, H.: Salicylate damage to the gastric mucosal barrier. New Eng. J. Med. 276: 1307–1312, 1967.
23. Willems, G., Vansteenkiste, Y., and Smets, P. H.: Effects of food ingestion on the cell proliferation kinetics in the canine fundic mucosa. Gastroenterology 61:323–327, 1971.
24. Stephens, F. O., Milverton, E. J., Hambly, C. K., and Vanderven, E. K.: The effect of food on aspirin induced gastrointestinal blood loss. Digestion 1:267–276, 1968.
25. Grossman, M., Matsumoto, K. K., and Lichter, R.: Fecal blood loss produced by oral and intravenous administration of various salicylates. Gastroenterology 40:383–388, 1961.
26. Brodie, D. A., and Hooke, K. F.: Effects of route of administration on the production of gastric hemorrhage in the rat by aspirin and sodium salicylate. Amer. J. Dig. Dis. 16:985–989, 1970.
27. Cooke, A. R., and Goulston, K.: Failure of intravenous aspirin to increase gastrointestinal blood loss. Brit. Med. J. 2:330–332, 1969.

Comment

Aspirin and the Stomach

Between 20 and 30 billion 0.33 gram tablets of aspirin are consumed in the U.S.A. annually. If a normal person takes 27 such tablets in a three-day period, he loses some 10 ml. more blood from his gut than he does during a nonaspirin control period.[1] Assuming that the effects of short-term experiments are also true of long-continued aspirin intake, and that blood loss increases linearly with amount of aspirin taken per day, one can derive a startling conclusion: annual aspirin consumption in the U.S.A. causes 10 billion milliliters of blood to go down the toilet per year. This is about twice the amount of blood used for transfusions in the U.S.A. annually. The benefits of an aspirin-less culture are unimaginable!

Ridiculous, isn't it? But this extrapolation of the undoubted fact that aspirin does cause a microscopic amount of gastrointestinal bleeding is not much more fantastic than the extrapolation that aspirin is a major cause of gross and clinically alarming blood loss from the gut. This extrapolation is, of course, supported by numerous retrospective analyses indicating that patients admitted to hospitals for gastrointestinal bleeding have taken more aspirin during a variable preadmission period than a control group. As a consequence, it is dogmatically asserted that aspirin commonly causes gastritis, that aspirin commonly causes gastroduodenal ulcer, and that aspirin commonly causes both of these lesions or even a "normal" stomach to bleed profusely. Trial lawyers are blandly advised in their professional journal that aspirin may be responsible when a patient vomits blood or has copious melena—with obvious implications for legal action.

We physicians often smile at what we consider the childish tendency of some of our patients to blame a variety of complaints on some easily identifiable but usually quite innocent culprit: "It must have been something I ate" . . . "I got my feet wet" . . . "The smell was choking me." The ready attribution of major gastrointestinal bleeding that is not easily explained otherwise to the intake of aspirin anywhere from 12 minutes to 12 days earlier shows that the medical profession is not immune to the same type of reasoning. A convenient whipping boy is a great source of comfort to us all.

Langman points out that there is no clear correlation between trends in aspirin consumption and the incidence of acute gastrointestinal bleeding. He also argues that on critical analysis the evidence accumulated by the various retrospective studies is far less overwhelming than one would suspect it to be in view of the frequent incrimination of the drug as a cause of clinically important gastrointestinal bleeding. And even Spiro, who has been known to say in private, "I hate aspirin" (personal communication), is not ready to label aspirin as "bad." He only goes so far as to say, "It is a bad drug for ulcer patients."

Yet the dogma of the sceptic is as bad as that of the enthusiast, and there are many reasons why, with respect to gastrointestinal bleeding, aspirin is suspect. After all, it does cause minute amounts of extra blood loss in most people who take the agent. Davenport's now famous studies show that aspirin in "acid" (pH below 3.5) gastric contents disrupts the gastric barrier sufficiently to permit back diffusion of potentially noxious hydrogen ions into the tissues of the stomach. Furthermore, although it is far from certain that aspirin can affect hemostatic mechanisms sufficiently in normal persons to cause any bleeding, the evidence is good that those who suffer from borderline coagulation abnormalities, and particularly those with deficient platelet function, may be susceptible to bleeding phenomena if they do take aspirin. Probably the population contains a small but definite number of people who have inapparent coagulation defects, and such people might be at risk if they take aspirin. Thus, it is very likely that once in a while aspirin does precipitate major gastrointestinal blood loss—either by its action on the stomach, by its action on the blood, or by a combination of these mechanisms.

All this adds up to the point of view that aspirin should be used with circumspection but not with alarm. Spiro's position is entirely tenable, and one might wish to include other types of patients, i.e., those in whom a peptic ulcer is not found but whose symptoms suggest that they have difficulty in handling their gastric secretions comfortably. Hence, why should not the occasional user of aspirin use a buffered preparation? And, let's face it, Alka-Seltzer is probably one of the most effectively buffered of aspirin preparations on the market. More regular aspirin users could be urged to take the medication with food. All such precautionary measures are entirely justified. But unjustified is such a fear of aspirin as a potential cause of major gastrointestinal bleeding as to lead to a blanket proscription of the drug. Indeed, our lawyer friends, instead of worrying whether a gastrointestinal bleeder might have been given aspirin, should be much more concerned from the viewpoint of questionable practice if a fear of its gastric effects causes the drug to be withheld from a patient who desperately requires the relief provided by this excellent analgesic.

1. Grossman, M., Matsumoto, K. K., and Lichter, R.: Fecal blood loss produced by oral and intravenous administration of various salicylates. Gastroenterology 40:383–388, 1961.

FRANZ J. INGELFINGER

20

Mechanisms That Prevent Gastroesophageal Reflux

THE IMPORTANCE OF THE ANATOMIC CONFIGURATION OF THE CARDIA IN PREVENTING GASTROESOPHAGEAL REFLUX
    by David B. Skinner

THE IMPORTANCE OF THE SPHINCTER AT THE GASTROESOPHAGEAL JUNCTION
    by Lauran D. Harris

COMMENT
    by Franz J. Ingelfinger

The Importance of the Anatomical Configuration of the Cardia in Preventing Gastroesophageal Reflux

DAVID B. SKINNER

The University of Chicago

Symptomatic gastroesophageal reflux and its complications are being recognized with increasing frequency. Failure to differentiate between hiatal hernia and reflux causes much confusion in diagnosis and therapy. It is well known that these are two separate conditions: hiatal hernia, the anatomical abnormality; and reflux, the physiological consequence of a malfunctioning cardia. While these conditions often coexist, each occurs without the other. Reflux causes the symptoms of heartburn and regurgitation and the complications of esophagitis, stricture, bleeding, and aspiration. A small hiatal hernia is usually inconsequential unless accompanied by reflux. Accordingly it must be asked whether anatomic rearrangements at the cardia within the capability of surgery can succeed in correcting the physiologic abnormality of reflux. Past experience indicates that the common operation of hiatal hernia repair often fails to control reflux. This has placed surgery for this condition in disrepute. Recently operations have been proposed and applied with the specific purpose of preventing reflux. Their success depends upon the correctness of observations and theories concerning factors which control reflux. It is the purpose of this essay to analyze these factors and to present evidence that anatomic relationships can be altered by surgery to restore physiological competency to the cardia.

Hiatal hernia is an extremely common finding, being observed in 10 to 60 per cent of upper gastrointestinal radiographic evaluations, depending upon the diagnostic criteria and the diligence employed by the radiologist in seeking this abnormality. No specific symptoms or complications can be attributed to the common, small, type I, sliding hiatal hernia unless reflux is present. Symptoms caused specifically by a hiatal hernia occur in patients with the unusual, large, or type II, parahiatal hernia which causes problems such as gastric obstruction, volvulus, strangulation, perforation, bleeding, gastritis, or acute intrathoracic gastric dilatation. These result directly from the anatomic presence of the hernia. Hiatal hernias of this type should be repaired to prevent such disastrous mechanical complications. Small hiatal hernias do not cause mechanical problems and are clinically insignificant unless gastroesophageal reflux coexists.

In our overweight, physically unfit, and anxiety ridden population, indigestion is a frequent complaint. This may result from a variety of causes, including reflux, duodenal or gastric ulcer, gastritis, biliary, pancreatic, or cardiac disease. To judge the clinical success of therapy for reflux, specific identification of reflux symptoms must be made. A story of substernal burning sensation (heartburn) and regurgitation of sour gastric contents elicited by stooping or lying flat and relieved by standing erect typically is caused by gastroesophageal reflux. While indigestion, postprandial fullness, belching, dysphagia, anginal-like chest pain, anemia, upper gastrointestinal bleeding, chronic cough, or hoarseness may all be caused by reflux, these complaints are not specific and cannot be attributed to reflux on symptomatic grounds alone. Nor will these complaints necessarily be relieved by therapy directed at reflux. Because of the frequency of such nonspecific complaints, objective means have been developed to diagnose reflux more precisely. Objective tests should be employed to evaluate the success of antireflux therapy since symptomatic results alone may be misleading.

Barium swallow examination offers the most accurate method for diagnosing hiatal hernia. A small hiatal hernia is clinically insignificant, so the pertinent question is how successful radiography is in diagnosing abnormal gastroesophageal reflux. My radiological colleagues, Drs. Margulies and Donner, state that approximately only 40 per cent of patients ultimately proved to have abnormal reflux will have reflux demonstrable during a standard or cineradiographic barium swallow evaluation. Clearly radiography is less than ideal for evaluating reflux. The addition of acid to barium as described by Donner and associates will provoke motility disorders visible during cineradiography in a large proportion of patients with symptomatic reflux.[1] However, the technique is based upon acid sensitivity of the esophagus, which is frequently present in patients with an incompetent cardia, but which may occur in patients who do not have reflux. The acid barium swallow is a useful screening test but cannot be regarded as definitive in diagnosing abnormal reflux.

Esophageal manometric studies provide useful information. The characteristics of the high pressure zone at the cardia can be measured by intraluminal pressure recordings. In patients with an incompetent cardia, the amplitude of pressure is frequently reduced. There is a significant statistical separation between the population of normal individuals and those with an incompetent cardia. Unfortunately the overlap in pressures at the cardia between the normal and abnormal is sufficiently broad to prevent manometry alone from being a reliable test for reflux in individual patients.[2] Manometry offers other important information such as detecting tertiary or spastic esophageal contractions which may be triggered by reflux and be the source of chest pain and dysphagia. Motility studies are useful in detecting aperistalsis and scleroderma, which are frequently associated with incompetency of the cardia. Manometry is also an excellent diagnostic method for identifying achalasia of the cardia, which may cause dysphagia and regurgitation of partially digested food. Thus, manometry should be performed in patients suspected of having an incompetent cardia but cannot be relied upon for diagnosis of this condition.

The most precise technique for diagnosing reflux is the direct measurement of pH in the esophagus 5 cm. above the cardia. Measurements are performed continuously under standardized conditions in which the patient has an acid load in the stomach and performs a series of respiratory and postural maneuvers in sequence. When we applied this technique to 91 normal subjects, only two had a "positive" test, i.e., more than two repeated drops in esophageal pH to less than 4.0.[2] Approximately 40 per cent of normal subjects will have one or two occasional episodes of pH drop during extreme respiratory and postural maneuvers. The remainder have no decreases in pH at all. But when we studied over 300 patients ultimately proved to have abnormal reflux, less than 1 per cent failed to demonstrate any drop in pH during the performance of the pH reflux test. In our expeience, detection of reflux with a pH probe 5 cm. above the cardia has proved much more accurate than the earlier technique of withdrawing the pH electrode across the cardia. During the latter maneuver most normal subjects have a sharp rise in pH over approximately a 1-cm. distance at the cardia, whereas most with an incompetent cardia will have a gradual rise in pH over a prolonged distance. However, false positive and false negative results from the pH electrode withdrawal test are frequently observed. The pH reflux test with the electrode fixed in the esophagus serves as the best standard currently available for assessing competency of the cardia.

Another frequently employed test of esophageal function is the acid perfusion test described by Bernstein and colleagues.[3] Acid and saline are alternately perfused into the esophagus. A positive test is recorded when a patient has his spontaneous symptoms reproduced by acid infusion and not by saline infusion. This test measures acid sensitivity of the esophagus and does not directly indicate an incompetent cardia. The acid perfusion test is most useful in patients with known reflux in whom one wishes to know whether atypical symptoms may be caused by the regurgitation of gastric contents into the esophagus.

The acid clearing test devised by Booth and associates constitutes the fourth of the esophageal function tests which we perform at one sitting.[2] In this study the pH electrode remains 5 cm. above the cardia, and a 15-cc. bolus of 0.1 N HCl is introduced into the esophagus 10 cm. above the electrode. The patient is asked to swallow at intervals. Normal subjects clear the acid bolus from the esophagus in less than 10 swallows. In patients with abnormal reflux, esophageal emptying is frequently delayed, permitting prolonged acid contact with the esophageal mucosa. Since esophagitis seems more likely to occur under these circumstances, an abnormal acid clearing test is a useful guide to the likelihood of esophagitis. A positive test is an indication for esophagoscopy in patients who also have a positive pH reflux test.

Esophagitis is a serious consequence of reflux and a precursor to stricture or bleeding. Careful analysis of symptoms and esophagoscopic findings shows that there is no correlation between the severity of symptoms and the presence of esophagitis. Esophagoscopy represents the only valid technique currently available for diagnosing esophagitis. Since esophagitis is an indication for vigorous therapy if the complications of stricture or bleeding are to be avoided, esophagoscopy should be performed in any patient with reflux demonstrated by radiography or a pH test in whom esophagitis is suspected on the basis of a prolonged acid clearing test, dysphagia, bleeding, or x-ray findings suggesting spasm or irregular mucosa. These objective techniques—radiography, manometry, the pH reflux test, the acid perfusion test, the acid clearing test, and esophagoscopy—form a solid basis for the evaluation of a patient's symptoms and assessment of the results of treatment designed to prevent reflux and its complications.

Since hiatal hernia does not necessarily cause reflux, and reflux may occur without a hiatal hernia, simple repair of a hiatal hernia is often insufficient to prevent further symptoms and complications of reflux. If the patient's symptoms or complications are severe enough to warrant surgery, the operation performed must be designed to alter the mechanisms which control reflux. For understanding of these factors, knowledge of the anatomy and physiology of the cardia is essential.[4]

The cardia or esophageal orifice of the stomach can be defined in several ways: as the junction of squamous and columnar epithelium, as the point where the tubular esophagus enters the pouch of the stomach, or as the junction between esophageal and gastric muscle layers. In considering factors which control reflux, the latter two definitions are more important than the precise location of the squamocolumnar junction. In normal individuals the point at which the tubular esophagus enters the stomach pouch can be determined by radiography. This point lies on the abdominal side of the esophageal hiatus in the diaphragm, and is believed to represent the junction of the innermost layer of gastric sling fibers and of the lower esophageal circular muscle. In patients with a widened hiatus, incompetent cardia, or hiatal hernia, this landmark is difficult to identify since the cardia takes on the appearance of an inverted funnel. Under these circumstances the difference in muscle contraction between stomach and esophagus following a swallow is a more reliable indicator of the position of the cardia. In patients with normal peristaltic progression, the junction between stomach and esophagus can be identified as that point at which the esophageal peristaltic wave stops. Normally this too is below the diaphragm.

Esophageal muscle is divided into two layers, an inner circular layer and an outer longitudinal layer. During normal swallowing these layers are coordinated so that a peristaltic wave progresses from the cricopharyngeal sphincter to the cardia. The lowermost segment of esophagus functions in a fashion different from the remainder of the organ. When studied by intraluminal pressure measurements, the resting tone in the normal distal esophagus is greater than gastric fundus or mid esophageal pressure. When a swallow or secondary peristaltic wave is initiated, intraluminal pressure in the distal esophageal segment falls to the level of gastric pressure and remains there until the peristaltic wave reaches the distal esophagus. Then the distal segment contracts, causing an elevation of pressure followed by a leveling off to the original resting tone. This specialized function of the distal esophagus is taken to represent a lower esophageal sphincter.

A sphincter muscle can be demonstrated at the cardia in some animal species, and esophageal manometric studies as just described suggest the presence of a sphincter mechanism in humans. However, no sphincter muscle can be conclusively identified by surgical or anatomic dissection in human beings. Thus, the concept of a human lower esophageal sphincter is proposed as a physiologic rather than anatomic barrier. The maintenance of a high pressure zone between the stomach and esophagus by such a sphincter is widely regarded as being one factor responsible for the prevention of gastroesophageal reflux.

Since the sphincter cannot be identified anatomically, controversy persists as to whether the high pressure zone is caused primarily by the distal esophageal muscle or represents a summation of forces applied externally to the cardia. This distinction has obvious therapeutic importance, since surgery may alter the external relationships of the cardia but is unlikely to increase intrinsic esophageal muscle tone. In favor of an intrinsic muscle function are the observations that the sphincter pressure drops promptly when a swallow is initiated and that the resting pressure can be altered by drugs such as gastrin, which elevates the pressure, and atropine, which reduces it. On the other hand, at least some of the pressure phenomena noted in the distal esophagus may be accounted for by mechanisms other than a specialized action of distal esophageal muscle. Johnson[5] and others offer evidence suggesting that opening of the cardia during a swallow is caused by the longitudinal muscle of the esophagus. This shortens the esophagus and would tend to draw the cardia upward from the positive pressure intra-abdominal environment into the less than atmospheric pressures of the thorax, which might account for a drop in pressure in the distal esophageal segment. Atropine has a generalized effect of reducing smooth muscle tension so that a fall in intraluminal pressure following administration of this drug cannot be taken as specific evidence for a sphincter muscle. In fact, reduction of the high pressure zone by atropine in normal humans does not cause an increase in reflux as measured by the pH electrode.[6] Observations by Castell and Harris[7] and by Cohen and Lipshutz[8] concerning the effects of gastrin on the high pressure zone are most interesting and do suggest a specific hormonally controlled function of the distal esophageal segment. Further substantiation and analysis of the effects of gastrin are required before the interpretation of those findings can be taken as proof of the role of intrinsic esophageal muscle in the control of reflux. The evidence to date does not conclusively support the contention that the high pressure zone and primary barrier to reflux mainly come from the distal esophageal muscle. Neither does the evidence clearly refute this theory.

To investigate this problem further, Chambers, Zarins, and I are studying pressure relationships on the inside and outside of the cardia and stomach in Rhesus monkeys. These animals are suitable for such investigations, as the anatomy and physiology of the cardia and lower esophagus are similar to those of humans. No identifiable muscle sphincter can be found in the lower esophagus, but a high pressure zone which functions like that of a human being is observed by manometric studies. In these animals simultaneous pressure recordings are made in the lumen of the stomach, the high pressure zone at the cardia and body of the esophagus, and on the outer surface of the stomach and cardia at points precisely opposite the intraluminal pressure catheters. Analyses of these five pressure recordings in 10 monkeys taken under resting conditions and with external pressure applied to the abdomen indicate that pressures recorded on the outside of the gastroesophageal junction exceed pressures on the outside or inside of the stomach in monkeys with a competent cardia. In monkeys in which reflux is induced, pressure on the outside of the cardia frequently is less than gastric pressure, so that the gradient of pressure between stomach and cardia is reversed. This difference between monkeys which reflux and those which do not is statistically significant. In both groups pressures recorded on the outside of the cardia generally are greater than pressures in the lumen at the same level. These findings suggest that the observation of a high pressure zone at the cardia may reflect the summation or vector of forces external to the gastroesophageal junction as well as whatever tone is generated by esophageal muscle. Thus, at least a portion of the high pressure zone at the cardia which is considered to be important in the control of reflux may result from the geometric configuration and relationships of the cardia as it enters the abdomen.

The esophageal hiatus of the diaphragm is a muscular tunnel 2 to 3 cm. long. While most frequently consisting of muscle fibers from the right crus, the margins of the hiatus may consist of fibers from both right and left origins of the diaphragm. The muscular margins of the hiatus are initially vertical as they arise from the vertebral bodies. Then the muscle becomes more horizontal as it crosses in front of the esophagus to insert into the central tendon of the diaphragm. This sling of diaphragmatic muscle around the lower esophagus has often been given a responsible role in the control of reflux, but its actual physiologic importance has never been clearly demonstrated. The fact that many patients have a hiatal hernia in which the distal esophagus is separated from the diaphragm and yet do not have an incompetent cardia is strong evidence against the importance of the muscular sling in controlling reflux.[9] Narrowing of the hiatal tunnel is the primary maneuver employed in simple hiatal hernia repair, but there are numerous reports indicating that this procedure alone frequently fails to control abnormal reflux in spite of correction of the herniation.

In addition to the esophagus, the vagus nerves pass through the hiatus, as do extensions of the endo-abdominal and endothoracic fascia which line both sides of the diaphragm. As these two extensions of fascia reach the esophageal hiatus they blend together and continue as the phrenoesophageal membrane which inserts into the muscle layers and submucosa of the esophagus. Careful autopsy dissections by Bombeck, Dillard and Nyhus[10] demonstrate that the major portion of this membrane arose from the endo-abdominal fascia in 46 of 56 cadavers. The fibroelastic fascicles join to the submucosal or intramuscular fibrous tissue of the esophagus 2 to 3 cm. above the upper margins of the hiatus and 3 to 5 cm. above the mucosal junction. These anatomic dissections suggest that the innermost layer of abdominal wall does not meet the cardia but rather joins the esophagus at some distance above the gastroesophageal junction. The lowermost segment of esophagus, or that portion associated with the high pressure zone, is an intraabdominal segment in normal individuals. This may be true even in patients with a hiatal hernia, as the hernia sac is lined by the extension of endo-abdominal fascia. Bombeck and associates offer evidence that patients with gastroesophageal reflux have an abnormally low or distal insertion of the phrenoesophageal membrane. This may cause a lack of transmission of abdominal pressures against the distal esophagus and possibly tend to draw the distal esophagus open when tension is placed on the abdominal wall. This theory can explain why some patients with a hiatal hernia have no reflux while others without a hernia do have abnormal reflux. Henderson[11] reports that reflux can be prevented in dogs in which the cardia has been excised if a 6-cm. tube is fashioned from the stomach and left below the diaphragm. If the junction of the tube with the stomach pouch is at the hiatus, free reflux occurs. The concept that control of reflux is at least partially achieved by an intra-abdominal segment of esophagus which is compressed by the greater than atmospheric pressures within the abdomen is widely accepted.

Another factor proposed as contributing to competency of the cardia is the angle of entry of the esophagus into the stomach. Suturing the gastric fundus around the lower esophagus causes the esophagus to enter the stomach at an acute angle, and distention of the stomach compresses the distal esophagus by a flap valve action. While this mechanism can be demonstrated to be effective under experimental conditions and is used in antireflux operations, it probably is not operative in the control of reflux in normal humans. Such a flap valve if normally present would make vomiting difficult or impossible. Evaluation of radiographic appearances of the normal cardia from multiple angles provides no convincing evidence of a flap valve in the normal human. With certain degrees of rotation, the entrance of the esophagus into the stomach can be made to appear as an acute angle, but this angle appears much more obtuse from other radiographic vantage points. The arrangement of mucosal folds at the cardia has been proposed as contributing to the control of reflux,[12] but convincing evidence for this in humans has not been presented.

Finally, the role of esophageal peristalsis in protection against reflux must be considered. A progressive peristaltic wave will quickly empty the esophagus of regurgitated acid material as demonstrated by the acid clearing test. In the normal human being, reflux probably occurs at times in everyone and effective esophageal peristalsis is a back-up mechanism to protect the lining of the esophagus from prolonged contact with transient episodes of regurgitation.

At the present time and based upon incomplete evidence, competency of the cardia in normal human beings should be considered to result from two mechanisms: extrinsic pressure generated against the intra-abdominal segment of esophagus, and an intrinsic specialized muscle function of the distal esophagus. Combined, these result in the high pressure zone, the amplitude of which is related statistically to competency of the cardia. The relative contribution of these two mechanisms is not known, and the role of other factors in preventing reflux cannot be excluded.

Considering the factors thought to control reflux, rational therapy can be given to strengthen these mechanisms. Medical therapy is based upon the use of antacids and postural maneuvers to keep gastric contents away from the cardia. Anticholinergic drugs are avoided so that the innervation of the esophagus remains intact, permitting effective peristalsis and maintenance of tone in the lower esophageal segment. The recent observations indicating that gastrin causes an increase in amplitude of the high pressure zone offers new therapeutic possibilities. In addition, these observations provide a new theoretical basis for the use of antacids to provide an alkaline environment in the stomach, which should cause more intrinsic gastrin production. In spite of intensive medical therapy there are a number of patients whose symptoms from reflux are not successfully controlled. Other patients suffer from reflux esophagitis of such severity as to warrant surgery when initially seen to protect them against stricture development or further bleeding. In such patients, surgical operations should be performed specifically to prevent reflux.

While medical therapy for reflux aims at improving competency of the cardia through posture and maneuvers directed at the intrinsic esophageal muscle, surgery obviously cannot strengthen the responses of the esophageal smooth muscle. The operations which are successful concentrate upon altering the anatomic relationships of the cardia to prevent reflux. As mentioned primarily, operations which simply repair a hiatal hernia such as those described by Sweet, or Harrington, or Allison are often unsuccessful in controlling reflux, although the actual recurrence rate of herniation is acceptably low in some series.[13, 14]

In 1955 Belsey[13] in Bristol, England, and Nissen[15] in Zurich, Switzerland, independently developed procedures specifically designed to prevent reflux by creating an exaggerated intra-abdominal segment of esophagus and an artificial flap valve mechanism by surrounding the distal esophagus with a partial or complete wrap of gastric fundus. In each of these repairs the reconstructed cardia is held in an intra-abdominal location by narrowing the diaphragmatic hiatus around the esophagus so that the bulky reconstruction cannot herniate back into the chest. About the same time, Collis[16] in Birmingham, England, developed an operation to prevent reflux by anchoring the cardia posteriorly to the pre-aortic fascia to hold a segment of distal esophagus within the abdomen. The pillars of the hiatus are approximated anteriorly around the esophageal segment to create a long intradiaphragmatic tunnel of esophagus. In 1962 Hill,[17] of Seattle, began to employ posterior gastropexy in the control of reflux. In this operation the gastroesophageal junction is anchored to the arcuate ligament overlying the aorta to restore a long segment of intra-abdominal esophagus. Subsequently Hill has modified his procedure to imbricate a portion of the gastric fundus around the intra-abdominal segment to "calibrate" the lumen of the cardia. The hiatus is narrowed with sutures posteriorly. These four operations designed specifically to prevent reflux have been evaluated in recent years. Each operation emphasizes rearrangement of the geometric and anatomic relationships of the cardia. Each emphasizes creation of an exaggerated intra-abdominal segment of esophagus, complete dissection of the cardia with division of the phrenoesophageal membrane, application of adjacent stomach or diaphragmatic muscle around the intra-abdominal segment of esophagus to create a compression or flap valve, and narrowing of the hiatus to maintain the position of the repair.

Evaluation of these operations provides clinical evidence of the success of the developers in analyzing the mechanisms controlling reflux. The operative mortality of approximately 1 per cent is similar for each procedure, and a success rate is reported for each in controlling symptomatic reflux and recurrent herniation or reflux by radiographic studies in more than 90 per cent of patients followed variable lengths of time up to eight years after operation.[13-17] In the only published report presenting the results of antireflux operations in patients followed more than 10 years, Orringer, Skinner and Belsey[18] found a recurrence rate of 15 per cent in 272 patients treated by the Belsey operation 10 to 15 years prior to evaluation. Since these results include the earliest cases operated upon and a number of patients with advanced esophagitis or stricture, it is expected that future long-term results will be at least as good or better than this figure.

As pointed out, assessments of symptoms and radiographic studies are not completely satisfactory ways to judge the diagnosis of reflux or its correction. To provide objective assessment of the effects of these operations, esophageal function tests have been applied by several investigators to patients before and after antireflux operations. We have done pH reflux tests in 72 patients treated by such operations. I or my associates performed a Collis repair in eight patients, reconstructed 15 by the Nissen technique, 32 by the Belsey technique, and 17 by the Hill technique. The pH reflux test demonstrated complete control of reflux in five of the Collis operations, but three patients who also received a vagotomy and gastric procedure had persistent abnormal reflux after surgery. All patients treated by the Nissen or Belsey procedures had normal pH reflux tests postoperatively. Thirteen who received the Hill type of operation had normal reflux tests, but four still had abnormal reflux, including two who also had vagotomy and a gastric procedure and two who had the posterior gastropexy only. In one patient of the latter group, repeat study performed six months later showed no reflux and the patient had become asymptomatic. Hill and associates[19] have reported the results of pH reflux tests before and after surgery in 60 patients operated upon by the posterior gastropexy technique and found that mild reflux was detected in 11 patients under the conditions of an acid load; two of these were symptomatic.

Several investigators have studied the effects of antireflux operations upon the lower esophageal high pressure zone. Lind et al.[20] reported a mean increase in the high pressure zone from 22.5 to 33.4 cm. of water following a modified Belsey repair in 16 patients. Moran and associates[24] reported an increase in the high pressure zone from 9.4 to 15.6 mm. Hg following a Nissen or Belsey type of repair. Csendes and Larrain[22] have recently reported pre- and postoperative measurements of the high pressure zone in 29 patients treated by the posterior gastropexy technique of Hill. The mean resting high pressure zone increased from 3.5 to 12.5 mm. Hg. Studies were repeated in some patients 16 months after surgery and demonstrated no decrease in pressure when compared to the results obtained shortly after surgery. Hill et al.[19] have reported a mean difference between the pre- and postoperative high pressure zone levels of 5.3 mm. Hg in 50 patients operated on by the posterior gastropexy technique. In three the pressures remained unchanged, and in seven there appeared to be a slight decrease in sphincter pressure following surgery.

Technically satisfactory pre- and postoperative manometric studies performed with constantly perfused catheters have been obtained in 36 of our own patients. In 20 treated by the Belsey technique, the high pressure zone averaged 4.0 mm. Hg (range 0 to 10) before surgery, and increased to an average of 7.8 mm. Hg (range 4 to 12) after operation. Increased pressures followed 17 of the 20 operations. Among eight patients receiving the Nissen operation, the high pressure zone preoperatively averaged 4.0 mm. Hg (range 0 to 10), and postoperatively averaged 12.3 mm. Hg (range 8 to 18); an increase was seen in each case. In eight patients treated by the Hill operation, preoperative pressures averaged 5.5 mm. Hg (range 0 to 10) and increased to an average of 7.8 mm. Hg (range 6 to 11) after repair. Increased pressure was noted after six of the eight operations. Vagotomy and a gastric procedure were performed concomitantly with five of the Hill operations. Among 11 other patients receiving vagotomy and a gastric procedure without a reconstruction of the cardia, there was no significant change in pressures compared before and after surgery.

These objective esophageal function studies performed before and after surgery demonstrate that gastroesophageal reflux can be prevented by anatomic and geometric rearrangements at the cardia in the vast majority of patients, who, in turn, are relieved of reflux symptoms. The antireflux operations cause a measurable increase in the high pressure zone at the cardia in most patients, and control of reflux is documented by the pH reflux test. Further studies are necessary before conclusive evidence is obtained to indicate which of these four rather similar techniques will be most successful. The technical approaches employed and possible side effects vary among them and must be considered in selecting the best procedure for an individual patient. However, it can be stated unequivocally at this time that surgical reconstruction by an antireflux operation of this type succeeds in increasing competency of the cardia. The mechanisms involved include establishment of an exaggerated intra-abdominal segment of esophagus, creation of an artificial flap valve by application of stomach or diaphragm to the distal esophagus, preservation of vagal nerve function to maintain innervation and function of the lower esophageal muscle segment, closure of the diaphragmatic hiatus to prevent recurrence of the herniation and destruction of the repair, and detachment of the phrenoesophageal membrane so that the new intra-abdominal segment of esophagus can be effectively attached to the diaphragm at a higher level. Recognition of these principles has given a physiologically sound and clinically satisfactory approach to surgical treatment of the patients with incompetency of the cardia.

References

1. Donner, M. W., Silbiger, M. L., Hookman, P., and Hendrix, T. R.: Acid barium swallows in the radiographic evaluation of clinical esophagitis. Radiology 87:220, 1966.
2. Skinner, D. B., and Booth, D, J.: Assessment of distal esophageal function in patients with hiatal hernia and/or gastroesophageal reflux. Ann. Surg. 172:627, 1970.
3. Bernstein, L. M., Fruin, R. C., and Pacini, R.: Differentiation of esophageal pain from angina pectoris: Role of the esophageal acid perfusion test. Medicine (Balt.) 41:143, 1962.
4. Skinner, D. B., Belsey, R. H. R., Hendrix, T. R., and Zuidema, G. D. (eds.): Gastroesophageal Reflux and Hiatal Hernia. Boston, Little, Brown and Company, 1972.
5. Johnson, H. D.: The Cardia and Hiatus Hernia. Springfield, Illinois, Charles C Thomas, 1968.
6. Skinner, D. B., and Camp, T. F., Jr.: Relation of esophageal reflux to lower esophageal sphincter pressures decreased by atropine. Gastroenterology 54:543, 1968.
7. Castell, D. O., and Harris, L. D.: Hormonal control of gastroesophageal sphincter strength. New Eng. J. Med. 282:866, 1970.
8. Cohen, S., and Lipshutz, W.: Hormonal control of lower esophageal sphincter competence: Interaction of gastrin and secretin. Gastroenterology 58:937, 1970.
9. Cohen, S., and Harris, L. D.: Does hiatus hernia affect competence of the gastroesophageal sphincter? New Eng. J. Med. 284:1053, 1971.

9a. Chambers, C. E., Zarins, C. K., Skinner, D. B., and Jones, E. L.: External compression of the cardia related to gastroesophageal reflux. Surg. Forum 23:396, 1972.
10. Bombeck, C. T., Dillard, D. H., and Nyhus, L. M.: Muscular anatomy of the gastroesophageal junction and role of phrenoesophageal ligament. Autopsy study of sphincter mechanism. Ann. Surg. 164:643, 1966.
11. Henderson, R. D.: Gastroesophageal junction in hiatus hernia. Canad. J. Surg. 15:63, 1972.
12. Botha, G. S. M.: *The Gastro-oesophageal Junction*. Boston, Little, Brown and Company, 1962.
13. Skinner, D. B., and Belsey, R. H. R.: Surgical management of esophageal reflux and hiatus hernia: Long-term results with 1,030 patients. J. Thorac. Cardiov. Surg. 53:33, 1967.
14. Urschel, H. C., Jr., and Paulson, D. L.: Gastroesophageal reflux and hiatal hernia. J. Thorac. Cardiov. Surg. 53:21, 1967.
15. Nissen, R.; Gastropexy and "fundoplication" in surgical treatment of hiatal hernia. Amer. J. Dig. Dis. 6:954, 1961.
16. Collis, J. L.: Review of surgical results in hiatus hernia. Thorax 16:114, 1961.
17. Hill, L. D.: An effective operation for hiatal hernia: An eight-year appraisal. Ann. Surg. 166:681, 1967.
18. Orringer, M. B., Skinner, D. B., and Belsey, R. H. R.: Long-term results of the Mark IV operation for hiatal hernia and analyses of recurrences and their treatment. J. Thorac. Cardiov. Surg. 63:25, 1972.
19. Hill, L. D.: Surgery and gastroesophageal reflux. Gastroenterology 63:183–185, 1972.
20. Lind, J. F., Burns, C. M., and MacDougall, J. T.: Physiological repair for hiatus hernia-manometric study. Arch. Surg. 91:233, 1965.
21. Moran, J. M., Pihl, C. O., Norton, R. A., and Rheinlander, H. F.: The hiatal hernia-reflux complex. Amer. J. Surg. 121:403, 1971.
22. Csendes, A., and Larrain, A.: The effect of posterior gastropexy on gastroesophageal sphincter pressure and symptomatic reflux in patients with hiatal hernia. Gastroenterology 63:19–24, 1972.

The Importance of the Sphincter at the Gastroesophageal Junction

LAURAN D. HARRIS

Boston University School of Medicine

Why, after all these years of study, are we still wondering what prevents gastroesophageal reflux? Surely we should be able to measure the relative contributions of the various factors theoretically capable of contributing to gastroesophageal competence and be done with it! To me, the key word in the previous sentence is the word *measure*. Without measurement, theories tend to flourish. Since gastroesophageal competence could not be measured, mechanisms of varying ingenuity explaining it have been postulated, attacked, and defended.

In 1969, however, a method for quantitating gastroesophageal competence was published.[1] The investigators defined gastroesophageal competence quite simply: the ability to keep gastric contents from entering the esophagus. Therefore, they measured the force (in grams) required to pull a 12-mm. Teflon sphere from the stomach into the esophagus. The result was a quantitative measurement of gastroesophageal competence, or the combined strength of the various factors theoretically capable of contributing to gastroesophageal competence. While this measurement was fairly straightforward, it was tedious and somewhat cumbersome. Therefore, this measurement of the strength of gastroesophageal competence was compared to intraluminal pressures measured at the gastroesophageal junction. An excellent correlation over a wide range was found when these two values were obtained essentially simultaneously. The correlation was equally good (and had the same slope and intercept) in patients who had a hiatus hernia and those who did not. Thus, an easily obtainable value—intraluminal pressure measured at the gastroesophageal junction—was shown to be a reliable quantitative index of the combined strength of all mechanisms responsible for gastroesophageal competence. However, only intraluminal pressures obtained by a system employing a continuous perfusion of the recording catheters were capable of providing this information; no correlation or only very poor and erratic correlation was found if other methods of measuring pressure in common use at that time were used.

Once this foundation had been laid, it became possible to measure the relative contributions of the various mechanisms postulated to be responsible for gastroesophageal competence. These mechanisms may be divided into two broad groups: (1) the lower esophageal sphincter (LES), and (2) extra-LES mechanisms. The latter group contains postulates ranging from the importance of compression of the terminal esophagus by surrounding structures or by positive intra-abdominal pressure to the importance of various angles and flap valves. Measuring the relative contribution of these broad groups is relatively easy; only group (1) (the LES) is operative in patients having the common axial or sliding hiatus hernia, while both group (1) and group (2) are operative in individuals without a hiatus hernia. Therefore, simply comparing strength of gastroesophageal competence in individuals with a hiatus hernia to that of individuals without a hiatus hernia will document the relative contribution of LES and extra-LES mechanisms. The results of such a study were absolutely clear-cut: there was no difference at all in the strength of gastroesophageal competence in individuals with and without a hiatus hernia.[2] This was true both for individuals having normal and for those having clinically weak or incompetent mechanisms. This study, of course, strongly suggested that the LES was solely responsible for gastroesophageal competence.

Other studies have approached the problem from slightly different angles. It has long been known that intraluminal pressures measured at the gastroesophageal junctional zone varied as intra-abdominal pressure varied.[3] The change in intraluminal pressure was simultaneous with and approximately equal to the change in intra-abdominal pressure, so change in intraluminal pressure was attributed to passive squeeze upon an intra-abdominal segment of esophagus. Since intraluminal pressure in the gastroesophageal junctional zone is a measure of the strength of gastroesophageal competence, any increase in intraluminal pressure contributed by an increase in surrounding intra-abdominal pressure would clearly represent a contribution by a group (2) (mechanical) mechanism. The first of a series of studies examining this effect in detail was published in 1966 by Lind and co-workers.[4] They found that change in intraluminal pressure measured in the gastroesophageal junctional zone was *not* just equal to change in intra-abdominal pressure, but rather exceeded it by some 60 per cent! For example, a mean increase in intra-abdominal pressure of 12.8 cm. H_2O was accomplished by a mean increase in intraluminal pressure measured from within the gastroesophageal junctional zone of 19.2 cm. H_2O. Even harder to reconcile with passive squeeze was the fact that the same thing was found in patients with a hiatus hernia, despite the fact that intrathoracic pressure surrounding the gastroesophageal junctional zone did not change!

Subsequent studies in hiatus hernia patients reported that the LES response to a given increase in intra-abdominal pressure was the same whether intrathoracic pressure surrounding the gastroesophageal junctional zone increased (as in a Valsalva maneuver), decreased (as in a Müller maneuver), or did not change (lifting the legs from the horizontal position while supine).[2] These studies concluded that the increase in LES pressure which accompanied an increase in intra-abdominal pressure was: (1) a property of the LES itself, (2) a real increase in the strength of gastroesophageal competence, and (3) not affected by changes in pressure surrounding the LES. Still further studies of this phenomenon not only completely eliminated any mechanical effects but also added a new dimension to our understanding of the mechanism of LES function.[5] The LES response to a given increase in intra-abdominal pressure was found to be linearly related to the initial or basal LES pressure. For example, the LES response to a standard increase in intra-abdominal pressure of 20 mm. Hg was about 10 mm. Hg (1:2) if initial LES pressure was 5 mm. Hg, about 40 mm. Hg (2:1) if initial LES pressure was 20 mm. Hg, and about 60 mm. Hg (3:1) if initial LES pressure was 30 mm. Hg. An initial LES pressure of about 10 mm. Hg was found to be the critical point in determining LES response; i.e., if initial LES pressure was below about 10 mm. Hg, the LES response to a change in intra-abdominal pressure was less than 1:1, but if initial LES pressure was greater than 10 mm. Hg the LES response to a given change in intra-abdominal pressure became progressively greater.

This ability of the LES to become stronger in response to an increase in intra-abdominal pressure is clearly an important mechanism for preventing gastroesophageal reflux. The fact that most patients with clinical evidence of gastroesophageal incompetence have initial LES pressures less than 10 mm. Hg (the level at which a 1:1 response is found) seems to emphasize this importance. How is the LES response to an increase in intra-abdominal pressure accomplished? Lind and his co-workers have suggested a reflex arc mediated by the vagus,[6,7] but they have not published the definitive studies necessary to prove that such a reflex arc exists. The presence of such a reflex arc, however, seems quite logical and fits the known facts.

None of the above studies produced even a shred of evidence suggesting that extra-LES or mechanical factors play any role at all in the maintenance of gastroesophageal competence. Rather, these studies showed that a highly sophisticated mechanism (possibly a vagally mediated reflex arc) exists which is capable of increasing the strength of the LES at the times that this increased strength is needed. The degree of this LES response is, in turn, modulated by basal LES strength! Obviously this is well beyond the capability of any of the crude mechanical systems which have been suggested. But there is still more. In 1969 studies were published which indicated that basal LES strength is profoundly affected (perhaps controlled) by the antral hormone gastrin.[8,9] Since then the picture has expanded remarkably so that other hormones (secretin, cholecystokinin-pancreozymin, glucagon, insulin) must now be added to the list of endogenously secreted agents capable of altering the strength of gastroesophageal competence.[10-14]

Thus, the mechanism for preventing gastroesophageal reflux is far more sophisticated and complex than we had suspected. Now that we are at least beginning to understand some of these mechanisms, the likelihood that we can learn to control gastroesophageal reflux pharmacologically seems considerably improved. We can now, for example, convert a perfectly normal LES to an incompetent one simply by putting 0.1 N HCl into the stomach (turning off endogenous gastrin production) or into the duodenum (turning on endogenous secretin production). We can then return this incompetent LES to normal by neutralizing gastric or duodenal contents. Incidentally, these swings from normal LES to incompetent LES and back to normal occur very rapidly, within a minute or so.

We can also, at least temporarily, convert the incompetent LES of a patient having severe clinical gastroesophageal reflux to normal or near-normal by alkalinizing the stomach (turning on endogenous gastrin production). At the risk of redundancy, I should perhaps mention that these effects are the same whether or not the patient has a hiatus hernia. Of course, alkalis have long been a mainstay of our medical mangement of gastroesophageal reflux. It is rather comforting to know, however, that we have not been just neutralizing refluxed material, but have actually been restoring the LES to normal or near-normal and preventing reflux! It is obviously impractical to keep the stomach continuously alkaline. However, I have no doubt that more physiologic—and more effective—medical management will be available in the near future.

Should mechanical factors still be considered at all seriously? Certainly those who stress the importance of mechanics will have trouble accepting the hormone effects just mentioned. The mechanically minded, however, do ask one question which I as a sphincter man have a bit of trouble with, "If mechanical factors are so unimportant, how do you explain the fact that patients with clinical gastroesophageal reflux and a hiatus hernia are improved after their hiatus is surgically repaired?" I have no serious doubt that some patients are clinically improved, or even that some apparently have an increase in LES strength.[15-17] (Just how many, I'm not really sure. It seems to me that a prospective study of patients randomly assigned to medical and surgical therapies is long overdue.) Frankly, I can't explain how surgery could possibly help anyone with LES incompetence. It has been shown that location of the LES above or below the diaphragm does not affect its strength. It has also been shown that neither the competent nor the incompetent LES is affected by surrounding pressure. Presence or absence of an acute angle of entry of esophagus into stomach has been shown to have no effect on LES strength. Yet these are "abnormalities" various surgical procedures have been designed to correct! Therefore, I have a few questions of my own: (1) How do you explain the apparent fact that some patients with clinical gastroesophageal reflux and a hiatus hernia seem to be improved after their hiatus hernia is surgically repaired? (2) What about patients with clinical gastroesophageal reflux who do *not* have a hiatus hernia? (3) What is the *minimal* surgical procedure necessary? (4) Does surgery affect basal endogenous gastrin or secretin or cholecystokinin-pancreozymin production? (5) Incidentally, just how good *is* surgery for gastroesophageal reflux?

To me, evidence is overwhelming that the LES is primarily—completely, in fact—responsible for gastroesophageal competence. Why have the various mechanical theories of gastroesophageal competence persisted for so long? One reason, perhaps, is that much of the evidence favoring the LES was published only recently, whereas the mechanical theories have been around for a long time and appear in most standard textbooks on the subject. In short, we have had time to become comfortable with the mechanical theories. Another reason, I suspect, has to do with hiatus hernia and its treatment. I cannot escape the impression that many consider surgery for hiatus hernia and the mechanical theories of gastroesophageal competence to be mutually dependent and therefore to be defended at all costs. Yet it seems to me that if hiatus hernia surgery works, it works whether or not the mechanical theories are correct. I also suspect that the energy expended defending an outmoded concept would be more than enough to devise a more effective treatment for gastroesophageal reflux.

References

1. Cohen, S., and Harris, L. D.: Lower esophageal sphincter pressure as an index of lower esophageal sphincter strength. Gastroenterology 58:157–162, 1970.
2. Cohen, S., and Harris, L. D.: Does hiatus hernia affect competence of the gastroesophageal sphincter? New Eng. J. Med. 284:1053–1056, 1971.
3. Fyke, F. E., Jr., Code, C. F., and Schlegel, J. F.: The gastroesophageal sphincter in healthy human beings. Gastroenterologia 86:135–150, 1956.
4. Lind, J. F., Warrian, W. G., and Wankling, W. J.: Responses of the gastroesophageal junctional zone to increases in abdominal pressure. Canad. J. Surg. 9:32–38, 1966.
5. Cohen, S., and Harris, L. D.: The adaptive response of the lower esophageal sphincter. (Abstract.) Clin. Res. 17:300, 1969.
6. Lind, J. F., Cotton, D. J., Blanchard, R., et al.: Effect of thoracic displacement and vagotomy on the canine gastroesophageal junctional zone. Gastroenterology 56:1078–1085, 1969.
7. Crispin, J. S., McIver, D. K., and Lind, J. F.: Manometric study of the effect of vagotomy on the gastroesophageal sphincter. Canad. J. Surg. 10:299–303, 1967.
8. Castell, D. O., and Harris, L. D.: The link between control of gastric acid secretion and control of lower esophageal sphincter strength. (Abstract.) Gastroenterology 56:1249, 1969.
9. Giles, G. R., Morson, M. C., Humphries, C., et al.: Action of gastrin on the lower esophageal sphincter in man. Gut 10:730–734, 1969.
10. Castell, D. O., and Harris, L. D.: Hormonal control of gastroesophageal sphincter strength. New Eng. J. Med. 282:886–889, 1970.
11. Cohen, S., and Lipshutz, W.: Hormonal regulation of human lower esophageal sphincter competence: The interaction of gastrin and secretin. J. Clin. Invest. 50:449–454, 1971.
12. Nebel, O., and Castell, D. O.: Lower esophageal sphincter pressure changes after food ingestion. (Abstract.) Gastroenterology 60:701, 1971.
13. Lipshutz, W., Hughes, W., and Cohen, S.: The genesis of lower esophageal sphincter pressure: Its identification through the use of gastrin antiserum. J. Clin. Invest. 51:522–529, 1972.
14. Cohen, S., and Harris, L. D.: The lower esophageal sphincter. Gastroenterology 63:1066–1073, 1972.
15. Lind, J. F., Burns, C. M., and MacDougall, J. T.: Physiologic repair for hiatus hernia—manometric study. Arch. Surg. 91:233–237, 1965.
16. Moran, J. M., Pihl, C. O., Norton, R. A., et al.: The hiatal hernia-reflux complex. Amer. J. Surg. 121:403–411, 1971.
17. Csendes, A., and Larrain, A.: Effect of posterior gastropexy on gastroesophageal sphincter pressure and symptomatic reflux in patients with hiatal hernia. Gastroenterology 63:19–24, 1972.

Comment

Mechanisms That Prevent Gastroesophageal Reflux

Each having unloaded a veritable battery of procedures to define that elusive gate mechanism at the gastroesophageal junction, Doctors Harris and Skinner appear to progress from puzzle to puzzle rather than from puzzle to solution. Harris frankly asks: If the lower esophageal sphincter is so all-important in preventing gastroesophageal reflux, why do the various manipulations described by Skinner appear reasonably successful in alleviating reflux esophagitis? Skinner argues that these manipulations, among other effects, raise intrasphincteric pressure to a moderate degree. Thus, unless the lower esophageal sphincter is an entirely mythical entity and merely reflects a concatenation of extra-esophageal pressures, Skinner must ask why the intrinsic muscle of the distal esophagus should perform better just because this segment and its adjoining gastroesophageal junction are reshaped, replaced, and battened down.

The point has often been made that new tests of esophageal function and malfunction proliferate like rabbits before those already available have been adequately validated and used. In addition, sound, well controlled studies on the effectiveness of the various types of hernia repair are extremely rare—in spite of volumes in praise of this or that technique or, more usually, modifications of this or that technique. The internist must, when the effects of a potentially useful drug are not self-evident, use properly controlled studies to determine the value of the agent. The surgical fraternity should do the same. And "properly controlled" means study groups defined by a standardized set of clinical and investigative criteria, randomization into treatment and control groups, a consistently performed operative procedure, and precisely defined follow-up studies, preferably carried out by some disinterested party. Perhaps all these requirements are impractical and they are asking for too much. But until such laborious evaluations have been performed it is unlikely that confident therapeutic advice can be given to the patient whose gastroesophageal reflux is so excessive as to give him trouble.

FRANZ J. INGELFINGER

21

Management of Gallstones, Particularly the Silent Variety

THE ADVANTAGES OF AN AGGRESSIVE SURGICAL APPROACH
   by Frank Glenn

ADVANTAGES OF A VARIED AND INDIVIDUALIZED APPROACH
   by Donald M. Small

COMMENT
   by Franz J. Ingelfinger

The Advantages of an Aggressive Surgical Approach

FRANK GLENN

Cornell University Medical College

Going back to the days when man first began to keep medical records, there is ample evidence that gallstones and biliary tract disease have long been recognized. Through the centuries correlation between the pathological changes that were present and the accompanying symptoms and disability has seldom been agreed upon. The authorities on divination, the soothsayers, and those given to prophesy were almost always at variance. Now thousands of years later and despite millions of words describing almost every imaginable facet of calculous biliary tract disease, there still persist areas of controversy. The "silent," asymptomatic gallstone is an example. Until a little more than a century ago biliary calculi found at autopsy without known symptoms that had been attributed to them were of little concern. Then with the development of surgery that moved rapidly after the introduction of ether anesthesia (1860) and somewhat later roentgenography with cholecystography, the silent calculi became of importance to pathologists, internists, and surgeons. Calculi were then suspect as not forever remaining silent. First pathologists and then surgeons observed that instead of being harmless they were occasionally the cause of death.

In this presentation I shall attempt to relate in sequence and without detail those innovations that resulted in surgery's becoming widely accepted for the treatment of biliary tract disease. These have evolved as anesthesia, roentgenography, chemotherapy, and antimicrobial agents have been developed as essentials in the surgeon's armamentarium. Operative procedures are adapted to the presenting situation. These are accomplished with less and less risk and indeed with minimal discomfort; the results are excellent. During this period the silent gallstone has come into increasing prominence. By 1945 there was general agreement among members of the medical profession that there was a greater incidence of silent gallstones than had been previously estimated. Furthermore, reports that many led to serious sequelae became common. Thus, the attitude that they were harmless or almost so was replaced by a realization that they caused acute cholecystitis and contributed to an extension of disease throughout the biliary tract with impairment of function and development of cirrhosis. If present for a long time there was often choledocholithiasis. The high correlation of cholelithiasis with carcinoma of the gallbladder was observed to be in the same proportion for both calculi with symptoms and those without. As the reader proceeds it will be obvious that the objective of this paper is to remove from the silent calculi the cloak of innocence and to reveal them as they really are—potential hazards to the well-being, health, and life span of their possessors.

It is readily understandable that in the era 1860 to 1880 asymptomatic gallstones were scarcely a problem because their presence was seldom known before operation or autopsy. Even then they were but an interesting but not unusual finding at postmortem examinations. Occasionally a patient was described who had died from a bile peritonitis secondary to perforation of an acute cholecystitis with calculi in the gallbladder. The role of the calculi in causing an obstructive acute cholecystitis seems to have escaped attention. With the advent of cholecystography, described by Graham and Cole,[1] and by Copher in 1928,[2] calculous biliary tract disease suddenly became a much more frequent diagnosis than previously. Roentgenography permitted a clear differential diagnosis between duodenal ulcer and cholelithiasis and demonstrated that they often occurred together. The entire field of surgery was then extending rapidly, and treatment of biliary tract disease was pursued with new vigor. With the increase in operations such as cholecystectomy and common duct exploration the relief of symptoms was gratifying. There was also evidence of interruption of the disease.

With this experience new concepts were set forth, and the indications for surgery were liberalized. Some even advocated operation during the first attack of acute cholecystitis in young women. Dr. Evarts Graham[3] contended that calculi in the gallbladder, regardless of symptoms or disability, was an indication for cholecystectomy. He believed that the risk for cholecystectomy was less than that of carcinoma developing in the gallbladder containing calculi. This attitude of a few in 1930 was in marked contrast to that of the preceding half century. Its evolution was gradual and its acceptance by the medical profession is still incomplete. A review of this development contributes to a better understanding of the factors involved in trends that have taken place.

Development of Surgical Treatment of Biliary Tract Disease

The reluctance to recommend surgery is well illustrated by Osler in his famous textbook.[4] In 1902 he wrote: "In the majority of the cases, gall-stones cause no symptoms. The gall-bladder will tolerate the presence of large numbers for an indefinite period of time, and post-mortem examinations show that they are present in 25 per cent of all women over sixty years of age." In the same text he stated that surgical treatment of the gallbladder was indicated under certain specific conditions: "(a) Repeated attacks of gall-stone colic . . . (b) The presence of a distended gall-bladder, associated with attacks of pain or with fever . . . (c) When a gall-stone is permanently lodged in the common duct."

By 1930 the demonstration of asymptomatic gallstones by cholecystography had become commonplace and the question of what should be done with them became a matter of controversy. Mason and Blackford[5] in 1932 cautioned against considering the demonstration of gallstones an indication for operation. However, one year later in an article published in the J.A.M.A. there is evidence of a marked change in Blackford's opinion. He states: "The patient with uncomplicated cholecystitis should be given a trial on medical treatment. If not markedly relieved promptly he should be operated on. In 1934 Musser[6] recommended that attacks of "biliary colic without evidence of infection" not be treated surgically. A slight departure from a completely nonsurgical attitude was voiced by Fitz[7] in 1942 when he wrote: "It is not harmful to follow patients with 'silent stones' for a time before advising surgery." This shift of attitude was not widely accepted by internists, as is evident from Christian's[8] statement:

"The decision for or against surgical treatment should be made in the course of repeated attacks, the single attack requires operation only in the unusual case of steadily increasing severity and evidence of severe infection. There are many patients in whom the symptoms are slight and for these surgical treatment is not indicated. . . . It is rare that cholecystectomy is advisable for the first attack, even though it is severe and typical. The present author has long followed the policy just stated: in his patients it has led to no serious consequences that would have been avoided by early cholecystectomy."

In 1945 H. E. Robertson[9] published his classic paper "Silent Gallstones." He concluded that the demonstration of silent gallstones in the living, and the disability and curtailment of life that had been observed to occur some time later in many patients with silent gallstones should alter the viewpoint of both internists and surgeons.

The decades since the turn of the century have brought about many changes that have contributed to the trend to treat all calculous biliary tract disease surgically. First of all, average life expectancy has increased from <50 to >70 years. Acute cholecystitis in those over 65 is recognized as a more serious problem than in those who are younger and more robust. Diagnoses are more accurate and unrelated conditions are recognized as important in preoperative evaluation and preparation. Better anesthesia and an understanding of water and electrolyte requirements have reduced the risk of surgery to an all time low. Thus, surgery is daily accomplished with less risk and less discomfort to patients; it is therefore more acceptable.

Reports on Studies of Incidence and Follow-up of Asymptomatic Gallstones

The actual prevalence of asymptomatic cholelithiasis is not known and not readily estimated. However, a report from the Copenhagen County Hospital in Denmark by Lund[10] in 1960 of a group of 526 patients with cholelithiasis may be indicative of their frequency. The patients were observed from five to 20 years (1936 to 1950), during which period 25 per cent died; only 14, or 10 per cent, of the deaths were ascribed to biliary tract disease. Between 35 and 50 per cent developed increased and severe symptoms or complications requiring surgery. An estimated 25 to 40 per cent remained relatively free of symptoms. For 100 of the 526 patients the gallstones were a chance finding on x-ray examination. The clinical course of patients following the diagnosis was similar regardless of whether or not previous symptoms had led to the diagnosis.

Truesdale[11] collected a group of 50 female patients in whom he discovered the gallbladder calculi during operation for a pelvic condition. Thirty-six of these patients with minimal or no symptoms were followed for 10 years. Of the 36, 12 underwent cholecystectomy because of symptoms, 12 were lost to follow-up, and 12 were closely observed; six of these developed symptoms that were considered by the patient to be tolerable and six remained symptom-free. Thus, six of the 24, or only one out of four remained undisturbed by the calculi. This is indeed a convincing bit of evidence that calculi are hazardous possessions.

Another report of significance was that of Comfort, Gray and Wilson[12] of the Mayo Clinic on 112 patients with an average age of 48.2 years when calculi were first diagnosed. Over a period of 14 to 23 years, 51 of the 112 (45.5 per cent) developed symptoms ascribed to the biliary tract. Of the 51, 24 (49 per cent) were treated by cholecystectomy. Karl A. Meyer[13] of Chicago in 1967 reported that of 1261 patients cared for by him and his associates over a six-year period 6 per cent were asymptomatic.

It is to be anticipated that in the not too distant future most of the people of the United States by the time they reach 50 will have had a cholecystogram. Medical records on these individuals should provide an increasing amount of data that will provide a firm statistical basis for prognosis. In the meantime, surgeons who see the complications of biliary tract disease among the elderly feel strongly that prophylactic cholecystectomy for silent stones is indicated, with the provisions mentioned previously. Many members of the medical profession remain little concerned about these untoward complications because they believe they seldom occur. Some emphasize that they are opposed to preventative surgery and cite instances of "well people" with a quiescent disease who have had catastrophic results of iatrogenic nature. Creditable case series of patients carefully evaluated and carefully prepared for elective cholecystectomy have been reported with a mortality rate of 0 to 0.3 per cent. Increasing reports of clinical experiences with an ever-diminishing risk strongly indicate that the best interests of the patient with silent gallstones are attained by cholecystectomy unless there is some contraindication. The proportional incidence of the serious complications of calculous biliary tract disease increases decade by decade after 50. The classic examples are acute obstructive cholecystitis, common duct obstruction, acute suppurative cholangitis, and carcinoma of the gallbladder. The morbidity of complications and the mortality rate following surgery for each of these is greater in the aged than among those who are younger. There is general agreement among surgeons that the greater proportion of these patients have had calculi for many years before any symptoms appeared. Sometimes their first manifestations were one of the four "serious" complications.

The experience with acute cholecystitis at The New York Hospital–Cornell Medical Center is pertinent (Table 1). It makes little difference whether or not the calculi in obstructive acute cholecystitis have been silent prior to the onset of

Table 1. *Acute Cholecystitis at The New York Hospital–Cornell Medical Center from September 1, 1932, to September 1, 1967*
1241(29)* patients

OPERATION AGE AND SEX	STONES NO. CASES	STONES DEATHS	NO STONES NO. CASES	NO STONES DEATHS	TOTAL NO. CASES	TOTAL DEATHS
Cholecystectomy						
Female						
Over 50 years	309	9	5	—	314	9
Under 50 years	381	1	11	—	392	1
Male						
Over 50 years	179	3	13	—	192	3
Under 50 years	146	1	14	1	160	2
	1015	14	43	1	1058	15
Cholecystostomy						
Female						
Over 50 years	66	4	12	3	78	7
Under 50 years	28	1	6	—	34	1
Male						
Over 50 years	48	5	14	—	62	5
Under 50 years	6	—	3	1	9	1
	148	10	35	4	183	14

* Number in parentheses indicates deaths.

this complication. The mortality as well as the morbidity of complications is greatest among those 50 years of age and older. From September 1, 1932, to September 1, 1967, there were a total of 1163 patients who underwent cholecystectomy or cholecystostomy for cholecystitis with cholelithiasis. Of the 602 patients 50 years of age and older there were 21 postoperative deaths, a mortality rate of 3.6 per cent, and among 561 patients under 50 years of age there were only three deaths, with a mortality rate of 0.5 per cent.

Acute Cholecystitis

The mortality rate of calculous biliary tract disease is concentrated largely among the elderly, those 65 and older. The specific conditions that account for these deaths are the complications of longstanding disease that has in many instances been well tolerated. Calculi in a gallbladder with sufficient changes in its wall to only slightly impair its physiological function may cause no symptoms over a period of years. The longer this situation exists the greater is the probability that an obstructive acute cholecystitis may occur. Age, debility, and longstanding biliary tract disease are conducive to the complications of acute cholecystitis, namely perforation and local and/or general peritonitis; these are common causes of resulting death. There are other sequelae in the patient with acute cholecystitis, such as cholecysto-enteric fistula, that occasionally result in intestinal obstruction caused by calculi (gallstone ileus). Another sequela of gallbladder calculi is that of choledocholithiasis. While this may result in an obstructive jaundice in the robust period of life with a relatively low morbidity of complications and a minimal operative mortality, it is a much more serious problem in the elderly.

Choledocholithiasis

Common duct calculi appear to be an ordinary sequela or complication of cholelithiasis. Calculi in the common duct are only occasionally found in patients with an acalculous gallbladder. The incidence is low in early life, gradually increases up to age 50, and then increases markedly each decade thereafter. An overall survey places the prevalence of choledocholithiasis at from 6 to 10 per cent of all patients operated upon for calculous biliary tract disease. For those over 75 the frequency is almost 50 per cent.

Whereas the demonstration of calculi in the gallbladder by cholecystography leaves no doubt as to their presence, Woolman and his associates[14] have called attention to the matter of nonvisualization of the gallbladder. In a series of 500 consecutive nonjaundiced patients subjected to cholecystectomy who had had cholecystograms attempted, they found the following: among 361 patients who had well visualized gallbladders, 12 patients, or 3 per cent, had common duct calculi, and among 139 patients with nonvisualization of the gallbladder, there were 15 patients, or 11 per cent, who had common duct calculi.

Elderly patients undergoing complete evaluation and without symptoms not infrequently have nonvisualization of the gallbladder on attempted oral cholecystography. Such a situation is an indication for intravenous cholangiography because of the likelihood of choledocholithiasis as well as cholelithiasis. A nonvisualized gallbladder almost always contains calculi and has a greater than 10 per cent chance of being accompanied by common duct calculi. Operation, cholecystectomy combined with operative cholangiography, is recommended unless there is some contraindication.

A complication of choledocholithiasis is acute obstructive suppurative cholangitis. It is associated with an operative mortality rate of 50 per cent. The onset is often sudden and so rapidly progressive that diagnosis is established only at autopsy. The history usually obtained on this group of patients reveals that many had no symptoms previously, or they had been forgotten.

Carcinoma of the Gallbladder

As a medical student clinical clerk I listened to Dr. Evarts Graham's contention that carcinoma of the gallbladder was almost always associated with cholelithiasis. It made no difference whether or not gallstones caused symptoms;

cholecystectomy was indicated and could be accomplished with less risk than that of developing carcinoma of the gallbladder. Many surgeons including myself have come to support this contention. However, a greater proportion of the medical profession give it little consideration and rarely discuss it with patients. A case can be made for its being a well justified indication by viewing the matter of calculous disease in perspective. It is very prevalent and causes much disability and contributes to reducing the life span. The total number of patients operated upon for biliary tract disease (90 to 95 per cent calculous) was estimated at 300,000 to 400,000 for 1971.[15] Another estimate believed to be reasonable is that 15 to 20 per cent of the adult population have or have had gallstones. Those who have interested themselves in study of cancer of the gallbladder are in general agreement that a fraction of 1 per cent of calculous gallbladders which have been removed also contain a malignant tumor. This varies with age, ranging up to 1.42 per cent frequency among the elderly according to the experience of Rhoads[16] at the University of Pennsylvania. Calculi are reported to be present in upwards of 90 per cent of patients with carcinoma of the gallbladder.

The prognosis in carcinoma of the gallbladder is very poor. Regardless of treatment accorded it, the life expectancy on an average is less than two years. Using the estimated figures of the American Cancer Society that 10,100 deaths in the United States during 1971 were due to cancer of the liver and biliary passages, one may conclude that 4000 to 5000 of these deaths were due to cancer of the gallbladder.[17] If 90 per cent of these occur in gallbladders with calculi, then cholecystectomy for cholelithiasis should reduce this number. In some case reviews it has been emphasized that a fair percentage of patients, up to 15 per cent, gave no history suggesting biliary tract disease until the onset of their terminal illness, which turned out to be carcinoma of the gallbladder with calculi. This varies among different segments of the population and in some is believed to be much greater. The prevalence of carcinoma of the gallbladder, usually associated with stress, is much higher among American Indians and Alaskan Indians than it is for the United States as a whole.

Coronary Heart Disease

Another situation in which gallstones may be silent occurs in individuals with coronary insufficiency. Anginal pains with electrocardiographic changes comparable with coronary heart disease have led to the patient's being treated for "heart disease." Stewart[18] and Patterson[19] have emphasized that pain due to biliary tract disease may be perceived by the patient as located in the precordial area and associated with a deep constrictive feeling within the chest. Conversely, pain of a severe nature in the right upper quadrant together with spasm of the right rectus muscle upon abdominal palpation has been demonstrated to be the result of myocardial ischemia due to coronary occlusion, without evidence of biliary tract disease.

Referred pain from the biliary tract can well be the result of impulses transmitted along the fifth to eleventh thoracic spinal segments, and that from the heart, somewhat higher, from the fifth thoracic to the fifth cervical spinal segments.

Because patients in the age group of 50 years and older often have disease of both the biliary tract and the heart, recognition of this overlap innervation becomes significant in differential diagnoses.[20] The patient and his physician are convinced that the symptoms are cardiac in origin. Episodes of pain are observed to be associated with changes in the electrocardiogram, further favoring the decision that the basic problem is in the heart. A number of patients have been reported who were relieved of their symptoms by cholecystectomy. Perhaps an equal or greater number have been operated upon without change. It should be stressed that the diagnosis of coronary heart disease is not a contraindication to cholecystectomy. Colcock and Perey[21] from the Lahey Clinic published a review of 1756 patients treated surgically for biliary tract disease between 1954 and 1958. Of this group of patients 9.5 per cent were without symptoms referable to the biliary tract. In this study in discussing the treatment to be accorded patients with gallstones who, in addition, have coronary heart disease, their policy is summed up as follows: "We advise any patient with cholelithiasis who has not had a recent coronary occlusion or who does not have severe angina on effort to have a cholecystectomy regardless of symptoms." Our experience at The New York Hospital–Cornell Medical Center over the past 20 years has rested on such a policy; it has been most satisfactory.

Factual Information for Patients with Asymptomatic Gallstones

A rather long (40 years) clinical experience with those having various diseases of the biliary tract leads me to urge that each patient be informed of the facts and the reasoning relative to his or her problem. How shall this be presented so that the patient may understand the basis for the advice given and also make his own decision without duress? For the surgeon who has been consulted it is important that the referring physician understand the objective and the risks involved together with the precautions to be taken in maintaining these at a minimum. There is some risk in all surgical procedures, and nothing can be more tragic for the individual patient than to sustain a fatal complication for a condition that has not caused symptoms. Thus, the patient, his internist, and his surgeon quite properly should discuss fully the proposed operation and its benefits and risks. In particular, any contraindications to operation require evaluation both as to the proposed procedure and their role should a complication of calculous biliary tract disease develop and render emergency operation mandatory. Details of these complications may not be appropriate in discussion with patients, but that there are several that may occur and be serious should be pointed out.

It is the surgeon's responsibility to present as clear and concise a picture of the patient's problem as he can. Emphasis should be placed upon the patient's reaching his own decision based upon the information provided by his medical advisors. They should not be adamant in their advice; they cannot know when and what sequelae may develop. However, they have the factual data that have been reported over the past several decades; thus, they know what may happen. The surgeon, with the facilities of a modern hospital available together with the attention to detail that he can provide, should be able to remove the gallbladder containing calculi with safety and minimal discomfort to the patient. Elective cholecystectomy for nonacute cholecystitis and cholelithiasis has been accomplished in the United States over the past two decades at an estimated mortality of less than 0.3 per cent. During this same period there have been several reports of a hundred or more patients undergoing cholecystectomy without a fatality.

Discussion

Underneath the factual data relative to silent gallstones that have been presented is my experience with patients in various stages of biliary tract disease. Included are those who had been advised to have a cholecystectomy for cholelithiasis or a choledochotomy for choledocholithiasis because of symptoms or disability and who have decided to await an increase in these manifestations. Many of them have been lost to my observation, some have remained well, and others have sustained such progress of their disease that operation became mandatory. As patients grow older various degrees of debility develop so that they tolerate operation less well. As the biliary tract disease causes increasing disability and symptoms, other systems sometimes may become impaired for one reason or another not always ascribable to age. The cardiovascular system is most often involved and, indeed, in some instances may be linked to calculous biliary tract disease.

It is among this group that are concentrated the majority of deaths and postoperative complications. In my opinion, most of these could have been prevented by operation years before. These patients are disturbing to the clinician whenever they are encountered. However, even more distressing to me have been those who were previously advised to have operation and later presented with an acute cholecystitis, perforation, or carcinoma of the gallbladder with metastases to the liver. It is then in retrospect that one regrets not having been more convincing in his counseling. One vivid example of this remains in my mind: A 34 year old mother of four children, who was demonstrated to have cholelithiasis by cholecystogram, soon thereafter began to have symptoms, which she tolerated for 21 years. Operation was precipitated by an attack of acute obstructive cholecystitis. The gallbladder when removed contained a small carcinoma, but there was no evidence of metastases. However, she died within a year of operation from diffuse spread of tumor.

As a surgeon long present in a community grows older he is more frequently requested by his colleagues to see patients in consultation who have a poor prognosis, either because of their disease or a complication of it. Not infrequently the situation is irretrievable. Those who requested the consultation are well aware that in all probability nothing will be contributed to either alleviation of symptoms or prolongation of life. Nevertheless, in the tradition of Oslerian consultation, all facets of the case are reviewed and anything that might be done is discussed. It is after such a consultation that retrospection sets in and the consultant asks himself the question: When in the patient's past could his terminal illness have been prevented? In calculous biliary tract disease the answer seems obvious. A cholecystectomy within a reasonable time after the gallstones were first demonstrated could have been done with little risk.

The matter of health has been and I trust will continue to be the primary responsibility of the individual. What decisions and actions are to be made are personal matters. The prerogatives are the individual's so long as they do not interfere with or jeopardize the well-being of another. Vaccination for smallpox has thus, until now, been properly mandatory. Cigarette smoking and its relation to cancer of the lung has become well established in recent decades. The accepted evidence has been widely publicized. The law provides for warning notices on packaged cigarettes. If the individual wishes to smoke cigarettes, surely it is his prerogative; the society of which he is a member has pointed out the hazard.

Calculous biliary tract disease is one of the major health problems in the United States. An estimated 15 to 20 per cent of the adult population have or have had gallstones. For 1969 the estimated total population was 202,711,000, with an estimated adult population of 154,811,000. Of operations performed, those upon the biliary tract rank fourth among the first 150 in our general hospitals. Tonsillectomy and adenoidectomy rank first, dilatation and curettage of the uterus second, and hernia repair third.[22]

A public well informed about a disease that involves so many should become increasingly interested in its prevention through research. Ways and means to prevent and/or cure calculous biliary tract disease will surely be brought about some time in the future. It is encouraging that over the past decade investigations directed at the formation of gallstones, and hopefully their prevention, have increased. The recent report from the Mayo Clinic[23] concerning decrease in the size of gallstones with the administration of chenodeoxycholic acid in four patients is certainly significant. Small,[24] one of the most diligent and productive workers, has stated that "from a long-term point of view and considering the considerable mortality and morbidity of gallbladder disease in the United States, it would seem important to try to develop a medical method for treating the so-called silent gallstone." I agree with Dr. Small and believe it should be evaluated among a group of selected young individuals with calculi. The editorial comment in the same issue of the *New England Journal of Medicine* that contained the Mayo report merits direct quote: "Before such therapy can be adopted and recommended, it is mandatory that controlled and long-term clinical trials be carried out to examine the effectiveness, indications for and safety of chenodeoxycholic acid therapy. Such clinical studies should begin at once."[25]

Conclusion

The demonstration of calculi in the gallbladder is considered by me to be an indication for cholecystectomy unless there exists some contraindication to definitive surgery. Surgery precludes the development of acute cholecystitis and its several complications and carcinoma of the gallbladder. In addition, it reduces the likelihood of choledocholithiasis and impairment of liver function that is associated with chronic longstanding cholecystitis. Among any large number of patients with asymptomatic cholelithiasis it is to be anticipated that there will be those with co-existing but unrelated disease that contraindicates cholecystectomy. A fair proportion of these may be able to tolerate a compromise procedure, cholecystostomy with cholelithotomy done under local anesthesia. Although stones may form in the gallbladder thereafter, still the hazard associated with cholelithiasis will have been reduced. The advancements of the past hundred years that have made cholecystectomy the procedure of choice are illustrated by the development of the surgical treatment of calculous biliary tract disease. The nature and magnitude of this condition and its ramifications have been presented.

The complications of acute cholecystitis, choledocholithiasis, and carcinoma of the gallbladder relate to disability and curtailment of life. The high incidence of coronary artery heart disease and its relation to symptoms in patients with cholelithiasis is briefly discussed as a diagnostic problem. The overall information supports and justifies cholecystectomy for asymptomatic gallstones. The clinical application of this policy requires judgment and flexibility in dealing with each patient. In this regard the guidance by the members of the medical profession should include careful instruction of the patient and his family with the information available. The acceptance or refusal of cholecystectomy is the patient's decision.

References

1. Graham, E. A., and Cole, W. H.: Roentgenologic examination of the gall bladder: Preliminary report of a new method utilizing the intravenous injection of tetraphenolphthalein. J.A.M.A. 82:613, 1924.
2. Graham, E. A., Cole, W. H., Copher, G. H., and Moore, S.: *Diseases of Gallbladder and Bile Ducts.* Philadelphia, Lea & Febiger, 1928.
3. Graham, E. A.: The prevention of carcinoma of the gallbladder. Ann. Surg. 93:317, 1931.
4. Osler, W.: *The Principles and Practice of Medicine.* New York, D. Appleton & Co., 1902, pp. 563 and 569.
5. Mason, J. T., and Blackford, J. M.: The conservative treatment of cholecystitis. J.A.M.A. 99:891, 1932.
5a. Blackford, J. M., King, R. L., and Sherwood, K. K.: Cholecystitis. J.A.M.A. 101:910, 1933.
6. Musser, J. H.: *Internal Medicine: Its Theory and Practice. In* Contributions by American Authors. 2nd ed. Philadelphia, Lea & Febiger, 1934.
7. Fitz, R.: Certain peculiarities of gallstone disease. J. Iowa Med. Soc. 32:483, 1942.
8. Christian, H. A.: *The Principles and Practice of Medicine.* New York, D. Appleton-Century Co., 1947, pp. 773–773(1).
9. Robertson, H. E.: Silent gallstones. Gastroenterology 5:345, 1945.
10. Lund, J.: Surgical indication in cholelithiasis. Ann. Surg. 151:153, 1960.
11. Truesdale, E. D.: Frequency and future of gallstones believed to be quiescent or symptomless. Ann. Surg. 119:232, 1944.
12. Comfort, M. W., Gray, H. K., and Wilson, J. M.: The silent gallstones: A 10 to 20 year follow-up study of 112 cases. Ann. Surg. 128:931, 1948.
13. Meyer, K. A., Capos, N. J., and Mittelpunkt, A. I.: Personal experiences with 1261 cases of acute and chronic cholecystitis with cholelithiasis. Surgery 61:661, 1967.
14. Woolman, G. L., Freeman, F. J., and Priestley, J. T.: Relationship of cholecystographic

visualization of the gallbladder to incidence of choledocholithiasis. Surgery 61:669, 1967.
15. PAS REPORTER. Personal Communication. Commission on Professional and Hospital Activities, Green Road, Ann Arbor, Mich.
16. Rhoads, J. E.: Liver, gallbladder and bile passages. *In* Harkins, H. N., Moyer, C. A., Rhoads, J. E., and Allen, J. G. (eds.): *Surgery, Principles and Practice*. Philadelphia, J. B. Lippincott Co., 1961, p. 726.
17. Cancer Facts & Figures 1971. New York, American Cancer Society, Inc., 1971, p. 5.
18. Stewart, H. J.: *Cardiac Therapy*. New York, Paul B. Hoeber, Inc., 1952, p. 368.
19. Patterson, H. A.: The relationship between gallstones and heart disease. Ann. Surg. 139: 683, 1954.
20. Glenn, F.: Pain in biliary tract disease. Surg. Gynec. & Obstet. 122:495, 1966.
21. Colcock, B. P., and Perey, B.: The treatment of cholelithiasis. Surg. Gynec. & Obstet. 117:529, 1963.
22. PAS REPORTER. Commission on Professional and Hospital Activities 9(12)1971. CPHA, Green Road, Ann Arbor, Mich.
23. Danziger, R. G., Hofmann, A. F., Schoenfield, L. J., and Thistle, J. L.: Dissolution of cholesterol gallstones by chenodeoxycholic acid. New Eng. J. Med. 286:1, 1972.
24. Small, D. M.: The formation of gallstones. Advances Intern. Med. 16:243, 1970.
25. Isselbacher, K. J.: A medical treatment for gallstones? (Editorial) New Eng. J. Med. 286:40, 1972.

Advantages of a Varied and Individualized Approach

DONALD M. SMALL

Boston University School of Medicine

"Gallstone disease" is classically included under "diseases of the gallbladder and bile ducts." Stones in the galbladder constitute the major manifestation of the disease, and the classic treatment has been surgical removal of the gallbladder and the stones. Recent advances concerning the etiology, pathogenesis, diagnosis, and treatment suggest that gallstones are usually the end product of an abnormal hepatic metabolism and that new modes of treatment are possible. Further, the indication for a specific therapeutic procedure should be re-evaluated in terms of (1) the type of gallstone disease, (2) the stage of the disease, and (3) the risk factors involved in the treatment.

Man is afflicted by two relatively common types of gallstone disease. One involves bile pigment metabolism and the other cholesterol and bile acid metabolism. Pigment stones are formed when excess unconjugated bile pigments are present in bile and precipitate to form insoluble polymer-like complexes with calcium and copper.[1,2] These stones are black, do not contain cholesterol and, as far as is known, cannot be dissolved in vivo nor in solutions of artificial bile. The source of excessive free pigment may involve increased hepatic secretion of bilirubin in diseases involving rapid hemoglobin breakdown or chemical alteration of conjugated bilirubin in the biliary tract or gallbladder by the action of deconjugating or other enzymes. Since little is known concerning the chemical and physical make-up of pigment stones, and nothing of the solubility of the precipitating molecules, one cannot discuss the earlier stages of this disease or predict from bile composition whether or not patients will develop the disease. One can, on epidemiologic grounds, suggest that patients with increased pigment production will tend to develop pigment stones.

Stages of Cholesterol Gallstone Disease

Cholesterol gallstone disease first manifests itself biochemically when the patient begins to secrete bile which results in gallbladder bile containing an excessive proportion of cholesterol relative to bile salts and phospholipids.[3-5] While all normal people may secrete such a bile occasionally or periodically, the potential gallstone patient probably secretes a bile whose mean daily bile composition contains excess cholesterol.[6] The gallbladder bile from these patients thus becomes supersaturated with cholesterol. If the level of supersaturation is very marked, precipitation of cholesterol may occur spontaneously. If only a moderate degree of supersaturation is present, nucleation may be necessary to initiate precipitation. Many small cholesterol crystals may flocculate to produce aggregates, or a single crystal may grow to form individual stones. The rate of growth will depend on, among other things, the degree of supersaturation—the greater, the more rapid the growth. Finally, stones once formed may block the cystic duct or the common duct and thus cause obstruction, cholecystitis, jaundice, and so forth.

Cholesterol gallstone disease can logically be subdivided into five stages (Table 1). Stage I involves the genetic, biochemical, or metabolic defect leading to the production of a bile with excess cholesterol relative to phospholipid and bile salt.

Stage II, the chemical stage, is the production of an abnormal supersaturated bile. By measuring gallbladder bile composition of samples obtained surgically[3-5] or duodenally[7, 8] and plotting them on triangular coordinates,[2, 9] one can compare the bile composition with an estimation of the maximum cholesterol solubility in bile.[9] Supersaturated biles contain more than the maximum cholesterol that can be solubilized under equilibrium conditions. Furthermore, the per cent saturation[6] may be estimated from observed bile composition and the maximum amount of cholesterol that bile could hold if fully saturated.* A bile 50 per cent saturated is unsaturated, whereas a bile 150 per cent saturated is highly supersaturated with cholesterol.

The physical stage (Stage III) involves the nucleation, flocculation, and precipitation of cholesterol from supersaturated bile. Stage IV involves the growth of the small crystals into macroscopic stones, and the final stage (Stage V) involves the production of clinical symptoms by the gallstone(s).

The diagnosis of cholesterol gallstone disease may now be made as early as Stage II. Thus, by passing the duodenal tube and collecting bile discharged from the gallbladder after a dose of cholecystokinin, bile can be examined microscopically and chemically.[7] If the gallbladder bile contains bile that is supersaturated by the criteria of Admirand and Small[9] but contains no crystals, the patient can be considered to have Stage II gallstone disease. While statistical proof is not yet available, I think that such patients will probably go on to form gallstones in the future. Stage III may be diagnosed by duodenal drainage which reveals abnormal bile containing cholesterol crystals in a patient who has a normal cholecystogram; Stage IV, by the finding of stones on cholecystography; and Stage V, by the presence of clinical signs and symptoms. The very earliest stage, presumably hepatic in location, has not yet been identified; however, it is possible that either genetic defects or enzyme abnormalities that can identify the potential gallstone patient may be found in the future.

---

* The degree of saturation has also been expressed as a ratio. This ratio, the "lithogenic index,"[10] is equal to the per cent saturation divided by 100. Thus, a bile 50 per cent saturated with cholesterol would have a lithogenic index of 0.5.

Table 1. Stages of Cholesterol Gallstone Formation

	STAGE I GENETIC-METABOLIC	STAGE II CHEMICAL	STAGE III PHYSICAL	STAGE IV GROWTH	STAGE V CLINICAL
Abnormality	See Table 2	Bile becomes supersaturated with cholesterol	Nucleation, flocculation, and precipitation of cholesterol crystals	Growth to macroscopic stones	Blockage of cystic duct, cholecystitis and/or jaundice
Diagnosis	See Table 2	Duodenal drainage shows gallbladder bile has excess cholesterol estimated from triangular plot[9] but no crystals by microscope	Duodenal drainage shows cholesterol crystals by microscope; no stones by cholecystography	Cholecystography reveals stones or nonfunctioning gallbladder. Usually cholesterol crystals and/or abnormal bile are found by duodenal drainage	Signs and symptoms; positive cholecystography
Therapeutic approach	Correction of genetic or metabolic defect	Reversion of bile to normal composition	Prevention of nucleation, flocculation, and precipitation	Disappearance of stones by dissolution or fragmentation or surgical removal of gallbladder and stones	Relief of obstruction and removal of gallbladder and stones

Logical Therapeutic Approach

Each stage in gallstone disease may be considered in terms of a logical therapeutic approach (Table 1). For instance, in Stage I, correction of the genetic or metabolic defect would prevent the other stages from occurring. The logical therapeutic approach to Stage II involves correcting the chemical defect, that is, reverting the bile to less than saturated levels. Thistle and Schoenfield[7] have shown that this is possible by administering the bile acid chenodeoxycholic acid (CDCA) for a period of four months. This approach represents a potential step toward the prevention of gallstone disease. If such therapy proves to be efficacious and safe,[11] then perhaps populations with epidemic gallstone disease such as the Indians of the American Southwest,[12] Central America, and South America could be treated preventively.

The therapeutic approach to the third stage of gallstone disease involves the prevention of the physical processes of nucleation, flocculation, and precipitation. Nucleation might be prevented in some patients by administration of small amounts of antinucleating substances which would be secreted into the bile. Under these circumstances it is theoretically possible to have a bile with a relatively high degree of supersaturation which would not nucleate and would thus be harmless. Further, flocculation of micro crystals might be prevented by stabilization of the crystalline surfaces. This also might be accomplished by the administration of small amounts of stabilizers which could be secreted into the bile. These are, of course, theoretical considerations but not altogether beyond possibility.

The growth stage (Stage IV) during which microscopic crystals enlarge to macroscopic stones might be attacked in several different ways as follows:

PERIOD OF ACTIVE GROWTH

During such a period, growth may occur by two distinct processes: The first is through growth of individual crystal nuclei by precipitation of excess cholesterol molecules on these nuclei. Therapy for this type of stone enlargement should be directed toward elimination of excess cholesterol from the bile, that is, reversion of bile composition to normal. The second process involves the agglomeration or sticking together of individual crystals. The therapeutic approach might be directed not only at reducing supersaturation but also at preventing agglomeration. There are several well known physicochemical techniques for preventing agglomeration of suspensions of colloids, solids, and crystals. For instance, applying a surface charge or layer of polyelectrolytes to a suspension of particles can effectively prevent flocculation and agglomeration. How to introduce such compounds into bile effectively may present some problems.

CONTINUED GROWTH OR STABLE STONES

Once the stones are well established and easily demonstrated by cholecystography they may continue to grow, remain stable, or slowly decrease in size.

Wolpers,[13] by performing repeated cholecystograms on many patients over a 20-year span, estimates that about 1 per cent of large solitary stones and about 7 per cent of multiple stones have totally dissolved. The asymptomatic patient might be followed with repeat cholecystograms after two to three years. If the stones are decreasing in size or numbers and no symptoms are present, the patient could be followed for another interval.

The approach to documented, uncomplicated, growing, or unchanging stones may be medical or surgical. The most direct method and most commonly used is to remove both the gallbladder and the stones. Cholecystectomy has been widely used, and recurrence of stones after uncomplicated cholecystectomy is probably rare. Lack of recurrence may perhaps be explained by the recent discovery that the presence of the gallbladder appears to be necessary to bring out the hepatic abnormality in some patients with gallstones.[5] Surgical mortality for this stage of disease is probably less than 1 per cent; nevertheless, since a controlled study concerning the fate of operated and medically followed "silent stone" patients is not available, one can argue successfully for either avenue of treatment.

The future therapy of the silent stone will not remain the exclusive province of the surgeon or the "wait-and-see" internist. The recent report of dissolution of stones by active medical therapy[14] opens a new field of clinical investigation which will, in the future, determine the effectiveness and safety of medical regimens. The basic aim of medical therapy for Stage IV is to cause the disappearance and to prevent the reappearance of stones without resorting to surgery. The decreasing size or number of stones can, like growth, occur as a result of two separate physical processes (I have here excluded passage of stones through the cystic and common duct): The first process, analogous to crystal growth, is crystal dissolution. Crystal dissolution depends on the net rate of removal of molecules of cholesterol from the crystal surface. While such factors as stone surface area, the rate of diffusion of cholesterol into bile, and the degree of stirring or agitation of bile in the gallbladder are significant, the most important factor is the degree of saturation of the gallbladder bile surrounding the stones. In general, the dissolution rate is proportional to the difference in concentration between a saturated solution and the dissolving solution. This is specifically true for gallstones in artificial bile.[15] This means that bile close to saturation will dissolve stones very slowly, whereas bile highly unsaturated will dissolve stones much more rapidly. Therefore, reversion of bile composition to one highly unsaturated should be a therapeutic goal. It must be remembered that once the stones have disappeared the patient still has Stage I disease. To prevent the patient from returning to Stage II and ultimately having a recurrence of stones, preventive therapy following dissolution must be considered.

The second major process is disintegration or fragmentation of stones. If stones were formed by agglomeration or have cracks in them, substances might be found which could cause them to become unglued. Smaller fragments would have a greater surface area for dissolution and might even be passed uneventfully if small enough. The recent experiments of Admirand and Way[16] with perfusion of sodium taurocholate into the common duct to "dissolve" retained stones may well be an instance of both disintegration and dissolution because of the rapidity of the effect.

The signs and symptoms which characterize the final stage (V) are often the result of cholecystitis or obstruction of the cystic or common ducts. Thus, this stage is probably best treated by relief of the obstruction if present and removal of the source of stones. Cholecystectomy appears to be the most rational mode of therapy for symptomatic gallstone disease of any etiology.

Pathophysiologic Classification of Cholesterol Stone Disease

Cholesterol gallstone disease is not, as the title implies, a single entity. At present there are probably at least five distinctly different types of cholesterol gallstone disease. The first four types are manifested by the hepatic secretion of an excess quantity of cholesterol *relative* to bile salt and phospholipid such that gallbladder bile in these patients becomes supersaturated with cholesterol. These four types all involve hepatic metabolism of cholesterol and bile salts in the liver and the enterohepatic circulation, while the fifth type involves a primary abnormality in the gallbladder or in gallbladder bile. The mechanism by which hepatic bile becomes supersaturated in the first four types may be quite different.

In order to understand the different mechanisms in the production of supersaturated bile we must look at the normal relation between the bile salt secretion rate and bile composition. In many animals,[6, 17, 18] and probably in man, there is a clear relationship between the per cent saturation of the bile and the bile salt secretion rate. By extrapolating animal data[6, 17, 18] and data from some humans[19-21] I have guessed at the normal relation between bile salt secretion rate and the per cent saturation of cholesterol in the secreted bile. This is illustrated schematically in Figure 1, in which the bile salt secretion rate, given in grams/day/70-kg. man, is plotted against the per cent saturation or the lithogenic index. The per cent saturation[6] and lithogenic index[10] were calculated from the cholesterol solubility data of Admirand and Small.[9] Normally at high bile salt secretion rates, biles are less than saturated with cholesterol.[20, 21] This is also true in several animal species.[6, 17, 18, 22] However, when bile salt secretion rate decreases the per cent cholesterol saturation begins to increase. A depressed bile salt secretion rate alone is enough to produce an abnormal gallbladder bile provided the mean secretion rate throughout 24 hours is quite low. Throughout the day biliary composition in normal man moves back and forth along the shaded curve.[5, 23] While he is eating, his bile salt secretion rate is high and his bile is not saturated with cholesterol. While he fasts, the secretion rate gradually diminishes as the bile salt pool is trapped in the gallbladder; thus, the bile tends to become more saturated. In about one of four "normal"* humans[5] hepatic bile collected at 6 A.M. after an overnight fast is supersaturated with cholesterol. Very shortly after feeding the bile composition becomes unsaturated as a result of the increased bile salt secretion rate.[5, 6, 23] Thus, even though some normal humans have a bile supersaturated

---

* The term "normal" here means patients without stones. "Normals" may include patients with Stages II or III disease. For a discussion of "normal" and "control" groups in gallstone disease see Reference 6.

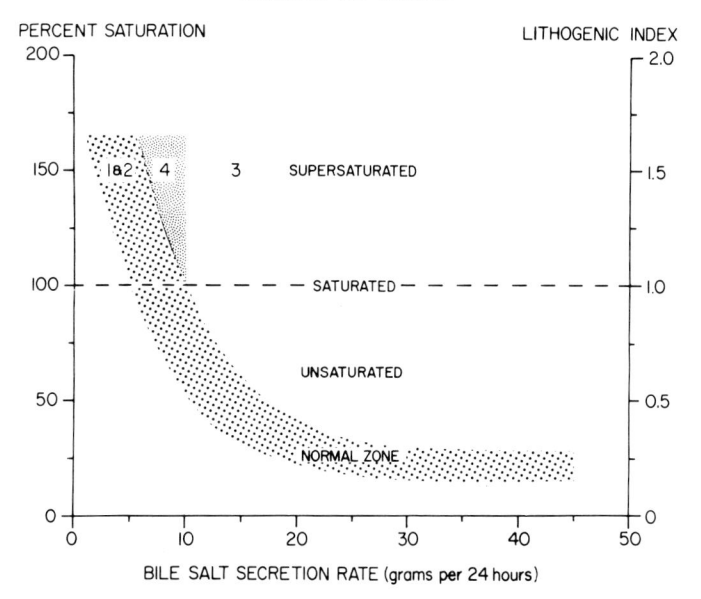

Figure 1. The probable relationship between bile salt secretion rate and cholesterol saturation in bile. The estimated normal relationship between bile salt secretion rate in grams per 24 hours per 70-kg. human is plotted against the per cent saturation of cholesterol in bile (left)[6] and the lithogenic index (right).[10] While the exact boundaries of each regions are not yet known, this figure will serve to illustrate the normal relationships and deviations which result in supersaturated bile. Bile composition in the normal human will fluctuate along the darkly shaded zone, depending on the hour-to-hour secretion rate. During fasting when the secretion rate is very low, a patient may even produce supersaturated bile for short periods of time. Nevertheless, in the normal subject the mean secretion rate over an average 24-hour period is high enough so that mean bile composition is unsaturated. Patients with Types 1 and 2 disease follow the normal relationship, but their mean secretion rate is so low that their mean bile composition falls into the supersaturated region. Patients with Type 3 have a normal overall 24-hour bile salt secretion rate, but the bile is supersaturated; thus, they secrete excessive cholesterol into the bile. Type 4 patients have both a low bile salt secretion rate and increased cholesterol secretion (stippled zone).

with cholesterol for short periods of time, because of a decreased bile salt secretion rate during fasting, it is my impression that this is not enough to produce stones. Small amounts of abnormal bile would probably mix with large amounts of normal bile in the gallbladder, giving a mean normal composition.* Although there may be some exceptions, I believe that the mean bile composition in the gallbladder must be supersaturated if cholesterol is to precipitate and stones form.

In animals,[24] and probably in normal man, the composition of gallbladder bile obtained after an overnight fast is an accurate reflection of the mean composition of bile secreted over the previous 24-hour period. The mean 24-hour bile salt secretion rate is the product of the total bile salt pool size in grams and the number of circulations of that pool per 24-hour period. Thus, a bile salt secretion rate may be low for two separate reasons: a decreased total bile salt pool size, or

---

* While the total solids may vary in different regions of the gallbladder, one cannot demonstrate a difference in the relative composition of bile taken from different levels of the gallbladder.[24]

a normal pool which circulates sluggishly. Recently techniques have become available for measuring bile acid pool sizes and rates of synthesis,[26] fecal excretion, and bile salt and biliary cholesterol secretion[27] in intact humans. By subtracting daily fecal bile acid loss from the bile salt secretion rate one can estimate the daily mean rate of hepatic return of bile salts. Very roughly the normal 70-kg. Caucasian without gallstones will have a total bile salt pool of 2.5 to 4.0 gm, will synthesize about 350 to 550 mg. of bile acid per 24 hours and will secrete 15 to 35 gm. of bile salt and 0.75 to 1.5 gm. of cholesterol per 24 hours. The number of circulations of the pool probably ranges between five and 15 per 24 hours. The mean hepatic return rate of bile salts is about 14-34 gm./24 hr. Our present knowledge of bile salt metabolism permits a tentative classification of cholesterol gallstone disease based on different mechanisms of production of supersaturated bile (Table 2 and Fig. 1).

Type 1. Excessive Bile Salt Loss

These patients are assumed to have a normal relationship between bile salt secretion rate and cholesterol saturation (Fig. 1). However, because of excessive bile salt loss such as occurs in ileectomy, ileal bypass, and certain kinds of ileal disease, or as might occur in an as yet undescribed disease of congenital loss of the ileal active transport system for bile salt, the bile salt pool drains out of the patient and the hepatic return rate decreases markedly. Bile salt synthesis responds by vigorously increasing to a maximal level. However, the increase in synthesis cannot totally make up for loss and the pool remains decreased and the bile salt secretion rate low; the bile becomes supersaturated. This mechanism probably accounts in part for the increased prevalence of gallstones in patients with ileectomy, ileal bypass, or ileal disease.[28, 29]

Recently Dowling, Bell, and White[30] found that gallbladder bile obtained by duodenal drainage from patients with ileal dysfunction but without gallstones was supersaturated with cholesterol. They appear to have identified Type 1 patients in Stage II.

Type 2. Oversensitive Bile Acid Feedback

Normally in monkeys,[17] and most probably in man, when hepatic return rate falls below a certain level, bile salt synthesis increases to augment the secretion rate and thus return it to normal. If the decreased hepatic return is the result of an increased loss, bile salt pool size and secretion rate can be maintained if the loss does not exceed the ability of the liver to compensate.[17] As a result of minor increases in bile salt loss such as occur with cholestyramine feeding or a small ileal resection bile salt secretion is maintained and bile composition remains unsaturated.

Vlahcevic et al.[26] have found in many Caucasian patients with gallstones a diminished pool size, and, assuming a normal and constant number of enterohepatic cycles of the pool, the calculated secretion rate of bile salts in these patients should also be quite low. Surprisingly, however, the synthetic rate is not increased but is normal or even low. Thus, if the secretion rate is low, the amount returning to the liver must also be low. Under normal circumstances hepatic

Table 2. *Classification of Cholesterol Stone Disease*

Type	BILE ACID Hepatic Return Rate	Synthetic Rate	Pool Size	Secretion Rate	CHOLESTEROL SECRETION RATE	PRIMARY DEFECT	EXAMPLES
1. Excessive bile salt loss	Decreased	Increased to maximum level	Decreased	Decreased	Normal to low	Loss of mechanisms to absorb bile salts results in decreased pool and bile salt secretion rate; synthesis cannot fully compensate loss	Ileectomy, ileal bypass, ileal disease, etc.; congenital loss of ileal active transport system of bile salts
2. Oversensitive bile acid feedback	Decreased	Normal to low	Decreased / Normal	Decreased due to small pool circulating normally / Decreased due to a normal pool circulating sluggishly	Normal to low	A relative depression in bile acid synthesis; decreased hepatic return rate excessively inhibits bile acid synthesis	Possibly some of the cholesterol stone cases in Caucasians
3. Excessive cholesterol secretion	Normal	Normal	Normal	Normal	High	Excessive cholesterol is secreted into bile despite normal bile salt secretion rate	Perhaps some of those patients with gallstones in whom bile acid pool size is within normal range; perhaps also obese patients with increased cholesterol synthesis
4. Mixed	Decreased	Normal to low	Decreased or normal	Decreased	High	Mixture of Types 2 and 3	American Indians[21] and perhaps many Caucasians
5. Primary extrahepatic gallstone disease						Absorption of bile salts and/or phospholipids or secretion of cholesterol by gallbladder; chemical alteration of normal hepatic bile in the gallbladder to produce supersaturated gallbladder bile; abnormalities of biliary dynamics	Primary cholecystitits, aseptic or bacterial; may secondarily complicate other types of gallstone disease, including pigment stone disease

synthesis should have increased, but in these patients the synthesis does not respond; it is as if there were an oversensitive feedback mechanism of bile acid synthesis in which relatively low rates of hepatic return are adequate to depress bile acid synthesis. The pathogenesis in Type 2 patients would be as follows: Assuming the patient starts with a normal secretion rate and pool size, as oversensitive feedback develops the patient undergoes a period of negative bile acid balance. Finally, a new steady state is reached characterized by a decreased pool size, a decreased bile salt secretion rate, and a decreased hepatic return. As a result of the decreased secretion rate, bile composition tends to become supersaturated (Fig. 1). The underlying mechanism for the abnormal sensitivity of synthesis to hepatic return is not yet known, but it is not a gross inability to respond to loss.[5]

I should emphasize that the actual secretion rate has not been measured in these patients with a small bile salt pool. It is possible that their bile salt secretion rate could be normal as the result of a small pool circulating rapidly. If this proves to be the case then a further etiology of gallstones must be entertained.

It should be noted that some of Vlahcevic's patients had a perfectly normal bile salt pool size.[26] Depressed secretion in these patients might be due to a sluggish circulation of the pool such as might occur if the gallbladder failed to function properly.

While oversensitive feedback inhibition may play a very important part in stone formation in many patients with gallstones, it is unlikely that this defect alone results in the majority of cases of gallstone disease.

TYPE 3. EXCESSIVE CHOLESTEROL SECRETION

There are some patients whose bile salt pools and estimated secretion rates appear to fall in a normal range however their bile is supersaturated (Fig. 1). Thus, one must assume that these patients have a cholesterol secretion rate above normal: in other words, even in the face of the normal bile salt secretion rate and pool size these patients secrete a bile containing more cholesterol than normal and, thus, their bile is supersaturated. Both Dr. S. Grundy (personal communication) and Dr. E. Shaffer in my laboratory (unpublished observations) have identified several Caucasian patients with gallstones with normal bile salt secretion rates but very high cholesterol secretion rates and lithogenic bile. It is possible that obesity, which increases the synthesis of cholesterol in man,[31] might augment cholesterol secretion into bile. Clofibrate and other similarly acting drugs which appear to mobilize cholesterol pools and increase biliary cholesterol secretion[32] might conceivably induce cholesterol stones in chronic users. Diet may be important in increasing biliary cholesterol. Qiuntao, Grundy, and Ahrens[33] showed that increased cholesterol absorption in certain patients results in increased cholesterol secretion in bile. Even total calorie ocnsumption may be implicated in increased cholesterol secretion, since Sarles et al.[34] noted an increased tendency toward supersaturation in patients fed high caloric diets.

TYPE 4. MIXED DEFECT

From the work of Grundy, Metzger, and Adler[21] it appears that the Indians of the American Southwest have a mixture of Type 2 and Type 3 defects. Most

Indians clearly have a decreased secretion rate and consequently a decreased hepatic return rate. However, their livers do not respond with increased bile acid synthesis; thus, they appear to have oversensitive bile acid feedbacks. In addition, the authors suggest that these patients also have an inordinately high cholesterol secretion rate. Hence, these people have two reasons for supersaturation of the bile. Grundy et al. reasonably postulate that there may be a defect in the conversion of cholesterol to bile acid in these patients resulting in excessive cholesterol secretion and inadequate synthesis of bile acid. This may implicate a defect in the 7 alpha hydroxylation of cholesterol, the rate-limiting reaction in bile acid synthesis from cholesterol, that in these patients which might well be genetic. More recently both Grundy (personal communication) and Dr. Shaffer in my laboratory have found Caucasians with mixed defect disease.

Type 5. Primary Extrahepatic Gallstone Disease

There are a number of possible mechanisms by which the gallbladder and bile ducts might be implicated in the formation of gallstone disease. First, primary cholecystitis might cause the gallbladder to absorb bile salts or even result in chemical degradation of bile salts and biliary lipids, thus converting a normal hepatic bile to supersaturation in the gallbladder.[2, 15] These mechanisms have not been looked for in man, but bile salt resorption in the gallbladder appears to be the cause of stones in mice fed cholesterol and cholic acid.[35] Certainly cholecystitis secondary to existing stones, by causing bile salt absorption or chemically altering biliary lipids, may make gallbladder bile composition even worse, or may result in the formation of cholesterol stones around existing pigment stones. More subtle defects may result from abnormal biliary dynamics. If, for instance, the cystic duct failed to open when the gallbladder contracted, cholecystitis might be produced. If the sphincter of Oddi failed to open when the gallbladder contracted, a condition of intermittent biliary obstruction would result. In the monkey intermittent biliary obstruction can readily produce decreased bile acid synthesis and secretion, accompanied by increased cholesterol secretion, and thus result in supersaturated bile. Thus, it is possible that abnormal biliary dynamics could lead to formation of gallstones.

A few comments are perhaps worthwhile concerning specific therapy for the different types of cholesterol stone disease:

Type 1 patients have an interrupted enterohepatic circulation[17] and are rapidly losing all the bile acids they synthesize into the distal bowel or through an ideostomy. One might attempt to increase the bile acid pool and secretion rate by feeding bile acids to these patients. However, since they lack normal mechanisms for bile salt absorption, this would result in even more bile salts entering the colon, and severe diarrhea might develop. An attempt to increase maximum hepatic synthesis might be made. Monkeys with interrupted enterohepatic circulations fed phenobarbital have a significant increase in the maximum synthesis rate and in the secretion of bile acids, but no increase in cholesterol secretion; thus, their bile becomes less saturated with cholesterol.[36] Phenobarbital treatment might be tested experimentally in these patients. At the present time, however, the most rational and effective therapy for stones in Type 1 patients is cholecystectomy or correction of any ileal defect if feasible.

Since patients with Type 2 disease have not lost their ability to resorb bile salts, one rational approach to therapy would be to attempt to increase the bile salt pool size and the secretion rate of bile salts. Danzinger et al.[14] administered CDCA to seven patients with cholesterol gallstones and demonstrated that the bile salt pool size increased and the bile composition tended to become less saturated with cholesterol in some of the patients. Over the course of two years the stones of four of these seven patients either diminished in size or disappeared. As a result of CDCA administration, both bile and body pool bile salt content became virtually entirely CDCA or its conjugates, and bile acid synthesis was almost completely depressed. Since bile acid and synthesis is controlled by the rate of hepatic return of bile salts, one can conclude that hepatic return must have been increased in these patients. While few short-term disadvantages to this therapy were found,[14] one should mention that the long-term risks of interfering with cholesterol and bile salt metabolism must be studied before this treatment can be recommended for general use.[11, 37] The potential hazards are at least three in relation to cholesterol metabolism: First, increasing the bile salt pool and secretion rate may well increase the quantity of dietary cholesterol absorbed from a given diet. Second, blocking of bile salt synthesis eliminates a major pathway to cholesterol excretion from the body. If cholesterol synthesis is not blocked to an equal extent, then one can expect an augmentation of the cholesterol pool first in the liver and then perhaps in the rest of the body. Salen and Meriwether[38] have fed CDCA in small amounts to patients with cerebrotendinoxanthomatosis, a rare disease involving the accumulation of cholestanol. CDCA suppressed the synthesis of cholestanol and, to some extent, the synthesis of cholestanol. However, it should be noted that during the treatment period the miscible pool of cholesterol did not decrease but, in fact, increased.

Third, converting the entire bile acid pool to chenodeoxycholic acid and its conjugates gives a greater substrate load to bacteria in the ileum and colon for production of toxic lithocolic acid. Under certain conditions of appropriate bacterial flora, intestinal pH, and in the presence of conjugated micelle-forming bile salts, appreciable quantities of lithocolic acid might be absorbed and cause liver damage. While only minor changes in the liver enzymes occurred during CDCA therapy in Danzinger's study,[14] this possibility needs to be studied over a longer period of time and in larger and more diverse groups of people. On the other hand, it is possible that feeding chenodeoxycholic acid might depress cholesterol synthesis to a great extent and, in fact, decrease the cholesterol pool. Only further careful clinical and laboratory experimentation will give us the answers to these potentially important problems.

Phenobarbital alters the metabolism of biliary lipids in the monkey[36] and is presently being tried on an experimental basis in patients with gallstones. This drug is an inducer of microsomal enzymes in the liver, and in the monkey has been shown to increase bile salt synthesis not only during a total bile fistula when synthesis is maximal but also in animals with an intact enterohepatic circulation. Bile acid synthesis was increased despite the fact that the rate of bile salt return to the liver was high enough to inhibit its synthesis completely. Thus, phenobarbital appears to alter the control mechanisms of bile salt synthesis. As a result, bile salt secretion and pool size were augmented but cholesterol secretion rate was unchanged. In phenobarbital-treated animals, bile thus became more unsaturated. Phenobarbital may enhance the conversion of bile salts from cholesterol.[36] While some of the side effects of phenobarbital ingestion may contraindicate use of this drug in some patients, the possible risk of giving CDCA mentioned previously[11, 37] would not be encountered in phenobarbital administration. In fact, the drug of choice for Types 2, 3, and 4 disease would be a drug that would enhance the synthesis of bile acid from cholesterol without enhancing cholesterol synthesis or pool size, thereby giving rise to a high unsaturated bile. If phenobarbital or a drug of similar action proves to be effective in Stages II to IV stone disease, further metabolic and toxicologic studies must, however, be carried out in humans. Though much is already known, phenobarbital cannot yet be recommended for treatment of gallstone disease.

At the present time there are really only two accepted modes of handling gallstone disease: one is cholecystectomy, the second is "wait and see." A third mode, active medical therapy, is in the clinically experimental stage and may offer a new therapeutic approach to the disease.

When does one operate? In my opinion, and without good statistics to back it up, one should operate if a patient has symptoms. Although there are no controlled studies on the probability that a patient who has had a single attack will have trouble again, in my opinion patients who have recently had an attack should probably have their gallstones removed. On the other hand, the patient who is discovered inadvertently by cholecystography or by flat plate of the abdomen to have gallstones and who has had no symptoms should probably be left alone or placed in an experimental group for the study of drug treatment. No important clinical study of the fate of patients with silent gallstones has ever been carried out. It is clear from many autopsy studies and studies in the Pima Indians[12] that somewhere between one half and two thirds of all people who have gallstones never know that they have them and probably never have any symptoms. In the Pima Indians, for instance, about two thirds of the men with gallstones have silent stones.[12] However, given 100 patients with silent gallstones in a given age and population group, one would like to know the incidence of symptoms and compare this with the risks of surgical treatment. It has been argued in the past, largely by surgeons, that patients who have silent gallstones will eventually have difficulties, and when they do that their surgical mortality will be greater and, ergo, they ought to be operated on prophylactically. On the other hand, it has also been argued[40] that if one considers not mortality but life years lost, operations on patients with silent gallstones may well cause a greater loss in years of life in a given group than letting the patients alone until they develop symptoms. The question has not been statistically settled, and with the present trend toward experimental medical treatment, this question may never be put to definitive test.

References

1. Maki, T.: Pathogenesis of calcium bilirubinate gallstone: Role of E. coli, β-glucuronidase and coagulation by inorganic ions, polyelectrolytes and agitation. Ann. Surg. *164:* 90–100, 1966.

2. Small, D. M.: Gallstones. New Eng. J. Med. 279:588–593, 1968.
3. Small, D. M., and Rapo, S.: Source of abnormal bile in patients with cholesterol gallstones. New Eng. J. Med. 279:53–57, 1968.
4. Vlahcevic, Z. R., Bell, C. C., Jr., and Swell, L.: Significance of the liver in the production of lithogenic bile in man. Gastroenterology 59:62–69, 1970.
5. Shaffer, E. A., Braasch, J. W., and Small, D. M.: Bile composition at and after surgery in normals and gallstone patients. New Eng. J. Med. 287:1317–1322, 1972.
6. Redinger, R. N., and Small, D. M.: Bile composition, bile salt metabolism and gallstones. Arch. Intern. Med. 130:618–630, 1972.
7. Thistle, J. L., and Schoenfield, L. J.: Lithogenic bile among young Indian women; lithogenic potential disease with chenodeoxycholic acid. New Eng. J. Med. 284:177, 1971.
8. Vlahcevic, Z. R., Bell, C. C., Jr., Juttijudate, P., et al.: Bile-rich duodenal fluid as an indicator of biliary lipid composition and its applicability to detection of lithogenic bile. Amer. J. Dig. Dis. 16:797–802, 1971.
9. Admirand, W. H., and Small, D. M.: The physicochemical basis of cholesterol gallstone formation in man. J. Clin. Invest. 47:1043–1052, 1968.
10. Metzger, A. L., Heymsfield, S., and Grundy, S. M.: The lithogenic index—a numerical expression for the relative lithogenicity of bile. Gastroenterology 62:499–501, 1972.
11. Small, D. M.: Prestone gallstone disease. Is therapy safe? New Eng. J. Med. 284:214–216, 1971.
12. Sampliner, R. E., Bennett, P. H., Comess, L. J., et al.: Gallbladder disease in Pima Indians: Demonstrations of high prevalence and early onset by cholecystography. New Eng. J. Med. 283:1358–1364, 1970.
13. Wolpers, C.: Personal communications.
14. Danzinger, R. G., Hofmann, A. F., Schoenfield, and Thistle, J. L.: Dissolution of cholesterol gallstones by chenodeoxycholic acid. New Eng. J. Med. 286:1–8, 1972.
15. Small, D. M.: The formation of gallstones. Advances Intern. Med. 16:243–264, 1970.
16. Admirand, W. H., and Way, L.: Medical treatment of retained gallstones. Trans. Amer. Ass. of Phys. 85:382–387, 1972.
17. Small, D. M., Dowling, R. H., and Redinger, R. N.: The enterohepatic circulation of bile salts. Arch. Intern. Med., 130:552–573, 1972.
18. Wheeler, H. O., and King, K. K.: Biliary excretion of lecithin and cholesterol in the dog. J. Clin. Invest. 51:1337–1350, 1972.
19. Thureborn, E.: Human hepatic bile. Acta Chir. Scan. Suppl. 303, 1962.
20. Nilsson, S., and Schersten, T.: Importance of bile acids for phospholipid secretion into human hepatic bile. Gastroenterology 57:625, 1969.
21. Grundy, S. M., Metzger, A. L., and Adler, R.: Pathogenesis of lithogenic bile in American Indian women with cholesterol gallstones. J. Clin. Invest. 51:3026, 1972.
22. McSherry, C. K., Javitt, N. B., de Carbalho, J. M., and Glenn, F.: Cholesterol gallstones and the chemical composition of bile in baboons. Ann. Surg. 173:569, 1972.
23. Metzger, A. L., Adler, R. Heymsfield, S., and Grundy, S. M.: Diurnal variation in biliary lipid composition. Possible role in cholesterol gallstone formation. New Eng. J. Med. 288:333–336, 1973.
24. Dowling, R. H., Mack, E., and Small, D. M.: Biliary lipid secretion and bile composition following acute and chronic interruption of the enterohepatic circulation in the Rhesus monkey. J. Clin. Invest. 50:1917–1926, 1971.
25. Tera, H.: Stratification of human gallbladder bile in vivo. Acta Chir. Scand. Suppl. 256, 1960.
26. Relationship of bile pool size to the formation of lithogenic bile in female Indians of the Southwest. Gastroenterology 62:78–83, 1972.
27. Grundy, S. M., and Metzger, A. L.: A physiological method for estimation of hepatic secretion of biliary lipids in man. Gastroenterology 62:1200-1217, 1972.
28. Heaton, K. W., and Read, A. E.: Gallstones in patients with disorders of the terminal ileum and disturbed bile salt metabolism. Brit. Med. J. 3:494–496, 1969.
29. Cohen, S., Kaplan, M., Gottlieb, L., and Patterson, J.: Liver disease and gallstones in regional enteritis. Gastroenterology 60:237–245, Feb. 1971.
30. Dowling, R. H., Bell, G. D., and White, J.: Lithogenic bile in patients with ileal dysfunction. Gut 13:415–420, 1972.
31. Miettinen, T. A.: Cholesterol production in obesity. Circulation 44:842, 1971.
32. Grundy, S. M., Ahrens, E. H., Jr., Salen, G., Schreibman, P. H., and Nestel, P. J.: Mechanisms of action of clofibrate on cholesterol metabolism in patients with hyperlipidemia. J. Lipid Res. 13:531, 1970.

33. Quintao, E., Grundy, S. M., and Ahrens, E. H.: Effects of dietary cholesterol on the regulation of total body cholesterol in man. J. Lipid Res. 12:233, 1971.
34. Sarles, H., Hauton, J., Planche, N. E., et al.: Diet, cholesterol gallstones, and composition of bile. Amer. J. Dig. Dis. 15:251–260, 1970.
35. Caldwell, F. T., Jr., and Levitsky, K.: Gallbladder and gallstone formation. Ann. Surg. 166:753–758, 1967.
36. Redinger, R. N., and Small, D. M.: Primate Biliary Physiology VIII: The effect of phenobarbital upon bile salt synthesis and pool size biliary lipid secretion and bile composition. J. Clin. Invest. 52:161–172, 1973.
37. Isselbacher, K. J.: A medical treatment for gallstones? New Eng. J. Med. 286:40–42, 1972.
38. Salen, G., and Meriwether, T.: Chenodeoxycholic acid (CDCA) inhibits sterol biosynthesis in cerebrotendinous xanthomatosis (CTX). Clin. Res. 20:465, 1972.
39. Redinger, R. N.: Beneficial effect of phenobarbital on lithogenic human bile. Clin. Res. 21:522, 1973.
40. Ingelfinger, F. J.: Diseases of the gallbladder and bile ducts. In Harrison, T. R., et al. (eds.): Principles of Internal Medicine. New York, McGraw-Hill Book Co., Inc., 1966, pp. 1083–1093.

Comment

Management of Gallstones, Particularly the Silent Variety

The treatment of gallstone disease may be drastically changed in the 1970's. Up to now, the options have been simple: surgery or no surgery. But with a possibility now arising that gallstones might be dissolved by medical methods, the ball game may indeed be brand new. Thus, the essays by Doctors Glenn and Small are most timely. In addition, although the focus of these controversialists is on the management of certain patients with gallstone disease, their broad approach to medical practice is also based on entirely different philosophies: the one depending on traditional empiricism, and the other invoking the rationalism of biochemistry and biophysics to support his respective opinion.

Dr. Glenn is a master surgeon who, on the basis of his experience, has written over 150 articles on diseases of the biliary tract. This experience, and that of his surgical colleagues, provides eloquent evidence of the effectiveness of surgery in relieving patients who suffer from gallstones and their complications. The number of failures has been small, and often, moreover, would probably have been far less had cholecystectomy been undertaken earlier. In the face of such apparent success, little need is perceived for considering alternative therapeutic approaches.

Dr. Small, an internist who has become a biophysicist, has been one of the major contributors to the knowledge that has recently accumulated concerning the pathogenesis of gallstones and their possible prevention and treatment by medical means. Dr. Small proceeds on the sound principle that the best treatment of a disease is based on a knowledge of the responsible mechanisms. Thus, Dr. Small's therapeutic plan is based on an extrapolation of phenomena demonstrable in the laboratory. Though rational, his program is still quite theoretical. Indeed, in contrast to Dr. Glenn's recommendations, those of Dr. Small are supported by extremely limited experience.

Dr. Small's view of gallstone management in the future, however, is not entirely without practical support. The report early in 1971[1] indicating that some cholesterol gallstones can be dissolved by having the patient take large amounts of chenodeoxycholic acid is being confirmed not only by further work at the Mayo Clinic but also by others.[2] But long-term effects of such therapy, and particularly the possibility of long-term adverse effects, will require careful and prolonged observations of patients who have essentially silent stones (most patients who have symptomatic stones will still be candidates for surgery) treated with chenodeoxycholic acid or other lithoclastic medical programs. Prospective studies of this type are already under way.

Other consequences of a possible medical managment of gallstone disease may be anticipated. If controlled prospective studies of medical therapeutic programs are to be undertaken, patients with asymptomatic stones will first have to be identified. Hence, cholecystography of high-risk but asymptomatic populations will presumably be necessary. If the clinical trials are then carried out as they should be, control groups selected by randomization will be created and observed over a period of time. Thus, objective data obtained by prospective methods will accumulate concerning the course of patients who have asymptomatic stones but who receive no treatment, either medical or surgical. At last some basis other than impression will be available to decide whether or not the patient with a silent stone is better off under aggressive management, surgical or medical, or whether, in terms of mortality, survival measured in patient years, morbidity, disability, and expense, the average patient with a silent cholesterol stone will do just as well if treated expectantly, i.e., observed until the appearance of symptoms signals the need for operative intervention.

References

1. Danzinger, R. G., Hofmann, A. F., Schoenfield, L. J., and Thistle, J. L.: Dissolution of cholesterol gallstones by chenodeoxycholic acid. New Eng. J. Med. 286:1–8, 1972.
2. Bell, G. D., Whitney, B., and Dowling, R. H.: Gallstone dissolution in man using chenodeoxycholic acid. Lancet 2:1213–1216, 1972.

FRANZ J. INGELFINGER

22

The Hepatotoxicity of Halothane

HALOTHANE HEPATITIS
   by Fenton Schaffner

EVIDENCE FOR HALOTHANE HEPATOTOXICITY IS EQUIVOCAL
   by B. R. Simpson, L. Strunin, and B. Walton

COMMENT
   by John P. Bunker

Halothane Hepatitis*

FENTON SCHAFFNER

Mount Sinai School of Medicine, New York

The association of the administration of volatile halogenated hydrocarbons for anesthesia and the subsequent development of hepatic injury dates back to early experiences with chloroform over 100 years ago. The introduction to anesthesiology of polyhalogenated hydrocarbons has reawakened interest in the relation of hepatic injury to anesthesia. Differences in assessment of the incidence, of the nature of the process, of the pathogenesis of the hepatic injury, and of the recommendations for the posture of the medical profession with regard to these drugs are reasons why the subject of "halothane hepatitis"[1] is included in this volume. The controversy is compounded by the increasing prevalence of viral hepatitis on one hand and nonspecific postoperative hepatic dysfunction on the other. The position represented in this paper is that halothane hepatitis, like other forms of drug-induced hepatitis, results from an immunologic reaction, most likely delayed hypersensitivity. The evidence to support this stand is marshaled in the description of the various aspects of halothane hepatitis.

The search between 1950 and 1960 for easily administered, well tolerated, and noninflammable anesthetic agents yielded three polyhalogenated hydrocarbons: halothane (2-bromo-2-chloro-1:1:1-trifluoroethane), fluroxene (2:2 2-trifluoroethyl vinyl ether), and methoxyflurane (2:2-dichloro-1:1 difluoroethyl methyl ether)[2] (Fig. 1). Halothane, first used in 1956 (in 1958 in the United States), found rapid and widespread acceptance. It does not irritate the respiratory tract and it inhibits laryngospasm, bronchospasm, and coughing, making intubation easy and its use in asthmatics safe. Smooth muscle elsewhere in the body is also relaxed, so that vasodilation is the rule except in the skin, and sphincter vasoconstriction does not occur. Also, vomiting does not develop. Furthermore, the physical properties of halothane permit it to be used with maximal oxygen supply even with profound anesthesia. Halothane, however, has two properties which may be factors in the development of adverse reactions involving

---

* The original observations described were made with support from U.S.P.H.S. Grant No. AM 03846, and Contract No. DA-39-193-MD-2822, U.S. Army Medical Research and Development Command.

1. 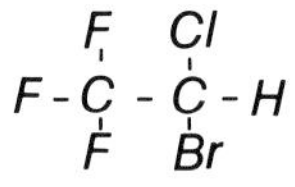 F-C(F,F) - C(Cl,Br) - H

2. 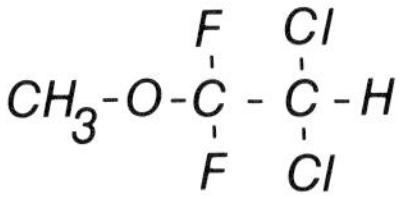 CH₃-O-C(F,F) - C(Cl,Cl) - H

3. 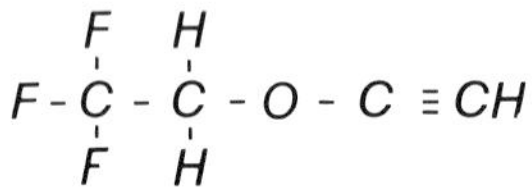 F-C(F,F) - C(H,H) - O - C ≡ CH

Figure 1. Structural formulas of: (1) halothane (1,1,1-trifluoro-2,2-bromochloroethane), (2) methoxyflurane (1,1-dichloro-2,2-difluoromethyl-ethyl ether), and (3) fluroxene (2,2,2-trifluoroethylvinyl ether).

the liver. First, halothane can cause arterial hypotension by virtue of: (1) a direct but complex effect on cardiac muscle, (2) sympathetic inhibition, (3) parasympathetic stimulation, and (4) inhibition of the response of the entire cardiovascular system to catecholamines.[4, 5] These circulatory changes decrease hepatic perfusion. Secondly, because halothane is a poor analgesic and because induction of anesthesia by halothane is slow, it must be given in combination with opiates, barbiturates, muscle relaxants, and other anesthetic agents. The use of such combinations can lead to drug interactions. So far, the advantages of halothane as an anesthetic agent have outweighed its disadvantages to such an extent that it remains the most widely used drug for this purpose throughout the world.

Halothane Metabolism

Before the picture of halothane hepatitis is described, the metabolism of the drug must be detailed as background for the understanding of possible pathogenetic pathways. The volatile halogenated anesthetics, except trichloroethylene, were thought to be inert[6] until labeled halothane was demonstrated to be metabolized by liver slices,[7] presumably by enzymatic dehalogenation.[8] About 20 per cent of the amount administered is metabolized in man.[9] Nontoxic and metabolically inert trifluoroacetate is the main and possibly only end product of this metabolism in rodents[10] and in man;[9] although trifluoroethanol may be an intermediate, at least in man,[11] no other intermediates have been identified. The trifluoroacetate is probably excreted as a glucuronide.[6] Carbon dioxide is not formed from halothane.[7] The rate of halothane metabolism in man is greatly influenced by both environmental and genetic factors, but the genetic control is less than that of the metabolism of several other drugs.[12] The metabolism occurs in the hepatic microsomes and is NADPH and oxygen dependent.[13] Halothane is bound to cytochrome P-450,[14] the hemoprotein in the endoplasmic reticulum responsible for most biotransformations. The drug induces the hepatocyte to enlarge the drug metabolizing enzyme system in rodents[11] and in man,[12, 15] but is not comparable to the effect of phenobarbital. (See next section.) Individual hepatocytes enlarge and more hepatocytes are formed, thereby enlarging the liver as a result of induction.[16] Halothane is dechlorinated more rapidly after phenobarbital pretreatment, but not after methylcholanthrene pretreatment,[13] because the latter substance possibly induces a modified or different cytochrome P-450.

Both methoxyflurane[13, 17] and fluroxene[18] are metabolized like halothane, except that the ether linkages are cleaved and the methyl or vinyl groups converted to CO_2. Pretreatment with phenobarbital increases not only the rate of dechlorination of these compounds, but also the rate of other cleavage. Administration of SKF-525A, an inhibitor of the drug metabolizing enzyme system, does not reduce the rate of biotransformation of fluroxene, but carbon tetrachloride which injures the endoplasmic reticulum inhibits anesthetic biotransformation. All the polyhalogenated anesthetics inhibit their own metabolism, and as anesthetic concentrations in blood increase, the amount extracted and metabolized by the liver diminishes,[7, 19] perhaps by as much as 50 per cent at anesthetic maintenance levels.[19]

Halothane as a Hepatotoxin

Although halothane is commonly referred to as a hepatotoxic drug, proof is lacking of its ability to injure hepatocytes directly (i.e., without some immunologic mechanism) to a clinically significant extent. However, biochemical pathways in different organelles of the hepatocyte are considerably altered by the drug. Some of these are reviewed, with particular attention to the endoplasmic reticulum and its drug metabolizing system.

Endoplasmic reticulum. During induction with phenobarbital, liver mass and the components of the hepatic microsomal biotransformation system in the endoplasmic reticulum increase in a parallel fashion. After halothane, liver mass increases,[16] but cytochrome P-450 and NADPH cytochrome C reductase are decreased, although much less so than after carbon tetrachloride.[20] The smooth endoplasmic reticulum is unchanged in intact animals exposed to halothane,[16, 20] but it is increased in the isolated perfused liver, whereas microsomal N-demethylation is inhibited.[21] Type I substrate metabolism (substrates presumably bound to the lipoprotein portion of the cytochrome P-450) decreases after exposure to halothane in vitro[21] as well as in vivo.[20] The inhibition of type I substrate metabolism appears to be noncompetitive,[22] i.e., increasing the concentration of substrate did not increase the inhibiting effect of the halothane. Methoxyflurane and fluroxene exert the same effect. The metabolism of type II substrates, those presumably bound to the heme of cytochrome P-450, is inhibited in a competitive fashion in vitro,[20] but no effect is noted in vivo.[22] Thus, halothane produces a hypoactive endoplasmic reticulum which can be an indication of liver cell injury.[23] The rough endoplasmic reticulum in the rat is not altered after single[20, 24] or multiple[16] exposures to halothane, and the synthesis of protein is normal, at least in the animals exposed once.[25]

The exposure to halothane of rats pretreated or "induced" with barbiturates has no effect on the amount and activity of the hepatic microsomal drug metabolizing system or on the ultrastructure of the hepatocyte.[20] Attempts have been made to reduce the drug metabolizing enzyme system prior to exposure to halothane by partial hepatectomy[27] or allyl alcohol intoxication,[28] but these treatments fail to enhance any possible subclinical toxicity.

Mitochondria. A single exposure to halothane does not change the ultrastructure of rat hepatocytes, but repeated exposures lead to breaks in outer membranes of hepatocellular mitochondria and herniations into the matrix of the inner membranes.[16] The membrane permeability of isolated mitochondria is altered by halothane; electron transport is decreased by low concentrations, while oxidative phosphorylation is uncoupled by high concentrations.[24] Oxidative phosphorylation is not affected in isolated perfused bovine livers exposed to halothane.[21]

Miscellaneous structural and functional derangements. The administration of halogenated anesthetic agents to rats increases the activity of the lysosomal enzymes, acid phosphatase, and beta glucuronidase in the liver and in the plasma.[29] Halothane increases the plasma activity of many other enzymes of hepatic and muscle origin.[30] None of the changes is so great as those produced by carbon tetrachloride, but all are greater than those produced by ether. Both halogenated and nonhalogenated hydrocarbon anesthetics increase serum glutamic pyruvic transaminase activity in two thirds of patients within five days; highest values are found after halothane.[31] Multiple halothane exposure reduces BSP clearance in perfused rat livers,[32] and somewhat increases the fat content in the liver of the intact rat.[33] Incorporation of acetate into fat by mammalian tissue cultures is accelerated by halothane.[26] Repeated exposure to halothane produces central necrosis with acidophilic cells in horses.[34]

Impurities in Halothane. Impurities arising in the manufacture of the anesthetic agents are considered toxic. The most important of these is dichlorohexafluorobutene,[35] but the amount present never exceeded a trace and could not account for any clinical signs or symptoms in man. Furthermore, it has long since been removed in the manufacturing process. The possibility of metabolites formed from splitting the carbon-fluorine bonds being toxic still exists but seems unlikely.[36] As previously mentioned, the major metabolite of halothane, trifluoroacetate, is metabolically inert and nontoxic.

Methoxyflurane renal toxicity. Special interest has been focused on methoxyflurane because it can produce increased oxalic acid excretion in the urine and polyuric acute renal failure within a day or two of anesthetic administration.[37-39] The oxalic acid may form by demethylation of the anesthetic, but a relation of this metabolism to renal tubular injury is not clear.

Prevalence and Epidemiology of Halothane Hepatitis

Accurate data are not available to indicate the overall frequency of halothane hepatitis. An early retrospective study in Canada put the figure at one case per 8000 anesthetics.[40] The larger retrospective study of the National Academy of Sciences–National Research Council indicated that the incidence would be 1:40,000.[41] Other studies suggested that the incidence might be as low as 1:800.[42] Data from England showed that without previous halothane exposure, hepatitis developed once in 600,000 exposures, but in repeat exposures within a month, the incidence rose to 1:22,000.[43] The statistics from Cardiff, Wales, suggested that the latter figure was about 1:6000. No data are available to indicate the relative incidence of fatal to nonfatal hepatitis, or the relative incidence of anicteric to icteric hepatitis.

Much of the collected data support the observation that repeated exposure greatly increases the incidence of halothane hepatitis.[43-46] Since the first episodes of halothane hepatitis, which were encountered shortly after the anesthetic was introduced,[47] reports of single cases or small groups of cases have been reported from all over the world every year, at least during the last 10 years;[48-56] most of these have occurred after repeated exposures. Some prospective and retrospective studies failed to uncover cases of halothane hepatitis, even with many multiple exposures,[57, 58] although retrospectively in one series[57] one case was found among 20,000 halothane anesthesias, and two cases in the other series[58] which, however, were not attributed to halothane.

Analysis of the causes of acute hepatic necrosis in recent years showed that about one fourth of the patients had been exposed to halothane, and many of these more than once.[59, 60]

People exposed to halothane in the course of their work may develop halothane hepatitis. This has occurred in anesthetists,[61-63] a laboratory technician,[64] and a worker in a halothane manufacturing plant.[44] Indeed, two of the anesthetists have been challenged with halothane, and they developed hepatic dysfunction.[61, 62]

Clinical and Laboratory Features of Halothane Hepatitis

The initial indication of halothane hepatitis is fever in the second postoperative week in the patient exposed to halothane only once.[44-46, 65, 66] Fever early in the first week seems to bear no relation to the type of anesthetic or the type of operation.[67] When halothane hepatitis develops in a patient exposed to halothane more than once, fever starts in the latter half of the first week. The onset of the fever is abrupt and is preceded by chills. It reaches up to 105°F. (40.5° C.), mainly in the late afternoon, only to subside at night and recur the next day. This hectic temperature course is associated with malaise, anorexia or nausea, often right upper quadrant pain, and occasionally a rash. It is followed by rapidly rising serum transaminase activity to levels over 1000 units in one to four days and by liver tenderness, usually with an increase in liver size. In previously exposed patients the transaminase activity rises soon after the temperature climbs. Jaundice, if it develops, appears within a day or two of the elevation of transaminase activity. Fever continues for several days after the onset of jaundice. The peak value of the serum bilirubin and that of alkaline phosphatase activity vary greatly from one patient to the next. Mild eosinophilia occurs in about half the patients, but other changes in the blood picture are not uniform. One instance of erythroid aplasia following halothane hepatitis similar to that seen after viral hepatitis has been reported.[68]

The peak of the disease is reached in a few days to one week. The patient either defervesces and regains his appetite and feeling of well-being rather promptly in the second week of illness, or develops signs of hepatic coma. In the latter case the liver shrinks and the patient dies at the end of the first week or during the second week of jaundice. Once coma has developed, the outlook is grim regardless of therapy, and the data collected in the Fulminant Hepatitis Surveillance Study[59] suggest that the mortality rate of patients in hepatic coma from halothane hepatitis is 95 per cent.

The laboratory feature, which heralds a poor outcome most clearly, is increasing prolongation of the prothrombin time. The peak level of bilirubin and of transaminase activity may be the same in survivors and in nonsurvivors.

The symptoms and signs, as well as the laboratory abnormalities, rapidly regress in the patients who recover, and no relapses occur. As in all instances of hepatitis, the more cholestasis that is present, the longer the illness tends to last.

Immunologic abnormalities have been detected in halothane hepatitis. Mitochondrial antibodies in serum, described by Doniach et al.[69] and found in high titer in primary biliary cirrhosis, are present in low titer in most patients with halothane hepatitis.[70] This is particularly true if the more sensitive but less specific method using rat stomach is employed. Similar antibodies are found in most patients with chlorpromazine jaundice, but not with hepatitis induced by alpha methyldopa. When lymphocytes of patients with halothane hepatitis are maintained as tissue cultures and then exposed to halothane, blastic transformation is induced.[71, 72] Lymphocytes from patients exposed to halothane but without hepatitis, and from patients with other liver diseases, will not react to halothane. Such stimulation of lymphocyte transformation is considered a sign of delayed hypersensitivity.

Pathology of Halothane Hepatitis

The structural changes seen in the liver with the light microscope are similar to those found in viral hepatitis,[44] with spotty necrosis in biopsy specimens and massive necrosis in fatal cases. Cholestasis varies from being severe and even the predominant finding in occasional patients to being absent in the anicteric ones. Clusters of macrophages and other mononuclear cells are scattered through the parenchyma as histiocytic nodules or small granulomas in some cases.[44, 73] Steatosis is sometimes more severe than in viral hepatitis, but this could result from the changes in nutrition associated with surgery. Eosinophils are in portal tracts and in areas of necrosis in about half the patients. Linear zones of parenchymal necrosis bridging the portal area and central vein are seen in nonfatal severe hepatitis, or in fatal cases when biopsies are done before autolysis is extensive. Central vein phlebitis is present in all survivors, and cholestasis is variable. Portal tracts are enlarged with a pleomorphic inflammatory infiltration and ductular proliferation.

Massive or centrolobular necrosis is conspicuous in patients who succumb within a week.[45] This may be the result of postmortal autolysis. Necrotic zones either contain numerous iron-laden, brown pigmented macrophages or are collapsed. Regeneration with many binucleated cells or two-cell-thick plates of hepatocytes is in the foreground after two weeks of illness.[44, 45] Central necrosis is uncommon in our material, even when biopsies are done early, and spotty necrosis is more typically found, as in viral hepatitis.

While light microscopic differences between viral and halothane hepatitis are uncertain, electron microscopic differences are clear-cut[44, 74, 75] (Fig. 2). The out-

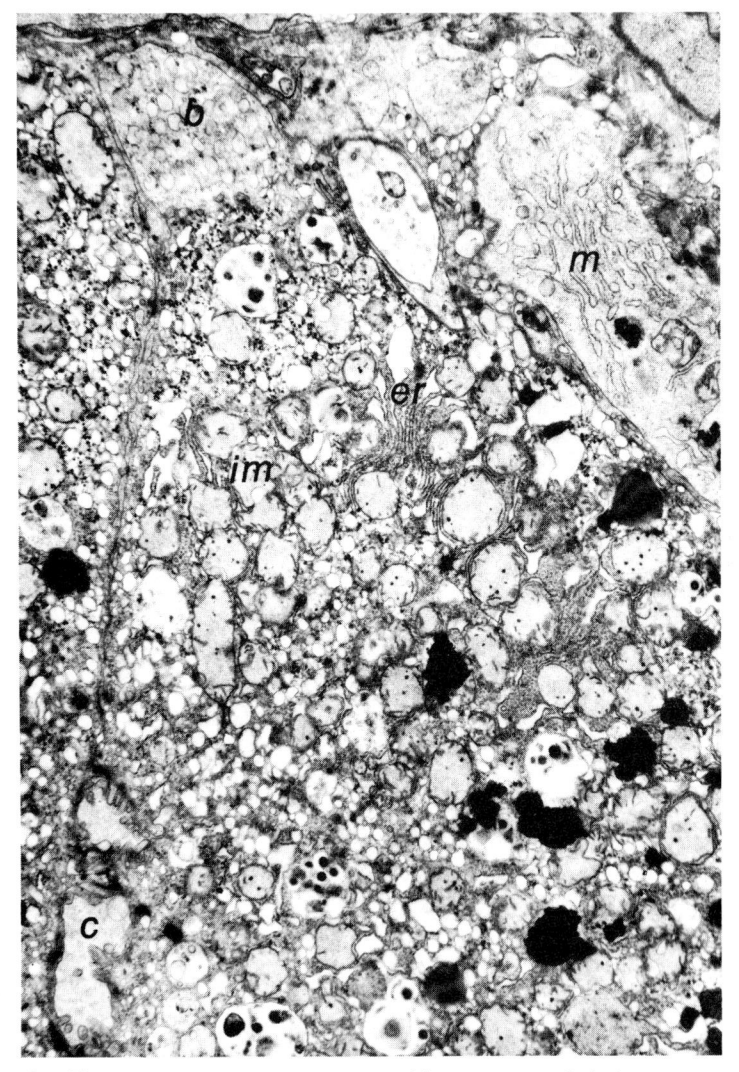

Figure 2. Electron microscopic appearance of hepatocyte in halothane hepatitis. *im* is a clump of mitochondria with interlocking membranes and invagination of one into another; *er* is intact rough exoplasmic reticulum; *c* is a dilated bile canaliculus; *b* is a bleb on the sinusoidal surface of the hepatocyte; and *m* is a mesenchymal cell, possibly a fibroblast in the space of Disse. The black clumps are lipofuscin pigment. (Osmium tetroxide fixation, lead citrate stain, x 12,000).

standing ultrastructural feature of halothane hepatitis is mitochondrial injury. The mitochondria vary greatly in size and their outer membranes show numerous breaks. Herniations of the intercrystal space into the matrix are numerous, as are interlocking of membranes of adjacent mitochondria. Similar changes have been seen in alcoholic liver disease and in various experimental toxic injuries, including repeated halothane administration to rats.[16] Injury to the endoplasmic reticulum and the formation of autophagic vacuoles are not so pronounced as in viral hepatitis.

Halothane and Pre-existing Liver Disease

Halothane is considered to be contraindicated as the anesthetic for patients with liver disease by some,[76] although there is no evidence that any hepatic drug reaction is more likely to occur in such patients.[77] Because good oxygenation is easily maintained with halothane, I think that it is the anesthetic of choice for cirrhotics undergoing shunt surgery. One presumptive case of mild halothane hepatitis developed under these circumstances at The Mount Sinai Hospital. Patients with acute viral hepatitis were exposed to halothane during surgery with no harmful effects.[78] Several patients who did develop postoperative hepatic dysfunction were found to have chronic hepatitis or cirrhosis.[79-81] It is not known whether the worsening of hepatic function in these patients was related (1) to halothane, (2) to the stress of surgery or the condition for which the surgery was performed, or (3) to aggravation of the pre-existing liver disease. Despite these last reports, no data contraindicate the use of halothane in patients with liver disease.

Methoxyflurane Hepatitis

Methoxyflurane produces the same picture of hepatitis that halothane does, but fewer cases have been reported.[44, 45, 48, 82-88] The clinical features of methoxyflurane hepatitis can be overshadowed by the appearance of polyuric renal failure mentioned before when hepatic and renal adverse effects occur together.[85, 86] Pathologically centrolobular necrosis appears to be more prominent than in halothane hepatitis.[82-84] The immunologic findings are similar to those in halothane hepatitis, with some cross reactivity between halothane and methoxyflurane as far as inducing blastic transformation of cultured lymphocytes.[71, 74]

Few cases of hepatic necrosis have been reported following fluroxene anesthesia.[45, 49] One patient had been taking phenobarbital and diphenylhydantoin, and the possibility of a drug interaction was raised.[89]

Differential Diagnosis

Halothane hepatitis must be separated from postoperative toxic[90] or cholestatic[91,92] jaundice, from viral hepatitis, and from obstructive jaundice, especially in those patients who have had upper abdominal surgery. Jaundice may develop within three days after surgery regardless of the type of anesthetic used, and without high temperatures or chills.[46] Usually this phenomenon occurs after abdominal operations, most often on the stomach or biliary tree. It was recognized long before halothane was discovered.[93, 94] The condition is benign in the majority of cases, although deaths occasionally occur, and in these shock and anoxia seem to play an important role, with extensive central necrosis the main histologic alteration. Indeed, in the National Halothane Study, severe central necrosis unrelated to a specific anesthetic was more frequent than the massive necrosis associated with halothane anesthesia.[95] The peak level of serum bilirubin varies in postoperative jaundice, and if many blood transfusions have been given, values over 15 mg. per 100 ml. may be reached.[92] Under these circumstances centrolobular cholestasis is seen in biopsy specimens. More often the serum bilirubin reaches a level of 7 to 8 mg. per 100 ml. by the third or fourth postoperative day, and then falls to normal within a week. The increases in the activities of serum alkaline phosphatase or the transaminases are not so great as the rise in bilirubin, although BSP retention is the rule. Possibly the defect is in the secretion of organic anions, as in the Dubin-Johnson syndrome, rather than liver cell injury or cholestasis. This idea is supported by the bland and nonspecific changes usually found in liver biopsy specimens. This complication of surgery is readily recognized by its oligosymptomatic onset soon after surgery, with hyperbilirubinemia being the severest abnormality and the course being short and benign.

The separation of halothane hepatitis from viral hepatitis is sometimes more difficult. The incubation period of viral hepatitis is longer, but the prodrome, onset, physical findings, laboratory abnormalities, and course may be indistinguishable. Hepatitis B (Australia) antigen supports the diagnosis of viral hepatitis. In the absence of this finding, challenging the cultured lymphocytes of the patients with halothane provides the strongest evidence for halothane hepatitis. Electron microscopic examination of liver biopsy specimens can provide presumptive evidence and may be useful in separating some of the different types of drug hepatitis.

When patients have undergone upper abdominal surgery, injury to the biliary system becomes a consideration in the differential diagnosis of postoperative jaundice. Ligation of the bile duct produces cholestasis with pruritus as the main clinical symptom and greatly increased activity of serum alkaline phosphatase as the main laboratory abnormality. Fever is late and results from complicating cholangitis.

The Controversy

Two factors account for the controversy or dilemma[96] now existing concerning the hepatitis following the use of halothane. The first is the low incidence recognized in all compiled data,[96, 97] which makes statistical association difficult, and the second is the concern that a useful and safe agent may have to be abandoned.

While the low incidence of halothane hepatitis cannot be questioned, and the principle of guilt by association must be avoided, guidelines were proposed for establishing a diagnosis of drug-induced hepatic damage.[98] Two basic clinical principles were proposed to establish the diagnosis: "(1) the abnormalities found are those produced by the drug in question, and (2) the hepatic abnormalities did not appear too soon after the initial dose of the drug or too long after the last dose." Halothane hepatitis probably fits the first principle, but the pathologists have not fully agreed, and their descriptions suffer from lack of uniformity. specifically, the opinion that viral and halothane hepatitis can be differentiated by light microscopy is not unanimous. The second principle is less controversial but is confused by the appearance of postoperative toxic jaundice or cholestasis, which is more common than halothane hepatitis. The association of such features as fever, rash, and arthritis with halothane hepatitis favors the diagnosis of drug jaundice, as long as Australia antigen remains absent. In the laboratory only eosinophilia is helpful when present. Structural differences, when present, are useful in separation from viral hepatitis. A positive challenge test represents direct and specific proof of drug-induced liver disease. This test has been carried out with halothane in intact individuals[61, 62] as well as with lymphocytes from sensitized persons.[99] The test on the intact patient is not recommended for general use because of the risk of inducing severe hepatitis.

On the whole, the case for halothane hepatitis is a convincing one. Many of the arguments in defense of halothane[96] are irrelevant or incorrect, such as criticism of the techniques for finding Australia antigen or the statement that halothane does not combine with proteins. It probably can combine with any lipoprotein and surely does with cytochrome P-450 in the liver. In fact, binding of halothane to the plasma membrane of the hepatocyte may be the initial step in creating the delayed hypersensitivity reaction which leads to the immunologic rejection and death of these cells. Statements that halothane is not a serious direct hepatotoxin, and that its metabolites also are harmless, seem to be agreed upon universally, despite the extreme metabolic and ultrastructural changes induced by the drug involving drug metabolism and energy production. Also, the opinion that halothane is more useful and safer than other anesthetic agents seems to be unanimous. Many unknowns remain, however. The short duration of halothane hypersensitivity[71] is curious, and exposure of normal persons to the drug has no effect on immunoglobulins.[100] Surgery, in general, depresses the immune response, even the cell mediated form, so that in the postoperative period lymphocytes are less likely to respond to mitogenic stimuli.[101] Therefore, the mild response which is noted has even greater significance.

A Personal Viewpoint

We have reviewed the problem of drug-induced liver disease four times in the past 13 years.[77, 102-104] During this time we have seen drugs taken off the market after they produced only a few cases of hepatitis (metahexamide, iproniazid, zoxazolamine), and we have seen drugs survive despite many instances of jaundice (arsenicals, chlorpromazine, contraceptives). Halothane has been associated with several hundred cases of hepatitis.

What recommendation should be offered? Because of the usefulness of the drug, halothane should not be withdrawn from the market. Whenever it is used, the benefit obtained must outweigh the risk. It should be avoided for all minor procedures, and it should not be used when repeated operations are necessary in a short period of time. An exception may be ophthalmologic procedures, in which postoperative vomiting may be responsible for loss of vision and this risk is greater than the risk of halothane hepatitis. Halothane is absolutely contraindicated in patients who have become febrile or jaundiced in the second week after previous exposure. One factor leading to the death of many patients has been surgical re-exploration to search for the cause of postoperative jaundice and fever. Such operations are often carried out again under halothane anesthesia, and death ensues in a few days. Another factor responsible for protracted morbidity and even mortality has been the overenthusiastic exhibition of antibiotics and intravenous fluids in the treatment of the febrile reaction. As stated in 1965,[98] "often patience on the part of physician and patient will resolve the issue." Patience and caution will provide the time necessary to uncover the mechanism of halothane hepatitis, but probably prevention will not be possible until the whole problem of delayed hypersensitivity is solved.

References

1. Tygstrup, N.: Halothane hepatitis. Lancet 2:466, 1963.
2. Price, H. L., and Dripps, R. D.: General anesthetics II. Volatile anesthetics: diethyl, ether, divinyl ether, chloroform, halothane, methoxyflurane, and other halogenated volatile anesthetics. *In* Goodman, L. S., and Gilman, A. (eds.): *The Pharmacological Basis of Therapeutics.* 4th ed. New York, The Macmillan Company, 1970, pp. 79–92.
3. Raventos, J.: The action of fluothane—a new volatile anesthetic. Brit. J. Pharmacol. *11:* 394–410, 1956.
4. Deutsch, S., Linde, H. W., Dripps, R. D., et al.: Circulatory and respiratory actions of halothane in normal man. Anesthesiology 23:631–638, 1962.
5. Price, H. L., Linde, H. W., and Morse, H. T.: Central nervous actions of halothane affecting the systemic circulation. Anesthesiology 24:770–778, 1963.
6. Brown, B. R. Jr., and Vandam, L. D.: A review of current advances in metabolism of inhalation anesthetics. Ann. N.Y. Acad. Sci. *179:*235–243, 1971.
7. Van Dyke, R. A., Chenoweth, M. B., and Van Poznak, A.: Metabolism of voltile anesthetics. 1. Conversion *in vivo* of several anesthetics to $C^{14}O_2$ and chloride. Biochem. Pharmacol. *13:*1239–1248, 1964.
8. Heppel, C. A., and Porterfield, V. T.: Enzymatic dehalogenation of certain brominated and chlorinated compounds. J. Biol. Chem. *176:*763–769, 1948.
9. Rehder, K., Forbes, J., Alter, H., et al.: Halothane biotransformation in man: A quantitative study. Anesthesiology 28:711–715, 1967.
10. Stier, A.: Trifluoracetic acid as a metabolite of halothane. Biochem. Pharmacol. *13:*1544, 1964.
11. Cascorbi, H. F., and Blake, D. A.: Trifluoroethanol and halothane biotransformation in man. Anesthesiology 35:493–495, 1971.
12. Cascorbi, H. F., Vesell, E. S., Blake, D. A., et al.: Halothane biotransformation in man. Ann. N.Y. Acad. Sci. *179:*244–248, 1971.
13. Van Dyke, R. A.: The metabolism of volatile anesthetics. III. Induction of dechlorinating and ether cleaving enzymes. J. Pharmacol. Exp. Ther. *154:*364–369, 966.
14. Van Dyke, R. R.: Metabolic pathways and anesthetic detoxification. *In* Fink, R. B. (ed.): *Toxicity of Anesthetics.* Baltimore, The Williams & Wilkins Company, 1968, pp. 61–64.
15. Cohen, E. N.: The metabolism of halothane-2 C^{14} in the mouse. Anesthesiology *31:*560–565, 1969.

16. Preis, C. Schaude, G., and Siess, M.: Histometrische Analyse der Lebervergrösserung nach chronischer Einwirkung von Barbituraten und Halothan. Naunyn Schmiedeberg Arch. Pharm. 254:489–504, 1966.
17. Berman, M. L., and Bochantin, J. F.: Nonspecific stimulation of drug metabolism in rats by methoxyflurane. Anesthesiology 32:500–506, 1970.
18. Blake, R. A., Rosman, R. S., Cascorbi, H. F., et al.: Biotransformation of fluroxene. 1. Metabolism in mice and dogs in vivo. Biochem. Pharmacol. 16:1237–1248, 1967.
19. Sawyer, D. C., Eger, E. I., II, Bahlman, S. H., et al.: Concentration dependence of hepatic halothane metabolism. Anesthesiology 34:230–234, 1971.
20. Davis, D. C., Schroeder, D. H., Gram, T. E., et al.: A comparison of the effects of halothane and CCl$_4$ on the hepatic drug metabolizing system. J. Pharmacol. Exp. Ther. 177:556–566, 1971.
21. Bombeck, C. T., Aoki, T. Smuckler, E. A., et al.: Effects of halothane, ether, and chloroform on the isolated, perfused, bovine liver. A comparative study. Amer. J. Surg. 117:91–107, 1969.
22. Brown, B. R., Jr.: The diphasic action of halothane on the oxidative metabolism in the liver: An in vitro study in the rat. Anesthesiology 35:241–246, 1971.
23. Hutterer, F., Klion, F. M., Wengraf, A., Schaffner, F., and Popper, H.: Hepatocellular adaptation and injury. Structural and biochemical changes following dieldrin and methyl butter yellow. Lab. Invest. 20:455–464, 1969.
24. Miller, R. N., and Hunter, F. E., Jr.: The effect of halothane on electron transport, oxidative phosphorylation, and swelling in rat liver mitochondria. Molec. Pharmacol. 6:67–77, 1970.
25. Scholler, K. L.: Der Einfluss von Halothan und Chloroform auf die Feinstruktur und Proteinsynthese der Rattenleber. Experientia 23:652–655, 1967.
26. Ishii, D. N., and Carbascio, A. N.: Some metabolic effects of halothane on mammalian tissue culture cells in vitro. Anesthesiology 34:427–438, 1971.
27. Almersjo, O.: Influence of halothane anesthesia on the normal liver and the liver subjected to partial hepatectomy or stimulated drug metabolism. Acta Chir. Scand. suppl. 416, 1971.
28. Scholler, K. L., and Schroeter, R.: Frage der Verstarkung des Allylalkoholschadens der Rattenlaber durch Halothan. Klin. Wschr. 46:207–208, 1968.
29. Serrou, B. C., Aldreté, J. A., and Schultz, R. L.: Effect of anesthetic drugs on lysosomal enzymes in the rat. Proc. Soc. Exp. Biol. Med. 137:1389–1971.
30. Zimmerman, H. J., Kendler, J., and Koff, R. S.: Intraperitoneal halothane administration: Evidence of hepatic and muscle injury. Proc. Soc. Exp. Biol. Med. 138:678–682, 1971.
31. Akdikmen, S. A., Flanagan, T. V., and Landmesser, C. M.: Comparative study of serum glutamic pyruvic transaminase changes following anesthesia with halothane, methoxyflurane, and other inhalation agents. Anesth. Analg. 45:819–825, 1966.
32. Biebuyk, J. F., Saunders, S. J., Harrison, G. G., et al.: Multiple halothane exposure and hepatic bromsulphthalein clearance. Brit. Med. J. 1:668–671, 1970.
33. Feise, G.: Gesamtfette und Triglyceride in der Leber nach Narkosen mit Halothan. Chloroform und Äther an der Ratte. Exp. Med. 147:190–196, 1968.
34. Gopinath, C., Jones, R. S., and Ford, E. J. H.: The effect of the repeated administration of halothane on the liver of the horse. J. Path. 102:107–114, 1970.
35. Cohen, E. N., Brewer, H. W., Belleville, J. W., et al.: The chemistry and toxicology of dichlorohexafluorobutene. Anesthesiology 26:140–153, 1965.
36. Goldman, P.: The carbon-fluorine bond in compounds of biological interest. Science 164:1123–1130, 1969.
37. Crandell, W. B., Pappas, S. G., and MacDonald, A.: Nephrotoxicity associated with methoxyflurane anesthesia. Anesthesiology 27:591–607, 1966.
38. Mazze, R. I., Shu, G. L., and Jackson, S. H.: Renal dysfunction associated with methoxyflurane anesthesia. J.A.M.A. 216:278–288, 1971.
39. Proctor, E. A., and Barton, F. L.: Polyuric acute renal failure after methoxyflurane and tetracycline. Brit. Med. J. 4:661, 1971.
40. Keéri-Szántó, M., and LaFleur, F.: Postanesthetic liver complications in a general hospital: A statistical study. Canad. Anaesth. Soc. J. 10:531–538, 1963.
41. Summary of the National Halothane Study. Possible association between halothane anesthesia and hepatic necrosis. J.A.M.A. 197:775–788, 1966.
42. Herber, R., and Specht, N. W.: Liver necrosis following anesthesia. Arch. Intern. Med. 115:266–272, 1965.

43. Mushin, W. W., Rosen, M., and Jones, E. V.: Post-halothane jaundice in relation to previous administration of halothane. Brit. Med. J. 3:18–21, 1971.
44. Klion, F. M., Schaffner, F., and Popper, H.: Hepatitis after exposure to halothane. Ann. Intern. Med. 71:467–477, 1969.
45. Peters, R. L., Edmondson, H. A., Reynolds, T. B., et al.: Hepatic necrosis associated with halothane anesthesia. Amer. J. Med. 47:748–764, 1969.
46. Sherlock, S.: Progress report: Halothane hepatitis. Gut 12:324–329, 1971.
47. Vertue, P. W., and Payne, K. W.: Postoperative death after fluothane. Anesthesiology 19:562–563, 1958.
48. Lindenbaum, J., and Leifer, E.: Hepatic necrosis associated with halothane anesthesia. New Eng. J. Med. 268:525–530, 1963.
49. Tornetta, F. J., and Tamaki, H. T.: Halothane jaundice and hepatotoxicity. J.A.M.A. 184: 658–660, 1963.
50. Rodgers, J. B., Mallory, G. K., and Davidson, C. S.: Massive liver cell necrosis: A retrospective study. Arch. Intern. Med. 114:637–646, 1964.
51. Klinge, O.: Toxische Hepatose bei Halothan-Narkose. Klin. Wschr. 43:1042–1049, 1965.
52. Morgenstern, L., Sacks, H. J., and Marmer, M. J.: Postoperative jaundice associated with halothane anesthesia. Surg. Gynec. Obstet. 121:728–732, 1965.
53. Griner, P. F.: Hepatitis after repeated exposure to halothane. Case report and brief review. Ann. Intern. Med. 65:753–757, 1966.
54. Wilbert, L., and Creutzfeldt, W.: Recurrent jaundice and fatal liver necrosis following a second administration of halothane. German Med. Monthly 12:360–362, 1967.
55. Nowill, W. K.: Death due to acute hepatic necrosis, secondary to administration of halothane anesthesia. Anesth. Analg. 49:355–362, 1970.
56. Sharpstone, P., Medley, D. R. K., and Williams, R.: Halothane hepatitis: Preventable disease? Brit. Med. J. 1:448–449, 1971.
57. DeBacker, L. J., and Longnecker, D. S.: Prospective and retrospective searches for liver necrosis following halothane anesthesia. J.A.M.A. 195:157–160, 1966.
58. Gronert, G. A., Schaner, P. J., and Gunther, R. C.: Multiple halothane anesthesia in the burn patient. J.A.M.A. 205:170–172, 1968.
59. Trey, C., Lipworth, L., Chalmers, T. C., et al.: Fuminant hepatic failure: Presumable contribution of halothane. New Eng. J. Med. 279:798–801, 1968.
60. Ritt, D. J., Whelan, G., Werner, D. J., et al.: Acute hepatic necrosis with stupor or coma, an analysis of 30 patients. Medicine 48:151–172, 1969.
61. Baifrage, S., Ahlgren, I., and Axelson, S.: Halothane hepatitis in an anesthetist. Lancet 2:1466–1467, 1966.
62. Klatskin, G., and Kimberg, D. V.: Recurrent hepatitis attributable to halothane sensitization in an anesthetist. New Eng. J. Med. 280:515–522, 1969.
63. Combes, B.: Halothane-induced liver damage: An entity. New Eng. J. Med. 280:558–559, 1969.
64. Johnston, C. I., and Mendelsohn, F.: Halothane hepatitis in a laboratory technician. Aust. New Zeal. J. Med. 2:171–173, 1971.
65. Trey, C., Lipworth, L., and Davidson, C. S.: The clinical syndrome of halothane hepatitis. Anesth. Analg. 48:1033–1042, 1969.
66. Hughes, M., and Powell, L. W.: Recurrent hepatitis in patients receiving multiple halothane anesthetics for radium treatment of carcinoma of the cervix uteri. Gastroenterology 58:790–797, 1970.
67. Dykes, M. H. M.: Unexplained postoperative fever; its value as a sign of halothane sensitization. J.A.M.A. 216:641–644, 1971.
68. Jurgensen, J. C., Abraham, J. P., and Hardy, W. W.: Erythroid aplasia after halothane hepatitis. Report of a case. Amer. J. Dig. Dis. 15:577–581, 1970.
69. Doniach, D., Roitt, I. M., Walker, J. G., et al.: Tissue antibodies in primary biliary cirrhosis, active chronic (lipoid) hepatitis, cryptogenic cirrhosis and other liver diseases and their clinical implications. Clin. Exp. Immun. 1:237–262, 1966.
70. Rodriguez, M., Paronetto, F., Schaffner, F., et al.: Antimitochondrial antibodies in jaundice following drug administration. J.A.M.A. 208:148–150, 1969.
71. Paronetto, F., and Popper, H.: Lymphocyte stimulation induced by halothane in patients with hepatitis following exposure to halothane. New Eng. J. Med. 283:277–280, 1970.
72. Lecky, J. H., and Cohen, P. J.: Hepatic dysfunction without jaundice following administration of halothane. Anesthesiology 33:371–372, 1970.
73. Dordal, E., Glagov, S., Orlando, R. A., et al.: Fatal halothane hepatitis with transient granulomas. New Eng. J. Med. 283:357–359, 1970.

74. Schaffner, F., and Paronetto, F.: Immunologic observations and electron microscopy of halothane-induced hepatic injury. *In* Smith, M., and Williams, R. (eds.): *Immunology of the Liver*. London, William Heinemann, Ltd., 1971, pp. 186–193.
75. Uzunalimoglu, B., Yardley, J. H., and Boitnott, J. K.: The liver in mild halothane hepatitis. Light and electron microscopic findings with special reference to the mononuclear cell infiltrate. Amer. J. Path. *61*:457–478, 1970.
76. Keown, K. K., and Bingham, H. G.: Halogen sensitization of liver. Anesth. Analg. *48*: 710–714, 1969.
77. Perez, V., Schaffner, F., and Popper, H.: Hepatic drug reactions. *In* Popper, H., and Schaffner, F. (eds.): *Progress in Liver Diseases*. 4th ed. New York, Grune & Stratton, 1972.
78. Hege, M. J. D.: Halothane anesthesia in a patient with acute hepatic disease. Anesthesia *32*:170–171, 1970.
79. Hofbauer, K., and Rissel, E.: Zur Frage der Leberschädigung nach Narkosen insbesondere nach Halothan. Acta Hepatosplen. *16*:112–119, 1969.
80. Lomanto, C., and Howland, W. S.: Problems in diagnosing halothane hepatitis. J.A.M.A. *214*:1257–1261, 1970.
81. Wilkinson, C.: Postanesthetic hepatic dysfunction. Arch. Surg. *101*:359–362, 1970.
82. Durkin, M. G., Brick, I. B., and Schreiner, G. E.: Fatal hepatic necrosis following penthane anesthesia. (Abstract.) Gastroenterology *50*:420, 1966.
83. Klein, N. C., and Jeffries, G. H.: Hepatotoxicity after methoxyflurane administration. J.A.M.A. *197*:1037–1039, 1966.
84. Lischner, M. W., MacNabb, G. M., and Galambos, J. T.: Fatal hepatic necrosis following surgery. Possible relation to methoxyflurane anesthesia. Arch. Intern. Med. *120*: 725–728, 1967.
85. Elkington, S. G., Goffinet, J. A., and Conn, H. O.: Renal and hepatic injury associated with methoxyflurane anesthesia. Ann. Intern. Med. *69*:1229–1236, 1968.
86. Panner, B. J., Freeman, R. B., Roth-Mayo, L. A., et al.: Toxicity following methoxyflurane anesthesia. 1. Clinical and pathological observations in two fatal cases. J.A.M.A. *214*:86–90, 1970.
87. Katz, S.: Hepatic coma associated with methoxyflurane anesthesia. Report of a case. Amer. J. Dig. Dis. *15*:733–739, 1970.
88. Brenner, A. I., and Kaplan, M. M.: Recurrent hepatitis due to methoxyflurane anesthesia. New Eng. J. Med. *284*:961–963, 1971.
89. Reynolds, E. S., Brown, B. R., Jr., and Vandam, L. D.: Massive hepatic necrosis after fluroxene anesthesia—a case of drug interaction? New Eng. J. Med. *286*:530–531, 1972.
90. Popper, H., and Schaffner, F.: *Liver: Structure and Function*. New York, Blakiston Division, McGraw-Hill Book Company, 1957, pp. 411–412.
91. Schmid, M., Hefti, M. L., Gattiker, R., et al.: Benign postoperative intrahepatic cholestasis. New Eng. J. Med. *272*:545–550, 1965.
92. Kantrowitz, P. A., Jones, W. A., Greenberger, N. J., et al.: Postoperative hyperbilirubinemia simulating obstructive jaundice. New Eng. J. Med. *276*:591–598, 1967.
93. Geller, W., and Tagnon, H. J.: Liver dysfunction following abdominal operations. The significance of postoperative hyperbilirubinemia. Arch. Intern. Med. *86*:908–916, 1950.
94. Sims, J. L., Morris, L. E., Orth, O. S., et al.: The influence of oxygen and carbon dioxide levels during anesthesia upon postsurgical hepatic damage. J. Lab. Clin. Med. *38*: 388–396, 1951.
95. Gall, E. A.: Report of the Pathology Panel, National Halothane Study. Anesthesiology *29*:233–248, 1968.
96. Simpson, B. R., Strunin, L., and Walton, B.: The halothane dilemma: A case for the defense. Brit. Med. J. *4*:96–100, 1971.
97. Bunker, J. P., and Blumenfeld, C. M.: Liver necrosis after halothane anesthesia. Cause or coincidence? New Eng. J. Med. *268*:531–534, 1963.
98. Schaffner, F.: Diagnosis of drug-induced hepatic damage. J.A.M.A. *191*:466–469, 1965.
99. Doniach, D.: Cell-mediated immunity in halothane hypersensitivity. New Eng. J. Med. *283*:315–316, 1970.
100. Cohen, P. J.: Response of human immunoglobulins to halothane anesthesia. (Abstract.) Fed. Proc. *31*:534, 1972.
101. Park, S. K., Brody, J. I., Wallace, H. A., et al.: Immunosuppressive effect of surgery. Lancet *1*:53–55, 1971.

102. Popper, H., and Schaffner, F.: Drug-induced hepatic injury. Ann. Intern. Med. 51:1230, 1959.
103. Popper, H., Rubin, E., Gardiol, D., et al.: Drug-induced liver disease: A penalty for progress. Arch. Intern. Med. 115:128–136, 1965.
104. Schaffner, F., and Raisfeld, I. H.: Drugs and the liver: A review of metabolism and adverse reactions. In Stollerman, G. H. (ed.): *Advances in Internal Medicine.* Vol. 15. Chicago, Year Book Medical Publishers, 1969. pp. 221–251.

Evidence for Halothane Hepatotoxicity Is Equivocal

B. R. SIMPSON, L. STRUNIN, and B. WALTON

The London Hospital and King's College Hospital, London

"When the dust passes, thou wilt see whether thou ridest a horse or an ass."

Even moderate opinion in the United States seems to have accepted the Klatskin and Kimberg report as proof of hypersensitivity to halothane.[1,2] At first sight the evidence of this case report is impressive, but it does not withstand careful scrutiny.

Klatskin and Kimberg[3] described the case history of an anesthesiologist who initially developed jaundice which was diagnosed as infectious hepatitis. During the following year he had relapses which appeared to be related to his practice as an anesthesiologist. When challenged with a subanesthetic dose of halothane, he developed severe aching in the legs, a shaking chill, fever and malaise—jaundice did not occur. His liver function returned to normal two weeks later. Klatskin and Kimberg stated "each of the relapses coincided with the patient's return to work and re-exposure to halothane." This is not the case. The data presented are liberally sprinkled with anomalies as follows: The relapse provoked by increased physical activity is suggestive of chronic active hepatitis.[4] For a patient who, on being "challenged" with halothane, developed symptoms within hours, it is strange to find that in January, 1963, he was at work for two weeks before a further relapse! Again, following treatment with prednisone from February to July, 1963, the anesthesiologist remained at work until December of that year without problems. Yet between January, 1966, and September, 1967, "symptoms and the functional abnormalities responded to prednisone, but promptly recurred whenever it was discontinued." It is of considerable interest that in January, 1964, the subject took up a post as an anesthesiologist in Florida for a period of two years without a further relapse occurring, "but was exposed to halothane only occasionally." However, halothane has been detected in the expired air[5, 6] and the blood of operating room personnel, and metabolites have been found in their urine. Furthermore, it is known that operating room air and the rubber tubing from anesthetic machines used to administer halothane contain measurable concentrations of halothane.[5, 7] Therefore, once halothane has been used in an operating area, the anesthesiologist is exposed to it even if he does not actually administer halothane himself. In December, 1965, he returned to his former home in New Jersey, and within weeks of taking up a new appointment in which he was using halothane regularly he had a three-week episode of high fever and dry cough accompanied by a further relapse; again, however, it must be pointed out that infection is known to aggravate chronic active hepatitis.[4]

Are the authors perhaps suggesting that hypersensitivity has now become a dose-related phenomenon? Or are they proposing a new syndrome of hypersensitivity which waxes and wanes to fit the facts of their case history? It would be hardly less facile to hypothesize that perhaps the anesthesiologist concerned was allergic to New Jersey!

The Klatskin and Kimberg case had been preceded by another report by Belfrage and his colleagues in 1966[8] of an ostensibly sensitive anesthetist. It was not possible to assess the reliability of the diagnosis made in this latter case as the short letter to The Lancet contained only a limited case history. The importance of comprehensive information can be illustrated by the case of the laboratory technician who was reported to have developed hypersensitivity to halothane as a result of repeated exposure to halothane while administering the agent to experimental animals.[9] We are currently examining this case in greater depth, and to date we have discovered that, at the relevant time, the technician was undergoing dental treatment from a dentist who resterilizes his own syringes and needles by boiling. The technician received some 16 local analgesic injections, 10 of them before the first attack of jaundice. Furthermore, serum from this patient, tested in the Clinical Laboratories of The London Hospital,[10] was positive for smooth muscle antibody (S.M.A.) at a dilution of 1 in 20. Up to the present, S.M.A. has not been described in association with "halothane hepatitis," but it is found in 87 per cent of patients suffering from viral hepatitis.[11]

To substantiate their diagnoses, both Belfrage and his colleagues, and Klatskin and Kimberg report ostensibly positive halothane challenges. The anesthesiologist involved in the former report, having been jaundiced two months previously, developed malaise, fever, myalgia, and abnormal liver function tests following halothane challenge. He did not become jaundiced, and three weeks later his liver function tests had returned to normal.

Similarly, the anesthesiologist in the Klatskin and Kimberg report was subjected to a subanesthetic dose of halothane for five minutes. Some four hours later he developed severe aching in the legs, a shaking chill, pyrexia, and malaise, but he also did not become jaundiced and two weeks later his liver function tests had returned to normal. The discrepancy between this response and his response to the many and prolonged exposures to subanesthetic concentrations of halothane in the operating room has already been discussed. Babior and Trey[12] have suggested that drug-induced hepatitis may be differentiated from relapsing viral hepatitis according to criteria listed in Table 1. Into which category do these two anesthesiologists appear to fit?

Table 1.

RECURRENT DRUG-INDUCED HEPATITIS	RELAPSE VIRAL HEPATITIS
Jaundice usual	Jaundice rare
Hepatitis subsides rapidly	Hepatitis of 2 to 3 weeks' duration

Furthermore, since the Klatskin and Kimberg subject relapsed after increasing physical activity, a respiratory infection, and transatlantic air travel, is it really surprising that he should also relapse nonspecifically to a halothane challenge after an overnight fast when unpremedicated, and aware that his career and perhaps the material welfare of his family depended on the result of the investigation to which he was to be subjected?

We therefore do not accept that hypersensitivity to halothane has been established either by the case histories referred to above or by evidence which will be discussed later in this paper. The possibility of a cause and effect relationship between halothane and postoperative liver dysfunction cannot be denied. We have, however, become increasingly uncomfortable about the quality of the evidence put forward to support this concept.

Many factors other than the anesthetic agent may be involved when a patient develops liver dysfunction following anesthesia and surgery. These include pre-existing liver disease or heart failure, concomitant drug therapy (e.g., antibiotics, diuretics, narcotics, steroids), hypoxia or hypotension, blood transfusion, and severe infection. In such circumstances it is hardly surprising that all anesthetic agents and techniques in common use have been incriminated.

Of particular interest is the report by Henderson and Gordon,[13] which indicated that the incidence of jaundice over the decade during which halothane was being introduced increased by a factor of four, *regardless of the anesthetic agent used*. This increase was attributed to the increasing complexity of surgical procedures and the more extensive use of blood transfusion and potentially hepatotoxic drugs, e.g., steroids and antibiotics. Perhaps this increase created the breeding ground for the post hoc ergo propter hoc line of reasoning which has linked a cause and effect relationship between halothane and the steady trickle of reports of liver damage following its introduction in 1956—the increasing number of reports correlating with the increasing use of the drug.

Nevertheless, these reports led to a number of retrospective surveys, the largest of which was the United States National Halothane Study.[14] This study reviewed retrospectively the incidence of fatal massive hepatic necrosis occurring within six weeks of anesthesia among some 850,000 patients undergoing surgery in 34 institutions, of whom about 250,000 had received halothane. Eighty-two cases of massive hepatic necrosis were recorded, but all but nine of these were considered by the expert panel to be explicable by factors other than the anesthetic agent. Seven of these nine "unexplained" cases had received halothane, of whom four had previously received the agent within six weeks of the final surgical procedure. However, four of the seven cases had previously been published, and two others were known to the participating institutions before the study began. Thus, this extensive review elicited only one new case of massive hepatic necrosis associated with halothane.

The overall incidence of massive hepatic necrosis in this study was approximately one in 10,000. This statistic is often misquoted as the incidence of halothane hepatitis;[15] however, at worst the true incidence of massive hepatic necrosis associated with halothane was seven out of 250,000 or about one in 35,000. Furthermore, the pre-existing knowledge of six of the seven cases may have further prejudiced the validity of even this statistic.

It is worth reiterating that only nine of the 82 cases of massive hepatic necrosis were felt to be attributable to the anesthetic agent, as this indicates that when severe liver damage occurs after anesthesia and surgery, in the great majority of cases the anesthetic agent will be involved only coincidentally.

In general terms the United States National Halothane Study exonerated halothane, but in fairness it must be pointed out that the opinion of the expert panel was by no means unanimous and the following caveat was issued: "Until the matter is finally settled, unexplained fever and jaundice in a specific patient following halothane administration might reasonably be considered a contraindication to its subsequent use in that patient." This statement has been repeated frequently since that time. For example, in 1971 Sherlock stated, "Unexplained postoperative fever is one of the most constant features indicative of liver damage related to halothane."[16] Furthermore, Sharpstone, Medley, and Williams[17] felt that the condition could have been avoided in 10 patients out of 11 with acute hepatitis following multiple anesthetics with halothane. Unexplained fever following the original exposure to halothane occurred in nine of these patients. However, over 60 per cent of postoperative patients developed pyrexia,[18,19] which in more than 50 per cent of such patients is unexplained.[20] Furthermore, postoperative pyrexia is as common after the use of other anesthetic agents as it is after halothane.[21] Analysis of the first 120 cases of postoperative jaundice investigated as part of a nationwide study in which we are currently involved shows that a variety of temperature patterns can be demonstrated after a previous halothane anesthetic, regardless of whether the cause is clear, e.g., massive hemolysis or stones in the common bile duct, or whether the cause is unexplained and therefore halothane might be suspected to be the cause. In particular it should be noted that a significant number of cases in the unexplained group were apyrexial after their previous halothane anesthetic (Table 2). Is it not time for this myth to be acknowledged?

With regard to the second caveat in the report on the United States National

Table 2. *London Hospital Survey of Pyrexias when Penultimate Postoperative Temperature Recorded*

	CAUSE OF JAUNDICE		APYREXIAL	"NORMAL" POST-OP. PYREXIA	PYREXIA CAUSE APPARENT	PYREXIA OF UNKNOWN ORIGIN
Patients with multiple halothane exposures	Clear	(15)	5	3	4	3
	Unexplained	(49)	22	6	11	10

° Total numbers in each group appear in brackets.

Halothane Study, a retrospective survey showed that of eight patients who were found to have become jaundiced after halothane anesthesia, four were again subjected to halothane anesthesia and in no instance did the jaundice recur.[22] From our interim data it would seem that when a patient who develops postoperative jaundice is submitted to further anesthesia and surgery it is not possible to predict the effect on liver function—regardless of the anesthetic agent or combination of agents used (Table 3). For example, the case history of one of the patients in our series reveals that a 58 year old woman developed a pyrexia of unknown origin following halothane anesthesia for a vulval biopsy. Eighteen days later she received thiopentone, suxamethonium, nitrous oxide, oxygen and d-tubocurarine for a radical vulvectomy, following which she developed fatal hepatic necrosis. The pathologist's report stated: "This is severe acute hepatitis, possibly of viral etiology, but again the changes are similar to those ascribed to halothane and other drugs." A further case history is of a patient who died following administration of three non-halothane anesthetics. Postmortem examination of the liver revealed a hepatitic picture. There is no logical support therefore for the postulate that halothane should be avoided if jaundice follows a previous use of halothane.

Halothane is now used in some 70 to 90 per cent of all anesthetics administered in countries in which it is readily available[23] and could therefore be expected to have been given to about 70 to 90 out of every 100 patients with postoperative hepatic necrosis, although extrapolating from the findings of the National Halothane Study, the drug is unlikely to have been directly involved as a cause. Since liver dysfunction after anesthesia and surgery has been demonstrated to be increasing, it is not surprising that despite the reassurance of the National Halothane Study, further studies, reviews, and leading articles have attempted to link the administration of halothane—particularly its multiple use—with liver dysfunction.

It is difficult to place the data from some of these studies in perspective; for example, Trey and his colleagues, who reported deaths from massive hepatic necrosis in 68 postoperative patients—61 of whom had received halothane—[21, 24] did not relate the number of patients who died with massive hepatic necrosis to the total number of patients who received halothane. Furthermore, 61 out of 68 correlates well with the percentage use of halothane. It must be stressed again that in the great majority of cases the agent itself will be only coincidentally involved.

Several of the surveys, including the fulminant hepatic necrosis surveillance

Table 3. *London Hospital Study of Patterns of Response to Multiple Anesthesia*

4 Patients	Halothane: Liver dysfunction
	Halothane: No liver dysfunction
2 Patients	Halothane: Liver dysfunction
	Non-halothane: Liver dysfunction
2 Patients	Non-halothane: Liver dysfunction
	Non-halothane: Liver dysfunction
1 Patient	Halothane X 2: Liver dysfunction
	Halothane: No liver dysfunction
	Halothane: Liver dysfunction

study of Trey,[24] depend on secondhand information. The risk inherent in relying on such reports is exemplified by a recent paper entitled, "Hepatic necrosis associated with halothane anesthesia"; perusal of the case histories in this paper reveals that two of the eight patients described did not, in fact, receive halothane.[25]

Hughes and Powell in 1970 reported six cases of severe liver damage in patients subjected to repeated halothane anesthesia and radiotherapy for carcinoma of the cervix within a period of two and a half years—an incidence of some 2 to 3 per cent.[26] Had this liver damage been directly related to the administration of halothane, one might reasonably have expected this to have been confirmed by other centers, halothane having been used up to the present time for approaching 100 million procedures. Furthermore, subsequent inquiry established that, in the institution concerned, syringes and needles were being resterilized by boiling. Similarly in 1968 an "outbreak" of halothane hepatitis occurred at the Royal Marsden Hospital, London, and nine cases were reported in one year. Inquiry established that at the time of the outbreak the patients concerned were among those from whom extra blood samples were being taken before, during, and after anesthesia by a doctor who became jaundiced, allegedly with viral hepatitis, around the same time. On the other hand, Samrah reported 400 patients with carcinoma of the cervix, all of whom received halothane anesthesia three times for radiotherapy without any evidence of liver dysfunction.[27]

Sharpstone and his colleagues[17] reported a series of 11 cases of postoperative jaundice in which nine patients had unexplained fever, and three had jaundice after previous halothane administration. All the patients became jaundiced after further administration of halothane, and six died of massive hepatic necrosis. Halothane was alleged to be responsible, although five of the patients had malignant disease, one had cholelithiasis with a subphrenic abscess, and one had cirrhosis of the liver. It is of particular interest that no less than five of the 11 patients described were suffering from malignant disease, as were at least five of the 15 patients with liver dysfunction following halothane anesthesia investigated by Paronetto and Popper.[28] Hepatitis is aggravated by a reduction in the immune responses such as occurs with malignancy.[29,30] Furthermore, Park et al.,[31] using the lymphocyte transformation test as an index of the immune responses, have demonstrated that the "normal" inhibition of immune responses following anesthesia and surgery is particularly protracted in patients with malignant disease. In addition, doubt has also been cast on the validity of one of the patients included in the report by Sharpstone and his colleagues (Patient 2),[17] whose liver function four days before his first anesthetic was reported as normal. However, laboratory investigations undertaken at a different hospital 14 days before the first anesthetic showed: W.B.C. 19,000 (eosinos. 3 per cent, monos. 7 per cent); E.S.R., 59 mm. in 1 hr. (Westergren); zinc sulfate turbidity, 5 units; alkaline phosphatase, 84 international K-A units per liter; aminotransferases: aspartate 23, alanine 28 IU/l.; serum proteins: total 8.6, albumin 4.4, globulin 4.2 gm/100 ml. (normal ranges for laboratory concerned: alkaline phosphatase, int. K-A units 20-90/l.; aminotransferases: aspartate 2-20, alanine 4.5-17 IU/l.).

Caution is, of course, necessary in the interpretation of these results in a patient with pyrexia of unknown origin, but when that patient subsequently died in hepatic failure it is difficult to justify the statement that "liver function had been normal before the first anesthetic." "Certainly nothing could be less controlled than a collection of isolated case reports."[32]

There remain a small number of cases for which no adequate explanation exists. Two groups of patients give cause for concern. First, overweight middle-aged patients, and second, patients subjected to multiple anesthetic exposures, often for minor surgical procedures. The latter concern was recently strengthened by Mushin and his colleagues,[23] who reported evidence which ostensibly showed that patients receiving halothane twice within a month are more likely to develop postoperative hepatic dysfunction. They reported a statistical comparison of three groups of patients: a control group of surgical patients, 54 patients reported to the Committee on Safety of Drugs (which collects reports of adverse reactions to drugs within the United Kingdom) during the period 1964-1969, and 74 patients from the literature. The latter two groups were patients who had become jaundiced after multiple administrations of halothane, and within these groups there was an apparent excess of patients who had received halothane twice within one month. Mushin and his colleagues concluded that "halothane should, if possible, be avoided in patients who have had it before, particularly if this was within the previous four weeks."

This study was based on the hypothesis that halothane hepatitis is a sensitization phenomenon, and therefore no clinical details of the patients were provided. It is important to note that all cases of jaundice associated with halothane reported to the Committee on Safety of Drugs were included. The acceptance of all these cases at face value must be considered naive, in view of the fact that adverse reactions are reported on a little yellow card, and if on the same yellow card the words *halothane* and *liver damage* appear, then the computer regurgitates this information as halothane hepatitis, regardless of any other information provided. The crux of the matter is, however, whether or not the jaundice in these cases was unexplained. The National Halothane Study[14] reported 82 cases of fatal postoperative massive hepatic necrosis, but in only nine of these did the expert panel decide that no alternative adequate explanation existed other than the anesthesia. These data suggest that only some 10 per cent of postoperative liver damage is likely to be attributable to the anesthetic agent. Similarly, in our own study, in many cases investigated, the jaundice may well be due to factors other than the anesthetic agent. It is unlikely, therefore, that all the cases reported to the Committee on Safety of Drugs were in fact unexplained, and the apparent excess figure of 68 per cent[23] of the total cases of jaundice reported or of patients who became jaundiced after two operations within a month—with an alleged cause and effect relationship with halothane—should be considerably reduced. In addition, the two groups of patients reported to the Committee and collected from the literature were limited to anesthetics repeated within 10 years, and it is therefore misleading to include in the calculations the 23 per cent of the control group who received their penultimate anesthetic more than ten years previously. Recalculation shows that 13 per cent of the control group, and not the 7 per cent stated, received two anesthetics within one month. Thus, the apparent excess of patients who became jaundiced after two operations within a month, with an alleged cause and effect relationship with halothane, may not exist. However, the high incidence of jaundice after operations repeated within a month remains a matter of concern.

A finding from the National Halothane Study[14] which perhaps has not received sufficient notice demonstrates that repeated low risk operations have an unexpectedly high mortality, regardless of the anesthetic agents used. Thus, frequently repeated operations, even of a minor nature, increase not only the risk of liver damage but also of death no matter what anesthetic agent is used. At the present time, therefore, there is no justification for the advice to refrain from repeated use of halothane within one month as suggested by Mushin and his colleagues, nor even three months as suggested by Lomanto and Howland.[33] The appropriate advice is to consider the possibility of postponing further operations in those patients most at risk, that is, patients who have shown evidence of unexplained liver dysfunction following their previous operations—regardless of the anesthetic agent used.

Klatskin[34] has listed the criteria which should be fulfilled by a drug if it is to be considered a direct hepatotoxin. These are summarized in Table 4. Halothane clearly fulfills none of these criteria. In recent times, therefore, controversy abiut halothane hepatitis has centered on four main themes: first, hypersensitivity to halothane; second, hypersensitivity to a macromolecule consisting of some hypothetic metabolite of halothane combined with a protein complex; third, hepatotoxicity of a halothane metabolite; and fourth, claims that halothane hepatitis can be differentiated from viral hepatitis.

The postulate of hypersensitivity to halothane has been advanced on the triad of clinical stigmata, the presence of antimitochondrial antibodies,[35] and the demonstration of lymphocyte transformation by halothane in patients with postoperative liver dysfunction.[28] As evidence of clinical stigmata, Doniach[36] quotes reports of "leukocytosis with eosinophilia, joint pains, rashes and bronchospasm . . . and in two cases abnormal lymphocytes similar to those seen in infectious mononucleosis have been noted in the peripheral blood." Halothane has been administered approaching 100 million times. Might it not be reasonable to expect more than two cases with abnormal lymphocytes if the relationship had been anything more than coincidental? References to joint pains, rashes, and bronchospasm are rare indeed and may have many causes. Furthermore, eosinophilia was not found in any of the 11 cases reported by Sharpstone and his colleagues.[17] Sherlock[37] includes malaise, fever, transient arthralgias, and rashes among the prodromal features of viral hepatitis, and it has been estimated that, in the United States alone, some 200 to 300 patients each year are likely to be subjected to anesthesia while incubating viral hepatitis.[38] Furthermore, subclinical viral hepatitis is about 12 times as common as overt disease,[39] so the population at hazard

Table 4. Criteria for Hepatotoxicity of a Drug

The Lesions:
1. Exhibit a distinctive histological pattern.
2. Vary in severity in direct relation to the dose.
3. Can be elicited in all individuals.
4. Are reproducible in animals.
5. Appear after a predictable and usually brief latent period following exposure.

may be considerably greater than even this figure suggests. Certainly the features mentioned by Doniach[36] have been reported occasionally in association with liver damage after halothane anesthesia, but is their relationship correlated or merely casual?

Antimitochondrial antibodies are found in a wide variety of liver diseases, e.g., primary biliary cirrhosis, active chronic hepatitis, cryptogenic cirrhosis, and chlordiazepoxide jaundice. It is possible that antimitochondrial antibodies may reflect an autoimmune response to liver damage, the implication being that liver damage releases tissue-specific antigen to which the subject may not have acquired full immunologic tolerance.

The initial report by Paronetto and Popper[28] of positive in vitro lymphocyte transformation in the presence of halothane in some patients with alleged halothane hepatitis has already been criticized.[40] As part of our study of postoperative jaundice we have repeated these tests on patients and physicians from our survey whose histories left us with the opinion that there was a high index of suspicion that halothane might be involved in the etiology of their hepatic dysfunction.[41] The responses obtained from our patients and physicians were not significantly different from the results obtained from a control group (Table 5). Thus, there is no evidence from these data to support the existence of cell-mediated hypersensitivity to halothane in our subjects, and previous work[28] has not been confirmed.

Before discussing the second and third postulates, a brief review will be presented of the new information which has become available on the metabolism of halothane. Seventy-five to 80 per cent of halothane is expired unchanged from the lungs. Trifluoroacetic acid (TFA) is the major metabolite in the liver (Table 6), and recently a second minor metabolite, trifluoroacetyl ethanolamide (TFAET) has been identified.[42, 43] The strong carbon-fluorine bond has been confirmed. Winrow and his colleagues[43] have recovered TFAET from mice dosed with TFA. Topham and Longshaw,[44] in rats and dogs, and Strunin and his colleagues,[45] in the isolated canine liver perfusion preparation, have demonstrated a progressive rise in unchanged halothane in bile during administration of halothane. TFA is present unconjugated in bile despite its small molecular weight, but neither TFAET nor other polar metabolites have been demonstrated in bile. TFA undergoes enterohepatic recirculation, which explains its long half-life in liver. The major urinary metabolite is TFA, with TFAET also present in small amounts. On

Table 5. *Preliminary Studies of Lymphocyte Transformation**

AGENT	CONCENTRATION ($\mu g./ml.$)	NORMAL SUBJECTS No.	Range	PATIENTS AND PHYSICIANS No.	Range
Phytohemagglutinin	10	11	19–349	14	22–341
Methoxyflurane	23 : 46	6	0.3–2.4	15	0.1–2.0
Diethyl ether	220 : 440	6	0.3–3.0	15	0.4–2.4
Trichloroethylene	22.5 : 45	6	0.3–1.8	15	0.3–2.1
Halothane	16 : 32	11	0.1–2.2	15	0.3–1.7

* Results expressed as index: transformation with antigen/transformation without antigen in each subject.

Table 6.

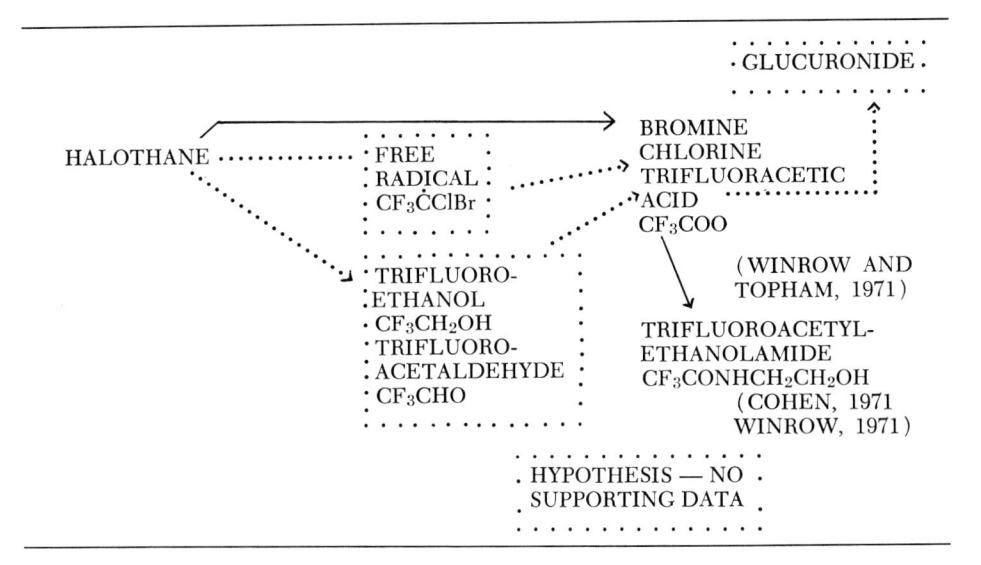

```
                                          ·········
                                          ·GLUCURONIDE·
                                          ·········
                                              ↑
                         ─────────→  BROMINE
HALOTHANE ············ ·FREE        CHLORINE
              ·.       ·RADICAL·  ········→ TRIFLUORACETIC
                ·.     ·CF₃ĊClBr·            ↗ACID        ·············
                  ·.   ·········            CF₃COO
                    ↳ ·TRIFLUORO-·                   (WINROW AND
                      ·ETHANOL                        TOPHAM, 1971)
                      ·CF₃CH₂OH   ·       ↓
                      ·TRIFLUORO-·        TRIFLUOROACETYL-
                      ·ACETALDEHYDE·      ETHANOLAMIDE
                      ·CF₃CHO     ·       CF₃CONHCH₂CH₂OH
                      ············         (COHEN, 1971
                                           WINROW, 1971)

                         ·················
                         · HYPOTHESIS — NO ·
                         · SUPPORTING DATA ·
                         ·················
```

the basis of chemical theory it has been suggested that trifluoroethanol (TFE) and trifluoroacetaldehyde (TF aldehyde) are possible intermediate metabolites. These substances, however, have not been identified in rat, mouse, guinea pig, cat, dog, marmoset, or man. Furthermore, following administration of trifluoroethanol in man, glucuronide was found in urine.[46] TFE glucuronide has never been found in man after anesthesia with halothane.

Let us turn then to the second postulate, that is, hypersensitivity to a halothane metabolite. Cohen[42] recently found two unidentified metabolites of high molecular weight in liver and argued that these could not be TFA or TFE because they were present after taking the liver to dryness, and both TFA and TFE are volatile.

Since then, however, Winrow and his colleagues[43] have deduced that at a pH of about 7, TFA would be present in liver as a nonvolatile acid salt. Appropriate extraction and recovery procedures by these workers have demonstrated these metabolites to be salts of TFA and TFAET. It is possible that Cohen was misled about the size of the molecules he isolated as a result of using a Sephadex column; it is generally accepted that polar low molecular weight compounds can produce misleading results in Sephadex columns. Rodriguez and his colleagues[35] demonstrated antimitochondrial antibodies in cases of alleged halothane hepatitis and postulated that a metabolite of halothane might form a stable complex with mitochondria. Schumer and his colleagues,[47] however, showed that halothane was not preferentially taken up by mitochondrial fractions of liver cells. There is, therefore, little supporting evidence for hypersensitivity to a halothane metabolite.

Turning now to the third postulate, that is, hepatotoxicity of a metabolite of halothane: if the causal agent were a normal metabolite it would be produced consistently and should fulfill the criteria laid down for a hepatotoxin. On the other hand, if an abnormal metabolite were involved one might expect a genetic or familial link to have been established—as with malignant hyperpyrexia—but none has been shown. The two major products of metabolism of halothane, TFA and TFAET, are nontoxic. The lethal dose of each is in excess of 2 gm./kg. orally in rats, and when death occurs the liver is not primarily involved. Furthermore, the pattern of metabolism does not vary from species to species. There is, therefore, at present little supporting evidence for hepatotoxicity of halothane metabolites.

It may well be that Klatskin's definition of a hepatotoxin is outmoded. Certainly clinical experience at centers such as Edinburgh and Newcastle in Great Britain indicates that liver damage resulting from administration of chloroform is neither consistent nor dose related. Brodie and his colleagues[48] demonstrated, *in rats*, that carbon tetrachloride incubated with liver supernate, NADPH, and oxygen was activated to a substance which readily oxidized glutathione in the presence of liver microsomes. This reaction was augmented when the microsomes were taken from rats pretreated with phenobarbitone. It is conceivable, therefore, that the mechanism by which liver damage is produced by chloroform and carbon tetrachloride is related to the capacity of metabolites of halogenated hydrocarbons containing a benzene ring to produce toxic epoxides, the characteristic centrilobular distribution of the lesions being explained by the fact that the smooth endoplasmic reticulum containing microsomal enzymes is concentrated in the central zone of liver lobules.

Considerable recent research has been aimed at attempts to find a causal mechanism for halothane hepatitis based on the acceptance that such an entity exists. In an elegant experiment Brown[49] demonstrated in vivo that, following enzyme induction, chloroform and halothane in anesthetic concentrations caused lipoperoxidation in hepatic microsomes, in contrast to fluroxene and diethyl ether, which did not. This observation, however, is unlikely to be of clinical significance since the pattern of centrilobular necrosis characteristic of chloroform-induced liver damage does not occur with halothane. Hughes and Lang[50] claim to have produced an animal model for liver damage by repeated doses of halothane in the guinea pig. Topham[51] has been unable to confirm their findings and, furthermore, he has demonstrated that 1 to 2 per cent halothane reduces blood pressure in guinea pigs by some 40 to 50 per cent. It would be interesting to see whether repeated periods of hypotension produce hepatic lesions similar to those demonstrated by Hughes and Lang.

Some recent attempts in this difficult field almost defy belief. Rosenberg and Wahlström[52] undertook an extensive immunologic investigation of alleged metabolites of halothane—which have never been shown to exist—combined with chicken globulin to demonstrate that these complexes were antigenic. Mathieu and his colleagues[53] conjugated trifluoroacetate and ethanolamine to guinea pig albumin and then demonstrated that these artificially produced complexes were immunogenic in the animals concerned. However, it has yet to be shown in man, or any other species, that such complexes occur naturally.

Sherlock[16] has claimed that halothane hepatitis can be differentiated from viral hepatitis on clinical, immunologic, and morbid anatomic grounds. We have already dealt with the clinical and immunologic aspects. The morbid anatomic differentiation appears to depend for recognition on "the experience of the pathologist," and it must be stressed that no pathologist or group of pathologists has attempted to differentiate halothane hepatitis from viral hepatitis without prior knowledge of the histories of the patients concerned. It is of further interest that authorities in the field of electron microscopy fail to agree on the expected findings in halothane hepatitis.[54-56] It would appear, therefore, that there is little justification at the present time for the statement that halothane hepatitis can be differentiated from viral hepatitis.

Let us now consider the evidence for an alternative hypothesis for postoperative jaundice. The incidence of viral hepatitis is unknown but increasing.[57] It is thought to be affecting an older age group; 80 per cent of the patients reported by Harville and Summerskill[29] were over 40 years of age, and this age group seems particularly associated with jaundice after anesthesia and surgery. As already mentioned, the ratio of overt to subclinical cases of viral hepatitis may be as high as 12:1,[39] and it has been estimated that in the United States alone some 200 to 300 patients each year are likely to be submitted to anesthesia while incubating viral hepatitis.[38]

It is now known that for both infectious and serum hepatitis oral or parenteral transmission is possible, and virus can be spread by nasopharyngeal secretions[58] and excreta.[59] Hepatitis association antigen (HAA) relates only to serum (long incubation) hepatitis.[60] Furthermore, hepatitis may occur without antigen,[61] antigen may be found only transiently,[62] the antigen may be bound by antibody,[62] and subspecies of HAA may not react with the antiserum.[62] A negative test for HAA does not, therefore, exclude serum hepatitis. Recently developed radioimmunoassay tests for HAA are considerably more sensitive, and Lander and his colleagues[63] have shown that some 10 to 15 per cent of the normal population in the United States have HAA antibodies in their serum. On the basis of an, as yet, small series of investigations in this country, Zuckerman[64] expects that comparable figures will pertain. No established test for infectious hepatitis exists, and other viruses may also cause hepatitis. It could be argued therefore that viral hepatitis cannot, at present, be excluded in any patient who develops jaundice after anesthesia and surgery.

We submit that the immunologic, metabolic, and viral data accumulated in recent months have tilted the scales sufficiently that the onus is now on the protagonists of halothane hepatitis to establish that viral disease is not involved when postoperative jaundice occurs. We will go further and state that many of us as anesthetists find that the interests of our patients are prejudiced by the social and medicolegal pressures resulting from ex cathedra statements by some of our physician colleagues. It is reasonable to expect a due sense of responsibility from these colleagues, and in the light of present evidence they should substantiate or withdraw.

Summary

At the present time there is no evidence to support the concept of a cause and effect relationship between halothane and postoperative jaundice following either single or multiple exposures. On the other hand, it is not possible to make a firm and categorical statement to the effect that halothane, or any other anesthetic agent, is never primarily involved when postoperative jaundice occurs.

Viral hepatitis cannot at present be ruled out in any individual case. Evidence suggests that the risks of postoperative liver damage, in common with the risk of death, rise precipitously if two exposures to anesthesia and surgery occur within a short period, regardless of the anesthetic agent used. This may relate to the known depression of immune responses engendered by exposure to anesthesia and surgery. In the light of this, how does one answer the question, "What anesthetic should be used in a patient who had a pyrexia of unknown origin or liver damage following a previous operation?" Operations of election should be postponed in order to lengthen the interval between the two periods of nonspecific stress. If surgery cannot be postponed, there is no logical reason for not using halothane. However, it is not possible to state categorically that if further halothane, or any other agent, is used in these circumstances, postoperative liver damage will not occur. Furthermore, if liver damage does occur, it will not be possible to state categorically that the anesthetic agent was culpable.

The choice of anesthesia must be in the best overall interests of the patient, and further detailed accurate information is required about cases of liver dysfunction following surgery and anesthesia before the mechanisms involved can be elucidated further.

References

1. Dykes, M. H. M., Gilbert, J. P., and McPeek, B.: Halothane in the United States. Brit. J. Anaesth. 44:925, 1972.
2. Little, D. M.: Editorial comment. Survey Anesthesiol. 16:449, 1972.
3. Klatskin, G., and Kimberg, D. V.: Recurrent hepatitis attributable to halothane sensitization in an anesthetist. New Eng. J. Med. 280:515, 1969.
4. Leevy, C. M., Tamburro, C. H., Sorrell, M. F., and Stone, R.: Hepatitis in the individual. J. Canad. Med. Ass. 106 (special issue):435, 1972.
5. Linde, H. W., and Bruce, D. L.: Halothane—occupational exposure. Anesthesiology 30: 363, 1969.
6. Hallen, B., Ehrner-Samuel, H., and Thomason, M.: Measurements of halothane in the atmosphere of an operating theatre and in expired air and blood of the personnel during routine anaesthetic work. Acta Anaesth. Scand. 14:17, 1970.
7. Dykes, M. H. M., and Laasberg, L. H.: Clinical implications of halothane contamination of the anesthetic circle. Anesthesiology 35:648, 1971.
8. Belfrage, S., Ahlgren, I., and Axelson, S.: Halothane hepatitis in an anaesthetist. Lancet 2:1466, 1966.
9. Johnston, C. I., and Mendelsohn, F.: Halothane hepatitis in a laboratory technician. Aust. New Zeal. J. Med. 2:171, 1971.
10. Perrin, J.: Personal communication, 1972.
11. Farrow, L. J., Holborow, E. J., Johnson, G. D., Lamb, S. G., Stewart, J. S., Taylor, P. E., and Zuckerman, A. J.: Autoantibodies and hepatitis associated antigen in acute infective hepatitis. Brit. Med. J. 2:693, 1970.
12. Babior, B. M., and Trey C.: In Dykes, M. H. M. (ed.): Anesthesia and the Liver. Boston, Little, Brown and Company, 1970, p. 337.
13. Henderson, J. C., and Gordon, R. A. The incidence of postoperative jaundice with special reference to halothane. Canad. Anaesth. Soc. J. 11:453, 1964.
14. Bunker, J. R., Forrest, W. H., Mosteller, F., and Vandam, L. D. (eds.): The National Halothane Study. A study of the possible association between anesthesia and postoperative hepatic necrosis. Washington, D.C., U.S. Government Printing Office, 1966.

15. Rosenberg, P. H.: Halothane hepatitis caused by halothane metabolites. Fluoride: Quart. J. Int. Soc. Fluoride Res. 5:106, 1972.
16. Sherlock, S.: Progress report. Halothane hepatitis. Gut 12:324, 1971.
17. Sharpstone, P., Medley, D. R. R., and Williams, R.: Halothane hepatitis—A preventable disease? Brit. Med. J. 1:448, 1971.
18. Klion, F. N., Schaffner, F., and Paronetto, F.: Clinical advances in diagnosis of halothane induced hepatitis. Gastroenterology 56:409, 1969.
19. Carney, F. M. T., and Van Dyke, R. A.: Halothane hepatitis—A critical review. Anesth. Analg. Curr. Res. 51:135, 1972.
20. Dykes, M. H. M.: Unexplained postoperative fever—Its value as a sign of halothane sensitization. J.A.M.A. 216:641, 1971.
21. Trey, C., Lipworth, L., Chalmers, T. C., Davidson, C. S., Gottlieb, L. S., Popper, H., and Saunders, S. J.: Fulminant hepatic failure. New Eng. J. Med. 279:798, 1968.
22. Dykes, M. H. M., Walzer, S. G., Slater, E. M., Gibson, J. H., and Ellis, D. S.: Acute parenchymatous hepatic disease following general anaesthesia. J.A.M.A. 193:339, 1965.
23. Mushin, W. W., Rosen, M., and Jones, E. V.: Post-halothane jaundice in relation to previous administration of halothane. Brit. Med. J. 1:18, 1971.
24. Trey, C., and Davidson, C. S.: Co-operative study of fulminant hepatitis. Clin. Res. 2: 462, 1969.
25. Peters, R. L., Edmonson, H. A., Reynolds, T. B., Meister, J. C., and Curphey, T. J.: Hepatic necrosis associated with halothane anesthesia. Amer. J. Med. 47:748, 1969.
26. Hughes, M., and Powell, L. W.: Recurrent hepatitis in patients receiving multiple halothane anesthetics for radium treatment of carcinoma of the cervix uteri. Gastroenterology 58:790, 1970.
27. Samrah, M. E.: Liver damage after halothane. Brit. Med. J. 2:1736, 1963.
28. Paronetto, F., and Popper, H.: Lymphocyte stimulation induced by halothane in patients with hepatitis following exposure to halothane. New Eng. J. Med. 283:277, 1970.
29. Harville, D. D., and Summerskill, W. H. J.: Surgery in acute hepatitis. Causes and effects. J.A.M.A. 184:257, 1963.
30. Fenster, L. F.: Viral hepatitis in the elderly. An analysis of 23 patients over 65 years of age. Gastroenterology 49:262, 1965.
31. Park, S. K., Wallace, H. A., Brody, J., and Blakemore, W. S.: Immunosuppressive effect of surgery. Lancet 1:53, 1971.
32. Dykes, M. H. M.: In Anesthesia and the Liver. Boston, Little, Brown and Company, 1970, p. 179.
33. Lomanto, C., and Howland, W. S.: Problems in diagnosing halothane hepatitis. J.A.M.A. 214:1257, 1970.
34. Klatskin, C.: Toxic and drug induced hepatitis. In Schiff, L. (ed.): *Diseases of the Liver*. 3rd ed. Philadelphia, J. B. Lippincott Co., 1969, p. 498.
35. Rodriguez, M., Paronetto, F., Schaffner, F., and Popper, H.: Antimitochondrial antibodies in jaundice following drug administration. J.A.M.A. 208:148, 1969.
36. Doniach, D.: Cell mediated immunity in halothane hypersensitivity. New Eng. J. Med. 283:315, 1970.
37. Sherlock, S.: *In Diseases of the Liver and Biliary System*. Oxford, Blackwell Scientific Publications, 1968.
38. Dykes, M. H. M., and Bunker, J. P.: Hepatotoxicity and anesthetics. Pharmacol. Physicians 4:1, 1970.
39. Eisenstein, A. B., Aach, R. A., Jacobsohn, W., and Goldman, A.: Infectious hepatitis in a general hospital. J.A.M.A. 185:171, 1963.
40. Bruce, D. L., and Raymon, F.: Test for halothane sensitivity. New Eng. J. Med. 286: 1218, 1972.
41. Walton, B., Dumonde, D. C., Williams, C., Jones, D., Strunin, J. M., Layton, J., Strunin, L., and Simpson, B. R.: Failure to demonstrate increased lymphocyte transformation in patients with postoperative jaundice and physicians with alleged halothane hypersensitivity. J.A.M.A., 1973.
42. Cohen, E. N.: Metabolism of volatile anesthetics. Anesthesiology 35:193, 1971.
43. Winrow, M., and Topham, J.: Unpublished data.
44. Topham, J., and Longshaw, S.: Studies with halothane 1. Distribution and excretion of halothane metabolites in animals. Anesthesiology 37:311, 1972.
45. Strunin, L., Strunin, J. M., and Simpson, B. R.: Unpublished data.

46. Cascorbi, H. F., and Blake, D. A.: Trifluoroethanol and halothane biotransformation in man. Anesthesiology 35:493, 1971.
47. Schumer, W., Erue, P. R., Obernolte, R. P., Bombeck, D. T., and Sandove, M. S.: The effect of inhalation of halogenated anesthetics on rat liver mitochondrial function. Anesthesiology 35:253, 1971.
48. Brodie, B. B., Cho, A. K., Krishna, G., and Reid, W. D.: Drug metabolism in man: Past, present, future. Ann. N.Y. Acad. Sci. 179:11, 1971.
49. Brown, B. R.: Hepatic microsomal lipoperoxidation and inhalation anesthetics. Anesthesiology 36:458, 1972.
50. Hughes, H. K., and Lang, C. M.: Hepatic necrosis produced by repeated administration of halothane to guinea pigs. Anesthesiology 36:466, 1972.
51. Topham, J.: Personal communication, 1972.
52. Rosenberg, P. H., and Wahlström, T.: Hapten function of halothane metabolites. Abstracts of papers presented at the Fifth World Congress on Anaesthesiology. Amsterdam, Excerpta Medica: Int. Congress Series 261:112, 1972.
53. Mathieu, A., di Padua, D., and Mills, J.: A test to avert halothane hepatitis? Med. World News 13:22, 1972.
54. Klion, F. M., Schaffner, F., and Popper, H.: Hepatitis after exposure to halothane. Ann. Intern. Med. 71:467, 1969.
55. Keeley, A. F., Trey, C., Marcon, N., Iseri, O. A., and Gottlieb, L. S.: Anicteric halothane hepatitis: Histologic and ultrastructural lesion associated with postoperative fever in two patients. Gastroenterology 58:965, 1970.
56. Uzunalimoglu, B., Yardley, J. H., and Boitnott, J. K.: The liver and mild halothane hepatitis. Amer. J. Path. 61:457, 1970.
57. McCollum, R. W.: Epidemiologic patterns of viral hepatitis. Amer. J. Med. 32:657, 1962.
58. Krugman, S., and Giles, J. P.: Viral hepatitis. J.A.M.A. 212:1019, 1970.
59. Chalmers, T. C., and Alter, H. J.: Management of the asymptomatic carrier of the hepatitis associated antigen. Tentative considerations of the clinical and public health aspects. New Eng. J. Med. 285:987, 1971.
60. Prince, A. M., Hargrove, R. L., Szmuness, W., Cherubim, C. E., Fontance, V. J., and Jeffries, G. H.: Immunological distinction between infectious and serum hepatitis. New Eng. J. Med. 282:987, 1970.
61. Blumberg, B. S., Sutnick, A., and London, W. T.: Australia antigen as a hepatitis virus. Amer. J. Med. 48:1, 1970.
62. Editorial: More about Australia antigen and hepatitis. Lancet 2:347, 1970.
63. Lander, J. J., Alter, H. J., and Purcell, R. H.: Frequency of antibody to hepatitis-associated antigen as measured by a new radioimmunoassay technique. J. Immunol 106:1166, 1971.
64. Zuckerman, A. J.: Personal communication, 1972.

Comment

The Hepatotoxicity of Halothane

If in debating a controversial subject, the object is to present extreme opposing positions, the authors of the foregoing papers on halothane hepatitis succeed admirably. These presentations read more like legal briefs than scientific monographs; indeed, these very issues are currently being widely argued before juries throughout the country.

As an example of how far apart are the respective authors' opinions, Schaffner would have us believe that there are several hundred known cases of halothane hepatitis, whereas Simpson and his colleagues suggest that there are none, or at least, none proved. Schaffner recounts in detail the evidence, much of it circumstantial, that there is a halothane-associated hepatic lesion, and he develops the by now well known thesis that the mechanism is one of delayed sensitization (a hypothesis for which, of course, he is largely responsible). Schaffner appears to entertain no other possible interpretation of the clinical data nor any other possible mechanism of action. Simpson and his associates systematically attempt to discredit this same body of evidence, which they do to their own obvious satisfaction. Where Schaffner sees no limitations to the data available, Simpson seems to see only limitations.

As a basis for debate the two papers are strong and useful. They contain almost all the arguments representing their respective polar positions. Unfortunately the line between hyperbole acceptable for purposes of debate and distortion of fact is occasionally blurred; this is true particularly in the sections on metabolism and cellular effects which include errors, incorrect references, and misquotes.

The heart of the controversy—the circumstance that makes controversy possible—is the fact that the clinical syndrome cannot be diagnosed with any certainty. Halothane hepatitis is clinically indistinguishable from viral hepatitis. Diagnostic criteria have been suggested by Schaffner and others, but their applicability or specificity have certainly not been established. Perhaps the best evidence that halothane hepatitis exists at all consists of the two anesthesiologists referred to in each paper who suffered from relapsing hepatitis, who recovered following removal from the operating room exposure to anesthetic agents, and each of whom suffered an acute relapse on subsequent deliberate "challenge" exposure to halothane. By questioning the validity of these two dramatic case reports, reports which have been widely accepted at face value, Simpson and his associates doubtless risk losing credibility in the eyes of "reasonable" physicians. Yet it is possible, as they suggest, that the relapse the two anesthesiologists suffered was simply a nonspecific response to stress. Indeed, I have often wondered what would have happened if they had been challenged with cyclopropane rather than halothane. But they were not; and therefore we have to live with the data, such as they are, and with the one to two dozen additional reasonably well documented patients who have suffered liver dysfunction or failure after the administration of halothane anesthesia on two or more occasions.

Simpson and his associates write these cases off as not passing the ultimate test of scientific proof. Unfortunately most of the practice of medicine is based upon less than perfect data and, indeed, the case for the existence of a halothane-induced hepatic lesion, rare though it may be, is better than most of the evidence on which we must act, on which we must make medical decisions.

In the matter of medical decisions, the authors again display a wide divergence of opinion. Schaffner expresses the opinion that "halothane is absolutely contraindicated in patients who have become febrile or jaundiced in the second week after previous exposure." Simpson and his colleagues, on the other hand, would impose no restraints on the use of halothane, for single or repeated procedures, and even if jaundice were to have been observed after a previous administration. To take this latter course would certainly be to fly in the face of a broad consensus on which most internists and anesthesiologists would agree—a consensus which Simpson himself ruefully acknowledges in his introduction. Neither advice is really very satisfactory; to accept Schaffner's proscription of the use of halothane in any patient who may have been "febrile in the second week after previous exposure" is tantamount to proscribing the second use of halothane in any patient, since almost all patients have some fever following any operation.*

The argument is thus reduced to whether halothane should ever be used on more than one occasion. Schaffner expresses an opinion widely held by internists that halothane "should not be used when repeated operations are necessary in a short period of time." The evidence offered by Schaffner and others in support of this pronouncement does not survive statistical scrutiny, as Simpson points out. (Simpson is correct in his interpretation of the mortality data of the National Halothane Study, which show that overall death rates rise rapidly with repeated surgery, regardless of anesthetic agent. Indeed, buried in the Final Report of the Study are data which show that overall death rates for two or more operations within six weeks were as low or lower when halothane was used for both as when any other anesthetics or combinations of anesthetics were used; this effect was equally true for low, mid, and high risk operations.)

If there is any point of potential agreement between Schaffner on the one hand and Simpson and his colleagues on the other, I believe it would be this: halothane should be used for specific indications. And if we, as anesthesiologists, have failed, it has been in not giving adequate attention to the definition of indica-

---

* Limiting attention to the second week is an interesting refinement of previous views; this may help to eliminate some false positives but, by excluding the first week, can conceivably miss some true positives.

tions for the use of halothane; and we have certainly failed to transmit our views to our medical colleagues. It is astonishing, in this regard, that Schaffner, a physician who has participated in the halothane dialogue throughout the past decade, expresses the opinion that halothane "should be avoided for all minor procedures," for it is in exactly such short, minor operations that the special advantages of halothane are most apt to be useful. I do not blame Dr. Schaffner for not coming to the operating room to observe first hand the advantages of this superb agent; but I do blame myself and my colleagues for our failure to educate him and other physicians.

Let us agree, then, that halothane should be used for specific indications—indications which should be fairly broad, and which I will not attempt to detail at this time. We should also agree that halothane should *not* be used when specifically contraindicated. Internists and anesthesiologists—Dr. Simpson and his colleagues apparently excepted—are almost unanimous in their agreement that halothane should not be used in a patient who has suffered liver damage following a previous exposure to halothane, and for which no reasonable explanation (multiple transfusions, biliary tract injury, cirrhosis, and so forth) is available. And I believe that Dr. Schaffner himself would accept the suggestion that fever "in the second week after previous exposure," rather than an absolute contraindication, be considered the basis for the most careful diagnostic scrutiny, whatever surgery or anesthetic is in prospect.

It seems likely that the next few years will see an elucidation of the mechanism of halothane-induced liver injury, assuming, as I think we must for the moment, that it exists at all. Or, perhaps, a better anesthetic drug will come along to replace halothane; none is available now. In the meantime, a moderate position would seem to be in order—halfway between the positions presented herein ought to be just about right.

JOHN P. BUNKER

23

The Treatment of Acute Granulocytic Leukemia

The Need for Aggressive Management
  by James F. Holland

The Tempered Approach
  by William H. Crosby

The Need for Aggressive Management

JAMES F. HOLLAND

Mount Sinai School of Medicine, New York

In any simplistic dichotomy of therapists, it is tempting to make the division between those who utilize the powder puff and those who employ the sledge hammer, as if these two types really existed and as if there were no middle ground. Although never having been accused of belonging to the "marshmallow" brigade, I do not advocate the use of any medication in practice, the toxic effect of which on some patients in a group is such as to outweigh the advantages for the remaining patients. In diseases in which therapy is not effective for nearly every patient, however, the costs (toxic effects) of treatment may well be manifest without corresponding individual benefit among the nonresponding patients. This is true for all types of therapy and mandates a consideration of therapeutic effects on groups of patients in addition to the effects on a single patient in question.

Acute myelocytic leukemia is the composite term for a fatal disorder characterized by neoplastic production of a progeny of limited heterogeneity from myeloid stem cells (whose relative degree of lack of maturation may characterize several subtypes of disease) together with deficient production of other normal progeny. The natural history of the disease from diagnosis to culmination is brief and frequented by infections and bleeding. Outriding cases that "do very well" without treatment are rare. They become the subject of anecdotal examples, because through repeated seeing, they are planted and even grow in the memory. Such cases of smouldering acute leukemia occur among the aged and are recognizable by a considerable maturation of the marrow infiltrate (or preservation of some normal-appearing marrow elements). They may be characterized by symptomatic anemia for several months before terminating in the more classic aggressive disease. More than 85 per cent of patients with acute myelocytic leukemia (AML) do not behave this way, however.[1]

Since it has been known for 20 years that remissions of AML can be produced with drug therapy, the choice of whether or not to treat would have seemed an easy one. Indeed, the most important influence determining survival in a particular patient is whether temporary remission of his disease can be accomplished by drug therapy.[1] Complete remission (an arbitrary definition, rather widely accepted, is reduction in tumor mass and restitution of normal hematopoiesis together with normal laboratory, physical, and symptomatic status) is associated with the longest survival times. Lesser degrees of amelioration evident as partial remission or improvement also impart survival advantage compared to those who do not improve (Fig. 1). The desideratum, then, is how most assuredly to achieve remission status for a particular patient.

The prognostication for individual patients with AML is difficult. If the physician knew in advance which drugs would be effective and which not, this essay would be superfluous. Such intelligent selection for the individual patient is not yet a captured art. It has been possible to grope toward this goal by formulation of therapeutic programs that are of progressively greater utility for groups of patients, however. Thus, discovery of treatment plans that elicit response in 50 per cent of all patients affords a randomly selected individual one chance in two of remission.

Certain characteristics of the patient or the disease have been recognized which modify response rate and survival during therapeutic trials in AML. Principal among these are age, performance status, and "extent of disease," manifest by certain hematologic values.[1] With each advancing decade the response rate decreases, although impressive therapeutic responses may occur in patients in their 70's[2] (Fig. 2). Survival shortens with each decade also, but more than by just the subtraction implied by fewer remissions (Fig. 3). Such commonplace

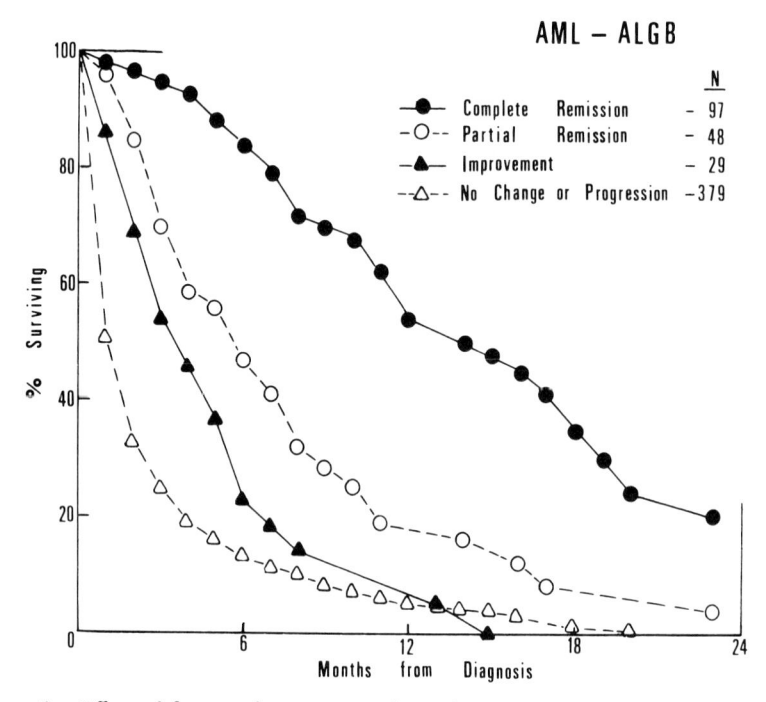

Figure 1. Effect of degree of response to chemotherapy on survival in patients with acute myelocytic leukemia. (From Ellison, R. R.: *In* Holland, J. F., and Frei, E., III (eds.): Cancer Medicine. Philadelphia, Lea & Febiger, 1973.)

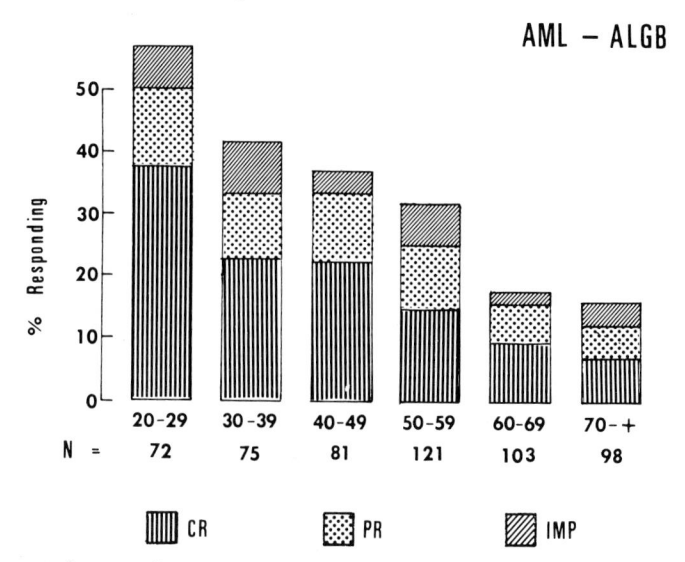

Figure 2. Influence of age on response rates to chemotherapy in patients with acute myelocytic leukemia. CR = complete remission; PR = partial remission; IMP = improvement. (From Ellison, R. R.: *In* Holland, J. F., and Frei, E., III (eds.): Cancer Medicine. Philadelphia, Lea & Febiger, 1973.)

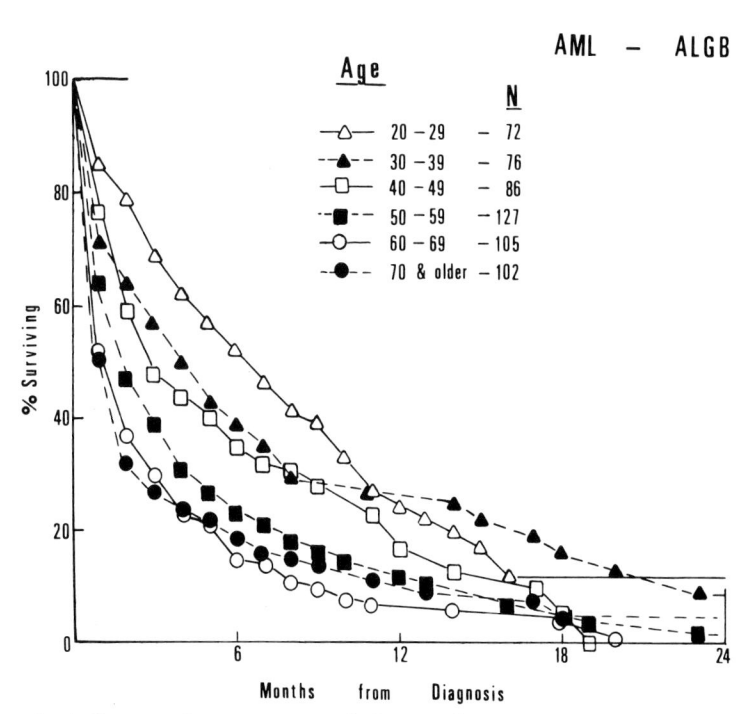

Figure 3. Influence of age on survival during chemotherapy of acute myelocytic leukemia. (From Ellison, R. R.: *In* Holland, J. F., and Frei, E., III (eds.): Cancer Medicine. Philadelphia, Lea & Febiger, 1973.)

phenomena of the disease and its treatment as sepsis, pneumonia, bleeding, anemia, fever, and drug toxicity precipitate fatal decompensation of normal organ function in the aged much more often than in the young. In most published studies the death rate in the first three months of clinical acute myelocytic leukemia is more than half among patients greater than 50 years of age. Such deaths are not a new phenomenon attributable to new treatment procedures. They have been recorded from many large series, including those using only single agents.[1]

Performance status influences prognosis, almost as a self-defining and self-fulfilling prophecy. Those who are ambulatory and able to care for themselves survive longer and have more remissions than those who present for treatment in a severely ill or bedridden status, with all that that impaired performance may imply about complicating illness, or virulent disease, and foreshortened opportunity to respond to therapy.[1] Extreme obesity in women has been reported to impair prognosis, perhaps more from difficulties in personal hygiene and care during severe illness than from pharmacologic considerations of drug dosage and distribution.[3]

Certain hematologic values have been found of favorable prognostic importance in AML:[1] a platelet count more than 100,000/cu. mm., a hemoglobin concentration more than 7 gm. per cent, and (particularly in those under 40) a leukocyte count less than 50,000/cu. mm. Auer rods convey a favorable prognosis for survival,[4] as does a hyperdiploid karyotype.[5] Cytologic differentiation into myeloblastic, monocytoid, or erythroblastic subtypes has not significantly affected response rate to modern drug regimens, and even promyelocytic leukemia, hitherto catastrophic, is therapeutically responsive to daunorubicin.[6]

Immunologic competence, measured by several nonroutine but simple clinical and laboratory parameters, has also been shown by Hersh and co-workers[7] to influence prognosis substantially.

A physician can do little about the natural determinants of prognosis (aside, perhaps, from public education) until the symptoms have disturbed the patient enough to cause him to seek medical aid. He can, however, make a correct diagnosis without delay and initiate the best possible treatment before the disease causes further disability or further compromise of normal organ function, thus jeopardizing eventual therapeutic benefit.

The patient and physician decisions at this point are critical, since the treatments that have been advocated are different in their values:

Supportive Care Only

No data exist of which I am aware that describe an *unselected* series of patients managed only by red blood cell transfusions, platelet transfusions, and antibiotics. Very rarely I have encountered an old patient with smouldering acute leukemia in whom anemia caused angina or congestive failure as the only significant clinical problem, and in whom for a few months only red cell transfusions seemed to be the best therapy to choose. When incipient granulocytopenia or incipient thrombocytopenia appear they premonish more difficult complications per se, and more difficulty during treatment; therapy directed at the neoplasm is prudent before spontaneous bleeding and infection occur.

"Gentle" Care

This pejorative term invites the concept that other treatment is rough or callous. It usually implies oral treatment with 6-mercaptopurine, and its advantages in outpatient management and minimum disruption to the family are cited. I believe this is so transient as to be illusory, for unfortunately only about 15 per cent of patients respond.[1]

Aggressive Care

The best possibility for the individual patient to survive the longest is to obtain a remission (Fig. 1). The nonremission state is complicated by all the clinical manifestations characteristic of untreated acute leukemia. The remission state at its worst may be punctuated by transient bouts of drug toxicity, but it is not the ordeal of florid acute leukemia. The remission state usually is compatible with normal home life and work, and for arranging one's affairs; it provides two to 24 months of additional "good time." The remission state at its best may be open-ended. Relapse-free survival exceeding five years has been documented in several patients by Burchenal[8] and Bernard et al.[9]

Induction of remission in AML in essentially every case in which it can be effected is accomplished sequentially: chemotherapeutic destruction of the leukemic infiltrate (and whatever normal differentiated cells are present), a phase of aplasia, and repopulation of the marrow with normal cells. During the latter part of the chemotherapeutic phase and the aplasia, thrombocytopenia and granulocytopenia are universal, fever may be hectic, and alimentary ulceration, sepsis, and pneumonia may occur. Maximum effort to support the patient during this time is required, for here, indeed, is the "valley of the shadow of death." No method of transforming leukemic cells to normal cells is known to me—nor do I believe this is a likely prospect. In today's state of knowledge one must anticipate and accept responsibility for the management of the aplastic crisis, for this is intrinsic to the initial management of AML. It is here that differences in philosophy and approach among different therapists are the most apparent. The aggressive approach admits of no reticence to act concerning the diagnosis and management of infection or bleeding, and it requires that each patient be treated with "intensive-care-unit" attention. Indeed, the resources to manage such a patient require excellence in nursing, laboratory, blood bank, and antibiotic resources, not to mention an alert and committed 24-hour-a-day house staff coverage. I have previously written that the care of patients with acute leukemia is not general medicine for the general internist; without the resources, the team, and the commitment, it is better to refer such patients to a leukemia center for their initial induction.[10] The primary physician will then more likely have opportunity to participate in the maintenance phase of the treatment.

Chemotherapy

Several regimens of aggressive chemotherapy appear to have ability to induce remission in 40 to 60 per cent of the patients tested. Variations within this range are not yet persuasively different one from another because of (1) lack of direct comparison, (2) different age distribution in the population studied, (3) slightly different definitions of response, (4) the referral nature of some institutions, which superimposes a selection factor on the patient material—only those well enough to travel present there, and (5) obscure policies of the basis for exclusions from study or analyses.

Several regimens have been reported by their proponents in ample detail to be used effectively, and they are listed in Table 1.

It is indispensable to the effective implementation of these regimens that the physician consider the marrow his primary criterion of response. The peripheral blood is satisfactory only as a positive indicator; abundant leukemic infiltration may persist in the marrow even when leukemic cells have disappeared from the periphery during leukopenia. Frequent marrow examination is necessary to gauge the need for more treatment.

Most of the regimens cited make use of intermittency of administration. This allows a concentrated exposure to chemotherapy with chance for normal tissue recovery. Immunologic responsiveness is depressed for only a minimum period during chemotherapy given in this fashion.[7] This preservation of immunologic function may be of value in abetting the antileukemic effects per se, as well as in protection against opportunistic infection.

Maintenance chemotherapy after remission has been induced can be accomplished by repetition of the intermittent courses used to induce remission, or by continuous medication at lower doses, with or without reinforcement treatments.

Table 1. *Selected Intensive Regimens of Chemotherapy in Acute Myelocytic Leukemia*

DRUGS		NO. PTS.	% REMISSIONS CR	Total	REFERENCE
1. Ara-C + 2-3 mg./kg./day	TG 2.5 mg./kg./day	36	42	53	Gee et al., 1969
2. Ara-C + 100 mg./m.²/d.	TG 2.5 mg./kg./d.	66	36	47	Carey et al., 1973
3. Ara-C + 110 mg./m.²/12 hr.	TG 90 mg./m.²/12 hr.	34	70		Dowling et al., 1972
4. DNR 60 mg./m.²/d.×5		39	43		Weil and Glidewell, 1973
5. DNR 60 mg./m.²/d.×3		61	58		
6. Ara-C + 100 mg./m.²/d.	DNR 45 mg./m.²/d.×2	60	22	37	Wiernik, 1972
7. Ara-C + 2 mg./kg./d.×5	DNR 1.5 mg./kg.	23	61		Crowther, et al., 1970
8. Ara-C + 100 mg./m.²/×d.	DNR 45 mg./m.²×2	63	33	54	Hoagland and Kyle, 1972
9. Ara-C + 50 mg./m.²/8 hr.×12	Cyt 50 mg./m.²/8 hr.×12	32	41		Bodey et al., 1970
10. Ara-C + 50 mg./m.²/8 hr.×12 +VCR 2 mg.×1	Cyt 50 mg./m.²/8 hr.×12 +Pred. 200 mg./m.²/×4	19	53		Bodey et al., 1970

Current Research

All the foregoing discussion and results are applicable to clinical chemotherapy in the practice of an experienced and committed physician. At the research level, even more intensive programs are under study. The value of atmospheric sterile filtration and barrier isolation to eliminate environmental contamination[11] appears established in prospective comparative studies with[12, 13] and without[12] nonabsorbable antibiotics. Thus, it may soon prove an economy of major importance to protect against the hazard of fatal sepsis during the aplastic drug-induced crisis by manipulating the environment. Such additional protection against infection should allow treatment programs of greater intensity and duration, with the minimum prospect of greater effect on patients with sensitive leukemic cells, and perhaps effects on more patients whose cells are relatively refractory.

Granulocytopenia is the principal determinant of bacterial infection. Its regular production early during chemotherapy has occasioned research over the past decade[14] to circumvent the disastrous consequences of septicemia in the presence of profound granulocytopenia. A controlled clinical trial demonstrating the value of repeated large granulocyte transfusions in controlling septicemia has recently been reported.[15] Djerassi's major simplification of methodology[16] holds promise of greater availability of this "retrieval" methodology. Assuming the effectiveness of granulocyte rescue is confirmed and extended, another tool to sustain life during the difficult chemotherapy of acute leukemia will be available. Thus, platelet transfusions, new antibiotics, environmental decontamination, and granulocyte rescue will assist in prolonging survival through the aplastic crisis.

Immunotherapy has been an intriguing clinical possibility for AML since the initial report of successful immunotherapy in acute lymphocytic leukemia by Mathe and colleagues.[17] The first reports of successful experimentation in this direction in AML have appeared from England where administration of BCG and x-irradiated allogeneic myeloblasts is undertaken in patients selected at random between their brief intensive courses of maintenance chemotherapy. An impressive and significant prolongation of remission time appears to have been produced.[18] Similar approaches using only MER (methanol extracted residue of tubercle bacilli) as an immunogen[19] or enzyme-treated leukemic cells[20] are currently under study elsewhere. In all these instances the investigators have shown in their experimental design full appreciation of the need to achieve maximal reduction of leukemic body burden before initiating immunotherapy.

Thus, a broad tide of research appears to be moving toward more intensive antileukemic treatment, with attempts to prevent or correct the life-threatening disorders which occur along the way.

The definition of conservative is often in dispute. Some consider that the term applies to those who perpetuate the old traditions, perserving the status quo with a minimum of new-fangled ideas. I believe that preservation of the maximum percentage of patients for the longest period of time is the proper definition. This will require the evolving concepts, new drugs, and new techniques that are the corpus of research aimed at control and cure of acute myelocytic leukemia.

References

1. Ellison, R. R.: Acute myelocytic leukemia. In Holland, J. F., and Frei, E., III (eds.): Cancer Medicine. Philadelphia, Lea & Febiger, 1973.
2. Lee, S. L., and Rosner, S.: Treatment of AGL. (Letters to the Editor.) Arch. Intern. Med. 123:205–206, 1969.
3. Wiernik, P. H., and Serpick, A. A.: Factors affecting remission and survival in adult acute nonlymphocytic leukemia (ANNL). Medicine 49:505–513, 1970.
4. Bennett, J. M., and Henderson, E. S.: The significance of Auer rods in acute granulocytic leukemia. XIII International Congress of Hematology. Abstract Volume, 191. Munich, Lehmann Verlag, 1970.
5. Hart, J. S., Trujillo, J. M., Freireich, E. J., George, S. L., and Frei, E., III.: Cytogenetic studies and clinical correlates in adults with acute leukemia. Ann. Intern. Med. 75:353, 1971.
6. Weil, M., and Glidewell, O. (For Acute Leukemia Group B): Daunorubicin in the therapy of acute granulocytic leukemia, Cancer Res. In press, 1973.
7. Hersh, E. M., Whitecar, J. P., Jr., McCredie, K. B., Bodey, G. P., Sr., and Freireich, E. J.: Chemotherapy, immunocompetence, immunosuppression, and prognosis in acute leukemia. New Eng. J. Med. 285:1211, 1971.
8. Burchenal, J. H.: Eventual control of clinical leukemia. In Dutcher, R. M., and Chieco-Bianchi (eds.): Proceedings of the Fifth International Symposium on Comparative Leukemia Research, Padua, 1971. Basel, S. Karger, 1972.
9. Bernard, J., Jacquillat, C., and Weil, M.: Treatment of the acute leukemias. Seminars in Hematology 9:181, 1972.
10. Holland, J. F.: Who should treat acute leukemia? J.A.M.A. 209:1511, 1969.
11. Bodey, G. P., Gehan, E. A., Freireich, E. J., and Frei, E., III: Protected environment–prophylactic antibiotic program in the chemotherapy of acute leukemia. Amer. J. Med. Sci. 262:138–151, 1971.
12. Yates, J. W., and Holland, J. F.: A controlled study of isolation and endogenous microbial suppression in acute myelocytic leukemia. Cancer. In press.
13. Levine, A. S., Siegel, S. E., Schreiber, A. D., Hauser, J., Preisler, H., Goldstein, I. M., Seidler, F., Simon, R., Perry, S., Bennett, J. E., and Henderson, E. S.: Protected environments and prophylactic antibiotics: A prospective controlled study of their utility in the therapy of acute leukemia. New Eng. J. Med. 288:477–483, 1973.
14. Freireich, E. J., Judson, G., and Levin, R. H.: Separation and collection of leukocytes. Cancer Res. 25:1516, 1965.
15. Graw, R. G., Jr., Herzig, G. P., Perry, S., and Henderson, E. S.: Normal granulocyte transfusion therapy: Treatment of septicemia due to gram negative bacteria. New Eng. J. Med. 287:367, 1972.
16. Djerassi, I., Kim, J. S., Suvansri, U., Mitrakul, C., and Ciesielka, W.: Continuous flow filtration—Leukophoresis. Transfusion 12:75, 1972.
17. Mathé, G., Amiel, J. L., Schwarzenberg, L., Schneider, M., Cattan, A., Schlumberger, J. R., Hayat, M., and De Vassal, F.: Active immunotherapy for acute lymphoblastic leukemia. Lancet 1:697, 1969.
18. Crowther, D., Powles, R., and Hamilton-Fairley, G.: Personal communication, 1972.
19. Izak, G., and Weiss, D.: Paper presented at Israel Society on Hematology, 1972.
20. Holland, J. F., and Bekesi, J. G.: Unpublished data, 1973.
21. Gee, T. S., Kou, P. Y., and Clarkson, B. D.: Treatment of adult acute leukemia with arabinosyl cytosine and thioguanine. Cancer 23:1019, 1969.
22. Carey, R. W., et al. (For Acute Leukemia Group B): Comparative study of cystosine arabinoside therapy alone and combined with thioguanine, mercaptopurine, or daunomycin in acute myelocytic leukemia. Submitted for publication, 1973.
23. Dowling, M. D., Gee, T. S., Lee, B. J., Clarkson, B. D., and Burchenal, J. H.: Treatment of acute non-lymphoblastic leukemia with arabinosyl cytosine (ara-C) and 6-thioguanine (TG) every 12 hours. Proc. Amer. Ass. Cancer Res. 13:21, 1972.
24. Wiernik, P.: Unpublished ALGB Protocol 7221. Personal communication, 1972.
25. Crowther, D., Bateman, C. J. T., Vartan, C. P., Whitehouse, J. M. A., Malpas, J. S., Hamilton Fairley, G., and Scott, R. B.: Combination chemotherapy using L-asparaginase, daunorubicin and cytosine arabinoside in adults with acute myelogenous leukemia. Brit. Med. J. 4:513, 1970.

26. Hoagland, C., and Kyle, R. A. (For Acute Leukemia Group B): Unpublished data, ALGB Minutes, December, 1972.
27. Bodey, G. P., Rodriguez, V., Hart, J., et al.: Therapy of acute leukemia with the combination of arabinosyl cytosine and cyclophosphamide. Cancer Chemother. Rep. *54:* 255–262, 1970.

The Tempered Approach

WILLIAM H. CROSBY

Scripps Clinic and Research Foundation, La Jolla, California

Illness was sometimes a central theme in the books of Thomas Mann. In *The Magic Mountain* it was tuberculosis; in *The Black Swan*, ovarian cancer; and in *Doctor Faustus*, syphilis. In other books the descriptions of physicians and episodes of illness or death are memorable examples of medical writing: childbirth in *Royal Highness*, the old steward's death of uremia in *Joseph*, and the death from lobar pneumonia of Consul Buddenbrooks's old widow. Here is a part of that report:

> The struggle began afresh. Was this a wrestling with death? Ah, no, for it had become a wrestling with life for death, on the part of the dying woman. "I want—," she panted, "I want—I cannot—let me sleep! Have mercy, gentlemen—let me sleep!"
>
> Frau Permaneder sobbed aloud as she listened, and Thomas groaned softly, clutching his head a moment with both hands. But the physicians knew their duty: they were obliged, under all circumstances, to preserve life just as long as possible; and a narcotic would have effected an unresisting and immediate giving-up of the ghost. Doctors were not made to bring death into the world, but to preserve life at any cost. There was a religious and moral basis for this law, which they had known once, though they did not have it in mind at the moment. So they strengthened the heart action by various devices, and even improved the breathing by causing the patient to retch.
>
> By five the struggle was at its height. The Frau Consul, erect in convulsions, with staring eyes, thrust wildly about her with her arms as though trying to clutch after some support or to reach the hands which she felt stretching toward her. She was answering constantly in every direction to voices which she alone heard, and which evidently became more numerous and urgent. Not only her dead husband and daughter, but her parents, parents-in-law, and other relatives who had passed before her into death, seemed to summon her; and she called them all by name—though the names were some of them not familiar to her children. "Yes," she cried, "yes, I am coming now—at once—a moment—I cannot—oh, let me sleep!"

That was a hundred years ago in Germany, from a book written in the 1890's. Since that time we have begun to change our attitudes toward suffering and death from immutable illness. And some of the immutability of illness has also changed. Today there are physicians who have not yet seen lobar pneumonia.

Today there are other problems and other reasons for contributing to patients' suffering. The American writer Peter de Vries has described the course of acute leukemia quite as poignantly as Thomas Mann described pneumonia. His book, *The Blood of the Lamb*, is the story of a teen-ager and her family and their experience with leukemia and the hematologists. It is a book that should be read by those who would learn about living and dying with leukemia from the other side. One of the child's family sums it up, "So death by leukemia is now a local instead of an express. Same run only a few more stops. But that's medicine; the art of prolonging disease."

The child's father describes her death.

> Once, later that afternoon, the smile parted her lips again, this time widely enough to show that her gums were dripping. The enemy was pouring out of every crevice at last. The sight of these royal children pitted against this bestiality had always consumed me with a fury so blind I had had often to turn my face away. . . .
>
> She went her way in the middle of the afternoon, borne from the dull watchers on a wave that broke and crashed beyond our sight. In that fathomless and timeless silence one does look rather wildly about for a clock, in a last attempt to fix the lost spirit in time. I had guessed what the hands would say. Three o'clock. The children were putting their schoolbooks away, and getting ready to go home.
>
> After some legal formalities I went into the room once more to say good-bye. I had once read a book in which the hero had complained, in a similar farewell taken of a woman, that it was like saying good-bye to a statue. I wished it were so now. She looked finally like some mangled flower, or like a bird that had been pelted to earth in a storm. I knew that under the sheet she would look as though she had been clubbed to death.

Those who treat leukemia will sense the beauty of that simile.

L. J. Witts has written, "De Vries's novel is already dated, because the outlook for children with acute leukaemia has improved so greatly since the period of which he was writing [late 1950's]. Now our hopes are centered not on palliation but on cure."[1] And thus Professor Witts himself subscribes to an attitude that de Vries calls "the sacred hoax to which we are one and all committed down to the gates of death; the hoax that Everything was Fine." De Vries's novel will be dated when acute leukemia has gone like lobar pneumonia, when kids with acute lymphocytic leukemia (ALL) live to 70 and when adults with acute granulocytic leukemia (AGL) can enjoy a significant and comfortable prolongation of life. The promise of the dawn of the chemotherapeutic era 25 years ago has not yet been realized. Hope as we may, the cure of leukemia is *not* at hand. The treatment of acute leukemia is a justified brutality, justified because it can in some cases prolong life, but a brutality nonetheless. The rigors of the theory of *total kill* applied to the treatment of acute leukemia must be witnessed to be appreciated. *However ineffectual our efforts, cure must be our aim, and to achieve it every cancer cell in the patient's body must be killed.*[2] This is the credo.

After 25 years of chemotherapy of leukemia one fact seems evident: the cancer cells are tougher than the patient. The persistent optimism that pervades the literature of acute leukemia seems almost equivalent to someone's saying, "We'll soon be flying. We have only to flap our arms a little faster." The one-in-a-thousand "cures" of acute leukemia must be due to the intervention of something besides chemotherapy.[3] To a great extent it has been the insistence upon cure as today's objective that has resulted in the severity of the chemotherapeutic regimens. The problem of AGL is especially grave, because here chemotherapy is applied with appalling harshness, although it seems to do very little good.

Before the era of chemotherapy, when antibacterials and transfusion were not so well developed as now, the median life expectancy with AGL was about five months and few patients lived longer than a year.[4] Chemotherapy, especially with 6-mercaptopurine (6-MP), began to produce some remissions, but the treatment was often destructive of the remnants of normal marrow so that many patients died promptly of aplastic anemia instead of eventually of AGL.[5] By the early 1960's the median life expectancy was three months in those clinics that employed the most sophisticated therapeutic plans, and by 1966 only 35 per cent of the patients were living three months after diagnosis.[6] At the same time complete remissions were being established in about 5 per cent of patients with AGL.[7] These few beautiful responses did much to obliterate the knowledge that chemotherapy was doing more harm than good. The gradual worsening of survival was a consequence of the gradual acceptance that remissions in AGL required the complete obliteration of the leukemic marrow. The increasing fatalities were a consequence of a calculated risk: one must wipe out the marrow to make way for the remission. (Those who achieved the good remissions said that the risk had been worth it. Besides, we told ourselves, we were learning something about leukemia and chemotherapy.) Although the program was called clinical investigation, no careful attempt was made to identify and analyze the iatrogenic deaths and treatment failures. Most therapists were satisfied to bear in mind that sepsis and hemorrhage, due respectively to agranulocytosis and thrombocytopenia, are sequelae not only of therapy, but also of the disease itself.

AGL is an uncommon disease. To accumulate comparable information from many clinics categorical leukemia groups were recruited (e.g., Acute Leukemia Group B) and provided with Federal funds. Rules and protocols were established. Over the years the protocols, reflecting the philosophy of total kill, the striving to cure, have become more and more strenuous. The rules of the categorical leukemia groups require that all patients with AGL be randomized into protocol studies. AGL is regarded as one disease, and no effort is made to stage the patients with a view to modifying therapy to fit the individual case. In 1968 I questioned this policy, pointing out evidence of the variability of the disease.[8] Some cases are rather inactive and, for a time at least, need no treatment. Others are refractory so that treatment causes much damage and no benefit. Some patients, especially the elderly, cannot tolerate the rigors of protocol therapy. Why not avoid rigorous therapy where injury is certain and the possibility of remission is remote?

Response to the proposal, even by those who read beyond the title, was singularly lacking in enthusiasm.[9-12] Chemotherapists tend to be "True Believers" and the proposal was a "Heresy." Besides, it was not well timed. Results were beginning to come in from two improvements in the therapy of AGL. The intensive harvesting of platelets was the salvation of many patients who might have died from bleeding during the induction phase of chemotherapy, and experiments with the use of cytosine arabinoside (ara-C) gave promise of an improved rate of remission. It was *a whole new ball game* in AGL. It was not the time to counsel moderation.

Now, five years later the score is in on the ara-C ball game. Although the chemotherapists have scored, AGL is still champ. The remission rate is 40 to 50 per cent, and median life expectancy after diagnosis has been extended to about 10 months, double the life span with no treatment at all.* The induction process

---

* Higher remission rates are achieved by eliminating from consideration those patients who die the first day or the first week or the first month or two.

has increased in strenuousness and duration. About one third of the patients do not survive it; among the elderly the decrement is two thirds. The period of drug-induced aplasia has extended hospitalization by weeks and months, and it is a miserable experience, with fever, infections, antibiotics, diarrhea, pain, hemorrhages, transfusions, fever. . . . Most of the remissions are brief; they average about four months. One patient may have three or four of them, each with its own "rounding of the Horn"—the aplastic crisis. Yet the brief remissions do count to improve the statistics and to extend, mathematically, the length of life. And there are also a few long, glorious, disease-free remissions, the come-on that brings us crapshooters back to the blanket. Confronted with an unpredicted long remission, even the keen, scientific, computer-lovin' leukemia fighter waxes anecdotal. *And today the Judge, bless his old heart, is feeling fine and fishing in Florida. If you have doubts about how to go with AGL in old people, just ask the Judge.* In that new AGL ball game the Judge was a winner, no doubt about it. But the remission rate in patients over 50 treated on the COAP* protocol is a meager 5 per cent. The losers are not available for comment.

The treatment of AGL in the categorical clinics has progressively increased to higher levels of intensity and cost, and the end is not in sight. For example, the recent availability of machines for creaming off white cells from blood donors via leukopheresis permits significant transfusions of granulocytes. Leukotransfusion will provide justification for yet another intensification of chemotherapy and another prop for the American Cancer Society's unconscionable advertisement. *We are Close to a Cure for Leukemia.* The message raises funds and hopes, both expendable.

Blessed with funds and equipment and skilled personnel, it is evident that the categorical clinics do possess some substantial advantages.[13] Other attributes are questionable (Table 1). At the present time their protocols probe at marginal refinements in the ara-C regimen. The cost of inducing a remission in AGL is probably in excess of $10,000.

Now to the question: Experience has reinforced the knowledge that many patients do not survive eight weeks of the induction process and that cure of AGL is not now a reality or even a hope. The time seems right to ask again about the treatment of AGL.

---

* This acronym stands for a combination of drugs, administered simultaneously, consisting of cyclophosphamide, Oncovin, ara-C and prednisone. There are alternative combinations such as TRAP and POMP and CART;[3] none is any better than COAP.

Table 1. *Treatment of AGL in the Categorical Clinics*

1. It is disease oriented more than patient oriented.
2. It is cure oriented more than survival oriented.
3. It is oriented toward length of life more than quality of life.
4. It is research oriented.
5. It is inflexible.
6. It is optimistic.
7. It is analyzed to accentuate success.
8. It is expensive.

Should the Elderly Be Treated Differently?

The attack rate of AGL increases with advancing age. At the same time the rate of remission decreases, even among those who can tolerate chemotherapy; also decreased is the ability of elderly patients to withstand the rigors of the antileukemia regimens. The optimism that activates the cure-oriented programs seems especially unrealistic in treating these elderly people with AGL. Surely in this situation the name of the game should be play-for-time, not shoot-to-cure.

The ethics of risk versus benefit require particular attention in clinical situations where, on the one hand, the treatment carries a certainty of severe morbidity and a high risk of death, yet, on the other hand, the disease is often catastrophic and average life expectancy is brief. Even a slim possibility of remission may entice both doctor and patient into accepting risks that are, on analysis, indefensible. In this situation, the analysis should not be avoided.

The danger to the elderly of rigorous chemotherapy is evident in a recently completed study.[13a] Seventy-one patients above the age of 50 were treated with ara-C. There were 11 remissions. Fifty-five patients (77 per cent) died during the induction period. Median survival of the 71 was an incredible two and a half weeks.

The play-for-time hypothesis seems worth testing. The staging of patients on the basis of age should not be unthinkable. To begin with, patients over 50 could be randomized, half into a standard contemporary protocol, say COAP, the other half treated by supportive therapy plus a moderate use of chemotherapy when the leukemia is aggressive. Each case should be scored not only for remission and survival, but also on the quality of survival.

Should Quality of Survival be Measured?

In addition to measuring the hematologic and physical changes stipulated by the protocols, some effort might be made to quantify suffering. We would better understand the cost of chemotherapy if we scored and recorded such factors as how many hours the patient is febrile; how many hours with intravenous tubing; how many days on "Life Island"; how long with nose packs; size and duration of mouth and anal ulcers; how many times vomited; suicide attempts; requests for euthanasia.

The quality of remission or post-therapy existence should also be quantified. Patterson[14] has proposed a classification of clinical response that includes factors in addition to the usual "Remission" and "No Remission" (Table 2). Patterson has also listed some aspects of treatment that he—and others—regard as *debatably* worthwhile.

1. Temporary gain at expense of long-term suffering or cost.
2. The improvement of one individual at great cost to public resources.
3. Subjective versus objective evaluation.
4. Contribution to medical knowledge.

Table 2. *The Quality of Survival with Classification of Clinical Response**

	DURATION (MONTHS)	SYMPTOMATIC AND/OR FUNCTIONAL IMPROVEMENT	USEFULNESS	COST
I	>12	Complete; no medication; full function; content	Taking responsibilities; enjoying life	Great saving
II	3-12	Controlled by oral medications and functionally adequate	Real, though limited	Some saving
III	<3	Controllable with or without better functions	Overall appraisal is positive	Tolerable expense
IV		Prolongation of life without improving symptoms or function Treatment worse than disease		

* After W. B. Patterson[14]

Is the Induction Phase of Chemotherapy Too Severe?

Is it necessary always to use the full dose of myelosuppressive drugs for initial induction? Patients vary in their susceptibility to the toxicity of the drugs. Leukemia varies in susceptibility. Remissions in some cases have been induced by 400 mg. of ara-C; others have required 4 gm.[15] Would anything but time be lost if the initial doses of ara-C were half the present standard? This would allow time to identify the very susceptible patients and the very susceptible leukemias. Osgood recommended that we approach chronic granulocytic leukemia (CGL) with gradually increasing doses until the right dose is established. This technique of "titration," as he called it, avoids the aplastic accidents that occur with regimens employing "loading" doses: starting with a toxic high dose and scaling down. A modified Osgood "titration" incorporated into the treatment of AGL might reduce the decimation that is a characteristic of induction with the current AGL protocols.

Should the Criteria of Complete Remission Be Revised?

Nowadays in the reports of leukemia therapy the criteria for "complete remission" of acute leukemia are seldom stipulated. There may be statements to the effect that *remission is considered complete when the blood and bone marrow have returned to normal*, but the definition of *normal* in this context is freighted with a certain undisclosed optimism. It is possible to obtain the official Criteria for Evaluating Acute Leukemia, a mimeographed sheet, from which one can learn that a man in an official complete remission of AGL may have as little as 12 gm. of hemoglobin; he may have only 2000 granulocytes and 100,000 platelets; his marrow may contain up to 5 per cent of myeloblasts or even a total of 10 per cent of myeloblasts plus promyelocytes.[16] These substandard standards increase the number of "complete remissions," but those who soften the criteria in this manner seem to lose sight of the objective of therapy, which is to improve patients, not statistics. The prospect is no less bleak for these additional remissions. Other forms of analysis also reflect this optimism. Should anyone be cheered by the news that patients who achieve remission survive longer than those who die during induction? If we convince ourselves that we are making progress down a blind alley, do we not divert effort from the seeking of other paths through the maze?

Do Treatment Failures Deserve Attention?

The literature of leukemia chemotherapy pays scant attention to treatment failures and adverse effects of the attempts to treat. The spectrum of improvement may be presented in as many as 10 hues of graduated brilliance, but no response is *No Response*.[17] Retrospective analysis and classification of treatment and iatrogenic deaths might yield information of prognostic value. To study what we do wrong is an important way of learning what to do right.

Can AGL Be Staged on the Basis of Morphology?

The diagnosis of acute leukemia depends upon microscopy of Romanowski-stained smears of blood and bone marrow. Subdivisions of acute leukemia are also attempted, but even the primary differentiation between AGL and ALL is not always possible. Experienced microscopists frequently cannot agree. The cases they cannot identify are called "undifferentiated" or "stem-cell" or "unclassified." But cases that one man calls typical may be called something else by another. The problem was effectively delineated 10 years ago by Lee et al.[18] on the basis of a series of 43 cases of acute leukemia, classified by the submitting microscopists as *typical myeloid, typical lymphatic,* and some *difficult*. As a blind exercise in diagnosis the slides were coded and sent to 13 institutions involved in protocol studies of acute leukemia. There were 381 replies. *Nine of 42 cases failed to get any agreed diagnosis, and only a minority of cases (13 of 42) won unanimous opinions. Of the total of 381 diagnostic reports, 116 (30.4 per cent) failed to be confirmed by a clear majority of other reports. Another measure of the degree of imprecision in cytologic classification was afforded by 12 institutions reviewing 33 slides which they had originally submitted. Ten of these 33 slides (30 per cent) were classified differently in the "blind" study.*

The 10 years since Lee's report have not improved the diagnosis of acute leukemia,[19] but very little effort has been made.

This confusion means, of course, that the reports of chemotherapy of AGL are contaminated with cases of ALL, and vice versa. Does the confusion compromise the value of the results? Does the presence of unrecognized AGL increase the rate of treatment failure among those believed to have ALL? Does the confusion compromise the safety of any patient? Perhaps the child with AGL should not have his brain irradiated, and perhaps the adult with ALL need not be treated to the point of complete aplasia. If staging on the basis of morphology is essential, if it is really important to be able to tell AGL from ALL, if it is necessary to be able finally to classify undifferentiated leukemia, should we not attempt to improve differential diagnosis? To this end should research in morphology be intensified? Should training be improved?

The subclassification of AGL, like the diagnosis, depends upon the judgment of microscopists. They agree that subgroups do exist: erythroleukemia, for example, and myelomonocytic leukemia, but few of them agree on the criteria for those categories. In many clinics about 20 per cent of AGL is called myelomonocytic.[20] In other clinics the proportion is 30 or 60 or 90 per cent.[11, 21, 22] Disparity also exists in the identification of erythroleukemia. Any attempt to stage AGL on a morphologic basis is pointless until the microscopists can resolve these patterns of certitude and chaos, individual certitude with chaos overall. This will require a study of morphology that no one at present seems willing to perform or fund. It will require agreement on differences strongly held by microscopists, but regarded by chemotherapists as of little importance.

The problem, if adequately investigated, would provide evidence concerning certain clinical impressions. Freireich,[23] for example, believes that erythroleukemia is resistant to treatment. To test this would require an agreement on the definition of erythroleukemia. Bailey et al.[15] have observed that a high leukocyte alkaline phosphatase (LAP) score in myelomonocytic leukemia is a bad prognostic factor. Here the agreement must be on the definition of myelomonocytic. Other morphologic abnormalities may have prognostic import: Auer rods, vacuoles, micromyeloblasts. Morphologic research in acute leukemia may provide insights into the disease. But if morphology became a basis for staging AGL it would complicate life for the chemotherapists. At present they are content to regard AGL as one and indivisible when randomizing cases for treatment and storing them in the computer afterward. And many microscopists, certain of their ability to diagnose and classify acute leukemia, remain confident that research directed toward improvement of performance is a waste.

Even available cytochemical methods can facilitate the identification of poorly differentiated cells.[24,25] To take full advantage of the state of the art the National Cancer Institute (NCI) might establish a reference laboratory to apply these unused techniques to the diagnosis and subclassification of acute leukemia and also to intensify research into the morphology of leukemic cells and leukemic tissues. This service could provide a more accurate and consistent diagnosis and could score the abnormal variables of each case (Auer bodies, microblasts, erythroblastosis, and so forth). If any prognostic attribute emerges it might then be determined to modify the therapy of such a patient to prolong his life or to prevent unnecessary suffering. The NCI service, by returning prompt and complete reports, would provide comparisons for the performance of each participating microscopist and a basis for one improvement of our hematologic training programs.

Is Chemotherapy the Way to Go?

In conclusion I would reiterate: *The extension of time spent in toxic reaction to chemotherapy is the aspect of the aggressive treatment of acute leukemia which has become truly repellent. As more effort is exerted to prolong the patient's life span to a point of statistical significance, the striving seems somehow to miss the point of life itself. By stepping up the aggressiveness of therapy, the injury and the agony of the patient are intensified and prolonged: the infections, the bleeding, the steroid side effects, the transfusion reactions, the isolation on Life Island. There must be some point of diminishing return in the escalation, and I suspect that in the chemotherapy of AGL we are well past that point.*[8]

References

1. Witts, L. J.: Personal view. Brit. Med. J. *1*:220, 1971.
2. Bodley Scott, R.: Cancer chemotherapy—the first twenty-five years. Brit. Med. J. *4*:259–265, 1970.
3. Spiers, A. S. D.: Chemotherapy of acute leukemia. Clin. Hematol. *1*:127–164, 1972.
4. Haut, A., Altman, S. J., Cartwright, G. E., and Wintrobe, M. M.: The influence of chemotherapy on survival in acute leukemia. Blood 10:875–895, 1955.
5. Witts, L. J.: Treatment of acute leukemia in adults. Brit. Med. J. *1*:1383–1389, 1966.
6. Holland, J. F.: Progress in the treatment of acute leukemia. *In* Yamada, K. (ed.): *Recent Advances in Acute Leukemia.* Kyoto, NISSHA, 1966, pp. 117–137.
7. Fairbanks, C. F., Shanbrom, E., Steinfeld, J. L., and Beutler, E.: Prolonged remissions in acute myelocytic leukemia. J.A.M.A. 204:574–579, 1968.
8. Crosby, W. H.: To treat or not to treat acute granulocytic leukemia. Arch. Intern. Med. 122:79–80, 1968; 123:206–207, 1969.
9. Lee, S. L., and Rosner, F.: Treatment of AGL. (Letter to editor.) Arch. Intern. Med. 123:205–206, 1969.
10. Dameshek, W.: Treatment of AGL. (Letter to editor.) Arch. Intern. Med. *123*:725–726, 1969.
11. Boggs, D. R., Wintrobe, M. M., and Cartwright, G. E.: To treat or not to treat acute granulocytic leukemia. Arch. Intern. Med. *123*:568–570, 1969.
12. Fairley, G. H: The treatment of acute myeloblastic leukemia. Brit. J. Haemat. 20:567–570, 1971.
13. Holland, J. F.: Who should treat acute leukemia? J.A.M.A. 209:1511–1513, 1969.
13a. Bickers, J. N., Gehan, E. A., Freireich, E. J., Coltman, C. A., Wilson, H. E., Hewlett, J. S., Stuckey, W. J., and Van Slyck, E. J.: Arabinosyl cytosine (NSC 63878) (ara-C) in acute leukemia in adults: Effect of schedule on therapeutic response. Arch. Intern. Med. In press.
14. Patterson, W. B.: Response to treatment as measured by the quality of survival. Symposium on Criteria of Response to Therapy. Sponsored by the Cancer Clinical Investigation Review Committee of the National Cancer Institute, Bethesda, January 24, 1972.
15. Bailey, C. C., Israels, M. C. G., Brown, M. J., Geary, C. G., Whittaker, J. A., and Weatherall, D. J.: Cytosine arabinoside in the treatment of acute myeloblastic leukemia. Lancet *1*:1268–1271, 1971.

16. Acute Leukemia Cooperative Group B: Criteria for Evaluating Acute Leukemia. Bethesda, National Cancer Institute, 1969.
17. Karnofsky, D. A.: Meaningful classification of therapeutic response to anticancer drugs. Clin. Pharmacol. Therap. 2:709–712, 1961.
18. Lee, S. L., Livings, D., James, C. W., Schroeder, L., Selawry, O., and Stickney, J. M.: Morphologic classification of acute leukemias. Cancer Chemother. Rep. 16:151–153, 1962.
19. Palmer, J. G.: Definition and classification of acute leukemia. North Carolina Med. J. In press.
20. Cutler, S. J., Axtell, L., and Heise, H.: Ten thousand cases of leukemia: 1940–62. J. Nat. Cancer Inst. 39:993–1026, 1967.
21. Wintrobe, M. M.: *Clinical Hematology.* 6th ed. Philadelphia, Lea & Febiger, 1967, p. 985.
22. Saarni, M. I., and Linman, J. W.: Myelomonocytic leukemia: Disorderly proliferation of all marrow cells. Cancer 27:1221–1230, 1971.
23. Bodey, G. P., and Freireich, E. J.: Acute leukemia. *In* Mengel, C. E., Frei, E., and Nachman, R. (eds.): *Hematology, Principles and Practice.* Chicago, Year Book Medical Publishers, 1972, p. 400.
24. Hayhoe, F. G. J., Quaglino, D., and Doll, R.: The cytology and cytochemistry of acute leukemia. Med. Res. Council Spec. Rep. No. 304, London, Her Majesty's Stationery Office, 1964.
25. Yam, L. T., Li, C. Y., and Crosby, W. H.: Cytochemical identification of monocytes and granulocytes. Amer. J. Clin. Path. 55:283–290, 1971.

24

Management of Disseminated Intravascular Coagulation

Heparin Should Be Used Cautiously and Selectively
    by James J. Corrigan, Jr.

Therapy of Clinically Significant Disseminated Intravascular Coagulation
    by Robert W. Colman, Stanley J. Robboy, and John D. Minna

Heparin Should be Used Cautiously and Selectively

JAMES J. CORRIGAN, JR.

University of Arizona Medical Center, Coagulation Research Laboratory

Although the focus of this article is to be on the management of patients with disseminated intravascular coagulation (DIC), certain basic concepts and the terminology used will be quickly reviewed. More detailed reviews have been published and are recommended for the interested reader.[1-5] DIC is a dynamic state in which the rate of conversion of the plasma protein fibrinogen to fibrin is accelerated. This occurs because the amount of thrombin generated exceeds homeostatic, physiologic limits. How this occurs in humans is speculative at the present time. However, in experimental animals various materials can elicit DIC; thus, it is not surprising that DIC in humans may have different etiologies (Table 1). Animal studies suggest that factors such as the quantitative amount of clot-promoting material (e.g., thromboplastin, endotoxin, particulate matter, and so forth), the functional capability of the reticuloendothelial system (RES), and the vascular flow are critical in determining the rate, duration, and extent of DIC. During this process of fibrin formation, other plasma coagulation factors are likewise consumed or depleted. Characteristically these are factor VIII (AHF), factor V, factor II (prothrombin), and the blood platelets in addition to fibrinogen. In response to fibrin formation the fibrinolytic mechanism is activated to produce plasmin which lyses the fibrin into soluble peptides called fibrinolytic split products (FSPs). The actual level of the plasma coagulation factors and platelets at any one point in time is the product of their rates of consumption (utilization) and production. Thus, in acute DIC, utilization of all factors and platelets far exceeds production rates in the majority of cases, and in chronic DIC states production may either not keep abreast or even exceed consumption in some or all of these factors. Nevertheless, in either acute or chronic DIC, if consumption exceeds production then the platelets and any of the coagulation factors may be reduced to below hemostatic levels, in which case the patient now manifests a bleeding state. Thus, other terms such as "consumption-coagulopathy," "defibrina-

Table 1. *Diseases in Which DIC Reportedly Occurs**

Infections	Shock
Bacterial	Pulmonary embolus
Viral	Lung surgery
Fungal	Snake bite
Rickettsial	Dissecting aneurysm
Protozoal	Thrombotic thrombocytopenic purpura
Abruptio placentae	Hemolytic uremic syndrome
Uterine rupture	Fat embolism
Fetal death in utero	Liver disease
Solid tumors	Open heart surgery
Acute leukemias	Respiratory distress syndrome of newborns
Polycythemia vera	Infants born of mothers with abruptio placentae
Purpura fulminans	CNS trauma
Hemolytic transfusion reactions	Trauma
	Renal homograft rejection
Allergic reactions	Cyanotic heart disease
Burns	Amniotic fluid embolism

*Not all-inclusive.

tion syndrome," and the "intravascular coagulation-fibrinolysis syndrome" have been used to describe DIC.

It should be pointed out that although patients with DIC are generating fibrin, they do not necessarily have diffuse intravascular thrombosis at autopsy. However, patients with diffuse or local thrombosis may have a consumption coagulopathy (Fig. 1). In DIC this may be due to the fibrinolytic mechanism lysing the fibrin before or as it is deposited in the blood vessels, or by the RES removing circulating activated coagulation products and fibrin. In any given case the major consequences of DIC can be (1) thrombosis, (2) bleeding, (3) both thrombosis and hemorrhage, or (4) none of these.

As noted previously, DIC is an acquired pathophysiologic state and it is a secondary event. There is always an underlying primary disease. As can be seen

TERMINOLOGY

Functional   *Anatomic*

Disseminated — — — — — — — — — — — — → Intravascular Thrombosis
Intravascular Coagulation

                         Consumption–Coagulopathy
                                    or
                         Defibrination Syndrome

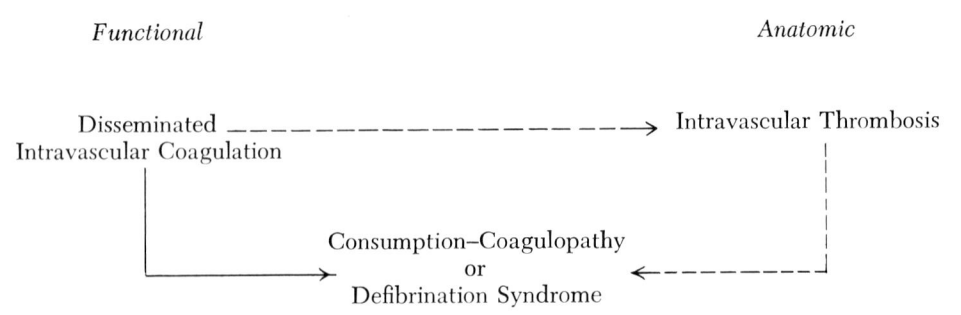

Figure 1. Intravascular coagulation implies activation of the coagulation mechanism. Intravascular thrombosis may result from intravascular coagulation. In both, when excessive amounts of plasma procoagulants and/or platelets are utilized in the process so that the amounts are below hemostatic levels, a hemorrhagic diathesis is produced and is called consumption-coagulopathy or defibrination syndrome.

from Table 1 there are numerous disease states in which DIC presumably occurs. Unfortunately a number of these have been reported only a few times, so that the true incidence is not known. For example, of all patients with giant hemangiomas, adenocarcinomas, and so forth, what percent have DIC? Larger series have been reported for some disorders (e.g., bacterial septicemia, purpura fulminans, abruptio placentae, and respiratory distress syndrome of prematures) from which frequency data can be found. Thus, a plethora of data are available for some and a paucity for others, which makes interpretation of the success or lack of success of management difficult.

Management of DIC

GENERAL CONSIDERATIONS

The management of any disease or pathologic process requires an accurate diagnosis. In the last five years there has been an enormous amount of literature on identifying clinical conditions with presumed DIC, as Table 1 attests. However, a number of these reports have had incomplete laboratory or anatomic data to support their case. Strict adherence to what constitutes DIC must be observed. It has become obvious that there are conditions which superficially look like DIC but are not, and management could be totally different. In those cases in which DIC is clearly operative, the plan of management is usually multifaceted. This consists of terminating the precipitating cause, replacing the depleted precoagulants and medically interrupting the DIC. The first of these is critical to the long-term successful management of DIC. It is clear that of paramount importance in the treatment of DIC is proper therapy for the underlying primary disease, e.g., antibiotics for septicemia, appropriate measures for combating shock, chemotherapy for malignancies, surgery or radiation therapy for giant hemangiomas, delivery for retained dead fetus, and so forth. There are now a number of reports which strongly suggest that prompt and adequate elimination of the primary disease will abolish DIC and anticoagulation may not be necessary. The next aim of management, especially in the patient who is bleeding, is the replacement of the coagulation factors or/and platelets to hemostatic levels. Depending on the need, this may be by the use of platelet concentrates, fresh or frozen plasma, cryoprecipitates, or fibrinogen. In some patients the treatment of the underlying disease may be inadequate or too slow, replacement therapy not effective, or the clinical setting may be such that the third aim of therapy must be considered, i.e., medically interrupting the DIC with anticoagulation.

HEPARIN THERAPY

RATIONALE

In experimental animals DIC can be elicited by a variety of agents, and in similarly treated animals it can be abolished with the anticoagulant heparin.[6]

Such data have been immediately carried over into the clinical setting. Since DIC is a fibrin-producing event, needing thrombin generation for its evolution, it would appear logical to treat this condition with anticoagulation. Heparin has been the drug of choice in view of its rapid onset of action, potent anticoagulating activity and ease of regulation and neutralization.[7-9] However, the indications for heparin therapy are not always clear.

INDICATIONS AND CONTRAINDICATIONS

Do all patients with DIC have to be treated with heparin? Do all patients with DIC have a favorable response to heparin? In the well documented case of DIC is heparin therapy harmless? The answer to each of these questions is probably no. The earlier enthusiasm for heparin therapy has been tempered as more experience has been gained. The data that suggest a beneficial effect of heparin have been clouded by the fact that in many cases the patients are receiving and responding to effective therapy of their underlying primary disease process. Thus, was it the heparin or was it the removal of the cause which abolished the DIC? Further, in certain clinical settings a hematologic response is being equated with overall clinical response. For example, it is obvious that heparin treatment of DIC in leukemia does not treat the leukemia, but in other clinical settings this is not clear. One such area is septic shock, in which some investigators suggest that DIC results from the shock and others propose that the DIC causes the shock. In the first instance heparin may not be useful, and in the second might be beneficial to the overall clinical course. In addition, the claims and counterclaims as to the usefulness of heparin in other clinical settings can now be explained in that not all patients with presumed DIC actually had DIC.

If heparin therapy is to be considered, the diagnosis of DIC must be established. This can be done only in the laboratory. Strict criteria must be followed, for patients may be bleeding or have thrombotic episodes and not have DIC. Because of this one cannot rely on coagulation screening tests (e.g., partial thromboplastin time or prothrombin time) to make this diagnosis. In the classic case of DIC the diagnosis is not difficult since it is characterized by hypofibrinogenemia, low levels of factors II, V, and VIII in plasma, fibrinolytic split products (FSPs) in the serum, and thrombocytopenia. Other supporting laboratory findings in DIC include the presence of fragmented red blood cells on the blood smear, and positive ethanol gelation, protamine precipitation, or staphylococcal clumping tests. If these laboratory determinations are not readily available, or if only one or two of the coagulation abnormalities exist, then one should exert caution in hastily diagnosing DIC. In such instances the clinical setting should be carefully evaluated and other laboratory aides used. For instance, in the absence of severe liver disease the finding of thrombocytopenia, hypofibrinogenemia, and FSPs is strong evidence for DIC. In addition, by using sequential coagulation factor studies or by determining the turnover rates of isotopically tagged platelets and fibrinogen, one can determine if excessive utilization exists. Another commonly used but potentially hazardous method is to give the patient a "trial" of heparin therapy and evaluate the hematologic and clinical response. Since the patient's underlying disease is being treated concomitantly, it is difficult to ascertain what produced the hematologic change and if indeed DIC was responsible. Moreover, heparin has protean effects, not just anticoagulation, which might influence the course.

Once the diagnosis is established it is the consequences of DIC which prompt the clinician to consider heparin therapy. In general, clinical indications for anticoagulation when there is laboratory evidence of DIC would appear to include: (1) patients who are bleeding due to severe consumption of platelets and plasma procoagulants and/or (2) patients with thrombosis. Bleeding as a clinical manifestation is easily recognized and is present in nearly all patients with DIC. It alerts the clinician that DIC may be present, and the severity allows him to make a decision as to the appropriate mode of therapy. On the other hand, thrombosis is usually not immediately obvious and, to make it more complex, actual incidence or frequency data are not available from a prospective study. Retrospective data, predominantly from postmortem studies, suggest that even though fibrin deposition is not uncommon, it is not always seen even in florid cases of DIC. The fact that reports are rare with regard to the long-term sequelae from thrombosis in DIC would suggest that either the fibrin is lysed and thus not deposited or, if deposited, results in no significant impairment in the majority of patients. However, more information is badly needed.

For interrupting DIC, aqueous heparin has been reported to be beneficial when used on either a continuous or intermittent intravenous schedule. In those patients with chronic DIC, subcutaneous heparin can be employed. Heparin must be given in anticoagulating concentrations. Since individual patients vary in their response and the response in the same patient may vary during the course of treatment, sequential coagulation evaluations must be performed in order to judge the effectiveness, or lack of it, of anticoagulant therapy. Although the whole blood clotting time, partial thromboplastin time, prothrombin time, and so forth, can be used to evaluate the heparin dose, specific coagulation factor assays and heparin assay of plasma are more desirable for judging the duration and effectiveness of therapy.

Can heparin therapy be harmful? One must take the conventional precautions and watch for the usual complications when heparin is used for DIC, as is done for its other uses (Tables 2 and 3).[10-17] Patients with DIC may have coexisting liver and/or renal disease but these are not contraindications to heparin. Usually, however, lower amounts are used when hepatic or renal dysfunction is present. Bleeding is the commonest and most significant complication of heparin therapy. Although the frequency of bleeding due to heparin in documented cases of DIC appears low, it should be emphasized that it does occur even at a time

Table 2. *Conditions That Indicate Caution in Using Heparin*

1. Presence of liver and/or kidney disease
2. Known blood dyscrasias
3. Neurocerebral injury
4. Age (newborns; > 60 years old)
5. Hemostatic defects not due to DIC
6. Incompatibilities of heparin and other drugs if admixed in intravenous infusion sets

Table 3. *Complications Resulting from Heparin Therapy*

A. Hemorrhage
   1. Due to overanticoagulation
   2. Due to underanticoagulation
   3. Not related to DIC (adrenal hemorrhage; heparin-induced thrombocytopenia)
B. Anaphylactic reactions
C. Osteoporosis
---

when laboratory data suggest that DIC is being brought under control. Some of such cases are due to obvious overdosage, but in others the laboratory tests have shown satisfactory or even suboptimal dosage at the time of bleeding. In some cases heparin induces thrombocytopenia, in which case the bleeding can be due to this, not just anticoagulation.

The most important caution to be exercised is in those patients who have defects in their hemostatic mechanism not due to DIC, in particular thrombocytopenia.[18] There are three conditions that may look like DIC and must be ruled out before heparin therapy is attempted. This can only be done by the use of specific studies in the laboratory since the usual coagulation screening tests are abnormal in each. Table 4 shows the similarities and dissimilarities between these entities and DIC. Patients with severe hepatocellular disease can usually be detected by clinical means and by derangement in the laboratory tests designed to test liver function. Pure systemic hyperfibrinolytic states, either primary or secondary, are rare but do exist. The third condition is seen in patients who are given massive blood volume replacement with coagulation factor–platelet-poor material.[19] In this situation dilutional changes can be quite profound, so that the levels of the platelets and/or certain plasma factors are below normal hemostatic levels. All coagulation factors and platelets are missing in dextrans, albumin solutions, and so-called plasma protein fractions. The labile factors (factors V and VIII) are low in outdated plasma and stored whole blood, and platelets are not present in fresh frozen plasma. From the available evidence heparin would be contraindicated in these conditions. Perhaps the most alarming has been the observation, both in vitro and in vivo, that the heparin-protamine neutralization mixture may in itself exert a procoagulant effect.[20,21] This suggests that heparin

Table 4. *Similarities and Dissimilarities Between DIC, Liver Disease, Hyperfibrinolysis, and Massive Volume Replacement*

	DIC	LIVER DISEASE	HYPERFIBRINOLYSIS	MASSIVE VOLUME REPLACEMENT
Platelets	↓	N to ↓	N	↓
Factor II	↓	↓	N	N to ↓
Factor V	↓	↓	↓	↓
Factor VIII	↓	N to ↑	↓	↓
Fibrinogen	↓	↓	↓	N to ↓
PTT	Abn	Abn	Abn	Abn
PT	Abn	Abn	Abn	Abn

↓ = reduced; N = normal; ↑ = elevated; Abn = abnormal.
PTT = Partial thromboplastin time; PT = Prothrombin time.

neutralization with protamine in DIC may be harmful. This observation needs further study for verification.

Specific Disease States

There are few controlled studies reported on heparin treatment of DIC. The data which have accumulated over the years suggest that at least five conditions have consistently responded to anticoagulant therapy. However, it must be appreciated that absolute control of DIC necessitates the effective removal of the underlying disease state and that anticoagulation may result in only a temporary cessation of DIC.

1. Diseases in which heparin is usually beneficial. Table 5 shows those diseases with DIC in which heparin therapy has been beneficial in most patients. In purpura fulminans, or postinfectious gangrene, heparin is strongly recommended.[22] Anticoagulant therapy in this rare but devastating condition can not only reduce morbidity but may also reduce mortality. Heparin is continued until all coagulation defects are normalized and until the disease process advances to the repair stage. Heparin therapy can then be stopped, but constant vigilance on the clinical course and sequential coagulation studies is necessary since these patients do have relapses. Patients with carcinomas and promyelocytic leukemia have documented episodes of bleeding and thrombosis secondary to DIC. Since adequate treatment of the primary disease in these two conditions may not be possible or the response to therapy delayed, heparin therapy should be used to control DIC and its consequences. Disseminated fibrin deposition does not appear to be a problem in the consumption-coagulopathy associated with giant hemangiomas. Heparin is indicated in this setting when a hemorrhagic diathesis appears. Removal or reduction in size of the hemangioma promptly abolishes DIC. In fetal death in utero the longer the dead fetus is carried the more likely it is that DIC will occur. It is clear that removal of the products of conception will abolish DIC, as it does in abruptio placentae, and heparin may not be needed. It is only when the consumption-coagulopathy is severe, i.e., when a bleeding state appears, that heparin may be indicated.[23]

2. Diseases in which the value of heparin is not clear. The vast majority of disease states shown on Table 1 belong in this category. Table 6 indicates some of the areas of active investigation. These are diseases in which DIC may be operative, but the value of heparin in either correcting the DIC or in influencing the total clinical course is not established.

Many studies have confirmed that patients with septic shock have DIC.[24,25] Our data have shown that adult and pediatric patients with bacterial infections without associated hypotension have evidence of an activated coagulation mech-

Table 5. *Diseases with DIC in Which Heparin Therapy Has Been Beneficial*

Carcinoma
Acute promyelocytic leukemia
Giant hemangioma
Fetal death in utero
Purpura fulminans

Table 6. *Major Conditions in Which the Efficacy of Heparin Has Yet To Be Delineated*

1. Bacterial infection
    a. Preshock
    b. Shock
2. Abruptio placentae
3. Respiratory distress syndrome of the newborn
4. Hemolytic-uremic syndrome and thrombotic thrombocytopenic purpura
5. Renal homograft rejection
6. Acute liver failure
7. Viral, rickettsial, and fungal infections

anism. This is manifested by elevations in fibrinogen concentration and in factor V and factor VIII activities. Furthermore, these same patients may have thrombocytopenia and abnormally prolonged prothrombin and partial thromboplastin times which are not due to DIC.[26,27] The hypotensive patient, on the other hand, regularly has the classic laboratory manifestations of DIC. As seen in our cases and reported by others, heparin therapy of septic shock has not significantly changed the mortality rate and is of questionable value in correcting the DIC if the hypotension is not corrected. In addition, we have seen five patients with septic shock and DIC who were not given heparin. All five had excellent clinical responses to antishock therapy and all had prompt cessation of the DIC concomitant with normalization of the cardiovascular status. These data strongly suggest that DIC in septicemia is highly dependent on blood stasis (hypotension) but they do not indicate what role DIC might have in changing reversible into refractory shock. More recent investigations are focusing on the preshock state to determine if heparin treatment, in very selected patients, may influence the subsequent onset of DIC or hypotension or both. These data are currently inconclusive, and no recommendations can be made at this time.

DIC is a well known occurrence in abruptio placentae. However, it probably occurs so rapidly and is of such short duration as not to allow heparinization to be effective. Claims and counterclaims regarding heparin are in the literature. It appears that until controlled studies are done, good prompt obstetric management without heparin can be effective therapy.[28]

DIC is found in 10 to 15 per cent of newborns with the respiratory distress syndrome. It has been also noted in some overwhelming viral and certain rickettsial and fungal infections. Heparin has been used in all these disorders, but the results are conflicting.

The role of DIC in thrombotic thrombocytopenic purpura, the hemolytic uremic syndrome and, more recently, acute liver failure has not been established.[29-32] Although heparin has been used, the data are not at all clear as to its efficacy. All three conditions represent potentially dangerous settings for anticoagulation. Until more data are forthcoming it would appear prudent not to use heparin in these clinical situations.

Another area that is receiving much study is the role of DIC in rapid renal homograft rejection.[33] The preliminary data suggest that DIC occurs, but the beneficial effect of heparin is in doubt.

Summary

Disseminated intravascular coagulation (consumption-coagulopathy, defibrination syndrome, intravascular coagulation–fibrinolysis syndrome) has been defined as a pathophysiologic state, always secondary to some underlying disease, in which the rate of conversion of fibrinogen to fibrin is accelerated. Specific laboratory criteria must be met to make this diagnosis. The consequences of DIC can be a hemorrhagic state, thrombosis, both bleeding and thrombosis, or none of these. Treatment consists primarily of removing the underlying disease process, replacing depleted coagulation factors and, in selected cases, medically interrupting the process with heparin. DIC associated with certain diseases has responded to heparin therapy; in others the data suggest no response, and in many both the role of DIC and the effect of heparin are not clear and require further study.

In those cases which have been judged as anticoagulant failures forthcoming data from controlled studies must consider: (1) Was the diagnosis of DIC accurate? (2) Were adequate amounts of heparin employed? and (3) Was the nature of the pathologic process which elicited the DIC such as to make it inaccessible to heparin therapy?

References

1. Deykin, D.: The clinical challenge of disseminated intravascular coagulation. New Eng. J. Med. 283:636–644, 1970.
2. Corrigan, J. J., Jr.: Disseminated intravascular coagulation (DIC): Diagnostic and therapeutic aspects. Med. Times 97:217–223, 1969.
3. Merskey, C., Johnson, A. J., Kleiner, G. J., and Wohl, H.: The defibrination syndrome: Clinical features and laboratory diagnosis. Brit. J. Haemat. 13:528–549, 1967.
4. Hjort, P. E., and Rapaport, S. I.: The Shwartzman reaction: Pathogenetic mechanisms and clinical manifestations. Ann. Rev. Med. 16:135–168, 1965.
5. Hathaway, W. E.: Care of the critically ill child: The problem of disseminated intravascular coagulation. Pediatrics 46:767–773, 1970.
6. Corrigan, J. J., Jr.: Effect of anticoagulating and non-anticoagulating concentrations of heparin on the generalized Shwartzman reaction. Thromb. Diath. Haemorrh. 24:136–145, 1970.
7. Engelberg, H.: *Heparin, Metabolism, Physiology and Clinical Application.* Springfield, Ill., Charles C Thomas, 1963.
8. McKay, D. G., and Müller-Berghaus, G.: Therapeutic implications of disseminated intravascular coagulation. Amer. J. Cardiol. 20:392–410, 1967.
9. Lasch, H. G.: Therapeutic aspects of disseminated intravascular coagulation. Thromb. Diath. Haemorrh. 36(Suppl.):281–293, 1969.
10. Fowler, T. J.: Some incompatibilities of intravenous admixtures. Amer. J. Hosp. Pharm. 24:450–457, 1967.
11. Walton, P. L., Ricketts, C. R., and Baugham, D. R.: Heterogeneity of heparin. Brit. J. Haemat. 12:310–325, 1966.
12. Zinn, W. J.: Side reactions of heparin in clinical practice. Amer. J. Cardiol. 14:36–38, 1964.
13. Jick, H., Sloane, D., Borda, I. T., and Shapiro, S.: Efficacy and toxicity of heparin in relation to age and sex. New Eng. J. Med. 279:284–286, 1968.
14. Pitney, W. R., Pettit, J. E., and Armstrong, L.: Control of heparin therapy. Brit. Med. J. 4:139–141, 1970.
15. McDonald, F. D., Myers, A. R., and Pardo, R.: Adrenal hemorrhage during anticoagulant therapy. J.A.M.A. 198:1052–1056, 1966.

16. Griffith, G. C., Nichols, G., Jr., Asher, J. D., and Flanagan, B.: Heparin osteoporosis. J.A.M.A. 193:91–94, 1965.
17. Cutcudache, C., Gorun, V., and Brailescu, G.: Coagulopathie de consommation au cours d'une réaction anaphylactique à l'héparine. Coagulation 4:19–24, 1971.
18. Natelson, E. A., Lynch, E. C., Alfrey, C. P., Jr., and Gross, J. B.: Heparin induced thrombocytopenia. An unexpected response to treatment of consumption-coagulopathy. Ann. Intern. Med. 71:1121–1125, 1969.
19. Miller, R. D., Robbins, T. O., Tong, M. J., and Barton, S. L.: Coagulation defects associated with massive blood transfusions. Ann. Surg. 174:794–801, 1971.
20. Godal, H. C.: Consumption of coagulation material by heparin. Lancet 2:50, 1970.
21. Castaneda, A. R., Gans, H., Weber, K. C., and Fox, I. J.: Heparin neutralization: Experimental and clinical studies. Surgery 62:686–697, 1967.
22. Hjort, P. R., Rapaport, S. I., and Jørgensen, L.: Purpura fulminans. Report of a case successfully treated with heparin and hydrocortisone. Review of 50 cases from the literature. Scand. J. Haemat. 1:169–192, 1964.
23. Lerner, R., Margolin, M., Slate, W. G., and Rosenfeld, H.: Heparin in the treatment of hypofibrinogenemia complicating fetal death in utero. Amer. J. Obstet. Gynec. 97: 373–378, 1967.
24. Corrigan, J. J., Jr., and Jordan, C. M.: Heparin therapy in septicemia with disseminated intravascular coagulation. Effect on mortality and on correction of hemostatic defects. New Eng. J. Med. 283:778–782, 1970.
25. Yoshikawa, T., Tanaka, K. R., and Guze, L. B.: Infection and disseminated intravascular coagulation. Medicine 50:237–258, 1971.
26. Corrigan, J. J., Jr., Ray, W. L., and May, N.: Changes in the blood coagulation system associated with septicemia. New Eng. J. Med. 279:851–856, 1968.
27. Goldenfarb, P. B., Zucker, S., Corrigan, J. J., Jr., and Cathey, M. H.: The coagulation mechanism in acute bacterial infection. Brit. J. Haemat. 18:643–652, 1970.
28. Pritchard, J. A.: Treatment of the defibrination syndromes of pregnancy. In Ratnoff, O. D. (ed.): *Treatment of Hemorrhagic Disorders*. New York, Harper and Row, 1966, pp. 175–196.
29. Lieberman, F.: Hemolytic uremic syndrome. J. Pediat. 80:1–16, 1972.
30. Clarkson, A. R., Lawrence, J. R., Meadows, R., and Seymour, A. E.: The haemolytic uraemic syndrome in adults. Quart. J. Med. 154:227–244, 1970.
31. Amorosi, E. L., and Ultmann, J. E.: Thrombotic thrombocytopenic purpura: Report of 16 cases and review of the literature. Medicine 45:139–159, 1966.
32. Rake, M. O., Shilkin, K. B., Flute, P. T., Lewis, M. L., and Williams, R.: Early and intensive therapy of intravascular coagulation in acute liver failure. Lancet 2:1215–1218, 1971.
33. Starzl, T. E., Boehmig, H. J., Amemiya, H., Wilson, C. B., Dixon, F. J., Giles, G. R., Simpson, K. M., and Halgrimson, C. G.: Clotting changes, including disseminated intravascular coagulation, during rapid renal-homograft rejection. New Eng. J. Med. 283:383–390, 1970.

Therapy of Clinically Significant Disseminated Intravascular Coagulation*

ROBERT W. COLMAN
Harvard Medical School

STANLEY J. ROBBOY
University of Pennsylvania School of Medicine

and JOHN D. MINNA
National Heart and Lung Institute

The proposition that heparin should be used in patients with clinically significant disseminated intravascular coagulation (DIC) has sparked a widely debated controversy. This paper, an argument in favor of heparin, presents our concepts about the biochemical pathogenesis of DIC, reasons why the actions of heparin should theoretically antagonize critical steps in this chemical sequence, a critique of cases in which failures or complications of heparin therapy have been reported and, lastly, our experience with heparin in a prospective study of 45 patients with clinically significant DIC.

If the possible consequences of the presence of thrombin in the systemic circulation are considered, many of the changes in plasma coagulation proteins and platelets can be understood and the role of heparin delineated. The actions of this enzyme result first in the proteolytic cleavage of fibrinogen to fibrin monomer and, thence, to the formation of fibrin. Thrombin also acts to convert coagulation factors V,[1] VIII, and XIII to forms which possess greater coagulant activity but less stability. To the extent to which thrombin is formed, its precursor, prothrombin, is utilized. Thrombin stoichiometrically combines with antithrombin III to form an inactive complex. Thrombin also acts to remove platelets from the

---

* From the Hematology Unit of the Medical Service, Department of Pathology of the Massachusetts General Hospital, the Departments of Medicine and Pathology, Harvard Medical School, and the Laboratory of Biochemical Genetics, National Heart & Lung Institute, National Institutes of Health. Supported in part by USPHS Grants HL-13206 and HL-11519, a Career Development Award, HL-48075 to Dr. Colman, and a Junior Faculty Fellowship from the American Cancer Society to Dr. Robboy.

circulation[2] by irreversibly aggregating the platelets at enzymatic concentrations much lower than that needed to clot fibrinogen. Thus, the actions of thrombin alone can account for the depletion of fibrinogen, prothrombin, factors V, VIII, XIII, antithrombin, and platelets. Once formed, thrombin acts via positive feedback reactions, accelerating its own formation. Not only does thrombin augment the activity of factors V and VIII, but it makes the phospholipid components of the platelet membrane more available[3] to form complexes with factors Xa and IXa, respectively.

Thrombin appears to convert plasminogen[4] to plasmin directly, thereby providing a critical link by which the fibrinolytic system might be physiologically activated during DIC. Plasmin has the capability to destroy the activity of many proteins that thrombin has already altered, i.e., factors V and VIII and fibrinogen. Also, in the process of digesting fibrinogen, fibrinogen degradation products (FDP) of characteristic weight and properties are produced that are pivotal to the hemorrhagic diathesis in DIC.[5,6] One of these fragments, Y, directly inhibits the action of thrombin on fibrinogen, while another fragment, D, is responsible for disordered fibrin polymerization frequently seen in DIC.

Since most of the characteristic clinical and laboratory findings of DIC can be conceptually regarded as results of thrombin activity, it would seem logical that the therapy of DIC should be focused toward blocking the actions of this proteolytic enzyme. The most potent, reliable, and effective antagonist of thrombin is heparin, a substance that occurs naturally in the liver and lung, but for which no physiological role is known. Further, heparin is not demonstrable in the systemic circulation, nor has any pathologic condition yet been uncovered for which excess heparin might be responsible. Heparin is a unique mucopolysaccharide with a high content of sulfate groups (2.5 per disaccharide unit). It is the strongest organic acid that occurs naturally and can be injected into man safely. It possesses the highest negative electric charge of any biologically active compound and can, therefore, interfere with a wide variety of biochemically important reactions in which proteins are involved. Although in vitro it inhibits more than 20 different enzyme systems, heparin has only two known in vivo functions: its activation of lipoprotein lipase, and its ability to serve as an anticoagulant. Heparin profoundly inhibits various stages of the coagulation system (Fig. 1). In concert with the plasma cofactor, antithrombin III, its cardinal action is the inhibition of thrombin. All actions of thrombin are inhibited, including fibrin monomer formation and the alteration of the activity of factors VIII, V, and XIII. Heparin also directly blocks the proteolytic activity of factor Xa.[7,8] Thus, theoretically heparin is an ideal drug to block the action of thrombin and, by inference, the syndrome of DIC.

Although heparin is effective in vitro as an antagonist of thrombin, what is its in vivo efficacy? Experimental disease models in animals suggest that heparin is capable of reversing or preventing the DIC produced by a variety of mechanisms. Thus, the decrease in platelet count, fibrinogen concentration, and appearance of fibrinogen degradation products that can be elicited by the slow intravenous injection of thrombin[9] or tissue thromboplastin into dogs can be blocked with heparin pretreatment. Pretreatment with heparin also prevents endotoxin-induced DIC in rabbits,[10] intravascular coagulation resulting from hemorrhagic

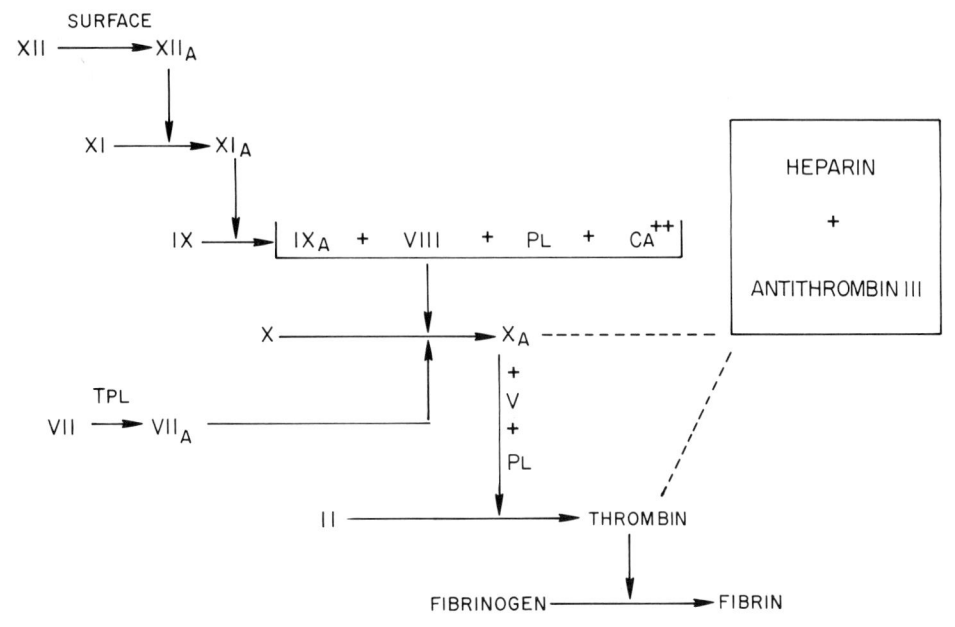

Figure 1. Sites of action of heparin in the plasma coagulation system indicated by dashed lines. The Roman numerals refer to the coagulation factor. Subscript A designates active form of protein. T_{PL} = tissue thromboplastin. P_L = phospholipid.

shock in dogs,[11] and DIC occurring in rabbits and monkeys after the infusion of epinephrine.[12] Perhaps most convincing is the experience with suckling mice and rats inoculated with the chickungunya virus, an organism responsible for hemorrhagic fever and DIC in man. Treatment with heparin corrected the thrombocytopenia, decreased factor V, prolonged prothrombin time in these animals, and reduced the incidence of hemorrhage by 50 per cent.[13]

These examples have given rise to the expectation that heparin may be of beneficial value in DIC in man, although such extrapolation is fraught with danger because of species variation, degree of clinical severity, and the ultimate pathogenetic mechanisms involved in producing DIC. The problems with species variations are well illustrated by an example in which renal cortical necrosis is produced easily with endotoxin injections in rabbits but not in dogs,[14] a discrepancy in the different activities of these fibrinolytic systems. Subclinical DIC occurs in certain diseases, notably alcoholic cirrhosis, renal disease, cancer, lymphoma, rheumatoid arthritis,[15] and systemic lupus erythematosus.[16] In cirrhosis, elevated FDP and accelerated fibrinogen turnover[17] are observed but hemorrhage or thrombosis is rarely manifested. Obviously no therapy is indicated when intravascular coagulation is neither clinically evident nor contributes to the morbidity of the disease process. Furthermore, DIC is not a primary disease, but rather a syndrome due to a wide variety of etiologies spanning all medical specialties, including surgery, obstetrics, internal medicine, and pediatrics. The most effective treatment of DIC must be treatment of the underlying disease. For example, in DIC due to abruptio placentae, delivery may be all that is necessary. Much of the controversy over the treatment of DIC stems from the erroneous belief that heparin is a panacea and should correct not only the effects of thrombin and plasmin as manifested by the DIC itself, but also the pathologic manifestations of the underlying disease. To understand this problem, some of the pathogenic mechanisms which trigger or accelerate the coagulation system should be considered.*

At least three types of injury activate the plasma coagulation system: (1) injury to the endothelial cell, which by exposing the underlying collagen activates Hageman factor and subsequently the intrinsic clotting system; (2) tissue injury which, by releasing tissue thromboplastin in the presence of factor VII, activates the extrinsic clotting system; and (3) red cell and/or platelet injury, which results in the exposure of phospholipids, components needed for the proper functioning of both the intrinsic and extrinsic clotting systems.

Activation of Hageman factor is an important central mechanism of the initiation of DIC, and in the induction of the pathological responses of the host to DIC. In viremia,[18] heat stroke,[19,20] meningococcemia,[21] and gram positive endotoxemia,[22] the endothelium may be injured or detached[23] and factor XII consequently activated.

Besides triggering the coagulation system, Hageman factor is responsible for the activation of at least three other proteolytic precursors present in plasma: prekallikrein,[24] plasminogen,[25] and the first component of complement.[26] Hageman factor (or its derivatives) catalyzes the transformation of plasma prekallikrein into kallikrein,[24] a consequence of which is the release of bradykinin, a potent peptide that lowers the blood pressure by vasodilation. Thus, in hypotensive septicemia, Hageman factor activation is responsible for both the DIC and the activated kallikrein system.[21] However, as heparin does not interfere with the kallikrein system, it therefore could not be expected to correct the hypotension. Thus, heparin may correct the hemostatic abnormalities, but it should not alter the mortality[27] which is consequent to the hypotension. It is clear that a Hageman factor inhibitor such as protamine might be far more efficacious in blocking not only the consumption-coagulopathy† but also the formation of bradykinin, which may contribute to the lethal hypotension. In the example of antigen-antibody reaction in hyperacute renal allograft rejection,[28] in which activation of Hageman factor, kallikrein, and fibrinolysis occur, heparin blocked intravascular coagulation and fibrin deposition, while termination of heparin therapy unmasked the DIC.[29] Although heparin may be expected to inhibit fibrin deposition, it would not prevent the vasculitis which is a direct consequence of the antibody-antigen reaction. In chronic renal allograft rejection, intravascular coagulation and fibrin deposition are localized to the graft[30] and the value of heparin is unknown.

Thromboplastic substances, which injured tissues release into the circulation, activate the extrinsic system of blood coagulation[31] and may be a second pathway triggering DIC. Several tumors commonly associated with DIC contain more thromboplastin than most other tissues,[32] and similar considerations may

---

* Further details are provided by the authors of this controversy in "Disseminated intravascular coagulation (DIC): An approach." Amer. J. Med. 52:679–689, 1972 and in *Disseminated Intravascular Coagulation in Man*. Springfield, Ill., Charles C Thomas, in press.

† Consumption-coagulopathy and DIC are used interchangeably.

explain the high incidence of DIC observed in leukemia[33] and with leukemic cell destruction consequent to chemotherapy.[34] Heparin may successfully correct plasma coagulation abnormalities but cannot alter the growth of the tumor or increase the platelet count, which may be depressed because of production defect.

In a third possible mechanism, injured red cells[35] and possibly platelets[36] release phospholipids known to accelerate blood coagulation. Examples of DIC in which rapid hemolysis may play a part are malaria,[37] microangiopathic hemolytic anemia,[38] and mismatched plasma[39] or blood[40] transfusions. In the case of microangiopathic hemolytic anemia, fibrin deposition in blood vessels is believed to be one of the causes of red cell fragmentation. As predicted, heparin therapy interrupted the vicious circle of fibrin deposition, red cell fragmentation, and consequent accelerated intravascular coagulation.[41] However, not all patients responded, since heparin probably cannot alter the primary vascular disease.

Despite the initial distrust of treating hemorrhage with an anticoagulant, increasing knowledge of the critical role of thrombin in DIC has led to the therapeutic use of heparin. Review of the literature suggests the value of heparin therapy in treating DIC secondary to a wide variety of diseases caused by a variety of pathogenic mechanisms. The evidence is of several types: (1) testimonials comprising single or at most several case reports of "success" which are, one hopes, not the result of spontaneous recovery coinciding temporarily with heparin therapy; (2) demonstrations of increased survival or decreased morbidity in a disease based on statistical analysis of similar and perhaps comparable patients; and (3) studies in which the chronic nature of the disease allows the use of the patient as his own control. All these approaches have their faults. The definitive double-blind study has not yet been performed. Nevertheless, since the use of heparin was first advocated 13 years ago,[42] this therapy has resulted in hemostasis and clinical improvement in a rather striking variety of diseases. To illustrate the panoply of underlying diseases in which DIC has been treated with heparin, we will attempt to sample these reports rather than to exhaustively list them.

Infectious diseases are among the most frequent causes of DIC, accounting for 40 per cent of cases in our series of 45 patients.[43] One of the now classic associations is fulminant meningococcemia. In one reported case[44] a patient who would have been expected to die because of adverse prognostic signs[45] was treated with heparin and improved; the low fibrinogen, factor V, and factor VIII returned to normal promptly. Although similar favorable responses to heparin have been reported,[46, 47] so have dissenting opinions. However, inspection of the data in one series, in which only two of eight patients survived,[48] disclosed that death occurred within 24 hours, a period probably too brief for heparin therapy to be effective.

That DIC occurs in other types of gram negative sepsis has only recently been recognized. Few cases have been treated with heparin. Of the 23 patients selected by Yoshikawa et al.[49] from the literature, almost all died. Of the two patients who received heparin, one died within hours, while the other survived, with reversal of both overt bleeding and acute renal failure. In the only large series reported, Corrigan and Jordan[27] concluded that "heparin does not appear to improve survival in patients with septicemia and associated hypotension but may improve coagulation defects." Yet, careful inspection of their data reveals that of 24 patients treated with heparin, 10, or 42 per cent, survived. Since no untreated group is reported, it is difficult to come to conclusions as to whether there is an effect on survival. Furthermore, the 14 patients who died survived an average of less than 24 hours after heparin therapy was begun (5.8 doses at 1 dose per 4 hours). The question of whether improvement can be expected in this short period is answered in part by these investigators' own data. In the 10 survivors, platelets took seven to 14 days to return to normal, while factor V and fibrinogen split products required 72 hours. Although the authors state that heparin does not correct the hypotension, there is no evidence yet that hypotension is in fact due to DIC. This suggests that effective therapy must be aimed at both the underlying disease and DIC.

DIC occurs commonly in certain viral infections,[18] especially the exanthematous diseases, including varicella, variola, rubella, and rubeola, and in arbor viruses. Virtually all the hemorrhagic fevers, including Thai, Bolivian, Argentine, and Philippine, implicate DIC as the most important mechanism of bleeding. In a large study of the effectiveness of heparin in Philippine hemorrhagic fever, only two of 20 patients developed recurrent bleeding, compared with seven in a control group.[18] Moreover, bleeding stopped sooner and platelet and fibrinogen levels recovered more rapidly.

Single instances of successful treatment of DIC with heparin have been reported in a protozoan infection, malaria,[39] and a rickettsial disease, scrub typhus.[51]

Another fascinating, although rare, cause of DIC is the postinfectious sequela, purpura fulminans. Survival in this disease was rare prior to the use of heparin.[42] Since then, at least seven patients have responded; new hemorrhagic necrotic lesions of the skin did not appear, and within 48 hours there was marked improvement, if not a return to normal, of the hemostatic mechanism. Although the cases are sporadic, heparin seems to be beneficial, since the fatality rate of the untreated cases is about 80 per cent.[52]

The method by which the effectiveness of heparin therapy is assessed has been to compare the number surviving with the expected mortality. This approach is fraught with uncertainty because of the variabilities by which cases are selected for therapy, the mode of heparin administration, and additional forms of concurrent therapy. Chronic DIC such as occurs in some carcinomas affords the possibility of using the patient as his own control. Thus, in a patient with metastatic carcinoma of the prostate with DIC[53] manifested by hemorrhage, hypofibrinogenemia and thrombocytopenia levels, and fibrinolysis (long thrombin time, rapid euglobulin lysis time, and elevated fibrin split products), heparin abolished, on four separate occasions, all evidence of the fibrinolysis. Not only is heparin frequently necessary in such cases, but other drugs which alter the hemostatic system are ineffective. The thrombotic complications of using epsilon aminocaproic acid (EACA) alone to control fibrinolysis are well known.[54] Mosesson et al.[55] reported a patient with DIC characterized by transient cerebral ischemic attacks associated with a low fibrinogen, low platelets, and cryofibrinogenemia, in whom carcinoma of the ovary eventually developed. After heparin treatment, the platelets and fibrinogen rose and the cryofibrinogenemia decreased; on stopping heparin, these changes reversed and cerebrovascular thrombosis ensued. Following several attempts to stop heparin, bishydroxycoumadin was substituted, but thrombophlebitis and pulmonary embolism developed. The antiplatelet agent dipyridamole failed to prevent a fall in fibrinogen and platelets. The patient remained on heparin for 18 months without thrombotic or hemorrhagic complications. Other types of carcinoma in which DIC responded to heparin included colon,[56] lung,[57] stomach,[58] and pancreas.[59] DIC has been successfully treated in leukemia of the stem cell,[60] myelocytic,[61] and promyelocytic[62] varieties. In the case of myelocytic leukemia, neither epsilon aminocaproic acid or fibrinogen was effective, whereas in the patient with promyelocytic leukemia, withdrawal of heparin resulted in a precipitous fall of fibrinogen.

Intrauterine fetal death is another example of chronic intravascular coagulation in which heparin has favorably altered a situation in which failure of hemostasis frequently occurs. The clinical picture is gradual depletion of fibrinogen and other coagulation factors, along with the appearance of cryofibrinogen[63] and fibrinogen split products,[64] probably due to release of thromboplastic substances derived from placental and fetal autolysis. This syndrome may lead only to a mild hemorrhagic tendency; then in association with delivery or some other surgical or traumatic event, severe bleeding ensues. In several patients[63, 64] heparin has reversed the coagulation abnormalities, with a rise in fibrinogen, platelets, and other clotting factors and a fall in cryofibrinogen and fibrinogen split products. The improvement allowed safe termination of pregnancy without the potential hazards of fibrinogen or transfusions. If severe bleeding has already ensued, rapid evacuation of the uterus is indicated. The chronic intravascular coagulation must be distinguished from the acute DIC of abruptio placentae,[65] in which pregnancy must be terminated rapidly. Heparin therapy may have no place in this self-limited acute problem, although together with replacement therapy (whole blood and fibrinogen) it has been used in seven to eight patients with good results.[62]

The third major pathogenic mechanism leading to DIC, phospholipid acceleration of blood coagulation, is caused by injury to red cells or platelets. Examples of this type are less common, making up about 10 per cent in a recent series.[43] In one patient with lupus erythematosus, platelet injury triggered DIC.[66] Chronic thrombocytopenic purpura and bilateral femoral vein thrombosis ensued. With heparin therapy the elevated fibrinogen split products returned to normal. Severe red cell injury due to hemolytic transfusion reaction is a well-known cause of DIC. Although bleeding ceased following heparin administration in two patients,[67] the role of therapy is uncertain because of the self-limited nature of the disease.

What are the risks when heparin therapy is given for DIC? The effects of heparin aside from its anticoagulant action are rare. Occasional hypersensitivity reactions ranging from nasal congestion and conjunctivitis to anaphylaxis with hypertension have been observed. Another serious side effect, osteoporosis and the consequent spontaneous fractures, requires doses of more than 15,000 units per day for at least six months. The mechanism explaining this phenomenon proposes that lysosomes become less stable and release hydrolytic enzymes that, in turn, destroy the supporting matrix of the bone. Alopecia occasionally occurs. Acute reversible thrombocytopenia attributed to transient sequestration has also been reported,[68] including once during DIC.[69] Despite the above, the main fear of heparin administration revolves about exaggeration of bleeding in a patient whose hemostatic system is already severely compromised. The problem should rather be viewed in terms of using a single drug—heparin—with an incidence of bleeding of 7.6 per cent[70] to treat a clinical state—DIC—in which the incidence of hemorrhage is 85 per cent.[43] In a patient with aspergillus-induced DIC, fatal bleeding was attributed to and occurred four hours after heparin therapy was initiated,[71] yet significantly the hemorrhage occurred at a time when heparin had not yet had time to correct the coagulation defects.

In a subsequent case of this disease, institution of heparin therapy on three separate occasions partially corrected the DIC.[72] Attributing the hemorrhage to heparin rather than to DIC within the first 24 hours of the initiation of therapy is highly speculative. If heparin were to prove to be effective therapy in DIC, the risks, although real, are probably acceptable.

We would now like to add our personal experience in the use of heparin therapy in a prospective study of clinically significant DIC. We evaluated 45 patients in whom the presence of 54 episodes of DIC was established on the basis of a hemorrhagic diathesis or thrombosis, a pattern of laboratory derangements, and the presence of fibrin thrombi. The details of the diagnostic criteria of the clinical and autopsy observations are presented elsewhere.[43, 73, 76]

All patients were treated with specific therapy, whenever possible, for their underlying disease. Although this was not a double-blind study, the effects of no therapy (i.e., neither heparin nor EACA), of heparin alone, of heparin plus EACA, and of EACA alone were assessed by the same criteria in 41 episodes of DIC. Patients who were not bleeding (four patients) were excluded.

To evaluate the response to therapy, ideally both clinical and laboratory changes should be documented. Thus, we insisted that in order to be considered to be "completely improved," bleeding should stop completely, acrocyanosis should disappear, or no new thromboses appear. All coagulation tests except the platelet count must improve, including a prothrombin time which returns to normal or demonstrates at least a 5-second fall, a fibrinogen which rises by at least 40 mg./100 ml., a fibrinogen split product titer which falls by a factor of at least fourfold, and a euglobulin lysis time which returns to normal. If these criteria were not met, a patient could be classified as partially improved if major bleeding stopped and at least two coagulation tests improved. Despite laboratory improvement, a patient was rated unchanged if bleeding or acrocyanosis was unchanged. If new bleeding, thrombosis, or acrocyanosis appeared and/or coagulation tests became more abnormal by the above criteria, the patient was scored worse. The results of therapy were regarded as indeterminate if death occurred in less than 24 hours after initiation of the therapy. Otherwise, the entire period of therapy was evaluated.

Fifty-four per cent of the heparin-treated patients improved completely (Table 1), and of these almost two-thirds (64 per cent) survived to leave the hospital. After an average of three days of heparin therapy, the fibrinogen had risen in 95 per cent of the patients, titer of FDP had fallen in 87 per cent, and the PT had improved in 67 per cent, while the platelet count had risen in only one third, and then only slightly.

Cessation of all major bleeding occurred in 79 per cent of the patients treated with heparin despite the correction of the underlying disease processes in only one third of the cases.

Although the initial prothrombin time, platelets, and fibrinogen were signifi-

Table 1. *Response to Therapy by Combined Clinical and Coagulation Criteria in Patients with Symptomatic DIC*

THERAPY	NUMBER OF PATIENTS	Improved Complete	Improved Partial	Unchanged	Worse	Indeterminate	NUMBER OF PATIENTS SURVIVING
Heparin	24	14	5	2	1	6	9
Heparin EACA	5	1	3	0	1	0	1
EACA	3	0	0	0	3	0	1
None	12	3	0	1	6	3	2

cantly different in patients whose bleeding stopped completely compared with those whose bleeding was unchanged or worse, these groups were not distinguished by other criteria (number of bleeding sites, fall in hematocrit, transfusion requirement) prior to therapy. Within three days, patients whose bleeding eventually stopped showed normalization of the prothrombin time (13.5 sec) and high levels of fibrinogen (314 mg./100 ml.) but variable changes in the platelet count. The FDP titer usually fell to normal within a day, but fell more slowly if a marked elevation was present at the outset. In the group with continued oozing, the prothrombin time and platelets fell and the fibrinogen levels rose, although the increment of change was significantly less than in the completely improved group. These data suggest that normal prothrombin time and fibrinogen levels must be achieved for improvement to occur. In contrast, the lack of an immediate platelet response is not an adverse prognostic sign; in many cases the platelet count did not rise for several weeks. Bone marrow depression due to infection, drugs, or metabolic derangement as well as myelophthisis might be important factors. Decreased numbers of megakaryocytes were uncommon, although the expected increase (seen, for example, in idiopathic thrombocytopenic purpura) was not observed. For these reasons a platelet count that does not rise rapidly may indicate a depressed bone marrow and does not rule out DIC.

Only one patient experienced a serious complication that might be attributed to heparin therapy. After five days of heparin therapy, a subdural hematoma appeared. This patient also had ongoing meningitis, a transfusion reaction, and multiple platelet transfusions, any of which may have played a role in the hematoma formation.

Of special interest are patients who, on the basis of their coagulation test values, might have been classified as having primary fibrinolysis. Four patients with five episodes with abnormal euglobulin lysis times, low plasminogen levels, and elevated titers of FDP were treated with heparin alone. All showed clinical and coagulation test improvement. All improved and two survived to leave the hospital. The results in five episodes of severe fibrinolysis in these four patients are shown in Figure 2. Heparin alone decreased fibrinogen split products and prothrombin time and normalized euglobulin lysis time. In each case the basic underlying disease remained unchanged. Thus, heparin therapy alone was associated with cessation of the manifestations of fibrinolysis.

Patients received heparin IV every four hours in doses ranging from 45 to

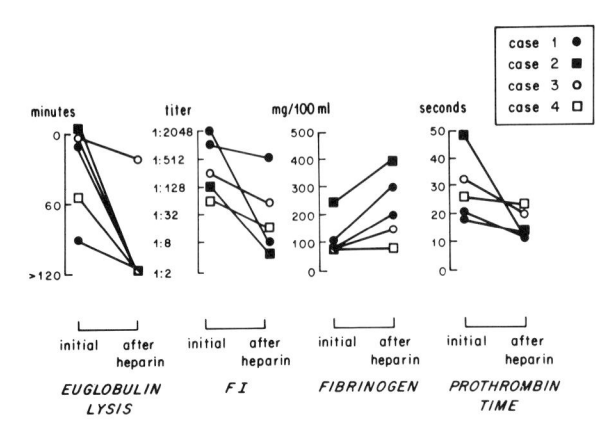

Figure 2. Response to heparin in four patients with severe fibrinolysis. The initial value of each of four laboratory tests at the time of diagnosis and the maximum response after heparin therapy are indicated. Number of the cases is arbitrary.

135 USP units/kg (0.36-1.1 mg./kg.). Although the fibrinogen rose 4.3-fold, the platelets and PT changed only slightly with increasing doses of heparin (Figure 3). The striking correlation of fibrinogen level with dose of heparin employed suggests a direct effect on normalizing fibrinogen turnover.

While our patients were not randomized into treatment groups, they received treatment of DIC within the same hospital (Table 2), with use of the same criteria for evaluation. In a comparison of the heparin-treated patients with those patients not receiving heparin (or EACA) but the same supportive therapy, the groups were similar in age, sex, and incidence of hypotension (approximately 50 per cent in both groups). The severity of bleeding as judged by fall in hemato crit, number of transfusions, and number of bleeding sites was comparable. There were relatively more patients with septicemic DIC in the heparin-treated group, and more of the carcinoma-leukemia DIC etiology in the untreated group. This sample bias is due in part to the more gradual onset of DIC in carcinoma, the severe thrombocytopenia and bleeding seen in leukemia, even when DIC is not present, and the lack of familiarity with the aggravation of DIC by chemotherapy

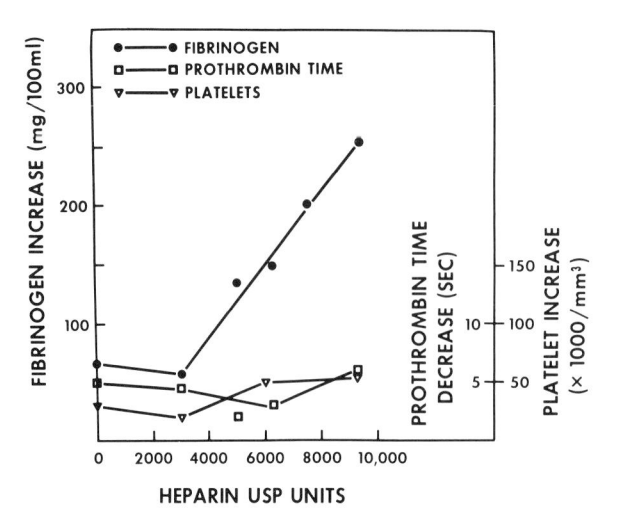

Figure 3. Response of fibrinogen, prothrombin time and platelet concentration to heparin therapy. The maximum change in each laboratory test for all patients treated with heparin is plotted versus the dose of heparin used in treatment.

Table 2. *Characteristics of Treatment Groups**

	HEPARIN	NONE
Number of patients	26	15
Age (average)	46	43
Sex (% males)	58	40
Hypotensive (%)	54	47
Septicemic (%)	69‡	27
Neoplastic	23‡	40
Prothrombin time (Sec)†	25	21
Platelets per µl.†	50,000	51,000
Fibrinogen mg.%†	132	118
FDP (ln₂)	7.5‡	4.8
Thrombin time (% abnormal)†	65	73
Euglobulin lysis time (% abn.)†	42	30
Survival (%)	37	17
Diminished bleeding (%)	68‡	31

*All patients included regardless of length of survival.
†Before therapy.
‡Statistically significant p <0.05.

delayed diagnosis and heparin therapy. The prothrombin time and platelet counts are comparable in the heparin therapy and no treatment group. After therapy the fibrinogen level was significantly higher in the heparin-treated patients. While the fraction of patients surviving among the heparin-treated patients was twice as great, it was not statistically significant because of the small number of patients. There was a significantly greater diminution of bleeding when one compares the heparinized with the nonheparinized patient groups. This was true even if the patients dying within 24 hours were included for comparison.

To obtain information on the influence of heparin on survival in DIC with a single etiology, the data on survival in pediatric, medical, and obstetric patients with septicemic DIC was obtained by pooling our series[13] with that of Corrigan and his associates,[27,77] Yoshikawa et al.,[49] and Najjar and Ahmad[48] (Table 3). If all patients are compared without regard to length of survival, the per cent survival is greater in the heparin-treated group, but not at a statistically significant level. However, when patients surviving for more than 24 hours are compared, the heparin-treated group has a statistically significant increased survival fraction

Table 3. *Survival in Septicemic Patients with DIC**

THERAPY		SURVIVED	DIED	TOTAL	% SURVIVING	x^2	P
		All patients regardless of length of survival					
Heparin		24	35	59	41	3.1	$<.10$
None		6	22	28	21		
	Total	30	57	87			
		All patients surviving more than 24 hours after initiating therapy					
Heparin		24	12	36	67		$<.02$
None		6	13	19	32	6.2	
	Total	30	25	55			

*Combined data from references 27, 43, 48, 49, and 77.

over the patients not receiving heparin. This is additional evidence suggesting that heparin requires a significant amount of time for clinical response.

Of the three patients in our series treated with epsilon aminocaproic acid therapy alone, all were classified as worse (Table 1). One patient developed increased bleeding, with a concomitant fall in platelets. In another the bleeding stopped; although the prothrombin time rose, the platelets and fibrinogen fell, and an anterior spinal artery thrombus developed. In a third no change in bleeding was noted, but further deterioration of platelets, fibrinogen, and prothrombin time occurred. In this patient, both before the EACA was begun and later when it was stopped, heparin therapy alone resulted in a rise in platelets and fibrinogen and a fall in prothrombin time.

Thus, patients receiving EACA alone showed either clinical or laboratory deterioration. Patients treated with heparin and EACA therapy did not respond so well as those treated with heparin alone (Table 1). Although there is insufficient data from our study to show whether heparin or heparin/EACA therapy is superior, our data suggest that heparin alone is sufficient, regardless of the severity of the associated fibrinolysis. Whether the fibrinolysis observed in our patients was "systemic" (due to a circulating fibrinolytic agent) or was secondary to multiple local sites of fibrinolytic activity is unknown. More important is the finding that fibrinolysis without DIC is rare, as first noted by Merskey et al.,[56] and because of this the therapeutic dilemma of heparin vs. EACA is, in practice, not a problem. For practical purposes, all fibrinolysis should be assumed to be secondary to DIC.

A vigorous attack on the underlying disease processes which initiated the DIC was undertaken in our study. Correction of hypotension, volume deficits, hypoxemia, acidosis, and sepsis and administration of appropriate pressor agents are crucial in the therapy of DIC. Replacement of clotting factors and fibrinogen with plasma and transfusion of platelets was occasionally necessary in critically bleeding patients. In three instances in which only the underlying disease was treated, neither heparin nor EACA was given and the outcome was successful (Table 1). In contrast, six patients with uncontrolled, recrudescent, or new underlying disease received no therapy and redeveloped or continued to exhibit DIC.

Forty per cent of the bleeding patients died or bled into vital structures (lungs and central nervous system). Thus, vigorous therapy of DIC in bleeding patients is indicated, and we believe this includes heparin.

There should be some optimism concerning the outcome of DIC. Half the patients stopped bleeding completely, and 74 per cent ceased all major bleeding. One fourth of the patients with bleeding and hypotension survived to leave the hospital. While the mortality rate of the patients who bled most severely was ultimately 100 per cent regardless of therapy, a large proportion of these survived with heparin therapy for more than four days after the onset of DIC, suggesting that there should be time to institute therapy against the underlying disease.

A strong rationale for the use of heparin is available from knowledge of the physiology of intravascular coagulation and study of experimental models. Evidence from previous investigators and our own experience suggests that heparin therapy results in improvement in coagulation tests and in cessation of bleeding.

The data suggest that a period of two or more days of heparin therapy is required for a beneficial clinical response to be manifested. This period probably represents the time for clearance of FDP and synthesis of clotting factors rather than control of the underlying disease. By combining data from several medical centers, we feel that the data suggest, but do not prove, that there is increased survival in patients with septicemic DIC who are treated with heparin. Further clinical research may help to define more clearly the pathogenesis of DIC and thus lead to new approaches to its therapy.

References

1. Colman, R. W.: The effects of proteolytic enzymes on bovine factor V. I. Kinetics of activation and inactivation by thrombin. Biochemistry 8:1438, 1969.
2. Mustard, J. F., and Packham, M. A.: Thromboembolism: A manifestation of the response of blood to injury. Circulation 42:1, 1970.
3. Hardisty, R. M., and Hutton, R. A.: Platelet aggregation and availability of platelet factor 3. Brit. J. Haemat. 12:764, 1966.
4. Engel, A., Alexander, B., and Pechet, L.: The activation of plasminogen by thrombin. Biochemistry 5:1543, 1966.
5. Marder, V. J., Shulman, N. R., and Carroll, W. R.: High molecular weight derivatives of human fibrinogen produced by plasmin. I. Physicochemical and immunological characterization. J. Biol. Chem. 244:2111, 1969.
6. Marder, V. J., and Shulman, N. R.: High molecular weight derivatives of human fibrinogen produced by plasmin. II. Mechanism of their anticoagulant activity. J. Biol. Chem. 244:2120, 1969.
7. Yin, E. T., Wessler, S., and Stoll, P. J.: Rabbit plasma inhibitor of the activated species of blood coagulation factor X. Purification and some properties. J. Biol. Chem. 246: 3694, 1971.
8. Yin, E. T., Wessler, S., and Stoll, P. J.: Biological properties of the naturally occurring plasma inhibitor to activated factor X. J. Biol. Chem. 246:3703, 1971.
9. Nordstrom, S.: Effects of fibrinolytic inhibitors and heparin on induced intravascular coagulation. Acta Physiol. Scand. 337(Suppl.):1, 1970.
10. Good, R. A., and Thomas, L.: Studies on the generalized Shwartzman reaction. IV. Prevention of local or generalized Shwartzman reaction with heparin. J. Exp. Med. 97:871, 1953.
11. Crowell, J. W., and Read, W. L.: In vivo coagulation. A probable cause of irreversible shock. Amer. J. Physiol. 183:565, 1955.
12. Whitaker, A. W., McKay, D. G., and Csavossy, I.: Studies of catecholamine shock. I Disseminated intravascular coagulation. Amer. J. Path. 56:153, 1969.
13. Weiss, H. J., Halstead, S. B., and Russ, S. B.: Hemorrhagic disease in rodents caused by chikungunya virus. I. Studies of hemostasis. Proc. Soc. Exp. Biol. Med. 119:427, 1965.
14. McKay, D. G.: *Disseminated Intravascular Coagulation: An Intermediary Mechanism of Disease.* New York, Harper & Row, 1965.
15. Thomas, D. P., Niewiarowski, S., Myers, A. R., Bloch, K. J., and Colman, R. W.: A comparative study of four methods for detecting fibrinogen degradation products in sera from patients with various diseases. New Eng. J. Med. 283:663, 1970.
16. Myers, A., Colman, R. W., and Bloch, K.: Fibrinogen degradation products in sera of patients with systemic lupus erythematosus. Arthritis Rheum. 12:318, 1969.
17. Tytgat, G. N., Collen, D., and Verstraete, M.: Metabolism of fibrinogen in cirrhosis of the liver. J. Clin. Invest. 50:1690, 1971.
18. McKay, D. G., and Margaretten, W.: Disseminated intravascular coagulation in virus diseases. Arch. Intern. Med. 120:129, 1967.
19. Sohal, R. S., Sun, S. C., Colcolough, H. L., and Burch, G. E.: Heat stroke. An electron microscopic study of endothelial cell damage and disseminated intravascular coagulation. Arch. Intern. Med. 122:43, 1968.

20. Bachmann, F.: Evidence for hypercoagulability in heat stroke. J. Clin. Invest. 46:1033, 1967.
21. Mason, J. W., Kleeberg, U., Dolan, P., and Colman, R. W.: Human plasma kallikrein and Hageman factor in endotoxin shock. Ann. Intern. Med. 73:545, 1970.
22. Thomas, L., Denney, F. W., and Floyd, J.: Studies on the generalized Shwartzman reaction. III. Lesions of the myocardium and coronary artery accompanying the reaction in rabbits prepared by infection with Group A staphylococci. J. Exp. Med. 92:751, 1953.
23. Gaynor, E., Bouvier, C. C., and Spaet, T. H.: Vascular lesions: Possible pathogenetic basis of the generalized Shwartzman reaction. Science 170:989, 1970.
24. Nasagawa, S., Takahashi, H., Koida, M., and Suzuki, T.: Partial purification of bovine plasma kallikrein, its activation by the Hageman factor. Biochem. Biophys. Res. Comm. 32:644, 1968.
25. Iatridis, S. G., and Ferguson, J. H.: Active Hageman factor: A plasma lysokinase of the human fibrinolytic system. J. Clin. Invest. 41:1277, 1962.
26. Donaldson, V. H.: Mechanisms of activation of C'1 esterase in hereditary angioneurotic edema plasma in vitro. The role of Hageman factor, a clot promoting agent. J. Exp. Med. 127:411, 1969.
27. Corrigan, J. J., Jr., and Jordan, C. M.: Heparin therapy in septicemia with disseminated intravascular coagulation. Effect on mortality and on correction of hemostatic defects. New Eng. J. Med. 283:778, 1970.
28. Starzl, T. E., Boehmig, H. J., Amemiya, H., Wilson, C. B., Dixon, F. J., Giles, G. R., Simpson, K. M., and Halgrimson, C. G.: Clotting changes, including disseminated intravascular coagulation, during rapid renal homograft rejection. New Eng. J. Med. 283:383, 1970.
29. Colman, R. W., Girey, G., Galvanek, E. G., and Busch, G.: Human renal allografts: The protective effects of heparin, kallikrein activation and fibrinolysis during hyperacute rejection. In von Kaulla, K. (ed.): Coagulation Problems in Transplanted Organs. Springfield, Ill., Charles C Thomas, 1972, p. 87.
30. Colman, R. W., Braun, W. E., Busch, D. J., Dammin, G. J., and Merrill, J. P.: Coagulation studies in hyperacute and other forms of renal allograft rejection. New Eng. J. Med. 281:685, 1969.
31. Fulton, L. D., and Page, E. W.: Nature of the refractory state following sublethal dose of human placental thromboplastin. Proc. Soc. Exp. Biol. Med. 68:594, 1968.
32. O'Meara, R. A.: Coagulative properties of cancers. Irish J. Med. Sci. 6:474, 1958.
33. Thomas, J. W., Hasselback, R. C., and Perry, W. H.: A study of the hemorrhagic diathesis in endemic and allied diseases. Canad. Med. Ass. J. 83:629, 1960.
34. Leavey, R. A., Kahn, S. B., and Brodsky, I.: Disseminated intravascular coagulation, a complication of chemotherapy in acute myelomonocytic leukemia. Cancer 26:142, 1970.
35. Pederson, J. H., Tebo, T. H., and Johnson, S. A.: Evidence for hemolysis in the initiation of hemostasis. Amer. J. Clin. Path. 48:62, 1967.
36. Evensen, S. A., and Jeremic, M.: Platelets and the triggering mechanism of intravascular coagulation. Brit. J. Haemat. 19:33, 1970.
37. Dennis, L. H., Eichelberger, J. W., Inman, M. M., and Conrad, M. E.: Depletion of coagulation factors in drug resistant Plasmodium falciparum malaria. Blood 29:113, 1967.
38. Brain, M. C.: Microangiopathic hemolytic anemia. Ann. Rev. Med. 21:133, 1970.
39. Lopas, H., Birndorf, N. I., and Robboy, S. J.: Experimental transfusion reactions and disseminated intravascular coagulation produced by incompatible plasma in monkeys. Transfusion 11:196, 1971.
40. Krevans, J. R., Jackson, D. P., Conley, C. L., and Hartman, R. C.: The nature of the hemorrhagic defect accompanying hemolytic transfusion reactions in man. Blood 12:834, 1957.
41. Brain, M. C., Baker, L. R. I., McBride, J. A., Rubenberg, M. L., and Cadie, J. V.: Treatment of patients with microangiopathic haemolytic anemia with heparin. Brit. J. Haemat. 15:603, 1968.
42. Little, J. R.: Purpura fulminans treated successfully with anticoagulants. Report of a case. J.A.M.A. 196:36, 1959.
43. Colman, R. W., Robboy, S. J., and Minna, J. D.: Disseminated intravascular coagulation (DIC): An approach. Amer. J. Med., 52:679, 1972.
44. Abildgaard, C. F., Corrigan, J. J., Seeler, R. A., Simeone, J. V., and Schulman, I.: Meningococcemia associated with intravascular coagulation. Pediatrics 40:78, 1967.

45. Stiehm, E. R., and Damrosch, D. S., Factors in the prognosis of meningococcal infection. J. Pediat. 68:457, 1966.
46. McGehee, W. G., Rapaport, S. I., and Hjort, P. E.: Intravascular coagulation in fulminant meningococcemia. Ann. Intern. Med. 67:250, 1967.
47. Winkelstein, A., Sangster, C. L., Caras, T. S., Berman, H. H., and West, W. L.: Fulminant meningococcemia and disseminated intravascular coagulation. Arch. Intern. Med. 124:55, 1969.
48. Najjar, S. S., and Ahmad, M.: Heparin therapy in fulminant meningococcemia. J. Pediat. 75:449, 1969.
49. Yoshikawa, T., Tanaka, K. R., and Guze, L. B.: Infection and disseminated intravascular coagulation. Medicine 50:237, 1971.
50. Clarkson, A. R., Sage, R. E., and Lawrence, J. R.: Consumption coagulopathy and acute renal failure due to gram negative septicemia after abortion. Complete recovery with heparin therapy. Ann. Intern. Med. 70:1191, 1969.
51. Chernof, D.: Hypofibrinogenemia in scrub typhus. Report of a case. New Eng. J. Med. 276:1195, 1967.
52. McKay, D. G., and Muller-Berghaus, G.: Therapeutic implications of disseminated intravascular coagulation. Amer. J. Cardiol. 20:392, 1967.
53. Straub, P. W., Reider, G., and Frick, P. G.: Hypofibrinogenaemia in metastatic carcinoma of the prostate: suppression of systemic fibrinolysis by heparin. J. Clin. Path. 20:152, 1967.
54. Charytan, C., and Purtilo, D.: Glomerular capillary thrombosis and acute renal failure after epsilon aminocaproic acid therapy. New Eng. J. Med. 280:1102, 1969.
55. Mosesson, M. W., Colman, R. W., and Sherry, S.: Chronic intravascular coagulation syndrome. New Eng. J. Med. 278:215, 1968.
56. Merskey, C. A., Johnson, A. J., Pert, J. H., and Wohl, H.: Pathogenesis of fibrinolysis in defibrination syndrome: Effect of heparin administration. Blood 24:701, 1964.
57. Johnson, A. J., and Merskey, C.: Diagnosis of diffuse intravascular clotting: Its relation to secondary fibrinolysis and treatment with heparin. Thromb. Diath. Haemorrh. 20 (Suppl.):161, 1966.
58. Verstraete, M., Amery, A., Vermyler, C., and Robyn, G.: Heparin treatment of bleeding. Lancet 1:446, 1963.
59. Godal, H. C., and Abildgaard, A.: The symptomatic effect of anticoagulant therapy in defibrination syndrome associated with demonstrable fibrin in plasma: A case report. Acta Med. Scand. 174:331, 1963.
60. Edson, J. R., Krivit, W., While, J. G., and Sharp, H. L.: Intravascular coagulation in acute stem cell leukemia successfully treated with heparin. J. Pediat. 71:342, 1967.
61. Baker, W. G., Bang, N. W., Nachman, R. L., Raafat, F., and Horowitz, H. I.: Hypofibrinogenemic hemorrhage in acute myelocytic leukemia treated with heparin. Ann. Intern. Med. 61:116, 1964.
62. Verstraete, M., Vermylen, C., Vermylen, J., and Vanderbroucke, J.: Excessive consumption of blood coagulation components as a cause of hemorrhagic diathesis. Amer. J. Med. 38:899, 1965.
63. Basu, H. K., and Williamson, G. F.: An unusual case of recurrent coagulation failure in pregnancy: Treatment with heparin. J. Obstet. Gynaec. Brit. Cwlth. 76:936, 1969.
64. Gallup, D. G., and Lucas, W. E.: Heparin treatment of consumption coagulopathy associated with intrauterine fetal death. Obstet. Gynec. 35:690, 1970.
65. Sutton, D. M., Hauser, R., Kulapongs, P., and Bachman, F.: Intravascular coagulation in abruptio placentae. Amer. J. Obstet. Gynec. 109:604, 1971.
66. Nossl, H. L., Niemetz, J., Waxman, S. A., and Spector, S. C.: Defibrination syndrome in a patient with chronic thrombocytopenic purpura. Amer. J. Med. 46:591, 1969.
67. Rock, R. C., Bovie, J. R., and Nemerson, Y.: Heparin treatment of intravascular coagulation accompanying hemolytic transfusion reactions. Transfusion 9:57, 1969.
68. Gollub, S., and Ulin, A. W.: Heparin induced thrombocytopenia in man. J. Lab. Clin. Med. 59:430, 1962.
69. Natelson, E. A., Lynch, E. C., Alfrey, C. P., and Gross, J. B.: Heparin induced thrombocytopenia: An unexpected response to treatment of consumption coagulopathy. Ann. Intern. Med. 71:1121, 1969.
70. Pitney, W. R., Pettit, J. E., and Armstrong, L.: Control of heparin therapy. Brit. Med. J. 4:139, 1970.
71. Doughten, R. M., and Pearson, H. A.: Disseminated intravascular coagulation associated with Aspergillus endocarditis. J. Pediat. 73:576, 1968.

72. Robboy, S. J., Salisbury, K., Ragsdale, B., Bobroff, L., Jacobson, B. M., and Colman, R. W.: Mechanism of aspergillus-induced microangiopathic hemolytic anemia. Arch. Intern. Med. *128*:790, 1971.
73. Robboy, S. J., Minna, J. D., and Colman, R. W.: Pathology of disseminated intravascular coagulation (DIC): Analysis of 26 cases. Hum. Path., *3*:327, 1972.
74. Robboy, S. J., Mihm, M., Minna, J. D., and Colman, R. W.: The skin in disseminated intravascular coagulation: Prospective analysis of 36 cases. Brit. J. Derm. *88*:221, 1973.
75. Robboy, S. J., Minna, J. D., Colman, R. W., Birndorf, N. I., and Lopas, H.: Pulmonary hemorrhage syndrome as a manifestation of disseminated intravascular coagulation: Analysis of 10 cases. Chest *63*:718, 1973.
76. Minna, J. D., Robboy, S. J., and Colman, R. W.: *Disseminated Intravascular Coagulation in Man*. Springfield, Ill., Charles C Thomas, in press.
77. Corrigan, J. J., Jr., Ray, W. L., and May, N.: Changes in the blood coagulation system associated with septicemia. New Eng. J. Med. *279*:851, 1968.

25

The Use of Steroids in Treating the Nephrotic Syndrome

Limited Role of Steroids in Managing the Nephrotic Syndrome
 by Douglas A. K. Black

The Advantages of Using Steroids in Some Patients with the Nephrotic Syndrome
 by Robert L. Vernier

Comment
 by Arnold S. Relman

Limited Role of Steroids in Managing the Nephrotic Syndrome

DOUGLAS A. K. BLACK

Royal Infirmary, Manchester, England

In some instances we know the etiology of a disorder with sufficient certainty to make us confident that we are treating the disease itself; at other times the means which we have available to arrest pathological sequences, and so to control symptoms, may make us feel that we can at least treat the patient, if not cure his disease. The distinction can be well made in relation to the nephrotic syndrome; with powerful diuretics we can override the factors conducing to salt and water retention, so that there is little excuse for allowing our patients to remain edematous, but can we have the same degree of confidence that we can arrest the disease process at the causal level by administering corticosteroids? The theme of this article is that we have been too ready to answer this question "Yes," and have overlooked, in our therapeutic zeal, the risks to the patient which are inherent in the long-term use of corticosteroids (henceforward to be referred to simply as "steroids"). Perhaps in many cases the long-term use of steroids is not a treatment for either the disease or the patient, but rather for the doctor himself, confronted with an unaccountably variable disorder and harassed by the importunities of distressed parents or other relatives.

Before considering the evidence bearing on the use of steroids, it is necessary to emphasize that I am not considering patients with unusual causes of the nephrotic syndrome—neither those in whom the use of steroids is probably beneficial (lupus nephritis) nor those in whom it is almost certainly harmful (amyloidosis, diabetic nephropathy)—but the great mass of nephrotic patients, some three quarters of the whole, in whom one or other form of primary glomerulonephritis is revealed by biopsy. At this same stage of reservations I should add that my own experience has been largely with adults who, in general, fare worse (with or without steroids) than children, the infantile nephrotic syndrome aside.

When steroids became generally available some 20 years ago, they were known to have anti-inflammatory and immunosuppressive actions. Whether nephritis was an inflammatory or an allergic disorder, it seemed reasonable to give the new drugs more or less empirically. The salt-retaining action of cortisone caused a transient increase in the edema; but it was soon noted that some patients with massive proteinuria entered into a striking clinical remission, sometimes during a short course of steroids, sometimes soon after its cessation. Similar remissions had, of course, been observed spontaneously and also following a variety of stresses such as exanthematous fevers or malarial inoculation; but there was little doubt that the incidence of steroid-associated remission was considerably higher than that of spontaneous remission, or remission induced by other means. The popularity of treatment with steroids was naturally increased when prednisolone and prednisone became available, with their greatly decreased tendency to cause salt retention. At the same time, evidence for an immunologic basis of glomerulonephritis was accumulating, fashioning a garment of etiologic respectability to cover the nakedness of empirical practice. It was noted, of course, that some remissions were followed by relapses; and this observation led first of all to repeated short courses, and later to long-term treatment with steroids. At this level it may not be unduly tendentious to discern a certain conflict of objectives. The clearly visible benefit, in a proportion of cases, was diminution in proteinuria, and this was worth having; but it was also claimed that there could be beneficent long-term effects of steroids in conserving renal function, a somewhat different matter. Moreover, in practice at least if not in explicitly formulated theory, steroids were continued on a long-term basis in patients in whom they were failing to suppress proteinuria, presumably for the sake of long-term preservation of renal function, any other basis being hard to see in these patients.

The advocacy of long-term steroids in the treatment of the nephrotic syndrome was particularly strong among pediatricians, with good reason, since a higher proportion of their patients remitted on steroid treatment, and also because the appetite of parents for any therapeutic intervention is stronger even than that of adult patients. If some patients failed to respond as they should have done, could this not be the effect of some neglected trick of dosage?—so regimens were devised which started with high doses, and then dropped to a lower level; or alternatively started low, and later increased; or occupied three, or perhaps four, days in each week. Devices of this order at least simplified the task of accounting for the poor results in other people's series; but it was less easy to account for one's own failures, or limited and relapsing successes.

Physicians who deal with adult patients are not inherently more critical than pediatricians; but as a group adult patients with the nephrotic syndrome are less responsive than children, so that the obduracy of their "material" more or less compelled the physicians looking after them to question the universal efficacy of steroid treatment. Also, their adult patients, some with hypertension, were more vulnerable to some of the dangers of long-term steroid medication. About 10 years ago my colleagues H. E. de Wardener and J. S. Robson discussed this problem with me, and we found ourselves united in doubt as to the overall efficacy of steroids, and especially long-term steroids, in adult patients with the nephrotic syndrome. From this foundation of honest doubt arose the design of a controlled prospective trial. We were fortunate in gaining the interest, and more importantly the participation, of a group of nephrologists, supported by the Medical Research Council. Professor M. L. Rosenheim was chairman of the group, and the subsequent trial was coordinated by Dr. (now Professor) Geoffrey Rose.

Why did we commit ourselves, and our colleagues, to a controlled prospective trial, which would clearly involve a number of years of effort? It had to be controlled, and randomized, because of the very considerable histologic and clinical diversity of patients with the nephrotic syndrome, a point to which I shall return later. It had to be prospective because of the inherent fallacy in comparing the fate of successive cohorts of patients over a period in which the general management of disease, and in particular the control of edema and of infection, had improved. It was indeed easy to show that patients who acquired the nephrotic syndrome during the period from 1955 to 1960, and had been treated with steroids, fared better than those who had acquired the syndrome during the years 1945 to 1950, but to identify the improved prospects of the later cohort with steroids alone, when they had also been preserved from the dangers of uncontrolled infection and edema, was surely unjustified.

Ethical objections were raised to the use of "controls," on the grounds that steroid treatment was of such undoubted value that it would be unjustifiable to withhold the treatment. Although the ultimate result of the trial casts doubt, to say the least, on this assertion, we were not of course aware of the outcome at the onset; so we had at the time little better defense than the counterassertion that in adults at least we were seeing some quite serious side effects of long-term steroids and that there was sufficient doubt in the matter not merely to justify, but to necessitate, a controlled trial. But we were not able to include children in the trial, and we had perforce, even in adults, to include an "escape clause," allowing the responsible clinician to give steroids (or withdraw them) if he felt his patient was being harmed. We did not, in the long run, suffer any material loss of patients from the trial through participants invoking the escape clause. A much more serious matter, accounting for the yield of only 125 patients from 19 centers over three and a half years, was the necessity of excluding from the trial all patients who had already been given steroids; in the prevailing practice at that time, even in adults, the majority of patients had already been given steroids before being referred to a renal center.

Another ethical issue raised by the trial was the value, as opposed to the risk, of renal biopsy. With a condition so histologically diverse as glomerulonephritis, a trial which did not include initial renal biopsy would have been meaningless. Again we could not anticipate the outcome of the trial, which has I think demonstrated the practical value of renal biopsy; but even on existing knowledge we judged that biopsy was justified, irrespective of its value in the trial. As it was, we made two errors of judgment on the histologic front. Believing that "membranous" histology would be commoner than "proliferative," we agreed to include in the proliferative group those patients whose glomeruli showed both membranous thickening and cellular proliferation. We were surprised by both the number and the diversity of the proliferative group, which is really quite heterogeneous in histology, though less so in responsiveness to steroids, or rather lack of responsiveness. We sent the tissue to two pathologists only; in a small minority of cases they disagreed, and we had to do some retrospective allocation. In later trials we have had three pathologists, so that disputes could always be settled by the wayward procedure of democracy.

Another objection which could legitimately be raised in relation to the trial design can be expressed thus, "Why did you not observe patients in successive periods 'on' and 'off' steroids, thus making each patient his own control, and indeed obviating the need for depriving *any* patient of the possible benefits of steroids?" The answer to this lies, I think, in the great clinical diversity of the nephrotic syndrome and in the possibility, already mentioned, of spontaneous remissions and relapses. When short courses of steroids are used it becomes apparent that some patients show a prompt reduction in proteinuria ("steroid-responsiveness"), while others show no such effect ("steroid-resistance"). If steroids are then stopped in the responsive group, the steroid-associated remission is then maintained in some patients, but in others relapse occurs; remission can again be induced in some of these patients by resuming steroids—a situation of "steroid-dependence." Not only do patients differ from one another in such respects, but the same patient may respond or fail to respond, at different times.

The results of the trial have been published,[3] and I do not propose to present them in detail, only to draw attention to the main conclusions and to mention certain criticisms which I have encountered after the event, in distinction to those difficulties already outlined which were apparent to us beforehand. Some of the conclusions have already been to some extent modified as we have learned more about other immunosuppressive agents, and perhaps in particular the effect of cyclophosphamide in prolonging a steroid-induced remission in children.[2] The general effectiveness of immunosuppressive agents other than steroids, reviewed by Cameron,[4] is also irrelevant to the present argument, as is the recent suggestion, based however on uncontrolled experience, that proliferative glomerulonephritis in adults may respond to combined prednisolone, azathioprine, and cyclophosphamide treatment.[5]

Findings of the Trial

In the group with minimal histologic change on light microscopy, proteinuria in a high proportion of steroid-treated patients disappeared or fell to low levels (<1 gm./day) promptly; in the control group proteinuria could fall ultimately to similarly low levels, but only after many months and in a smaller proportion of patients. This phenomenon of prompt disappearance of proteinuria was not encountered in patients with established abnormalities in gross glomerular histology, whether these were membranous, proliferative, or both.

There was, moreover, a suggestion, at no time reaching statistical significance, that creatinine concentrations in serum were lower in the steroid-treated patients, a finding consistent with better-maintained renal excretory function. This suggestion was similar in the minimum-change group to that in the entire series.

On the credit side, then, we have the clear-cut effect on proteinuria in one group, and the overall suggestion of better-maintained renal function (the latter quite undramatic, e.g., 1.0 mg./100 ml. of creatinine as against 1.3 mg./100 ml. in the control group of minimal change patients at four years from onset). To offset these modest gains, the actual mortality was somewhat higher in the steroid-treated group than in the control group, including patients on long-term dialysis among the "mortality" in each group. The actual figures at a follow-up period between two and four years were 21 out of 61 patients in the prednisone-treated group, and 15 of 64 patients in the control group. In crude consistency with the trend of apparent excretory renal function as judged by serum creatinine in the survivors, there were 12 deaths from renal failure in the control group and only seven in the prednisone group. This advantage to the prednisone group is more than outweighed by the nonrenal deaths in that same group, some of which were due to causes such as hypertension, thrombosis, and infection, which could well have been aggravated by steroids. A further important point is that mortality from nonrenal causes clustered in the group of older patients and those with pre-existing hypertension.

Deductions

If steroids are given as a matter of routine to adult patients with the nephrotic syndrome, the likelihood is that more than half the patients (those with established glomerular changes) will have little prospect of tangible benefit; renal biopsy is of value in identifying those patients (with minimal lesions) who are likely to benefit, at least in terms of a prompt reduction in proteinuria. Renal biopsy is more specific in identifying probable steroid-responsiveness than are tests for selectivity of proteinuria. It does, of course, carry more risk than tests for selectivity, but there is the fringe benefit of detecting some unusual, and possibly remediable, cause of the nephrotic syndrome, such as amyloidosis or renal-vein thrombosis.

It could be argued that the best test of steroid responsiveness is to give a short course of steroids, but even the risks of a short course may not be entirely negligible in patients made vulnerable by age or hypertension. In the majority of steroid-responders, the response in terms of proteinuria is apparent in less than six weeks, and courses of steroids longer than this are hard to justify in the non-responder. Even in those who make an encouraging response in terms of proteinuria, the risks of long-term steroid therapy still have to be weighed against the benefits, which in this group seem more likely than in nephrotics generally. Age and hypertension are the main identifiable contraindications in nephrotics particularly, but to these would have to be added the general contraindications to long-term steroids discussed in Section 18. Even in responsive and dependent patients, it may well be better to attempt to induce a lasting remission by adding cyclophosphamide to the steroid course than to prolong steroid dosage indefinitely.

Criticism of the Trial Regimen

Since our main interest was in long-term use of steroids, the regimen in the first three weeks was not narrowly limited, but had to be in excess of 20 mg./day of prednisone. Thereafter the dose had to be in the range of 20 to 30 mg. of prednisone daily. Once begun, the protocol had to be maintained for the five and a half years of the trial. I have met three main criticisms:

1. We gave too little prednisone to reveal its benefits.
2. We gave too much, thus accounting for the high incidence of side effects.
3. We should have given it on alternate days.

The first two of these do not entirely cancel out. There would have been merit in a trial of several dose levels, but our access to patients was so limited by the necessary exclusion of those who had already been given steroids that we could not have found the necessary number to increase the subgroups. The desirability of giving alternate-day, rather than daily, steroids is now fairly generally recognized;[1] but this was not so in 1962, at least not by us. If we were starting again, we would adopt this protocol.

Conclusion

I am conscious of having leaned heavily on the conclusions of a trial which is no doubt imperfect in some ways, but is the only one of its kind of which I am aware. There is nothing facile about multicenter clinical trials, and possibly those who live with them acquire a bias to prefer them to random impressions, usually more respectably presented as "my own experience." By way of corrective summary, I indicate in Figure 1 my present approach to the therapy of the

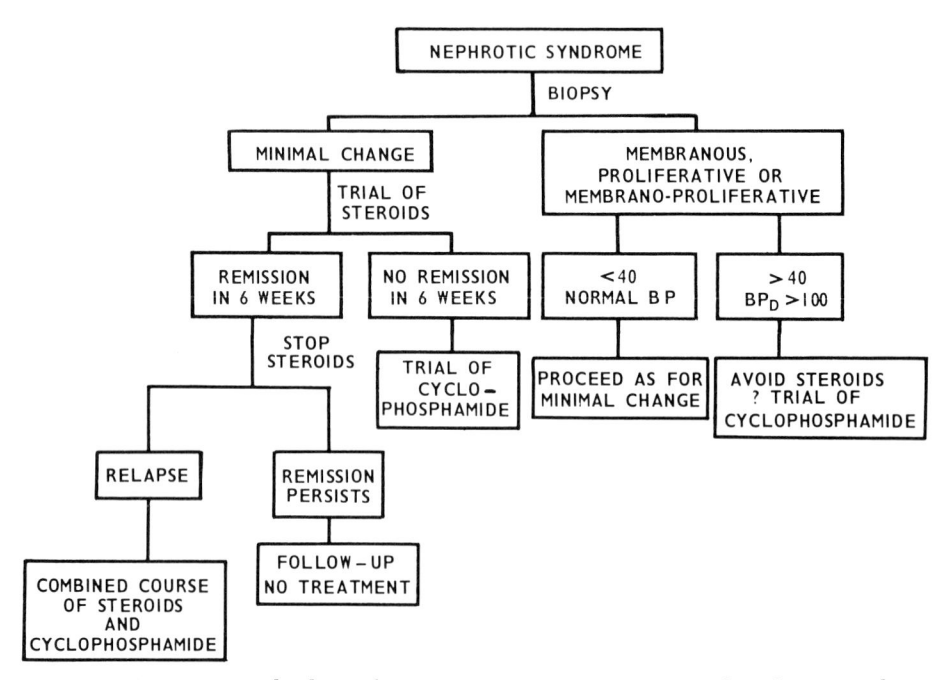

Figure 1. Operational scheme for immunosuppressive treatment of nephrotic syndrome.

nephrotic syndrome, when based on glomerulonephritis. I hope it is negativistic only in the comparatively limited role which it accords to steroids, even though it does not specifically mention the use of diuretics and antibiotics, which to me seem at least as important in the therapy of the nephrotic patient as the use of steroids.

What I see as the relative failure of steroids in nephrotic patients has little or no bearing on the likelihood of an immunologic basis for glomerulonephritis. Not only may the original immunologic insult be long buried under secondary changes, but it may never have been of the type which responds to steroids. My bias against steroids (as it must seem to many, and of course the nature of this dialogue tends to accentuate the expression of bias, I hope entertainingly) cannot be quantitatively transferred to the care of childhood nephritis. But neither, on the other hand, is the adult experience devoid of relevance. From time to time I see children who look like old people and have had to give up schooling because of their appearance or because of broken bones and stunted growth; if I then find that the urine is still loaded with protein, after many months of steroid medication, I am perhaps entitled to ask just what the steroids are supposed to be achieving.

References

1. Ackerman, G. L., and Nolan, C. M.: Adrenocortical responsiveness after alternate-day corticosteroid therapy. New Eng. J. Med. 278:405, 1968.
2. Barratt, T. M., and Soothill, J. F.: Controlled trial of cyclophosphamide in steroid-sensitive relapsing nephrotic syndrome of childhood. Lancet 2:479, 1970.
3. Black, D. A. K., Rose, G. A., and Brewer, D. B.: Controlled trial of prednisone in adult patients with the nephrotic syndrome. Brit. Med. J. 3:421, 1970.
4. Cameron, J. S.: Immunosuppressant agents in the treatment of glomerulonephritis. Part 2. Cytotoxic drugs. J. Roy. Coll. Phys. Lond. 5:301, 1971.
5. Mukherjee, A. P.: Combined prednisolone, azathioprine and cyclophosphamide treatment for persistent proliferative glomerulonephritis in adults. Lancet 2:1350, 1971.

The Advantages of Using Steroids in Some Patients with the Nephrotic Syndrome

ROBERT L. VERNIER

University of Minnesota School of Medicine

Steroids (adrenocortical steroids) have now been used for 20 years in the treatment of the nephrotic syndrome. Unfortunately the mechanism by which these complex compounds frequently modify the pathophysiology and induce remission of all signs and symptoms remains unknown.

The early trials of steroid therapy of the nephrotic syndrome were in children[1] and resulted in a high frequency of complete remissions of this difficult disease. The first retrospective comparative analyses of the longer term benefits of steroid therapy[2] suggested significantly improved survival of steroid-treated patients, although the incidence of complications was also high. As improved modes of therapy evolved, complications of therapy were less common and steroids became the foundation of management of the nephrotic syndrome.[3] Unfortunately very few controlled trials have been designed to evaluate the therapy, and those available have been criticized because of the relatively low dose of steroids utilized in the trial, or on the basis of disagreement with criteria for patient selection and comparison.

Much of the disagreement and confusion resulted from failure of physicians to fully appreciate, until recently, the multiple different and complex pathological changes associated with the nephrotic syndrome. Improved understanding of the histopathology, immunology, and ultrastructural characteristics of the nephrotic syndrome, resulting from wide application of the percutaneous renal biopsy technique, now provides a rational basis for evaluation of steroid therapy and other treatment methods. It is clear that no treatment protocol which ignores these considerations can provide meaningful comparative information, since the clinical manifestations of nephrotic syndromes of diverse kind may be very similar.

When appropriate clinical, pathological, and immunologic correllates are considered, the case for use of steroid therapy in the management of the nephrotic syndrome is readily justified.

Analysis of the histology of kidney specimens from children presenting with the nephrotic syndrome revealed that the majority showed little or no glomerular pathology.[4] Strong correlates were demonstrated between minimal glomerular pathology, negative immunofluorescent studies for deposition of immune globulins, and complete remissions following steroid therapy.[5] These early analyses have been confirmed by many studies in larger groups of children from around the world. In a recent study of 145 children by White et al.,[6] 90 per cent of patients with onset between one and six years of age and 97 per cent of those who were steroid responsive (complete remission) demonstrated minimal glomerular pathology. One of the reports of the International Cooperative Study[7] reveals that 77 per cent of 127 children under 16 years of age had minimal pathology and 95 per cent of these were steroid responsive.

In contrast to these findings, only 9 per cent[6] and 12 per cent,[7] respectively, of the patients with glomerular proliferative, focal sclerotic, or membranous lesions were steroid responsive in the studies cited above.

A recent analysis of 406 children with a nephrotic syndrome by Habib and Kleinknecht[8] revealed minimal glomerular abnormalities in 209 (51.5 per cent). Of these children 181 were treated with steroids and 111 (62 per cent) had a complete remission, while 41 (22 per cent) additional children had a partial remission. It is hoped that terminology such as minimal lesion (or idiopathic) nephrotic syndrome will replace other terms such as lipoid nephrosis, since the former connotes a useful concept in the management of involved patients.

The incidence of minimal lesion nephrotic syndrome is clearly different in adults as compared to children. In a recent review Hopper et al.[9] found that 31 (25 per cent) of 125 adults had this morphology by light and electron microscopy. Their review of 29 published adult series revealed an incidence of between 0 and 43 per cent, but they felt that their observed incidence was not different from that reported in most large series. "Cure," defined as a steroid-induced remission and freedom from proteinuria for one year or longer, occurred in 74 per cent of this group.

Reports of several other series of adult patients have indicated a much lower steroid response rate and frequency of prolonged remission. At least two important variables, the specific lesion treated and the dose of drug, deserve consideration in an attempt to reconcile the large differences of opinion held by various groups.

Some nephrologists have continued to use classification terminology and concepts such as Ellis Type 2 nephritis, which includes minimal lesion (idiopathic) nephrotic syndrome, various forms of proliferative glomerulonephritis, and membranous glomerulonephritis. Wider use of renal biopsy, light microscopy, and routine staining procedures readily identifies those patients with proliferative and those with moderate to severe membranous glomerulonephritis. However, early membranous glomerulonephritis continues to be confused with minimal lesion disease, and the distinction may not be readily accomplished unless special stains such as the silver impregnation methods, immunofluorescent microscopy, and electron microscopy are used. Since membranous nephropathy is a major lesion found in adults with nephrotic syndrome, and since patients with this lesion rarely if ever respond to steroid or other available therapy, their identification is essential when comparisons of treatment series is considered. These concepts are illustrated and further discussed by Churg et al.[10] and Hopper et al.[9] and others.

Because of variability in patient selection and completeness of study of patients in various series, it is difficult to generalize and to develop an acceptable classification-treatment concept. Table 1 is an attempt to reconcile the data available from the literature of the past 20 years and to summarize the foregoing statements.

Recent studies of large series of children with the nephrotic syndrome have identified a subpopulation of patients with a morphologic glomerular lesion termed focal sclerosis. Churg et al.[11] recognized this abnormality in 12 of 127 patients (9 per cent). The lesion was characterized by focal and segmental sclerosis of one or two lobules of isolated glomerular tufts. Many other glomeruli were normal or showed minimal abnormalities. These focal sclerotic lesions were also recognized by Dr. Arnold Rich in autopsy tissue many years ago, and it was he that called attention to their prevalence in juxtamedullary glomeruli, as compared to cortical glomeruli. These lesions are uncommon in most patients and thus are readily missed in a biopsy specimen which is not large or which does not include the corticomedullary junction. The lesion is of great importance with regard to steroid therapy, since patients with this lesion rarely respond to treatment.[7] The relationship of the lesion to minimal change disease and the prevalence of the lesion among adults with the nephrotic syndrome are not known. The majority of patients with this lesion appear to develop renal insufficiency slowly.

The optimal dose of steroid therapy in the nephrotic syndrome is not known. Clinical practice varies widely, and since the therapy is entirely empirical and toxic, it is not surprising that differing opinions exist. The lack of controlled comparative trials of various dosage schedules leaves the clinician to his own resources, and he must weigh the risk-benefit considerations and develop a treatment

Table 1. *Principal Morphologic Lesions of Nephrotic Syndrome and Response to Optimal* Steroid Therapy*

| | PER CENT INCIDENCE || PER CENT RESPONSE ||
	Children	Adults	Children	Adults
Minimal lesion (idiopathic)	70–80	20–30	75–90	50–75
Membranous nephropathy†	1–5	10–25	0	0
Proliferative glomerulonephritis (includes focal sclerosis)	10–15	30–40	5–10	0–5
Nephrotic syndrome in: Diabetes mellitus, amyloid, lupus erythematosus, anaphylactoid purpura, etc.	5–10	20–25	0–5	0–5

*Optimal dose steroid therapy: children, 2 mg./kg./day; adults, greater than 80 mg./day;[9] for period of at least one month.

†Recognition requires use of silver staining methods, fluorescent microscopy, and/or electron microscopy. (See text.)

plan which is satisfactory. Pediatricians have advocated rather high dose therapy (2 mg./kg. to an upper limit of 80-90 mg./day) for about one month. Toxicity is certainly cumulative, and the merits of lower dose, longer term therapy, as compared to the above approach, have recently been discussed by Hopper et al.[9] These authors recommend at least 80 mg. prednisone per day, at weekly intervals, to as much as 150 mg. per day, for a total duration of therapy of at least one month in adults with a minimal lesion nephrotic syndrome. The patients in this series are defined by the criteria discussed previously, including light, fluorescent, and electron microscopy of kidney biopsy specimens. It is important to recall that the "cure" rate in this series of adult patients was 74 per cent, comparable to the experience from many pediatric centers with a similarly defined population. The data of Hopper et al.[9] suggest that lower dose (20-40 mg./day) prednisone therapy in adults with the minimal lesion nephrotic syndrome is inadequate therapy.

Any degree of enthusiasm for steroid therapy is dampened by consideration of the frequency of relapses in patients who respond initially. Siegel et al.[12] found that relapses of the disease occurred in 51 of 61 (84 per cent) young children followed for an average of 13.7 years. A relapsing course was evident early, and complete and permanent remission was likely when relapse did not occur within three years. In spite of multiple relapses (average about one per year for the first year and 0.6 per year for the subsequent nine years) the 51 relapsing patients had, for the most part, grown and thrived while receiving steroid therapy for relapse. Forty-one per cent (25 patients) were well, 22 were continuing to experience relapse, and of these only three appeared to be steroid resistant. Four children died at five, six, seven and nine years after onset; three of renal failure, even though they had initially been entirely steroid responsive.

A similar relapsing course is typical of adults with the steroid-responsive, minimal lesion, idiopathic nephrotic syndrome.[9] Various treatment programs have been advocated to minimize the relapse rate, including prolonged low dose steroid therapy, treatment three days of each week, and every other day. Again no controlled observations are available to provide guidance regarding the value of any of these approaches, although they are widely employed.

Alternative or additive approaches with antimetabolic, immunosuppressive, and cytotoxic drugs have also been recommended for relapsing patients and for steroid-resistant cases of the nephrotic syndrome. Although Barratt and Soothill[13] have presented controlled observations of the benefits of cyclophosphamide in children with relapsing nephrotic syndrome, the gonadal toxicity and other toxicity of this compound raise serious questions regarding the efficacy of this approach. None of the other programs advocated have been shown to have significant merit.

The most discouraging factor in modifying attitudes regarding the use and value of steroids in the management of the nephrotic syndrome is the certain knowledge that a better approach should become available. The scientist-physician must be discontent, recognizing that this treatment is entirely empirical. We have no knowledge of the mechanism of action of steroids in this disease, and since we also have very imperfect knowledge of the pathogenesis of the disease, a more rational approach is not likely to evolve until improved understanding of the mechanism is acquired through research.

In spite of all these difficulties, steroid therapy has greatly improved the quality of life and the survival in patients with the appropriately diagnosed idiopathic minimal lesion nephrotic syndrome. Inappropriate (by present criteria) application of this toxic therapy has undoubtedly increased the mortality and morbidity of this syndrome in the past. It is hoped that these considerations will assist in resolving the controversy, will direct attention to more appropriate selection of patients for treatment with these drugs, and will stimulate interest in support of research which may ultimately provide an improved solution of this difficult medical problem.

References

1. Barnett, H. L., McNamara, H., McCrory, W., Forman, C. W., Rapoport, M., Michie, A. J., and Barbero, G.: The effects of ACTH and cortisone on the nephrotic syndrome. Amer. J. Dis. Child. 80:519, 1950.
2. Riley, C. M., and Seaglione, P. R.: Current management of nephroses: Statistical evaluation and a proposed approach to therapy. Pediatrics 23:561, 1959.
3. Baratt, M.: Cytotoxic agents in childhood glomerulonephritis. Arch. Dis. Child. 47:159–161, 1972.
4. Vernier, R. L., Farquhar, M. G., Brunson, J. G., and Good, R. A.: Chronic renal disease in children. Correlation of clinical findings with morphologic characteristics seen by light and electron microscopy. Amer. J. Dis. Child. 96:306, 1958.
5. Drummond, K. N., Michael, A. F., Good, R. A., and Vernier, R. L.: The nephrotic syndrome of childhood: Immunologic, clinical, and pathologic correlations. J. Clin. Invest. 45:620, 1966.
6. White, R. H. R., Glasgow, E. F., and Mills, R. J.: Clinicopathological study of the nephrotic syndrome in children. Lancet 1:1353, 1970.
7. Abramowicz, M., Barnett, H. L., Edelmann, C. M., Jr., Greifer, I., Kobayashi, O., Arneil, G. C., Barron, B. A., Gordillo, P. G., Hallman, N., and Tiddens, H. A.: Controlled trial of azathioprine in children with nephrotic syndrome. A report of the International Study of Kidney Disease in Children. Lancet 1:959, 1970.
8. Habib, R., and Kleinknecht, C.: The primary nephrotic syndrome of childhood. Classification and clinicopathologic study of 406 cases. In Sonnes, S. C. (ed.): Pathology Annual. New York, Appleton-Century-Crofts, Inc., 1971, pp. 417–472.
9. Hopper, J., Jr., Ryan, P., Lee, J. C., and Rosenau, W.: Lipoid nephrosis in 31 adult patients: Renal biopsy study by light, electron, and fluorescent microscopy with experience in treatment. Medicine 49:321, 1970.
10. Churg, J., Grishman, E., Goldstein, M. H., Yunis, S. L., and Porush, J. G.: Idiopathic nephrotic syndrome in adults. A study and classification based on renal biopsies. New Eng. J. Med. 272:165, 1965.
11. Churg, J., Habib, R., and White, R. H. R.: Pathology of the nephrotic syndrome in children. A report for the International Study of Kidney Disease in Children. Lancet 1:959, 1970.
12. Siegel, N. J., Goldberg, B., Krassner, L. S., and Hayslett, J. P.: Long-term follow-up of children with steroid-responsive nephrotic syndrome. J. Pediat. 81:251, 1972.
13. Barratt, T. M., and Soothill, J. F.: Controlled trial of cyclophosphamide in steroid-sensitive relapsing nephrotic syndrome of childhood. Lancet 2:479, 1970.

Comment

The Use of Steroids in Treating the Nephrotic Syndrome

Steroids have been used in the treatment of the nephrotic syndrome for more than two decades, but there is still considerable uncertainty about their value. Much of the initial difference of opinion undoubtedly resulted from a failure to identify and separate the various forms of renal lesions and systemic pathological processes associated with the nephrotic syndrome, each with its own natural history and response to therapy.

Age also has a major influence on results. From the beginning of the steroid era, therapeutic results have always been much better in children than in adults. This is largely because children have a higher frequency of "nil disease" ("lipoid nephrosis"), a form of nephrotic syndrome that appears to be more benign and far more responsive to therapy than the membranous and proliferative types of glomerulonephritis, which comprise the majority of the cases of idiopathic nephrotic syndrome in adults. The results are so good in children, as explained by Dr. Vernier, that no one has ever done a properly controlled study to compare concurrently managed groups of children with and without steroids. Thus, most pediatric nephrologists remain convinced that steroids at least hasten the remission of lipoid nephrosis in children and many—including Dr. Vernier—evidently believe that the long-term morbidity and mortality of the disease are improved.

Black argues that, while the use of steroids in children may be justified by the high rate of success and the relatively low incidence of therapeutic complications, the value of steroid therapy in adults with idiopathic nephrotic syndrome— even those with nil disease—cannot be taken for granted. Because of such doubts, he and his British colleagues undertook a controlled, prospective multi-institutional trial of prednisone in adult patients with the nephrotic syndrome,[1] the results of which have led him and many others to take a skeptical view of this form of therapy.

The details of this study—the only one of its kind published so far—are worth close scrutiny. The conclusions were that steroids probably accelerate the disappearance of proteinuria in nil disease and may even favorably influence the deterioration of renal function in those with membranous or proliferative lesions, but the overall effect of steroids on mortality was unfavorable because of an increased incidence of nonrenal deaths among the treated groups. Most of these excess deaths were, in fact, due to probable complications of the therapy itself. I believe, however, that the dosage schedule chosen for the treated group was not optimal, and this defect casts serious doubts on the significance of the conclusions. An average dose of approximately 30 mg. per day was administered continuously for no less than six months, and in many cases for much longer periods. This daily dosage level is probably not quite high enough to obtain the best therapeutic results, and yet more than sufficient to induce all the complications of hyperadrenalism. Other studies[2,3] have shown that higher initial doses produce better results and that undesirable side effects of prolonged therapy can be avoided by using intermittent rather than continuous administration.

Despite his skepticism about the value of steroids, Black's suggested "operational scheme for immunosuppressive treatment of nephrotic syndrome" indicates that he is evidently willing to give steroids a six-week trial in all adults with nil disease and in those with membranous or proliferative lesions who are under the age of 40 and have normal blood pressure. For those patients who do not meet the latter criteria, and for all those who are resistant to steroids or relapse after therapy, Black now favors a trial of cyclophosphamide.

These recommendations are probably not far from the current consensus on both sides of the Atlantic, although some students, I among them, would feel that he may still be too conservative in his indications for the use of steroids. There is suggestive evidence that long-term, intermittent therapy with steroids is relatively safe in most nephrotic adults with early stages of membranous and proliferative nephritis, and that such therapy may be of value in preserving renal function even when there is only partial improvement in proteinuria.[2] This is a possibility that deserves a careful prospective controlled trial. It would also seem worthwhile to explore the alternative or concomitant use of other immunosuppressive agents such as cyclophosphamide. Such trials are tedious and expensive but, given the present unsatisfactory state of our knowledge about the therapy of idiopathic nephrotic syndrome, there seems to be no better way of establishing the facts.

References

1. Black, D. A. K., Rose, G., and Brewer, D. B.: Controlled trial of prednisone in adult patients with the nephrotic syndrome. Brit. Med. J. 3:421, 1970.
2. Miller, R. B., Harrington, J. T., Ramos, C. P., et al.: Long term results of steroid therapy in adults with idiopathic nephrotic syndrome. Amer. J. Med. 46:919, 1969.
3. Hopper, J., Jr., Ryan, P., Lee, J. C., and Rosenau, W.: Lipoid nephrosis in 31 adult patients: Renal biopsy study by light, electron, and fluorescence microscopy with experience in treatment. Medicine 49:321, 1970.

ARNOLD S. RELMAN

26

Treatment of Uremia

Dialysis as a Definitive Treatment for End Stage Uremia
  by Stanley Shaldon

The Indications for Renal Transplantation
  by John R. Merrill

Comment
  by Arnold S. Relman

Dialysis as a Definitive Treatment for End Stage Uremia

STANLEY SHALDON

The National Kidney Centre, London, England

Controversy exists where disagreement and uncertainty flourish. Today no aspect of therapeutics can be more controversial than the treatment of terminal uremia.

Although most physicians now accept hemodialysis as a worthwhile alternative to certain death and a satisfactory form of substitution therapy for irreversible renal failure, the objectives of such treatment and its duration remain highly controversial.

I believe that hemodialysis is the treatment of choice for all sufferers of chronic renal failure, with the exception of certain fortunate individuals who possess an identical twin or sibling whom HLA cross matching shows to have identical antigens (a so-called full house cross match); in this case the treatment of choice would be transplant from a living related donor. I do not consider that survival rates for transplants from other living or cadaver donors justify renal transplantation when adequate dialysis facilities are available. In fact, cadaver transplantation compares very unfavorably with adequate dialysis, as judged by a recent comprehensive survey in Europe based on over 6000 patients.[1] Seventy-eight per cent of patients treated by hemodialysis at home were alive after five years compared with 68 per cent of patients who had had transplants from living donors and 41 per cent who had received cadaver kidneys (Figure 1). Furthermore, investigation of the quality of life assessed by the degree of rehabilitation revealed that after two years' treatment 95 per cent of home dialysis survivors were able to work full or part time, compared to 90 per cent of transplant survivors. This would indicate that in spite of the inadequacies of dialysis treatment, the practical assessment of its value by standards other than survival showed it to permit a better quality of life than that enjoyed by grafted patients who had functioning grafts beyond the time of highest mortality, i.e., the first two years (the group with "successful transplants"). These results would tend to confirm an earlier statement made in 1965, "It does not seem unreasonable to postulate that in the

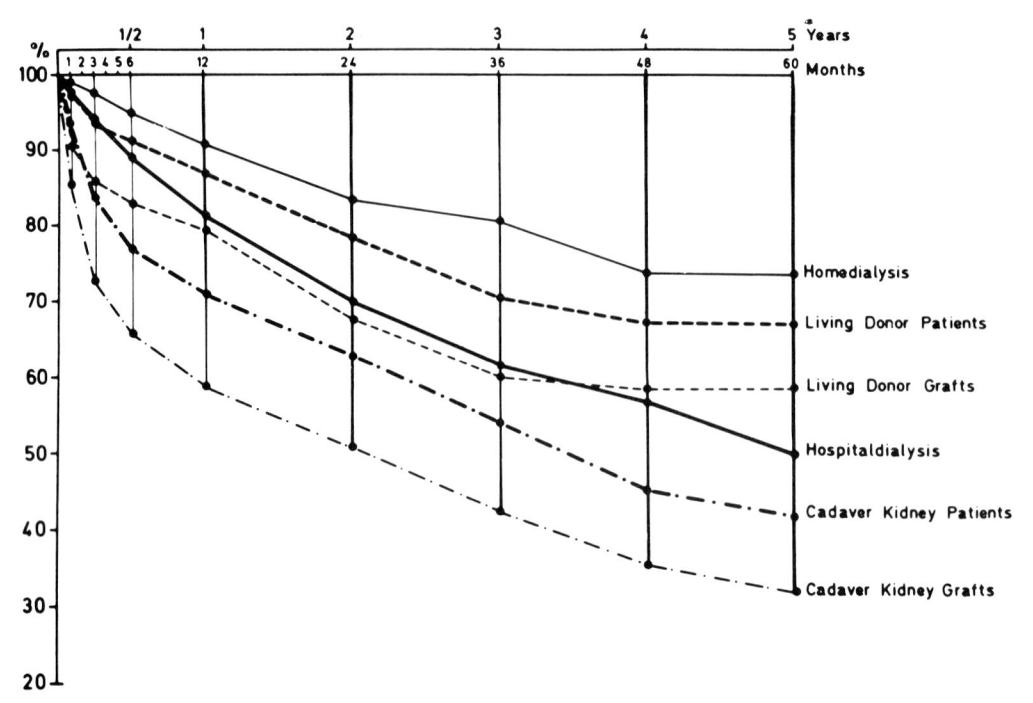

Figure 1. Cumulative survival of dialysis and transplantation in Europe over past five years.[1] (Published by permission of the Editors of the European Dialysis and Transplant Association and Pitman Medical Publishing Company, Ltd., London.)

next decade chronic dialysis will become the insulin of the 'chronic nephritic.' "[2]

However, many arguments are raised against the policy whereby patients receive hemodialysis as an indefinite form of treatment. The most cogent argument is cost effectiveness; that is to say, while hemodialysis facilities remain limited and vastly inadequate for the ever-increasing demand, greater efforts must be made to use cadaver transplantation as a substitute, because transplantation offers the potential of more treatment facilities for more people.

This problem has not as yet been effectively resolved. It is true that where a combined dialysis and transplant program is instituted, the intake of new patients can be increased per year[3] compared with a fixed capacity when a hospital offers only dialysis facilities. However, the evolution of home dialysis[4-6] in 1964 and its clear superiority as a method of treatment over all other forms of renal substitution therapy would suggest that the expansion of home dialysis is the logical step for the provision of adequate facilities for treatment of terminal uremia. The disturbing feature about home dialysis has been the dependence upon hospital-based centers of patients who, in theory, are receiving a domestic form of treatment. The failure to integrate home dialysis into domestic medicine under general practitioner care may be responsible for the ever-incrasing reluctance of hospital dialysis units to expand their home patient program beyond a fixed number. Many factors have been responsible for this failure, including poor training methods, badly manufactured equipment, poor industrial and technical servicing of such equipment, and total lack of cooperation between the hospital-based nephrologist and the general practitioner. Most of these problems are remediable if the impetus is there to find the solution.[7, 8]

Nevertheless, the price of home dialysis units indicates that substantial reductions in running costs will be necessary to achieve competitive cost effectiveness with transplantation. With this view in mind, research into reuse of membranes and the development of an automated recycling system built into the dialyzing apparatus[9] now offer the prospect of considerable reductions in cost and, even more important, a shortening in the tedious procedures currently involved in preparation for, and termination of, the individual treatment. If one can achieve a 10-minute start-up time and five-minute termination in any bedroom without a whole host of ancillary modifications to the house, together with the reuse of the dialyzer for periods of up to 100 dialyses, then the cost and labor involved in achieving home dialysis will be reduced to about 25 per cent of their present level. Furthermore, such improvements would open the way to schedules of more frequent dialysis and the prospect of an unrestricted dietary intake.

A second argument against dialysis as a long-term therapeutic modality is that the level of health of the dialyzed individual is less than that of a patient with a functioning grafted kidney. This statement, although superficially true, requires careful examination. First, dialysis patients survive longer, and although it is argued that in the event of failure of a graft one may readily return to dialysis, patient survival after regrafting has shown twice as high a mortality compared with the first graft, and only 15 per cent regrafted kidneys function at three years, at least according to the 1971 European Dialysis and Transplant Association survey.[1] The problems of resistance to infection, the effects of long-term steroid and immunosuppressive therapy, together with the possibility of antibody formation to previous grafts, all seem to be factors responsible for raising of the odds against survival or rehabilitation to a satisfactory quality of life. And so the moral dilemma arises of whether one should advise a well adjusted dialysis patient to accept an alternative because his health will be improved, although statistically he will stand a greater chance of dying.

The question of health as opposed to survival is clearly fundamental to my claim that dialysis can be an adequate form of treatment in its own right. If every terminal uremic could achieve a state of health comparable to that of the well stabilized insulin-dependent diabetic, then would anyone prescribe a transplant for such a patient? The answer is probably no. Between 1966 and 1971 only 23 cases of pancreatic transplantation have been reported for diabetics and no patient survived more than one year.[10] It would seem appropriate, therefore, to consider the major problems that attend substitution therapy for terminal uremia when dialysis alone is provided.

Frequency of Dialysis

The key to better health in the dialyzed patient may be related to more frequent periods of treatment. This is not surprising if one considers that the natural kidney functions continuously for 168 hours each week. The history of regular dialysis supports this hypothesis; 12 years ago a dialysis treatment was given once every 14 days, and today many patients receive dialysis four times per week. More frequent dialysis treatments may be possible by applying them when the patient sleeps, and 6- to 8-hour schedules are then easily compatible with normal living activities. Such a goal can be achieved when patients sleep during unattended overnight hemodialysis in their own homes, a concept introduced in 1964. However, many patients do not sleep well under such conditions, and an alternative approach has recently been developed based on the concept that both duration of use and surface area of the dialyzer are factors in the control of the uremia. Thus, by doubling the surface area, one could hope to halve the time on dialysis per treatment schedule.[11] This "square meter-hour" hypothesis remains to be proved; it implies an increase in the extracorporeal blood volume if treatment times are shortened and the surface area of the dialyzer is increased. The writer feels that a more physiological approach is to use dialysis during sleep on a 5- to 7-night basis, and that this method will, in the end, prove more effective. However, to achieve this goal, reuse and simplification of dialysis equipment will be essential.

A further major problem in this area lies in obtaining repeated and frequent access to the blood stream. The original technique involved use of subcutaneous indwelling cannulas surgically inserted in a peripheral artery and vein in either the arm or leg. These cannulas were exteriorized and joined by a detachable bridge. This Quinton-Scribner shunt, although of great value, invariably went wrong and required further surgery. It also presented hazards commonly associated with indwelling prosthetic materials in the blood stream, e.g., thrombosis, embolus, and infection. It has largely been superseded by the Cimino arteriovenous fistula created surgically between a peripheral artery and vein in the upper limb to produce enlargement of the superficial veins of the arm. Access to the blood stream is achieved by repeated venipuncture. With the use of adequate surgical technique these fistulas can now be made to last indefinitely and may be punctured up to five times per week. Further surgery seems unnecessary, and the incidence of complications requiring medical or surgical assistance because of malfunction has been considerably reduced in comparison with the Quinton-Scribner shunt. The Cimino technique therefore offers the possibility of frequent access to the blood stream without the encumbrance of a prosthetic device remaining within the body during the time the patient is not receiving treatment. In addition, the patient is free to indulge fully in any physical activity, which he was precluded from doing with the prosthetic shunt.

A research program involving seven-hour dialysis schedules overnight five times per week, with automated reuse of the dialyzer together with an unrestricted diet, has been undertaken for six months in two patients. Adequate control of blood pressure on an unlimited salt intake, improvement in hematocrit from 15 to 40 per cent, the disappearance of skin pigmentation, and perhaps most interestingly the complete resolution of renal bone disease with restoration of parathyroid hormone secretion rates to normal have occurred during this program of intensive dialysis. A detailed analysis of the improvement in health will now be attempted to indicate the future potential of adequate renal dialysis when it is provided on a routine basis with a frequency that this research program indicates is feasible.

Avoiding the Complications of Dialysis

Anemia

The abnormality which probably affects dialysis patients most is chronic anemia. The problem of anemia seems largely resolvable by a policy of non-transfusion.[12] The result of this is that the patient drops his hematocrit (HCT) to a stable level; provided he then receives iron replacement therapy, the HCT will rise with time as the ensuing iron deficiency associated with repeated blood loss is reversed and the inhibitory effect of transfusion on endogenous erythropoiesis is avoided. The addition of parenteral testosterone[13] has enabled the mean HCT of dialysis patients to rise above 30 per cent. When used with a dialysis schedule of four to five times per week and an increase in the total number of hours of treatment per week, testosterone can produce a normal HCT even in the bilaterally nephrectomized patient.[14] Alternatively, when the number of dialyses and the time per week are reduced but testosterone is continued on an unaltered dosage, a drop in HCT can be produced, suggesting that the action of testosterone is complemented by intensive dialysis (Figure 2). This evidence indicates that more frequent and more prolonged dialysis may offer the key to better health.

"Renal" Bone Disease

One of the most distressing long-term complications of dialysis is the progressive development of bone disease, with consequent fractures and associated metastatic calcification and arterial disease, resulting in mortality from coronary artery thrombosis and cerebrovascular accidents. The solution to this problem is as yet uncertain, but encouraging observations have been made when plasma phosphate levels were kept continuously below 4.0 mg. per cent and the patient was put into positive calcium balance by keeping the calcium level in the dialysis fluid at 7.0 mg. per cent (3.5 mEq./L.). Under these conditions, which often require dialysis five times per week, parathyroid hormone secretion rates have been seen to return to normal and "renal" bone disease can be contained. The danger of this particular approach, however, lies in the fact that when the serum calcium levels rise as a result of the dialysate's calcium content of 3.5 mEq./L., metastatic calcification will occur unless the phosphate level in the blood is controlled. It would seem that the solution to the problem of "renal" bone disease is partially dependent on more frequent dialysis, although phosphate binders in the gut such as aluminium hydroxide are also helpful in controlling increased inorganic plasma phosphate levels.

Growth

Pediatric dialysis has been evolving as a specialty over the past three years, particularly because of the reluctance of many pediatricians to subject young

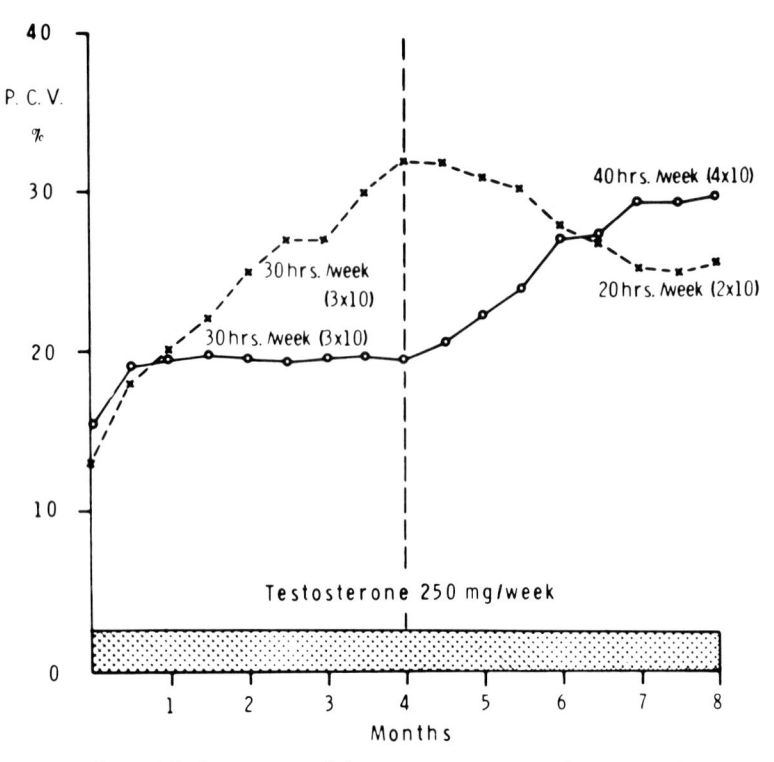

Figure 2. Effect of dialysis time and frequency on HCT with constant I.M. testosterone dosage.

patients to transplantation and subsequent high steroid dosage. One of the major anxieties in preadolescent dialysis patients is the question of growth. Growth and progression through puberty have, however, been attained during dialysis provided the calorie intake of the patient has been adequate.[15, 16] It would therefore appear that the possibility of pediatric renal disease being treated by dialysis without transplantation offers distinct possibilities.

GONADAL FUNCTION

Ovulation has been shown to occur in well dialyzed female patients, and there is now on record one successful pregnancy in a patient who was treated by dialysis throughout the full term of pregnancy and delivered a normal child.[17] Male infertility has previously been reported in dialysis patients, but recent evidence suggests that with more frequent dialysis spermatogenesis may be maintained at a normal rate. There are several reports of male dialysis patients who have fathered children.[18]

HYPERTENSION AND HEART FAILURE

The problem of hypertensive renal disease has to a large extent been resolved over the years, and it is clear that when the salt and water balance of the patient are held within normal limits by some degree of sodium restriction, blood pressure can usually be controlled in up to 90 per cent of patients. In the research program mentioned earlier, where sodium balance is controlled by a five times per week dialysis schedule, unlimited salt is permitted. However, on more restricted dialysis schedules excellent blood pressure control for long periods of time has also been reported on numerous occasions.[19] Heart failure as a clinical entity is more often attributable to excessive blood volume owing to water retention rather than to any positively identified disease of the heart muscle, but there is increasing evidence that genuine myocardial degeneration associated with coronary artery disease has occurred in older patients. Bilateral nephrectomy is indicated to control severe malignant hypertension in about 10 per cent of uremics in whom frequent dialysis has failed to control the blood pressure. The disadvantage of bilateral nephrectomy has been that with the removal of both kidneys one has to contend with a higher degree of anemia but, as was previously mentioned, this is treatable with more intensive dialysis and adequate amounts of testosterone.

Hepatitis

The spread of hepatitis in dialysis units, with deaths among staff members and relatives of patients over the past six years, has impeded the recruitment of staff for dialysis units and may be one of the biggest factors precluding the expansion of this form of treatment.[20] It would appear that the vast majority of dialysis patients are abnormal in their immune response to infection with Australia-antigen associated hepatitis virus and consequently remain chronic carriers. The result is that by the very nature of the treatment, both dialysis patients and the staff caring for them are exposed to contaminated blood, thus accounting for the epidemic outbreaks of hepatitis reported with ever-increasing frequency in dialysis units throughout the world. The risk of contracting hepatitis in transplant units has been substantiated, and deaths of several surgeons operating on Australia-antigen positive cases have been reported. It would seem that a possible way of dealing with this dilemma would be to promote the expansion of home dialysis so that Australia-antigen positive patients can be isolated in their own homes.

Conclusion

The arguments that I have presented to justify the claim that dialysis should be the definitive treatment of choice for the patient with terminal uremia are stimulated by a basic philosophic concept, and the future alone may determine its validity. The basis of my belief is that with the present state of our technical knowledge it is clear that a man-made device is capable of restoring a patient to virtually normal health. Although the demand for treatment is enormous, facilities for treatment inadequate, and cost high, my basic credo is that a man-made device is within man's reach and that future developments will lessen costs and heighten patient acceptance. The ultimate hope for transplantation, on the other hand, lies in finding a method by which the fundamental natural reaction of the body to a foreign substance can be altered.

References

1. Parsons, F. M., Brunner, F. P., Gurland, H. J., and Harlen, H.: Combined report on regular dialysis and transplantation in Europe. Proceedings of the European Dialysis and Transplant Association 8:3, 1971. London, Pitman Medical Publishing Company, Ltd.
2. Shaldon, S.: Long-term dialysis as a substitute for kidney function. The scientific basis for medicine. Annual Reviews, The Athlone Press, University of London, 1966, p. 201.
3. Farrow, S. C., Fisher, D. H. J., and Johnson, D. B.: Statistical approach to planning on integrated haemodialysis/transplantation programme. Brit. Med. J. 2:671, 1971.
4. Merrill, J. P., Schupak, E., Cameron, E., and Hampers, C. L.: Hemodialysis in the home. J.A.M.A. 190:468, 1964.
5. Curtis, F. K., Cole, J. J., Fellows, B. J., Tyler, L. L., and Scribner, B. H.: Hemodialysis in the home. Trans. Amer. Soc. Artif. Intern. Organs 11:7, 1965.
6. Baillod, R. A., Comty, C., Ilahi, M., Konotey-Ahulu, F. I. D., Sevitt, L., and Shaldon, S.: Overnight haemodialysis in the home. Proceedings of the European Dialysis and Transplant Association 2:99, 1965. Amsterdam, Excerpta Medica Foundation.
7. Shaldon, S.: Independence in maintenance haemodialysis. Lancet 1:520, 1968.
8. Rae, A. I., Marr, T. A., Stevry, R. E., Gothberg, L. A., and Davidson, R. C.: Hemodialysis in the home. J.A.M.A. 208(1):92, 1968.
9. Shaldon, S.: Automated Dialyser Reuse. In preparation.
10. Pancreatic transplantation. (Editorial.) Brit. Med. J. 1:326. 1972.
11. Babb, L. A., Popovich, R. P., Christopher, T. G., and Scriber, B. H.: The genesis of the square meter-hour hypothesis. Trans. Amer. Soc. Artif. Intern. Organs 17:81, 1971.
12. Crockett, R. E., Baillod, R. A., Lee, B. N., Moorhead, J. F., Stevenson, C. H., Varghese, Z., and Shaldon, S.: Maintenance of fifty patients on intermittent haemodialysis without blood transfusion. Proceedings of the European Dialysis and Transplant Association 4:17, 1967. Amsterdam, Excerpta Medica Foundation.
13. Shaldon, S., Koch, K. M., Oppermann, F., Patyna, W. D., and Schoeppe, W. E.: Testosterone therapy for anaemia in maintenance dialysis. Brit. Med. J. 3:212–215, 1971.
14. Shaldon, S., Patyna, W. D., Kaltwasser, P., Werner, E., Koch, K.M., and Schoeppe, W. E.: The use of testosterone in bilateral nephrectomized dialysis patients. Trans. Amer. Soc. Artif. Intern. Organs 17:104, 1971.
15. Shaldon, S., Shaldon, J., McInnes, S., McDonald, H., and Oag, D.: Long term maintenance domestic haemodialysis in children. Proceedings of the European Dialysis and Transplant Association 6:145, 1969. London, Pitman Medical Publishing Company, Ltd.
16. Simmons, J. M., Wilson, C. J., Potter, D. E., and Holliday, N. A.: Calorie intake and linear growth of children on haemodialysis. New Eng. J. Med. 285:653, 1971.
17. Confortini, P., Galanti, G., Ancona, G., Giongo, A., Bruschi, E., and Lorenzini, E.: Full term pregnancy and successful delivery in a patient on chronic haemodialysis. Proceedings of the European Dialysis and Transplant Association. 8:74, 1971. London, Pitman Medical Publishing Company, Ltd.
18. Elstein, M., Smith, E. K. M., and Curtis, J. R.: Reproductive potential of patients treated by maintenance haemodialysis. Brit. Med. J. 2:734, 1969.
19. Ledingham, J. M.: Blood pressure regulation in renal failure. J. Roy. Coll. Phys. London 5:103, 1971.
20. Hepatitis in dialysis units. (Editorial.) Brit. Med. J. 4:255, 1970.

The Indications for Renal Transplantation

JOHN R. MERRILL

Harvard Medical School

Homer Smith[1] in his essay *De Urina* quotes the Danish writer Isak Dinesen (the Baroness von Blixen), who describes an Arab sailing along the coast of Africa by starlight and speculating, "What is man when you think upon him but a minutely set, ingenious machine for turning, with infinite artfulness, the red wine of Shiraz into urine?" Unquestionably the part of man which most effectively transforms the red wine to urine is the kidney, and man has yet to devise a "minutely set, ingenious machine" to rival it in efficacy.

In the event of failure of this "ingenious machine," two forms of replacement therapy are available, hemodialysis and kidney transplantation. It is the purpose of this essay to consider and compare these two modalities.

Background

The development of the artificial kidney as a practical therapeutic tool for the treatment of renal failure in the early 50's[2] made possible the first attempts at kidney transplantation.[3] Because of the ability to maintain terminally ill uremic patients, heroic therapeutic attempts at transplantation became justified. In 1954 the first successful kidney transplant between identical twins was accomplished. In 1959, with the successful transplantation of a kidney between nonidentical twins, the era of true renal allografts dawned, to be followed shortly thereafter by transplantation of a cadaver kidney in a patient who survived for more than one year. The world experience with human kidney transplantation of all kinds now includes more than 10,000 such operations recorded in the International Transplantation Registry.

During the years when physicians and surgeons were struggling with the problem of allografts, dialysis too was making progress. Perhaps the most significant milestone in this progress was the development of an arteriovenous shunt which made continual access to artery and vein possible, thus eliminating the repeated cut downs and cannulation which had previously limited dialysis to eight or 10 procedures. With the advent of this technique and more sophisticated types of artificial kidneys, maintenance of life in patients with terminal renal failure, indeed in bilaterally nephrectomized patients, became possible for an indefinite period in many instances. Dialysis and transplantation have continued to be utilized in conjunction since; until very recently it was not deemed medically feasible to transplant a kidney into an individual whose renal failure had not progressed to the point where he required dialysis to keep him alive. For a good many years these two forms of treatment were considered inseparable partners.

Which Form of Therapy?

Recently, however, some controversy has arisen as to whether one or the other might not be considered the "preferred" form of therapy. There is, indeed, a school of thought which considers the partners not only separate but even separate and *un*equal. Stated in simpler terms, it has been suggested that because of the complications of transplantation and the relatively unsatisfactory success rate of cadaver kidney transplantation that chronic dialysis might be the "preferred" form of rehabilitation of the terminal uremic patient. In my opinion this form of generalization has no merit. It is a medieval and specious argument which has no pertinence to real life unless each case is considered on its own merits.

Let us consider for a moment the reasons for such a statement; they are simple and straightforward. In the terms of our legal brethren, res ipsa loquitur. One has only to talk to an identical twin who has been treated with dialysis for a six- or eight-month period and then gone on to have a successful kidney transplant which has functioned normally for two years or more. Can one really believe that there is any question in the mind of this patient or that of the observer as to which is the more effective and satisfying form of treatment? Should there be any question either that a normally functioning kidney sustains life more effectively than even the most effective form of hemodialysis?

The Practical Problems of Both Dialysis and Transplantation

With few exceptions we still have no clear idea about the cause of the signs and symptoms of "uremia." Although dialysis ameliorates a good many of these, it fails to do so in an important number of aspects: (1) Certainly anemia remains a problem.[4] (2) Neuropathy may fail to progress or even improve slightly with adequate dialysis, but it is clear that a successfully functioning transplant ameliorates the anemia and neuropathy[5] of uremia far better than even the most successful forms of dialysis. (3) Bone disease, particularly aseptic necrosis of the hip, is a major source of difficulty, even in post-transplant patients, but it can be shown that such bone disease begins before transplantation, although it certainly may be hastened by the use of steroids in the post-transplant period. (4) Dialysis in children does not permit normal growth, whereas successful transplantation does. (5) In most patients on dialysis, sodium and water restriction are necessary to prevent hypertension and congestive heart failure. This is not true in a patient with a successfully functioning transplant. (6) Murawski has pointed out very clearly in his excellent study on psychologic testing in patients before and after dialysis that "as a group the dialyzed patients do not achieve normal levels until transplanted."[6] It is equally clear to those of us who have followed a number of dialyzed patients over a period of years that although many of them do well, less than 50 per cent are totally "normal," and more subtle neurologic, psychologic, and biochemical evaluations reveal abnormalities even in the absence of symptoms. Again, this is not true in the patient with a normally functioning transplanted kidney. Studies of Parsons[7] give further evidence for this. Parsons has found, as have we, evidence of "malnutrition" even in well dialyzed patients and has demonstrated a reduction in serum levels of essential amino acids which resembles that produced by kwashiorkor. Finally, recovery of menses and female reproductive function, absent during dialysis, has occurred after successful renal transplantation.

On the other hand, it can and should be argued that not all transplanted kidneys function normally. It is pertinent to compare survival rates. The one-year survival rate for patients begun on a chronic dialysis program in the United States is between 78 and 92 per cent. Stated in another fashion, between 22 and 8 per cent of patients on chronic dialysis are lost each year. The one-year success rate for identical twin transplants is 98 per cent and is marred only by an occasional technical failure. Between siblings who are good tissue matches ("A" matches) the one-year success rate is some 95 per cent and does not further decline after two years. Between less well matched siblings it is 85 to 90 per cent. Transplants between parent and child average about an 85 per cent one-year survival, but this declines after two years to some 75 per cent (here we are talking about survival of the kidney, not the patient). The survival of transplanted cadaver kidneys is about 65 per cent at one year and declines to some 50 per cent at two years. Therefore, in comparing renal transplantation with dialysis, one must identify the source of the kidney and the degree of tissue compatibility. Further, in those individuals who receive transplanted kidneys from donors who are poor matches, the amount of immunosuppressive therapy, i.e., azathioprine and prednisone, predisposes to infection, to bone disease, to gastrointestinal ulceration, Cushingoid facies, hyperglycemia, and aseptic necrosis of the hip.

Psychologic problems are not uncommon in the dialyzed patient and have been well documented by a number of observers. Equally common, however, are psychiatric problems, usually related to fear of rejection, in the first six to nine months after transplantation.[9] The fact remains, nevertheless, that a normally functioning transplanted kidney is always a more successful form of therapy for uremia than the best form of dialysis. Furthermore, it is considerably cheaper after the first year.

It is possible to predict survival in sibling to sibling transplants by the degree of histocompatibility which can be measured preoperatively, and this is generally true of parent to child transplants. Unfortunately our ability to test all the antigens in unrelated donor recipient transplant pairs is at the present time inadequate, and our techniques for prediction on this basis are considerably less accurate. If one then compares the overall statistics of 50 per cent two-year cadaver kidney survival and adds to this comparison the complications in the post-transplant period which have been outlined above, it is not unreasonable to suppose that a patient who is doing well and leading a happy productive life on a home dialysis program should continue this program rather than undergo the rigors and uncertainties of cadaver kidney transplantation. This cannot be said, however, if he has an "A" match sibling who is able and willing to donate a kidney.

Not "Either Or"

Nevertheless, as I have suggested, the argument as to which is to be preferred is irrelevant since these two modalities can and should be utilized together. Dialysis, of course, is an adjunct to transplantation as a holding action for patients awaiting cadaver transplants or in preparation for a related transplant. Should the transplant fail, the patient can always be returned to dialysis. Second and even third transplants have succeeded where a first has failed, and it seems likely that, as our techniques for evaluating tissue compatibility between unrelated donors improves, we shall be able to select better matches even from this source. In this sense, then, dialysis is a means of keeping alive and in good health a large pool of uremic patients until a kidney with a predictably good chance of transplantation success becomes available from a cadaver source. Efforts at the creation of organ banks, organ sharing, and the transport of kidneys across the state lines and even between countries have already been undertaken, and the success rate of this kind of cooperative endeavor should improve greatly as our ability to predict tissue compatibility between unrelated donor recipient pairs improves.

It might be argued that a patient who is doing well on dialysis should not be exposed to the possible risks to life at this time inherent in the transplantation procedure. We hew to the philosophy that the patient should be saved even if the kidney is lost, and the result of this approach is shown in statistics that document the fact that the survival rate in the combined effort (transplantation and dialysis) does not affect the survival rate of dialysis alone.

The fact that 50 per cent of cadaver kidneys fail within a two-year period is disappointing. However, it must be remembered that this also means that the other 50 per cent do well for two years or more. If the risk to life of cadaver-kidney transplantation is not greater than that of remaining on dialysis, these odds might well be worth taking. The return to dialysis of 50 per cent of cadaver recipients within a period of two years has led at least one expert in hemodialysis to label transplantation of cadaver kidney as a "vacation from dialysis." However, the 50 per cent chance that this vacation might be considerably prolonged makes the prospect attractive and certainly reasonable to some patients.

Even from the economic point of view, there are some gains to be realized from a two-year vacation. The cost of an initially successful kidney transplant plus the cost of clinic visits and rehospitalization can be estimated at some $7000. This is to be compared with the cost of the cheapest form of artificial kidney treatment home dialysis, which amounts to some $16,000 over the first two-year period.

There are two other reasons why transplantation should at least be considered early in the course of hemodialysis. The first is that many patients on dialysis require blood transfusions. Blood transfusions contain platelets and white cells which in turn contain human tissue antigens similar to those contained in the kidney. Many of these patients thus become sensitized to human tissue antigens and thus immune to the renal tissue of a prospective donor. Many such individuals can be shown to be presensitized to more than 80 per cent of all the prospective kidney donors tested. Thus, they become "nontransplantable" in the present state of our knowledge, since transplantation of a kidney to a recipient already sensitized to tissues of the donor results in sudden and dramatic destruction of the graft ("hyperacute rejection"). It is true that not all dialysis patients become sensitized by transfusion. There appear to be "responders" and "nonresponders." Furthermore, the use of frozen blood appears to be diminishing this risk. Nevertheless, the chance of presensitization should be carefully weighed against the chances of failure of a cadaver transplant kidney before committing the patient permanently and irrevocably to dialysis. Secondly, there is a high incidence of Type 4 hyperlipidemia in uremic patients, even those who are well dialyzed.[10] Furthermore, the mortality among dialyzed patients is largely attributed to atherosclerotic vascular disease. These two facts suggest that vascular disease may progress at an accelerated rate in the dialyzed patient, particularly one whose blood pressure is not under control. Transplantation has been shown to arrest, but in many instances not to reverse, such atherosclerotic vascular disease, and thus one might expect a successfully transplanted patient who developed vascular disease during the dialysis period to suffer a vascular accident even after he obtains a normally functioning kidney. This hazard was clearly demonstrated by the first successful kidney transplant. The first identical twin who received a kidney transplant in 1954 following a period of severe renal failure and malignant hypertension died of a myocardial infarction at the age of 29, some seven years after transplantation.

My own experience with dialysis, beginning in 1948, and with transplantation of the kidney, beginning in 1950, is large and varied, and I write with some conviction when I say that these two modalities should be used together, that the most successful kidney transplantation is far and away more effective than the most successful form of hemodialysis, and that ultimately our ability to predict tissue compatibility in unrelated donor recipient pairs plus the organization of large and effective "organ sharing" plans will improve the results even in this area to the point where the amount of immunosuppression needed will make cadaver transplantation a less hazardous and more effective form of therapy and, thus, preferable in most instances to dialysis.

Conclusions

No less a scientific figure than Homer Smith stated in the early days of hemodialysis that the artificial kidney was of little use in the treatment of uremia since it removed only urea and everyone knew that urea was not important in the genesis of uremia. At the time of this statement the artificial kidney was a huge, ungainly contraption comprising a web of poles and tubes in the center of which rotated a grotesque barrel with spirals of blood-filled cellophane on its surface. Certainly Smith can be forgiven his incredulity after the sight of such a monstrosity. Nevertheless, even at that time those with experience with this awkward device were well aware of the clinical improvement with the artificial kidney itself. It is important, therefore, to have some personal experience in both areas in order to adequately compare them. They can and should be used conjointly. The advantages and disadvantages of each must be weighed for each individual patient. On balance, however, there is no question that kidney transplants between related individuals are more likely to produce a healthier individual than the best chronic dialysis program. For cadaver transplants whose success at the present time is of a lower order of magnitude, transplantation should be considered, and in most cases is worth the 50 per cent chance that the patient may do well for more than two years. Equally important, however, is the realization, which can come only from familiarity with both fields, of what the future holds in each area. Unquestionably a normally functioning kidney will be possible for a greater number of individuals when the present horizons for immunosuppressive therapy and tissue matching are crossed. Given a life with a single, normally functioning transplanted kidney to be compared with a life as a patient who must undergo dialysis three times a week, the argument as to which is the "preferred" form of therapy seems futile. Since we must deal with the present, however, it is critically important to emphasize that these two modalities, at least in the foreseeable future, must be used together and by physicians familiar with both forms of treatment and willing and able to cooperate with each other in seeking the optimum combination of therapy for the well-being of the patient.

References

1. Smith, H.: De urina. (Essay.) Kaiser Foundation Med. Bull. 6:1, 1958.
2. Merrill, J. P., Thorn, G. W., Walter, C. W., Callahan, E. J., III, and Smith, L. H., Jr.: The use of an artificial kidney. I. Technique. J. Clin. Invest. 29:412, 1950.
3. Hume, D. M., Merrill, J. P., Miller, B. F., and Thorn, G. W.: Experience with renal homotransplantation in the human. Report of 9 cases. J. Clin. Invest. 34:327, 1955.
4. Kominami, N., Lowrie, E. G., Ianhez, L. E., Sharen, A., Hampers, C. L., Merrill, J. P., and Lange, R. D.: The effect of total nephrectomy on hematopoiesis in patients undergoing chronic hemodialysis. J. Lab. Clin. Med. 78:524 (1971).
5. Asbury, A. K.: Recovery from uremic neuropathy. (Editorial.) New Eng. J. Med. 284:21, 1971.
6. Bluemle, L. W., Colletti, R. B., and Krueger, K. K.: Proceedings of the Workshop on Behavioral Bioassays in Uremia. Artificial Kidney-Chronic Uremia Program of the National Institute of Arthritis and Metabolic Diseases, P. H. S. Pub. No. NIH 72–37. Bethesda, Maryland, Department of Health, Education, and Welfare, 1970.
7. Young, G. A., and Parsons, F. M.: Plasma amino acid imbalance in patients with chronic renal failure on intermittent dialysis. Clin. Chim. Acta 27:491–496, 1970.
8. Merkatz, I. R., Schwartz, G. H., David, D. S., Stenzel, K. H., Riggio, R. R., and Whitsell, J. C.: Resumption of female reproductive function following renal transplantation. J.A.M.A. 216:11, 1971.
9. Beard, B. H.: The quality of life before and after renal transplantation. Dis. Nerv. Syst. 22(1):24–31, 1971.
10. Bagdade, J. D.: Lipemia, a sequela of chronic renal failure and hemodialysis. Amer. J. Clin. Nutr. 21:426, 1968.

Comment

Treatment of Uremia

The decade of the 1960's has seen a dramatic change in the therapy of end stage chronic renal disease. The development of effective techniques for chronic hemodialysis and the advent of successful transplantation of renal allografts from living or cadaver donors have made possible the rehabilitation of many patients who, only a few years earlier, would surely have died of uremia.

But these extraordinary advances have brought with them a host of new problems. The new techniques are terribly expensive. They make great demands on patients and their families, as well as on their physicians. They are by no means always successful, and often a patient is not completely rehabilitated but must endure a protracted period of incapacitation resulting from the complications of partially treated uremia.

One of the most difficult decisions facing the physician is: Which patients should be dialyzed and which transplanted? The two essays in this chapter deal with this issue in a forthright manner. They agree on some points: (1) Homotransplantation is the treatment of choice when the patient is lucky enough to have an identical twin or a sibling with closely matched tissue antigens. (2) A patient doing well on a home dialysis program should continue on this regimen rather than risk a cadaver transplant. Beyond this, however, Shaldon and Merrill diverge sharply in their general philosophies.

Merrill points out that a successful transplant restores a uremic patient to essentially normal health, while even the most successful of current dialysis programs still leaves the patient with serious health problems plus the burden of a confining, highly expensive therapy. Shaldon, on the other hand, looks forward to the day when night-time dialysis, at least five times weekly, will result in nearly total rehabilitation, and when advances in technology will greatly lower costs. He argues that survival statistics are better with hemodialysis than with cadaver kidney transplants, and he expresses doubt as to whether the problem of immune rejection with cadaver transplants will ever be solved. Merrill recognizes that at present only 50 per cent of cadaver transplants are functioning after two years, but points out that there need be no increase in mortality since a patient whose transplant fails can easily be returned to dialysis therapy. He believes that continued progress will be made in solving the rejection problem, and he looks forward to the day when organ banks, better tissue typing, and more effective control of the rejection reaction will result in uniformly successful cadaver transplants.

Regardless of the present relative merits of dialysis and cadaver transplants, it seems clear to me that Merrill is correct when he says that "the argument as to which is to be preferred is irrelevant since these two modalities can and should be utilized together." Dialysis is, of course, an essential adjunct to transplantation and is the modality which is used to sustain life if and when the transplant fails. Cadaver transplantation, on the other hand, can be viewed as an opportunity to escape from the constraints, expense, and disability of dialysis, when the dialysis patient is not doing well. If it is acceptable to the patient that his escape is likely to be only temporary, and if the patient's life is not jeopardized by heroic efforts to prevent rejection, there would appear to be good reason in many cases to recommend a cadaver transplant.

Neither dialysis nor cadaver transplantation has yet been fully perfected. If the problem of rejection is eventually solved, then there is no doubt that cadaver transplantation will be the preferred therapy. If not, and if the techniques of dialysis can be improved enough to prevent the complications and minimize the expense of present methods, then dialysis may well become the prime mode of therapy. In the long run, of course, the optimal solution to the problem of uremia will be the development of new methods for the prevention or cure of all those forms of renal disease that ultimately lead to terminal renal failure.

ARNOLD S. RELMAN

27

Immunologic Mechanisms in the Pathogenesis of Glomerular Diseases

THE IMPORTANCE OF IMMUNOLOGIC MECHANISMS
    by Curtis B. Wilson and Frank J. Dixon

AN EVALUATION OF IMMUNOLOGIC MECHANISMS
    by Robert T. McCluskey and Paul D. Leber

COMMENT
    by Arnold S. Relman

The Importance of Immunologic Mechanisms*

CURTIS B. WILSON and FRANK J. DIXON

Department of Experimental Pathology, Scripps Clinic and Research Foundation

Human glomerulonephritis is commonly induced by antigen-antibody reactions, with the ensuing glomerular injury mediated via humoral and cellular pathways. Beginning around 1900, investigations in animals led to the identification of two distinct immunologic mechanisms of immune glomerular injury.[1] Both mechanisms have been found in human glomerulonephritis and require the reaction of specific antibodies either with antigens in the glomerular basement membrane (GBM) or with nonglomerular antigens in the circulation to form nephritogenic immune complexes. Although cellular sensitization may accompany antibody formation, there is little morphologic or experimental evidence to implicate sensitized cells, prominent in delayed-type hypersensitivity and transplantation rejection, in the causation of either of these immunologic forms of glomerulonephritis.

Immunofluorescent techniques can be used to identify immunoglobulin and complement in glomeruli and have gained wide acceptance in distinguishing the two major immunopathogenic mechanisms of glomerular injury. When kidneys with glomerular damage either from animals subjected to experimental immunologic manipulations or from patients with glomerulonephritis are overlaid with fluoresceinated antibodies and examined by ultraviolet microscopy, one of two distinctive patterns of immunoglobulin and/or complement deposition is generally identified (Fig. 1). In the first mechanism, which involves antibodies specific for structural antigens of the GBM itself, immunofluorescent studies reveal smooth, continuous linear deposits of immunoglobulin and, frequently, complement

---

* This is Publication No. 593 from the Department of Experimental Pathology, Scripps Clinic and Research Foundation, 476 Prospect Street, La Jolla, California 92037. The work was supported by United States Public Health Service Contract PH-43-68-621, United States Public Health Service Grant AI-07007 and the Atomic Energy Commission Contract AT(04-3)-410.

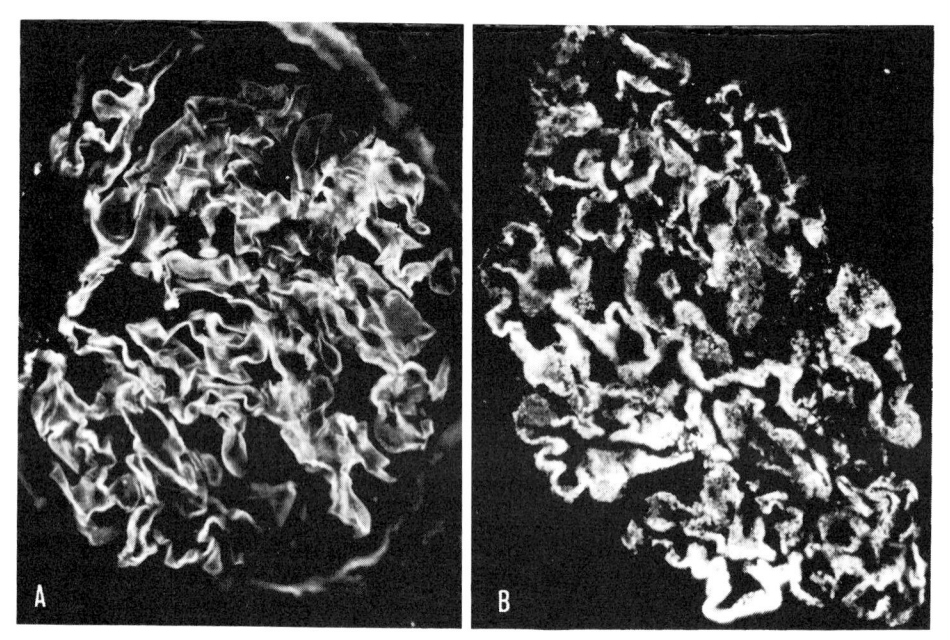

Figure 1. A, Smooth, linear deposits of immunoglobulin (anti-GBM antibody) are seen along the GBM of a glomerulus from a patient with Goodpasture's syndrome. Deposits are also present along Bowman's capsule. B, Irregular, granular deposits of immunoglobulin (presumed immune complexes) are present along the GBM of a patient with nephrotic syndrome and membranous glomerulonephritis. Complement (C1q, 3, 4, 5 and 6) could be identified in an identical pattern. (Stained with fluoresceinated rabbit anti-human IgG, original magnification X 250.)

along the entire distribution of the GBM. This immunopathogenic mechanism has been termed anti-glomerular basement membrane or anti-GBM nephritis. The second mechanism, that of antibodies reacting with nonglomerular antigens to form circulating immune complexes, causes, as would be expected, a very different and easily distinguishable immunofluorescent staining pattern. Since the circulating immune complexes are discrete aggregates which randomly deposit in the glomerular filter, probably in part related to its physiological filtering function, they appear as scattered, irregular, ofttimes granular deposits of immunoglobulin, complement, and, if sought, antigen along the GBM. These deposits can also be visualized with the electron microscope, where they appear as electron dense masses in subendothelial, intramembranous or, most characteristically, subepithelial, positions along the GBM. These electron dense deposits have been shown to contain immunoglobulin, complement, and streptococcal antigen(s) in poststreptococcal glomerulonephritic patients.[2]

The mediators responsible for immunologic injury have been identified in experimental animal models of glomerular injury in which each of several interrelated mechanisms has been altered selectively.[3] Although such studies have not been done in man, similar systems are part of immunologic inflammatory responses, and implication of equivalent processes in human glomerular injury seems justified. When antibody reacts with a specific antigen, molecular alterations in the immunoglobulin molecule occur which are recognized by the C1q portion of the first component of complement. Through a series of steps, many enzymatic, the complement cascade is activated, with release of biologically active products, some of which are chemotactic for polymorphonuclear leukocytes. Polymorphonuclear leukocytes thus attracted to the site of antigen-antibody interaction are probably retained there by another feature of complement activation, namely, immune adherence. Proteolytic enzymes released from the lysosomes of the polymorphonuclear leukocytes are capable of producing structural damage to the surrounding glomerular substrate, including the GBM. Polymorphonuclear cells also accumulate in glomeruli in human glomerulonephritis[4] and are known to contain proteases, collagenase, and elastase which would be capable of producing structural damage. Manipulation of these injury pathways may in the future provide therapeutic benefits to man.

Additional and/or alternative pathways of immunologic injury are probably also involved, since in about one-third of human anti-GMB glomerulonephritides complement cannot be detected in glomeruli. Acute experimental glomerular injury also occurs without the participation of complement or polymorphonuclear leukocytes after administration of avian and some mammalian nephrotoxic (anti-GBM) sera in animals. Likewise, in experimental acute serum sickness, neither complement nor polymorphonuclear leukocytes[5] are necessary for the production of glomerular lesions which heal rapidly without leaving permanent structural damage, reminiscent of the course of acute poststreptococcal glomerulonephritis in most patients. Kinins and vasoactive amines activated or released during immune reactions are being investigated for their possible contributory roles in this type of glomerular injury.

The recently described complement "bypass" system,[6] a series of serum proteins capable of activating the third component of complement (C3) and the remaining terminal components in the absence of antigen-antibody reactions, may provide an alternate pathway of glomerular injury. This mechanism, probably related to the properdin system, may be involved in hypocomplementemic membranoproliferative glomerulonephritis,[7] seen most commonly in children. Although heavy deposits of C3, sometimes accompanied by properdin,[8] are identified by immunofluorescence in glomeruli of these patients, immunoglobulins may not be found.[9] Factors yet to be identified but capable of activating C3 have been reported in the sera of these patients.[10] If in fact such bypass complement activation can be nephritogenic but not initiated by an antibody-antigen reaction, then such a form of nephritis would not be truly immunologic in origin even though its mediator system, complement, is traditionally considered an immunologic process.

Anti-GBM Nephritis

The nephrotoxicity of heterologous antikidney antibodies was discovered in 1900 by Lindemann. Subsequent investigations led to the recognition of two phases of injury in this experimental model of nephritis. The first was due to the direct toxic effects of the heterologous antibody (heterologous phase) and the second occurred when the recipient produced and deposited antibodies to the heterologous antibody protein bound to its glomeruli (autologous phase). The immunogen(s) required for the production of nephrotoxic sera resides in the GBM, making this type of sera in reality an anti-GBM antibody. This model of immunologic glomerular injury has served well in establishing the mechanisms of action of anti-GBM antibodies and has provided a means to manipulate the mediation pathways of such injury. Recently heterologous antilymphocyte globulin preparations used in immunosuppressive therapy for renal homografts have often been shown to contain GBM reactive antibodies.[11] These antibodies can produce fatal glomerulonephritis in subhuman primates and almost certainly have a similar potential in humans. Local absorption of the GBM reactive antibodies by muscle vasculature after intramuscular injection and concomitant chemical immunosuppressive therapy have probably minimized their nephrotoxic effects in man.

In 1962 Steblay[12] produced autologous anti-GBM antibodies and fatal nephritis in sheep after injection of GBM in adjuvant, providing an animal model of spontaneous human anti-GBM nephritis. In sheep made nephritic by this technique, linear immunofluorescent deposits of anti-GBM antibodies can be identified, and circulating anti-GBM antibodies which accumulate after bilateral nephrectomy can be used to transfer the disease to normal sheep, thereby directly demonstrating the nephrotoxicity of such antibodies.[13]

Anti-GBM antibodies demonstrable in human kidneys by direct immunofluorescence were shown to be responsible for the production of human glomerulonephritis in experiments similar to those described above in sheep by Lerner, Glassock, and Dixon in 1967.[14] These investigators were able to remove or elute anti-GBM antibodies from homogenized human kidneys by treatment in acid pH. The isolated anti-GBM antibodies reacted with normal human GBM and transferred nephritis to subhuman primates. The ultimate demonstration of the nephrotoxicity of these anti-GBM antibodies came when anti-GBM nephritis was accidentally transferred to a renal homograft placed in a patient in whom circulating anti-GBM antibodies were demonstrated after nephrectomy.

A common immunologic etiology is suggested when hemorrhagic pulmonary disease accompanies anti-GBM nephritis (Goodpasture's syndrome). Antibodies which are capable of combining with the GBM can be eluted from the lungs of these patients.[15] Studies with anti-GBM antibodies eluted from the kidneys of patients with anti-GBM nephritis, when those with and without Goodpasture's syndrome are compared, have demonstrated a broader basement membrane specificity in the Goodpasture's eluates, both in various human tissues and among other species.[16]

There can be little doubt about the role of anti-GBM antibodies in the production of human glomerulonephritis. The incidence of anti-GBM nephritis is not firmly established but would appear to be about 5 per cent in the general glomerulonephritic population. A 10 per cent incidence has been found among patients treated in a military hospital.[*] Little is known regarding the events which trigger human autologous anti-GBM antibody production. Its coincident

---

[*] J. J. McPhaul, Jr., M.D., personal communication.

appearance with influenza A2 virus infection[17] and following hydrocarbon solvent inhalation[18] suggests that immunogenic alterations of pulmonary basement membranes may be involved. The demonstration of potentially nephritogenic[19] circulating antigens identical to those of the GBM and their presence in normal urine[20] indicate another possible antigenic source.

Immune Complex Nephritis

Von Pirquet in 1911 recognized that there was a relationship between the host immune response to foreign serum protein, the coexistence of antigen and antibody in the circulation, and the development of serum sickness, a condition often accompanied by glomerular injury.[21] Later investigations by Dixon culminating in the early 1960's[22-24] convincingly established that tissue deposition of immune complexes of antigen and antibody, which formed in the circulation when antibody production had been elicited after introduction of a foreign antigen, was the cause of both the glomerulonephritic and arteritic lesions seen in serum sickness. Specifically, these studies demonstrated that antibody production was required; injury occurred only when complexes of antigen and antibody were deposited in tissue, and neither antigen nor antibody alone was injurious. Subsequent investigations have shown that immune complex size, the immunologic release of vasoactive amines with alteration of vascular (glomerular) permeability, and the functional state of the mesangium may influence glomerular deposition of immune complexes.[25, 26] Antibody from the circulation may continue to interact with and accumulate on previously deposited immune complexes, influencing their final composition and possibly their phlogogenicity. Quantitative studies in rabbits with chronic nephritis induced by daily injection of foreign serum protein antigens in amounts to balance antibody production have shown that about 0.5 per cent of the injected antigen deposits in the kidney in immune complex form, while the remaining immune complexes are apparently removed by phagocytic cells throughout the body.[26] The etiologic role of immune complex deposition in tissue injury has been further shown by the specific ability of excessive antigen administration to cause dissolution of glomerular bound immune complexes with improvement in the glomerular lesions.

Approximately 78 per cent of kidneys from patients with clinical and morphologic evidence of glomerulonephritis contain granular glomerular deposits of immunoglobulin and complement identifiable by immunofluorescence. The pattern of this deposition is identical with that seen in animals with experimental immune complex nephritis. This observation has led to the widely held idea that most human glomerulonephritides result from glomerular deposition of circulating immune complexes.

The histologic picture of human kidneys with granular immune complex deposits varies widely and has been a source of concern to some investigators in applying a single pathogenic mechanism. This should not be troublesome. In chronic nephritis induced in rabbits by daily administration of antigen, the entire spectrum of recognized glomerulonephritic pathologic alterations can be observed, although the etiologic agent and pathogenic mechanism are identical.[27] Simple proliferative changes, isolated membranous thickening of the GBM, or any combination of these may be observed, as well as necrotizing, crescent-forming, fulminant nephritis. Glomerular pathology appears to be much more influenced by the intensity and tempo of the immunologic reaction and the host response to it than by the nature of the inciting antigen. Thus, evaluation of the routine histologic alterations of the kidney is of little value in determining etiology.

The list of proven examples of human immune complex nephritis continues to grow; however, the etiologic agent(s) remains unidentified in the majority of human glomerulonephritides with granular glomerular deposits of immunoglobulins and complement.

Lupus nephritis is probably the clearest example of human immune complex glomerulonephritis. Circulating antibodies specific for nuclear antigens, especially DNA, can be shown to fluctuate with amelioration or exacerbation of disease, the latter being accompanied by the appearance of immune complexes and, occasionally, free DNA in the circulation.[28] Immune complexes composed of DNA, anti-DNA antibody and complement can be demonstrated in the kidneys of such patients, and anti-DNA antibodies can be eluted from the kidney.[29-32] The variable renal pathology of patients with lupus nephritis caused by similar antigen-antibody systems again attests to the fact that morphologic changes do not correlate with etiologic agents or pathogenic mechanisms. Current investigations are directed toward identification of other antigen-antibody systems in this disease with anti-immunoglobulin autoantibodies drawing considerable attention.

Glomerular deposits of thyroglobulin antithyroglobulin complexes have been identified by immunofluorescence and/or elution of specific antibodies from glomerular deposits in the glomerulonephritis that sometimes occurs in patients with thyroiditis.* Thus, a second immune complex glomerulonephritis with an endogenous antigen is known.

Exogenous or foreign antigens, frequently of microbial origin, have also been implicated in glomerular immune complex deposits of direct immunofluorescence and/or elution of specific antibody. By using these techniques, streptococcal antigen in poststreptococcal glomerulonephritis,[33] staphylococcal antigen in hydrocephalic patients with glomerulonephritis secondary to infected ventriculoatrial shunts,[34] plasmodial antigen in malarial nephrosis,[35] and viral antigen in the glomerulonephritis of patients with Australian antigen positive hepatitis[36] have been identified. Many laboratories are now attempting to increase this list, and certainly numerous other examples will soon be forthcoming. One difficulty in identifying the antigenic content of glomerular immune complexes is exemplified in the courses of acute serum sickness in rabbits[37] and poststreptococcal glomerulonephritis in man.[33] In both instances the antigenic content of immune complexes can be identified by immunofluorescence for only a few days after deposition. In experimental acute serum sickness, radio-labeled antigen can be shown to persist even after its identification by immunofluorescence is blocked by continued deposition of antibody from the circulation. A similar situation probably

---

* D. Koffler, M.D., personal communication; R. S. Schwartz, M.D., personal communication.

occurs in poststreptococcal glomerulonephritis and may obscure antigenic identification in many other human immune complex glomerulonephritides.

The incidence of immunologically induced glomerulonephritis demonstrated by immunofluorescence varies, depending upon the patient population studied and, although often not commented upon, the stage of the renal disease at the time of study. In late stage glomerulonephritis the immunologic deposits may well be obliterated along with morphologic evidence of preceding pathogenic events. During the past two years we have used immunofluorescence to study kidneys from approximately 500 glomerulonephritic patients, many from transplantation centers and transplantation-oriented nephrology groups. The patterns of immunoglobulin and/or complement deposition were typical of the characteristic patterns of anti-GBM antibody in 5 per cent and of immune complex glomerulonephritis in 78 per cent of these patients. An additional 5 per cent had immunoglobulin and/or complement present in atypical distributions. The remaining patients had no immunoglobulin or complement deposits that were apparent by immunofluorescence. Some of these negative findings may be caused by inadequate sampling as revealed when larger tissue sections are examined, whereas others reflect the late stage of glomerular damage. An infrequent, yet to be described alternative injury mechanism cannot be excluded in the rest.

Occasional patients with suspected "nonimmunologic" renal disease, such as diabetic glomerulosclerosis, nephrosclerosis, or pyelonephritis, have been found to have deposits of immunoglobulin and/or complement by means of immunofluorescence.[38] Observations of this type should not distract from the implication of immunologic processes in glomerulonephritis but should focus attention on possible immune mechanisms in the causation of these other forms of renal disease, the pathogenic mechanisms of which are only poorly understood. Also, when immunoglobulin and/or complement deposits are identified in presumed "nonimmunologic" renal disease, evidence is not available to exclude the possibility that an immunologic insult has been superimposed on the course of a so-called "nonimmunologic" disease.

At the time of this writing it is reasonable to say that the vast majority of human glomerulonephritides are induced by one of the two well defined immunologic mechanisms described herein. It remains now to identify the events responsible for the induction of autologous anti-GBM antibody formation and to identify the etiologic agent in the majority of immune complex glomerulonephritides.

References

1. Unanue, E. R., and Dixon, F. J.: Experimental glomerulonephritis: Immunological events and pathogenetic mechanisms. Advances Immunol. 6:1, 1967.
2. Andres, G. A., Accinni, L., Hsu, K. C., Zabriskie, J. B., and Seegal, B. C.: Electron microscopic studies of human glomerulonephritis with ferritin-conjugated antibody. J. Exp. Med. 123:399, 1966.
3. Cochrane, C. G.: Immunologic tissue injury mediated by neutrophilic leukocytes. Advances Immunol. 9:97, 1968.
4. Burkholder, P. M.: Ultrastructural demonstration of injury and perforation of glomerular capillary basement membrane in acute proliferative glomerulonephritis. Amer. J. Path. 56:251, 1969.

5. Henson, P. M., and Cochrane, C. G.: Antigen-antibody complexes, platelets and increased vascular permeability. In Movat, H. Z. (ed.): *Cellular and Humoral Mechanisms in Anaphylaxis and Allergy*. Basel, S. Karger, 1969, p. 129.
6. Götze, O., and Müller-Eberhard, H. J.: The C3-activator system: An alternate pathway of complement activation. J. Exp. Med. *134*:90s, 1971.
7. West, C. D., McAdams, A. J., McConville, J. M., Davis, M. C., and Holland, N.H.: Hypocomplementemic and normocomplementemic persistent (chronic) glomerulonephritis; clinical and pathological characteristics. J. Pediat. *67*:1089, 1965.
8. Westberg, N. G., Naff, G. B., Boyer, J. T., and Michael, A. F.: Glomerular deposition of properdin in acute and chronic glomerulonephritis with hypocomplementemia. J. Clin. Invest. *59*:642, 1971.
9. Herdman, R. C., Pickering, R. J., Michael, A. F., Vernier, R. L., Fish, A. J., Gewurz, H., and Good, R. A.: Chronic glomerulonephritis associated with low serum complement activity (chronic hypocomplementemic glomerulonephritis). Medicine *49*:207, 1970.
10. Vallota, E. H., Forristal, J., Spitzer, R. E., Davis, N. D., and West, C. D.: Characteristics of a non-complement-dependent C3-reactive complex formed from factors in nephritic and normal serum. J. Exp. Med. *131*:1306, 1970.
11. Wilson, C. B., Dixon, F. J., Fortner, J. G., and Cerilli, J.: Glomerular basement membrane reactive antibodies in anti-lymphocyte globulin. J. Clin. Invest. *50*:1525, 1971.
12. Steblay, R. W.: Glomerulonephritis induced in sheep by injections of heterologous glomerular basement membrane and Freund's complete adjuvant. J. Exp. Med. *116*:253, 1962.
13. Lerner, R., and Dixon, F. J.: Transfer of ovine experimental allergic glomerulonephritis (EAG) with serum. J. Exp. Med. *124*:431, 1966.
14. Lerner, R., Glassock, R. J., and Dixon, F. J.: The role of anti-glomerular basement membrane antibody in the pathogenesis of human glomerulonephritis. J. Exp. Med. *126*: 989, 1967.
15. Koffler, D., Sandson, J., Carr, R., and Kunkel, H. G.: Immunologic studies concerning the pulmonary lesions in Goodpasture's syndrome. Amer. J. Path. *54*:293, 1969.
16. McPhaul, J. J., Jr., and Dixon, F. J.: Characterization of human anti-glomerular basement membrane antibodies eluted from glomerulonephritic kidneys. J. Clin. Invest. *49*:308, 1970.
17. Wilson, C. B., and Smith, R. C.: Goodpasture's syndrome associated with influenza A2 virus infection. Ann. Intern. Med. *76*:91, 1972.
18. Beirne, G. J., and Brennan, J. T.: Anti-glomerular basement membrane antibody mediated glomerulonephritis associated with chronic exposure to hydrocarbon solvents. Arch. Environ. Health. In press.
19. Lerner, R., and Dixon, F. J.: The induction of acute glomerulonephritis in rabbits with soluble antigens isolated from normal homologous and autologous urine. J. Immunol. *100*:1277, 1968.
20. McPhaul, J. J., Jr., and Dixon, F. J.: Immunoreactive basement membrane antigens in normal human urine and serum. J. Exp. Med. *130*:1395, 1969.
21. Von Pirquet, C. E.: Allergy. Arch. Intern. Med. *7*:259, 1911.
22. Dixon, F. J., Vazquez, J. J., Weigle, W. O., and Cochrane, C. G.: Pathogenesis of serum sickness. A.M.A. Arch. Path. *65*:18, 1958.
23. Dixon, F. J.: Tissue injury produced by antigen-antibody complexes. In *Second International Symposium on Immunopathology*, Basel, Benno Schwabe and Company, 1962, p. 71.
24. Dixon, F. J.: The role of antigen-antibody complexes in disease. Harvey Lect., *58*:21, 1963.
25. Henson, P. M., and Cochrane, C. G.: Acute immune complex disease in rabbits. The role of complement and of a leukocyte-dependent release of vasoactive amines from platelets. J. Exp. Med. *133*:554, 1971.
26. Wilson, C. B., and Dixon, F. J.: Quantitation of acute and chronic serum sickness in the rabbit. J. Exp. Med. *134*:7s, 1971.
27. Dixon, F. J., Feldman, J. D., and Vazquez, J.: Experimental glomerulonephritis. The pathogenesis of a laboratory model resembling the spectrum of human glomerulonephritis. J. Exp. Med. *113*:899, 1961.
28. Koffler, D., Agnello, V., Thoburn, R., and Kunkel, H. G.: Systemic lupus erythematosus: Prototype of immune complex nephritis in man. J. Exp. Med. *134*:169s, 1971.
29. Tan, E. M., Schur, P. H., and Kunkel, H. G.: DNA in the serum of patients with systemic lupus erythematosus (SLE). J. Clin. Invest. *44*:1104, 1965.

30. Tan, E. M., Schur, P. H., Carr, R. I., and Kunkel, H. G.: Deoxyribonucleic acid (DNA) and antibodies to DNA in the serum of patients with systemic lupus erythematosus. J. Clin. Invest. 45:1732, 1966.
31. Paronetto, F., and Koffler, D.: Immunofluorescent localization of immunoglobulins, complement, and fibrinogen in human disease. I. Systemic lupus erythematosus. J. Clin. Invest. 44:1657, 1965.
32. Koffler, D., Schur, P. H., and Kunkel, H. G.: Immunological studies concerning the nephritis of systemic lupus erythematosus. J. Exp. Med. 126:607, 1967.
33. Treser, G., Sermar, M., Ty, A., Sagel, I., Franklin, M. A., and Lange, K.: Partial characterization of antigenic streptococcal plasma membrane components in acute glomerulonephritis. J. Clin. Invest. 49:762, 1970.
34. Kaufman, D. B., and McIntosh, R.: The pathogenesis of the renal lesion in a patient with streptococcal disease, infected ventriculoatrial shunt, cryoglobulinemia and nephritis. Amer. J. Med. 50:262, 1971.
35. Ward, P. A., and Kibukamusoke, J. W.: Evidence for soluble immune complexes in the pathogenesis of the glomerulonephritis of quartan malaria. Lancet 1:283, 1969.
36. Combes, B., Stastny, R., Shorey, J., Eigenbrodt, E. H., Barrero, A., Hull, A. R., and Carter, N. W.: Glomerulonephritis with deposition of Australian antigen-antibody complexes in glomerular basement membrane. Lancet 2:234, 1971.
37. Wilson, C. B., and Dixon, F. J.: Antigen quantitation in experimental immune complex glomerulonephritis. I. Acute serum sickness. J. Immunol. 105:279, 1970.
38. Gallo, G. R.: Elution studies in kidneys with linear deposition of immunoglobulin in glomeruli. Amer. J. Path. 61:377, 1970.

An Evaluation of Immunologic Mechanisms*

ROBERT T. McCLUSKEY and PAUL D. LEBER

Children's Hospital Medical Center, Boston

The suggestion that glomerular disease may result from hypersensitivity mechanisms is not new. It has been known for many years that acute poststreptococcal glomerulonephritis is accompanied by a marked decrease in the serum hemolytic complement activity. The latent period between the infection and apparent onset of renal disease, the absence of streptococci in glomeruli, and the demonstration that glomerulonephritis could be produced experimentally by injection of foreign serum or nephrotoxic antibodies were also used as arguments favoring hypersensitivity mechanisms. During the past 15 years two major developments have served to expand greatly our knowledge of glomerular diseases and to strengthen the belief that many forms are immunologically mediated. One development has been the study of renal biopsies, especially by immunofluorescence and electron microscopy, which, in addition to providing insight into pathogenic mechanisms, has led to a considerable increase in the number of recognized forms of glomerulonephritis (Table 1). The second factor has been the extensive investigation of experimental models of immunologically induced glomerular diseases. Many of the conclusions about immunopathogenetic mechanisms in human disease rest on information derived from these models.

Experimental Immunologic Glomerular Disease

Two major forms of immunologically induced glomerular disease are recognized, namely, immune complex glomerulonephritis and anti-glomerular basement membrane antibody (anti-GBM) disease. Immune complex glomerulonephritis results primarily from deposition in glomeruli of immune complexes

---

* Supported in part by USPHS Grant #AI 10,780.

Table 1. *Classification of Glomerulonephritis*

I. Diseases presumed or known to result from immunologic mechanisms
   A. Immune complex glomerulonephritis
      1. Diseases of known etiology
         Poststreptococcal glomerulonephritis*
         Glomerulonephritis associated with other bacterial infections:
            staphylococcal; pneumococcal; bacterial endocarditis; shunt
            infections; secondary syphilis
         Glomerulonephritis associated with malaria*
      2. Glomerular diseases associated with systemic diseases of
         unknown etiology
         Lupus nephritis†
         Nephritis with anaphylactoid purpura
         Nephritis in periarteritis nodosa
         Nephritis in idiopathic "mixed" cryoglobulinemia‡
      3. Primary glomerular diseases of unknown etiology
         Membranous glomerulonephritis
         Membranoproliferative glomerulonephritis
         IgA IgG nephropathy (Berger)
         Some cases classified as focal glomerulonephritis
         Some cases classified as rapidly progressive glomerulonephritis
         Some cases classified as chronic sclerosing glomerulonephritis
         Unclassified glomerular diseases
   B. Anti-glomerular basement membrane (anti-GBM) antibody diseases
      1. Glomerulonephritis associated with Goodpasture's syndrome
      2. Some cases classified as rapidly progressive or chronic
         glomerulonephritis
II. Diseases without impressive evidence of immunologic mechanisms
   A. Most cases of chronic sclerosing glomerulonephritis
   B. Some cases of focal glomerulonephritis
   C. Lipoid nephrosis§ (childhood nephrosis, "minimal disease")
   D. Unclassified glomerular diseases

---

*Antigen may have been identified in glomerular deposits.
†Antigen (DNA) definitely identified in glomerular deposits.
‡Antigen presumed to be altered IgG, complexed with IgM.
§Although not generally classified as a form of glomerulonephritis, it is included here for convenience.

formed in the circulation.[1] Although the factors responsible for localization of complexes in glomeruli are not completely understood, in a general way it is thought that certain complexes become trapped along or within the basement membrane or in mesangial regions because of their physical properties (such as size or solubility). However, at most, only a small fraction of circulating complexes accumulate in glomeruli, the bulk being removed by the reticuloendothelial system. Once complexes lodge in glomeruli, free antibody or antigen derived from the circulation may combine with unreacted sites in the deposits, which generally results in an increase in their size. In addition, other serum factors, such as complement components or rheumatoid factor, may interact with the deposited complexes. The way in which complexes bring about glomerular damage is only poorly understood and will not be discussed here. (See references 1 and 2 for review.)

A variety of antigens can be used to induce immune complex glomerulonephritis, including foreign serum proteins (serum sickness), viral antigenic material, and even certain autologous antigens. In addition to experimentally induced models, immune complexes have been shown to be responsible for the glomerular lesions seen in certain spontaneous diseases of animals, including chronic viral infections, and in certain strains of New Zealand mice (NZB/W).

Immune complexes may produce a variety of morphologic forms of experimental glomerular disease, including acute proliferative or necrotizing diseases, as well as chronic disease with proliferative, membranous, and sclerosing changes. The type of glomerular injury depends upon a number of factors, such as the species studied, the amount and duration of antigen administration, the intensity of the antibody response, the antigen itself, and the operation of secondary pathogenic mechanisms. Although there is no pathognomonic histologic picture, immune complex diseases exhibit highly characteristic features by immunofluorescence, namely, irregular or granular accumulation of immunoglobulins, complement components, and antigen within glomeruli. These materials may be seen within or along either side of the basement membrane or in mesangial regions. Generally, corresponding dense granular deposits are seen by electron microscopy.

The second major form of immunologically induced glomerular disease, experimental anti-GBM disease, can be produced in two major forms: one, by administration of heterologous anti-GBM antibodies (Masugi or nephrotoxic serum nephritis), and two, by immunization of certain species with heterologous GBM preparations, which results in the formation of autoantibodies directed against the GBM (Steblay nephritis).[3] Both forms are typically severe, rapidly progressive, proliferative glomerular diseases, characterized by conspicuous crescent formation. However, again the histologic features are not unique and the most distinctive picture is seen in immunofluorescence preparations, in which completely continuous, smooth ("linear") staining for IgG and complement is seen along the glomerular basement membrane. Electron microscopy usually fails to reveal significant deposits.

Human Glomerular Diseases

In considering the basis of glomerular diseases, it is helpful to attempt to distinguish between etiologic factors and pathogenetic mechanisms. Although usage differs somewhat, the designations immune complex and anti-GBM disease would best be used to refer to the basic pathogenetic mechanisms responsible for the glomerular damage, and etiology to those factors which initiate the formation of immune complexes in the circulation or of autoantibodies directed against the GBM. In these terms, the etiology of an immune complex disease includes more than the antigen involved. In some experimental forms the etiology is fairly simple; for example, in acute serum sickness the major etiologic factor is the intravenous injection of antigen. However, the nature and the intensity of the antibody response, which may be under genetic control, also determine whether or not disease will develop. In other situations the etiologic factors are even more diverse; in NZB mice, for example, they include genetic factors (which influence the immune response) and viral infection. Under pathogenesis one can consider not only the primary mechanisms, that is, the accumulation in glomeruli of immune complexes or anti-GBM antibody, but also secondary mechanisms that may come into play, such as generation of chemotactic factors, release of leukocyte lysosomal enzymes, or initiation of coagulation. It should be apparent that it may be possible to establish conclusively either of the two major pathogenic mechanisms without being able to identify underlying etiologic factors. Conversely, the major etiologic factor may be apparent and the pathogenesis not understood.

One of the main reasons for the belief that many forms of glomerulonephritis in man result from immunologic mechanisms is provided by immunofluorescence observations. In many conditions, conspicuous, irregular, or granular accumulation of immunoglobulins and complement are found in glomeruli, and in these instances it appears justifiable to suspect an immune complex pathogenesis (Table 1). In a considerably smaller number of cases, typical "linear" staining for immunoglobulins and complement is found, suggesting anti-GBM disease (Table 1). However, ever since the first report describing the presence of gamma globulin in diseased glomeruli, the suggestion has been made that this merely represents secondary nonspecific accumulation of plasma proteins in damaged glomeruli. Accordingly the question may be asked: What constitutes sufficient evidence to establish with reasonable certainty either major type of immunopathogenic mechanism? In the case of suspected immune complex disease, two lines of evidence are most important: First, it should be shown that a significant percentage of the immunoglobulin deposited in glomeruli represents antibody of a given specificity. This can be demonstrated with immunoglobulin eluted from glomeruli, provided the antigen is known and available. Second, the corresponding antigen should be demonstrated within glomeruli by immunofluorescence in the same location as immunoglobulin and complement. In experimental studies it has been found that this may require partial elution of the antibody to uncover reactive antigenic sites. While these findings would establish beyond any reasonable doubt an immune complex pathogenesis, it would be of additional value to show that immune complexes of the same specificity as found in glomeruli are present in the circulation. If complexes themselves cannot be demonstrated, the finding of free antibody at certain times and free antigen at other times provides essentially the same evidence.

In situations in which it is not possible to obtain sufficient material for elution studies, the demonstration of antigenic material within glomeruli by immunofluorescence, although not conclusive, can be considered as strong evidence for the presence of immune complexes, provided there are other reasons to implicate that antigen. This situation will be considered in connection with poststreptococcal glomerulonephritis and nephritis in mixed cryoglobulinemia.

In the absence of such evidence, the conclusion that a glomerular disease is due to immune complexes must be considered tentative. However, if there is an established experimental model that very closely resembles the human disease, especially in terms of immunofluorescence and electron microscopic findings, the presumption may be very strong that the disease has an immune complex pathogenesis.

In order to prove that a glomerular disease is due to anti-GBM antibodies, it should be shown that immunoglobulin eluted from glomeruli can react with glomerular basement membrane in vitro, as shown by immunofluorescence. Of almost equal weight would be the demonstration of circulating anti-GBM antibodies in a patient with glomerular disease and typical "linear" staining.* Another kind of evidence that has been obtained in a few cases, but which is hardly practical, is the demonstration that immunoglobulins eluted from human glomeruli localize in glomeruli with a typical "linear" distribution following intravenous injection into a nonhuman primate.

Using these criteria, which human glomerular diseases have been conclusively shown to be due to immunologic mechanisms? Among those suspected of being due to immune complexes, only in lupus nephritis can the evidence be considered conclusive (and even here the story is not complete). In addition, some evidence for the presence of antigen in glomeruli has been obtained in poststreptococcal nephritis, malarial nephritis, and nephritis in idiopathic mixed cryoglobulinemia. An anti-GBM pathogenesis has been conclusively established in a relatively small number of patients classified as having rapidly progressive glomerulonephritis or Goodpasture's syndrome.

With the exception of a handful of cases, in which a particular antigen may have been identified in glomeruli, the evidence for an immune complex pathogenesis in all the other forms listed under IA in Table 1 can only be considered tentative.

IMMUNE COMPLEX GLOMERULONEPHRITIS

DISEASES OF KNOWN ETIOLOGY

Poststreptococcal glomerulonephritis. Acute poststreptococcal glomerulonephritis has long been considered to be an immunologically mediated disease. This view has been considerably strengthened by the immunofluorescence demonstration of granular deposits of immunoglobulins and complement along the glomerular basement membrane and to a lesser extent in mesangial regions. These findings not only support an immune complex pathogenesis, but they virtually eliminate the possibility that anti-GBM antibodies are responsible, since if that were the case, typical linear staining for IgG and C3 should be found. An anti-GBM mechanism has been suggested because it has been shown experimentally that streptococcal infection may lead to the formation of antibodies that cross react with the glomerular basement membrane.[4] (For further discussion on this point see the section on anti-GBM disease, rapidly progressive glomerulonephritis.)

In most respects acute glomerulonephritis is faithfully reproduced in the

---

*In some circumstances, serum anti-GBM activity may be detected by passive hemagglutination even when no linear glomerular staining is present.[3a] It appears that the affinity of the anti-GBM in these instances is low and that probably, therefore, it plays no primary pathogenetic role. Indeed, the presence of low affinity circulating anti-GBM occurs in association with massive renal injury (i.e., cortical necrosis) and in association with other forms of renal injury in which other pathogenetic mechanisms are presumed to operate. It is thus more than likely that they represent autoantibodies whose formation is provoked by the release or alteration of antigen from damaged kidney. It nevertheless remains a possibility that these antibodies may secondarily contribute to renal injury.

model of acute "one shot" serum sickness. Both are characterized by diffuse proliferative changes, by granular accumulation of immunoglobulins and complement, and by electron-dense deposits on the epithelial side of the basement membrane. Both forms usually go on to complete recovery, although this occurs much more slowly in the human disease. Although these considerations indicate that poststreptococcal glomerulonephritis is almost certainly a form of acute immune complex disease, the nature of the antigen has yet to be established. Obviously the first question to be answered is whether or not the antigen is of streptococcal origin, and evidence concerning this point is controversial. Three groups have reported the demonstration by immunofluorescence of streptococcal antigens within glomeruli using fluorescein-labeled rabbit antisera to Type 12 streptococci;[5-7] two groups have reported that they were unable to find such material.[8,9] Zabriskie[10] has presented arguments that favor acceptance of the positive rather than the negative results. First, in order to obtain positive results, it may be necessary to study biopsies obtained very early, presumably because the antigen is degraded or rapidly becomes saturated with antibody; most biopsies studied have not been obtained in the first days of the disease. Second, the streptococcal antisera employed in the negative studies may have been inadequate to detect the relevant antigen. While these arguments are reasonable, they do not prove that the positive results are valid, especially in view of the vagaries of the immunofluorescence technique. Moreover, there is a significant obstacle to accepting the claims that streptococcal antigens have been demonstrated within glomeruli, namely, that the material has been observed principally in mesangial regions and not in deposits along the basement membrane, where immunoglobulins are typically found. While the failure to find streptococcal antigens within deposits could, as suggested above, be accounted for by saturation of antigenic sites, the frequent absence of immunoglobulin in mesangial areas, which supposedly contain significant amounts of streptococcal antigen, would be difficult to explain. Treser et al.[11] have used another approach and claim to have demonstrated streptococcal material within glomeruli. Fluorescein-labeled IgG fractions of sera obtained from patients recovering from acute poststreptococcal glomerulonephritis were reported to stain material in glomeruli in biopsies obtained early in the disease. Moreover, it was reported that absorption of the sera with certain Group A streptococci prevented the staining. These interesting results await confirmation.

Beyond this, even among those who have reported positive results, there is a difference of opinion as to the nature of the streptococcal antigen. Treser et al.[11] have concluded that the material is part of the cell membrane. In contrast, Zabriskie[10] has presented evidence that the antigen is present in the cell wall.

Since poststreptococcal glomerulonephritis is rarely fatal, it has not been possible to obtain sufficient renal tissue to permit elution studies, which might reveal whether the immunoglobulin deposited in glomeruli contains a high percentage of antibodies directed against streptococcal material.

If the complexes that appear to be responsible for the glomerular disease do not contain streptococcal antigens, what alternative exists? One possibility, which has been proposed by Kaufman and McIntosh,[12] is that they represent autologous immune complexes. According to this hypothesis, the streptococcal infection results in alteration of some circulating autologous material, rendering it immunogenic to the host. In support of this, McIntosh has presented evidence that circulating complexes composed of altered autologous IgG and antibody directed against it are present in some patients. It remains to be demonstrated, however, that these complexes are of pathogenic significance and, beyond that, to determine whether they initiate the glomerular disease, rather than being of secondary importance.

Nothing definite is known about secondary pathogenic mechanisms in acute glomerulonephritis. The presence of neutrophils, components, and fibrin[8] in glomeruli suggests these factors may be involved. However, in the experimental model that most closely resembles the human disease, namely, acute "one shot" serum sickness in the rabbit, neither the complement system, leukocytes, nor the coagulation system appears necessary for the development of glomerular lesions. It should be noted, however, that neutrophil accumulation is often more conspicuous in the human disease.

Thus, although available evidence indicates that poststreptococcal glomerulonephritis is an acute immune complex disease, there is uncertainty concerning the nature of the antigen and ignorance of secondary pathogenic mechanisms. Unfortunately there appears to be no entirely satisfactory experimental model in which these questions could be more easily explored. In any case, if the glomerular disease is in fact due to immune complexes, it must be presumed that these complexes possess certain distinctive properties which render them extremely efficient in producing glomerular disease, since in many other situations, including other types of infection, where complexes are formed in the circulation, glomerular disease is either mild or absent.

GLOMERULAR DISEASE ASSOCIATED WITH OTHER BACTERIAL INFECTIONS

It seems possible that immune complexes are largely or entirely responsible for the glomerular lesions seen in some patients with certain massive bacterial infections, such as endocarditis, and infected ventriculoatrial shunts. A priori, this explanation appears attractive because of the prolonged release of bacterial antigens into the circulation in these conditions. However, supporting evidence is rather meager and consists largely of the finding by immunofluorescence of glomerular deposits of immunoglobulins and/or complement. Demonstration of antigenic material within glomeruli by immunofluorescence has apparently been claimed in only a single case, namely, in a patient with an infected shunt.[13] More complete evidence, as might be provided by elution studies, has not been reported.

In a few patients with the nephrotic syndrome occurring in secondary syphilis, granular deposits of immunoglobulins and complement have been found in glomeruli, suggesting an immune complex mechanism.[14] Further supporting evidence is lacking. Moreover, it has not even been established beyond question that the glomerular lesions are due to syphilis, although the rapid disappearance of evidence of renal disease following penicillin therapy strongly supports the relationship.

There is fairly impressive although not conclusive evidence that a form of glomerulonephritis seen in association with quartan malaria is due to immune complexes containing malarial antigens.[15]

GLOMERULAR DISEASE ASSOCIATED WITH SYSTEMIC DISEASES OF UNKNOWN CAUSE

Lupus nephritis. Among the glomerular diseases associated with systemic diseases of unknown cause (Table 1), lupus nephritis has been most thoroughly studied. In fact, of all human glomerular diseases it is in lupus nephritis that the most convincing evidence for an immune complex pathogenesis has been obtained. In lupus nephritis the glomeruli invariably show irregular or granular deposits of immunoglobulins and complement, either within mesangial regions or along the basement membrane. Corresponding dense deposits are seen by electron microscopy. Studies of glomerular eluates have shown that the deposited immunoglobulins do not represent a cross section of circulating antibodies, but instead show a selective concentration of antinuclear antibodies, especially antinative DNA.[16, 17] Since in some patients DNA is demonstrable in the circulation at certain times and anti-DNA at others, complex formation must be occurring intermittently within the circulation.[17] Moreover, in most patients with SLE there is a correlation between the presence and titer of circulating antinative DNA antibodies and disease activity. Finally, DNA itself has been demonstrated by immunofluorescence within glomeruli.[17]

Thus, the evidence favoring a role for DNA antinative DNA complexes in the pathogenesis of lupus nephritis appears unassailable. It seems likely that other complexes also participate; in addition to antinative DNA, antibodies against single-stranded DNA, as well as rheumatoid factors (that is, IgM antibody against IgG), have been demonstrated within glomeruli in some cases.[18] Nevertheless, complexes containing native DNA appear to be of major importance. Two general possibilities can be suggested to account for this situation: one, DNA may be one of the few autologous antigens that gain access to the circulation in appropriate form and amounts, or two, DNA anti-DNA complexes possess distinctive physical properties that cause them to be readily arrested within glomeruli.

As in other glomerular diseases, there is no direct evidence concerning secondary pathogenic mechanisms in lupus nephritis. However, the presence of readily demonstrable complement components within glomeruli and the correlation between depression of circulating complement and disease activity point to a role for this system. The presence of fibrin[8] and leukocytes in glomeruli in some cases suggests these factors may also participate.

Although the primary pathogenetic mechanism responsible for lupus nephritis has been uncovered, the etiology of the disease SLE is unknown. Based in part on studies of NZB/w mice, in which a remarkably similar spontaneous disease occurs, it is now widely believed that the disease will be shown to depend upon a genetically determined derangement of the immune system, manifested by excessive antibody production to certain antigens, including viral antigens, some of which stimulate antibodies that cross react with autologous antigens. In support of the latter possibility, evidence has been obtained indicating that anti-RNA antibodies in lupus may be induced by viral nucleic acid.[19] The finding of "tubular structures" by electron microscopy in tissues of many patients with SLE has been cited as evidence of viral infection. However, it is not certain that these structures do in fact represent viral material, rather than a manifestation of cell injury.[20]

Nephritis in anaphylactoid purpura. Evidence supporting the possibility that the nephritis of anaphylactoid purpura may have an immune complex pathogenesis consists almost entirely of the finding by immunofluorescence of immunoglobulins and complement in glomeruli, generally in mesangial regions. There is no information concerning the nature of the putative antigen or antigens.

Nephritis in periarteritis nodosa. Periarteritis nodosa* is generally considered to be the prototype of immune complex disease. However, the evidence supporting this view is in most cases surprisingly meager. A major reason for the belief that the arteritis is due to hypersensitivity has been provided by the resemblance of the arterial lesions to those of acute serum sickness in rabbits, as emphasized by Rich and Gregory.[21] Further support of a similar nature comes from the fact that in SLE, where circulating complexes are known to be of pathogenic significance, arteritis is sometimes found. Beyond the belief that the disease has an immunologic basis, it is widely thought that many cases are due to hypersensitivity to certain drugs. This belief stems from a paper by Rich,[22] in which he reported that seven patients who had received sulfonamides were found at autopsy to have necrotizing arterial lesions. However, six of these patients had also received foreign serum, and on the basis of the nature of the autopsy findings and the clinical picture it seems likely that these patients died of the infectious process for which they were given serum and that at least in six patients the arterial lesions resulted from serum sickness and were unrelated to sulfonamides. In fact, this was the interpretation that Rich himself favored. Since then, a number of sporadic reports have linked certain drugs with periarteritis nodosa, but it is not clear that the associations are statistically significant. Moreover, it is likely that in some instances the patients were treated with the drug in question because they had signs and symptoms resulting from periarteritis nodosa. As far as we are aware, there is no convincing evidence either in man or in experimental animals that a simple drug can initiate necrotizing arteritis† through an immune complex mechanism‡ or proliferative and necrotizing glomerulonephritis (which is the kind of lesion seen in some cases of periarteritis nodosa). Confusion on this point has arisen because certain drugs, such as penicillin, may lead to hypersensitivity reactions that resemble true serum sickness in man (i.e., the disease that follows administration of large amounts of foreign serum), with fever, urticaria, arthralgia, and lymph node enlargement. However, it seems unlikely the lesions in these drug reactions are exclusively or even principally due to circulating immune

---

* It seems likely that the term "periarteritis nodosa" encompasses a variety of diseases, even after excluding known conditions in which arteritis may occur, such as SLE, rheumatoid arthritis, and possibly poststreptococcal glomerulonephritis.

† It is true that in certain drug reactions in man, inflammation of small dermal vessels may be seen, but these are generally venules and the lesions do not resemble those seen in cases classified as periarteritis nodosa.

‡ A possible exception is seen in hydralazine- or procainamide-induced lupus-like disease. However, it is not entirely clear that such patients exhibit necrotizing arteritis or glomerulonephritis. Moreover, pressor agents may induce arterial necrosis, when administered in large amounts, presumably as the result of intense vasospasm.

complexes. Furthermore, present evidence indicates that the renal lesions associated with hypersensitivity reactions to certain drugs, such as methicillin or penicillin, consist of an interstitial nephritis without arterial or glomerular lesions.[23]

Immunofluorescence findings have been variable in periarteritis; in some cases gamma globulins and complement components have been found within glomerular and arterial lesions,[24] whereas in others these materials were absent,[25] although fibrin was readily demonstrable. The failure to demonstrate immunoglobulin and complement does not exclude the possibility that immune complexes initiated the lesions, since they may have been rapidly degraded. On the other hand, the significance of positive findings in arterial lesions is not clear; it would be surprising if various plasma proteins, including immunoglobulins and complement components, failed to gain access to the kind of necrotic lesions seen in periarteritis. Whether they are demonstrable by immunofluorescence may depend on the extent to which they become denatured or aggregated and thus resist removal by the washings employed in the immunofluorescence procedure. Indeed, it has been shown that immunoglobulin is demonstrable in the fibrinoid arterial and arteriolar lesions seen in rats with adrenal regenerative hypertension.[26] In contrast with glomerular disease, it is not feasible to elute immunoglobulin from arterial lesions in order to study the content of antibodies of various specificities.

Recently Gocke et al.[27] have presented findings that indicate that some cases of periarteritis nodosa may be due to complexes containing Australia (Au) antigen. Six of 16 patients with polyarteritis nodosa were found to have chronic Australia antiginemia. This is a considerably higher incidence than in normal individuals. In two patients Au antigen was demonstrated in blood vessel walls, in association with IgM and BIC. Although these findings are impressive, they require confirmation by further studies.

We regard the evidence favoring an immune complex pathogenesis in periarteritis nodosa as largely indirect. Although we have emphasized the difficulties in providing conclusive evidence for this mechanism, it remains the most appealing possibility. Evidence concerning etiologic factors is almost entirely lacking, except in a few cases that may be produced by Au antigenic material. It seems likely that various etiologic factors will be implicated.

Idiopathic mixed cryoglobulinemia. Another condition (which is not widely recognized) in which immune complexes are the likely cause of vascular injury and renal disease is essential mixed cryoglobulinemia.

This condition was first delineated by Meltzer et al.,[28] who identified a distinctive group of nine patients among 29 in whom they found circulating cryoglobulins. Although there were features that overlapped with other diseases, especially rheumatoid arthritis and SLE, the condition appeared sufficiently distinctive to warrant classification as a separate entity. The serum of these patients formed a cryoprecipitate containing both IgG and IgM. The IgM component possessed rheumatoid factor activity. Clinically the patients presented with a fairly typical picture, with weakness, arthralgias, purpura, splenomegaly, and lymphadenopathy. Three of the patients developed rapidly progressive and fatal renal disease. At autopsy a characteristic, but not unique, form of diffuse proliferative glomerulonephritis was present in all three; necrotizing vasculitis was found in two. One patient was studied by immunofluorescence and was found to have granular deposits in glomeruli containing both IgG and IgM. On the basis of these observations Meltzer and his associates[28] proposed that the renal and vascular lesions were produced by the deposition at these sites of circulating complexes containing altered autologous IgG combined with an IgM antibody.

Since this publication a relatively small number* of cases of idiopathic mixed cryoglobulinemia with glomerulonephritis have been reported.[29, 30] In general, the clinical and pathologic features were similar to those just described, but it has been learned that the glomerular disease is not always fatal. In addition, electron microscopic studies have shown dense granular deposits within and along the basement membrane.

The immunofluorescence and electron microscopic findings are characteristic of immune complex glomerulonephritis. Moreover, the presence of both IgM and IgG within glomeruli supports the view that circulating complexes formed of these proteins are responsible. However, studies of the antibody specificity of immunoglobulins eluted from glomeruli have not been reported and crucial proof is thus lacking. The etiology of the condition is unknown.

Mixed cryoglobulins may be seen in association with a variety of diseases, such as SLE or rheumatoid arthritis, often without evidence of glomerular disease. Thus, it appears that only certain kinds of mixed cryoglobulins possess the kind of physical properties that cause them to lodge in glomeruli; these properties have yet to be defined. In addition to initiating glomerular disease, such complexes may play a contributory role in certain conditions, such as lupus nephritis or possibly in poststreptococcal glomerulonephritis.

Primary Glomerular Diseases of Unknown Etiology

The conditions listed under this heading are considered as possible immune complex diseases because of the finding of irregular or granular deposits of immunoglobulins and complement within glomeruli. However, only one form, membranous glomerulonephritis, is very closely reproduced in experimental models, namely, in rats with autologous immune complex disease and in some rabbits with chronic serum sickness. The presumption is very strong therefore that membranous nephritis is a form of chronic immune complex disease. In a handful of cases classified as membranous nephritis, evidence has been obtained that the antigen may be thyroglobulin, tumor specific antigens,[31] or Australia antigens. These findings indicate that membranous nephritis has diverse etiologies.

In the other conditions listed under the heading of primary glomerular disease there is no clue as to etiologic agents or the nature of the putative antigen. Although not strictly relevant to the present discussion, it is worth emphasizing that a large percentage of glomerular disease cannot be classified at present, even in morphologic terms; in some of these, immunofluorescence findings suggest an immune complex pathogenesis.

---

* It is not known whether the lack of larger reported series of patients reflects the rarity of the condition or the failure to recognize it. Although the condition is fairly typical, cryoprecipitates may be missed, since they frequently require 24 hours or more to form.

Anti-GBM disease

It is thoroughly documented that some cases of human glomerular disease are due to anti-GBM antibodies,[32,33] notably in most patients with Goodpasture's syndrome and in some cases classified as rapidly progressive glomerulonephritis.* Conclusive evidence of anti-GBM disease consists of showing "linear" accumulation of immunoglobulins and complement in glomeruli and demonstration that anti-GBM antibodies are present in the circulation or in glomerular eluates. The finding of typical "linear" staining for immunoglobulin cannot by itself be considered conclusive evidence of anti-GBM disease, since apparently nonspecific "linear" accumulation of immunoglobulin may occur in some situations, especially in diabetes.[34]

It should be emphasized that established anti-GBM disease in man is distinctly uncommon. Early estimates[32] that this mechanism might account for about one third of human glomerulonephritis grossly overestimated its frequency.

There is no direct evidence concerning the etiology of human anti-GBM disease. Two general possibilities are worth considering, based on experimental observations: first, that anti-GBM antibody formation is stimulated by autologous basement membrane material, possibly altered in some way so as to render it immunogenic; or second, that an exogenous agent with cross reacting determinants is responsible. The second possibility is suggested by the observation that streptococcal infection in rabbits may induce anti-GBM antibodies. Although it appears that poststreptococcal glomerulonephritis is an immune complex disease, the *remote possibility remains* that on *extremely rare occasions* streptococcal infection might initiate anti-GBM disease, which would appear clinically as rapidly progressive glomerulonephritis.[33] Evidence supporting this might be obtained if it could be shown that anti-GBM activity in serum or eluates could be absorbed with streptococcal material. There is no evidence for or against the possibility that other infectious agents might stimulate anti-GBM antibody formation.

Concerning secondary pathogenic mechanisms in anti-GBM disease, it appears from experimental observations that accumulation of fibrin in Bowman's space is an important, if not essential factor in crescent formation.[35] However, even if this be true in man, it may be difficult or impossible to obtain a beneficial effect through anticoagulant therapy, since the disease generally progresses so rapidly to an irreversible state.

Two possibilities have received relatively little attention: one, that structures other than glomeruli may be directly damaged by immunologic mechanisms, and two, that delayed sensitivity may play a pathogenic role in certain forms of renal disease. Concerning the first possibility, experimental models exist in which tubular damage results from deposition of autologous immune complexes in tubular basement membranes[36] or from autoantibodies directed against the tubular basement membrane (TBM).[37,38] Either form may occur in the absence of glomerular disease. There is evidence that deposits of immune complexes within tubular basement membranes may be seen in man,[39] and suggestive evi-

---

* Some cases so classified have granular deposits, suggesting an immune complex pathogenesis. In others, immunoglobulins are not found at all.

dence that anti-TBM disease may also occur. However, the incidence and possible functional significance of immunologically induced tubular disease in man remains to be evaluated. Concerning the role of delayed sensitivity in renal disease, it would appear to be unnecessary on the basis of present evidence to invoke such a mechanism in the pathogenesis of glomerular diseases. However, it is reasonable to suspect that interstitial mononuclear cell infiltration, which is seen in many renal diseases, may in some instances represent a cell-mediated reaction, either to exogenous or autologous antigens. Unfortunately entirely satisfactory models of cell-mediated renal disease are not available at present.

Diseases Without Impressive Evidence of Immunologic Mechanisms (Table 1)

In a number of human diseases, most of which are included under the general heading glomerulonephritis, immunoglobulins and complement either are not found in glomeruli or are found in trivial amounts. Although these observations do not definitely exclude immunologic mechanisms, for the most part there is no other substantial reason to involve such mechanisms. One condition, lipoid nephrosis, deserves special comment. In patients classified as having lipoid nephrosis, the major classes of immunoglobulins (IgG, IgM, and IgA) and complement are generally absent or inconspicuous. However, recently Gerber and Paronetto[40] reported that untreated patients frequently show conspicuous deposits of IgE. These observations await confirmation, and even if they are confirmed their pathogenic significance would remain to be evaluated.

Another observation that has been used to support an immunologic basis for lipoid nephrosis is the fact that most patients with this condition respond to corticosteroid therapy. However, corticosteroids are not particularly effective immunosuppressive agents in man and are known to exert other in vivo effects, such as anti-inflammatory actions or effects on cell membranes. Their mode of action in lipoid nephrosis is unknown.

Conclusion

Although we have called this paper "An Evaluation of Immunologic Mechanisms," we have for the most part really been considering the question: how convincing is the evidence for the *operation* of certain experimentally well defined immunologic mechanisms in human renal diseases? We have assumed that if either of the two major immunopathogenetic mechanisms is at work, all the glomerular damage can be presumed to depend ultimately upon this mechanism. For example, we believe that the glomerular lesions in lupus nephritis are due to accumulation of immune complexes and that, even if it should be shown that viral infection plays an important role in the production of the disease SLE, it will be unlikely that viruses contribute to the glomerular damage in any way except by leading to the formation of immune complexes. This formulation appears justifiable on the whole, because in experimental models glomerular lesions similar to those seen in man are clearly attributable to the basic mechanisms outlined above.

However, several important questions remain. Most important is the identification of etiologic agents, that is, of factors that initiate the formation of complexes in the circulation or of anti-GBM antibodies. Almost no progress has been made in this area, except for a handful of cases in which certain antigens may have been implicated, and with the exception of the recognition that malaria is responsible for a form of glomerulonephritis presumably due to immune complexes. However, in a negative sense we have advanced somewhat, since it is now clear that most forms of chronic glomerulonephritis previously thought to result from poststreptococcal glomerulonephritis are of unknown etiology. No evidence is available concerning factors responsible for the stimulation of anti-GBM antibodies in man.

Another problem is that the factors responsible for the localization of complexes in glomeruli are largely unknown. It is clear that, at most, only a very tiny fraction of complexes that are formed in the circulation accumulate in glomeruli. Although there is evidence from experimental work that neither very small nor very large complexes localize in glomeruli, the precise physical properties that enable certain complexes to arrest in glomeruli are not known. It has been shown experimentally that host mechanisms, such as release of vasoactive amines into the circulation, may facilitate glomerular localization of complexes. However, these observations have been made in acute serum sickness, and to what extent they apply to other forms of immune complex diseases, and to those occurring in man, is not certain.

Finally, there is little direct information concerning the mechanisms by which deposited immune complexes or anti-GBM antibodies produce glomerular damage. In fact, even in experimental models information is surprisingly scanty and derived principally from two models, acute serum sickness and nephrotoxic serum nephritis; and only in the latter has a pathogenic role of the complement system, coagulation, or neutrophils been established.[3]

Thus, although progress has been made in identification of immunologic mechanisms in human renal diseases, the kind of knowledge that might lead to prevention or effective treatment has so far eluded detection.

References

1. Leber, P. D., and McCluskey, R. T.: Immune complex diseases. In Zweifach, B., Grant, L., and McCluskey, R. T. (eds.): *The Inflammatory Process*. 2nd ed. New York, Academic Press. In press.
2. Immune complexes and disease. (This is a supplemental issue, summarizing a symposium on immune complex disease.) J. Exp. Med. *134*:1, 1971.
3. McCluskey, R. T., and Vassalli, P.: Experimental glomerular disease. In Rouiller, C., and Muller, A. I. (eds.): The Kidney. Vol. II. New York, Academic Press, 1969, pp. 83-198.
3a. Mahieu, P., Dardenne, M., and Bach, J. F.: Detection of humoral and cell mediated immunity to kidney basement membranes in human renal diseases. Amer. J. Med. 53:185, 1972.

4. Markowitz, A. S., and Lange, C. F.: Streptococcal related glomerulonephriitis I. Isolation, immunochemistry and comparative chemistry of soluble fractions from type 12 nephritogenic streptococci and human glomeruli. J. Immunol. 92:565, 1964.
5. Seegal, B. C., Andres, G. A., Hsu, K. C., and Zabriskie, J. B.: Studies on the pathogenesis of acute and progressive glomerulonephritis in man by immunofluorescein and immunoferritin. Fed. Proc. 24(Pt. I):100, 1965.
6. Michael, A. F., Jr., Drummond, K. M., Good, R. A., and Vernier, R. L.: Acute poststreptococcal glomerulonephritis: Immune deposit disease. J. Clin. Invest. 45:237, 1966.
7. Treser, G., and Lange, K.: Personal communication. Cited by Zabriskie, J. B.: J. Exp. Med. 134:180s, 1971.
8. McCluskey, R. T., Vassalli, P., Gallo, G., and Baldwin, D. S.: An immunofluorescent study of pathogenic mechanisms in glomerular diseases. New Eng. J. Med. 274:695, 1966.
9. Feldman, J. O., Mardinig, M. R., and Shuler, S. E.: Immunology and morphology of acute poststreptococcal glomerulonephritis. Lab. Invest. 15:283, 1966.
10. Zabriskie, J. B.: The role of streptococci in human glomerulonephritis. J. Exp. Med. 134:180, 1971.
11. Treser, G., Semar, M., Ty, A., Sagel, I., Franklin, M. A., and Lange, K.: Partial characterization of antigenic streptococcal plasma membrane components in acute glomerulonephritis. J. Clin. Invest. 49:762, 1970.
12. Barnett, E. V., Bluestone, R., Cracchiolo, A., Goldberg, L. S., Kantor, G. L., and McIntosh, R. M.: Cryoglobulinemia and disease. (UCLA Conference.) Ann. Intern. Med. 73:95, 1970.
13. Kaufman, D. B., and McIntosh, R.: The pathogenesis of the renal lesion in a patient with streptococcal disease, infected ventriculoatrial shunt, cryoglobulinemia and nephritis. Amer. J. Med. 50:262, 1971.
14. Bhorade, M. S., Carag, H. B., Lee, H. J., Potter, E. V., and Dunea, G.: Nephropathy of secondary syphilis. A clinical and pathological spectrum. J.A.M.A. 216:1159, 1971.
15. Hendrickse, R. G., Glasgow, E. F., Adeniyi, A., White, R. H. R., Edington, G. M., and Houba, V.: Quartan malarial nephrotic syndrome, collaborative clinicopathological study in Nigerian children. Lancet 1:1143, 1972.
16. Krishman, C., and Kaplan, M. H.: Immunopathologic studies of systemic lupus erythematosus. II Antinuclear reaction of gamma globulin eluted from homogenates and isolated glomeruli of kidneys from patients with lupus nephritis. J. Clin. Invest. 46:569, 1967.
17. Koffler, D., Agnello, R., Thoburn, R., and Kunkel, H. G.: Systemic lupus erythematosus: Prototype of immune complex nephritis in man. J. Exp. Med. 134:169s, 1971.
18. Agnello, V., Koffler, D., Eisenberg, J. W., Winchester, R. J., and Kunkel, H. G.: C1q precipitins in the sera of patients with systemic lupus erythematosus and other hypocomplementemic states, characterization of high and low molecular weight types. J. Exp. Med. 134:228s, 1971.
19. Talal, N.: Antibodies binding ³H-reovirus RNA in systemic lupus erythematosus Clin. Immunol. Immunopath. 1:230, 1973.
20. Andres, G. A., Spiele, H., and McCluskey, R. T.: Virus-like structures in systemic lupus erythematosus. In Schwartz, R. (ed.): *Progress in Clinical Immunology*. New York, Grune & Stratton, 1:23, 1972.
21. Rich, A. R., and Gregory, J. E.: The experimental demonstration that periarteritis nodosa is a manifestation of hypersensitivity. Bull. Johns Hopkins Hosp. 72:65, 1943.
22. Rich, A. R.: Role of hypersensitivity in periarteritis as indicated by 7 cases developing during serum sickness and sulfonamide therapy. Bull. Johns Hopkins Hosp. 71:123, 1942.
23. Baldwin, D. S., Levine, B., McCluskey, R. T., and Gallo, G. R.: Renal failure and interstitial nephritis due to penicillin and methicillin. New Eng. J. Med. 279:1245, 1968.
24. Paranetto, F., and Strauss, L.: Immunocytochemical observations in periarteritis nodosa. Ann. Intern. Med. 56:289, 1962.
25. Gallo, G.: Personal communication.
26. Group, C.: Personal communication.
27. Gocke, D. J., Hsu, K., Morgan, C., Bombardieri, S., Lockshin, M., and Christian, C: L.: Vasculitis in association with Australia antigen. J. Exp. Med. 134:330s, 1972.
28. Meltzer, M., Franklin, E. C., Elias, K., McCluskey, R. T., and Cooper, N.: Cryoglobulinemia. II. Cryoglobulins with rheumatoid factor activity: A clinical and laboratory study. Amer. J. Med. 40:837, 1966.

29. Baldwin, D. S., and McCluskey, R. T.: Renal involvement in systemic lupus erythematosus, periarteritis nodosa, scleroderma and cryoglobulinemia. *In* Becker, E. L. (ed.): *Structural Basis of Renal Disease*. New York, Hoeber Division, Harper and Row, 1968.
30. Verroust, P., Mery, J. P., Morel-Maroger, L., Clauvel, J. P., and Richet, G.: Glomerular lesions in monoclonal gammopathies and mixed essential cryoglobulinemias IgG-IgM. *In* Hamburger, Crosnier, and Maxwell (eds.): *Advances in Nephrology*. Vol. 1. Chicago, Year Book Medical Publishers, 1971, pp. 61–194.
31. Lewis, M. G., Loughridge, L. W., and Phillips, T. M.: Immunological studies in nephrotic syndrome associated with extrarenal malignant disease. Lancet 2:134, 1971.
32. Lerner, R. A., Glassock, R. J., and Dixon, F. J.: The role of antiglomerular basement membrane antibody in the pathogenesis of human glomerulonephritis. J. Exp. Med. *126*: 898, 1967.
33. Lewis, E. J., Cavallo, T., Harrington, J. T., and Cotran, R. S.: An immunopathologic study of rapidly progressive glomerulonephritis in the adult. Human Path. 2:185, 1971.
34. Gallo, G.: Elution studies in kidneys with linear deposition of immunoglobulin in glomeruli. Amer. J. Path. *61*:377, 1970.
35. Vassalli, P., and McCluskey, R. T.: The pathogenic role of the coagulation process in rabbit Masugi nephritis. Amer. J. Path. *45*:677, 1964.
36. Klassen, J., McCluskey, R. T., and Milgrom, F.: Nonglomerular renal disease produced in rabbits by immunization with homologous kidney. Amer. J. Path. 63:333, 1971.
37. Steblay, R. W., and Rudosky, U.: Renal tubular disease and autoantibodies against tubular basement membrane induced in guinea pigs. J. Immunol. *107*:589, 1971.
38. Sugisaki, T., Andres, G. A., Klassen, J., Milgrom, F., and McCluskey, R. T.: Immunopathological study of autoimmune tubular and interstitial renal disease in BN rats. Lab. Invest. In press.
39. Klassen, J., Andres, G. A., Brennan, J. C., and McCluskey, R. T.: An immunologic renal tubular lesion in man. Clin. Immunol. Immunopath. *1*:69, 1972.
40. Gerber, M. A., and Paronetto, F.: IgE in glomeruli of patients with nephrotic syndrome. Lancet *1*:1097, 1971.

Comment

Immunologic Mechanisms in the Pathogenesis of Glomerular Diseases

Only the most hardened skeptic could fail to be impressed by the evidence that immunologic mechanisms play a role in at least some forms of human glomerulonephritis. The controversy concerns not the existence of such mechanisms, but rather their incidence and pathogenetic significance.

Wilson and Dixon evidently are convinced that the deposition of immune complexes in glomeruli accounts for the great majority of human glomerulonephritides, and that anti-glomerular basement membrane (anti-GBM) reactions account for most of the remainder. McCluskey and Leber, on the other hand, take a more cautious position, suggesting that anti-GBM nephritis is relatively rare, and that immune complex deposition has been proved to be of primary importance in only a limited number of clinical types of nephritis.

Both essays agree that immunofluorescence microscopy demonstrates immune proteins in the glomeruli of many patients with glomerular diseases, but they disagree as to what this proves. In order to establish the primary deposition of antigen-antibody complexes, as distinguished from a purely nonspecific accumulation of plasma proteins in damaged glomeruli, McCluskey and Leber would like to see specific antigen and antibody eluted from the glomerular lesions or identified in the circulation. Similarly, to prove anti-GBM nephritis, they would require the elution of specific anti-GBM antibodies from the glomerular lesions or the demonstration of specific antibodies in the circulation. Wilson and Dixon, extrapolating from animal experiments and from those few types of human disease in which an immunologic mechanism seems well established (e.g., lupus nephritis, Goodpasture's syndrome, and poststreptococcal glomerulonephritis), are prepared to accept the presence of diffuse granular or linear deposits of immunoglobulin as prima facie evidence of an immunologic mechanism in a wide variety of other glomerular disease.

This is a question that gives every promise of yielding soon to continued and intensive investigation. In the meanwhile, however, I tend to agree with the more conservative and cautious position taken by McCluskey and Leber. Immune proteins have been demonstrated in the glomeruli of so many diverse renal lesions, including such unlikely immunologic diseases as diabetic glomerulosclerosis and renal vein thrombosis, that the significance of these findings needs to be carefully evaluated. It is possible, as Wilson and Dixon suggest, that we shall need to revise our ideas about the pathogenesis of these "nonimmunologic" renal diseases, or that an immunologic insult has been superimposed on the course of an initially nonimmunologic disease. It is also possible, however, that the unique structure and function of the glomerulus results in the nonspecific accumulation of circulating immune proteins under a variety of conditions that may have nothing to do with immunologic mechanisms.

Pending the elucidation of the questions discussed by these essays, one can only hope for more and better information about the correlation between clinical findings and light, electron, and immunofluorescence microscopy. We are particularly in need of statistically valid quantitative surveys, upon which reliable estimates of frequency and a rational system of classification can be based.

ARNOLD S. RELMAN

28

Evaluation of Carcinoembryonic Antigen in Diagnosis of Cancer of the Colon

EVALUATION OF CARCINOEMBRYONIC ANTIGEN IN DIAGNOSIS OF CANCER OF THE COLON
   by Jeffrey J. Collins and Paul H. Black

COMMENT
   by Phil Gold and Samuel O. Freedman

Evaluation of Carcinoembryonic Antigen in Diagnosis of Cancer of the Colon

JEFFREY J. COLLINS and PAUL H. BLACK

Harvard Medical School

The carcinoembryonic antigen (CEA) of the human digestive system is an antigenic specificity* which has been found to be closely associated with adenocarcinoma of the colon. CEA was originally described and characterized by Gold and his colleagues in an extensive series of studies commencing in 1965. Initial investigations demonstrated the presence of this new antigenic determinant in all tumors of the colon obtained from unrelated patients and its absence in control colonic tissue from the same patients.[1] Subsequently the antigenic reactivity was detected in all adenocarcinomas of the adult digestive system (with a gradient of decreasing concentration as one moved up the gastrointestinal tract), yet the antigen was absent in the corresponding normal tissue.[2] Of additional interest was the finding that only normal fetal gut, liver, and pancreas taken between two and six months' gestation contained CEA, while these fetal tissues were devoid of the antigen during the third trimester of pregnancy. The term "carcinoembryonic antigen" was derived from this distribution pattern, which in turn was interpreted as reflecting the presence of this determinant only in tissues originating from (or part of) the embryonic entoderm.[2]

At the present time there is little direct information relating to the mechanism of the appearance of CEA in certain human neoplasms. Similarly, the mechanism(s) responsible for the presence of fetal substances, antigenic or otherwise, in a wide variety of naturally occuring[3-11] and experimentally induced[12-22] tumor cells remains to be delineated. Nevertheless, despite the paucity

---

* We mean by "antigenic specificity" a particular moiety(s) on an antigen which is responsible for its specificity, and the site(s) to which the immune response is primarily directed. It is used synonymously in this article with "antigenic determinant." With some antigens (and possibly CEA) there may be more than one determinant on the molecule.

of relevant data, it has generally been presumed that the reappearance of fetal antigens or other embryonic products in cancer cells is due to a derepression of host-cell genes, normally expressed during embryogenesis, but "turned off" in the adult organism. Gold has suggested that such a mechanism, which he called "derepressive-dedifferentiation," is responsible for the presence of CEA in human digestive system tumors.[2] However, studies of cell surface alterations in virus-transformed cells[23-26] suggest that an equally appropriate mechanism would involve the uncovering or redistribution of surface antigens or sites not normally exposed in the adult tissue (so-called cryptic sites).[25] This is a particularly attractive hypothesis in the case of CEA since the antigen has been shown to be a glycoprotein[27] which is localized to the cell surface.[28, 29] However, initial attempts to expose CEA on normal colon cells by treatment with various surface-active enzymes have been unsuccessful.[30]

Whether CEA plays any role in tumor immunity is not known at present. In fact, investigations of its immunogenicity have produced conflicting results. Initial studies by Gold,[31] utilizing a hemagglutination assay, demonstrated the presence of anti-CEA antibodies in the sera of a majority of pregnant women and patients with nonmetastatic digestive system tumors. However, subsequent investigations by others have failed to confirm the presence of autoantibodies specific for CEA in sera from patients bearing such neoplasms.[32, 33] Utilizing the "in vitro" colony inhibition test, results have been obtained which indicate that CEA is capable of eliciting specific cell-mediated immunity in patients bearing colon carcinomas.[34] A similar interpretation was proposed to account for the positive delayed hypersensitivity skin tests achieved with crude colonic tumor extracts in patients with colonic cancers.[35] The specificity of these reactions, however, is made questionable by the inability of purified CEA to induce similar skin reactions or to transform lymphocytes from patients with the appropriate tumors.[35, 36]

Despite the uncertainties concerning the mechanism of appearance of CEA and its role in tumor immunity, it has become increasingly clear that CEA may have great practical clinical value as a prognostic and/or diagnostic tool in the treatment of digestive system tumors. This potential use stems from the ability to detect circulating CEA in the sera or plasma of appropriate cancer patients. Gold and his colleagues first reported the presence of CEA in the sera of patients bearing colon and rectal tumors, utilizing a sensitive radioimmunoassay technique.[37] Furthermore, preliminary results suggested that by monitoring the level of circulating CEA after tumor resection one could obtain an early indication of regrowth or of previously undetected metastases, as reflected by a rising CEA titer. In considering the clinical significance of CEA as a diagnostic and/or prognostic tool one must determine as definitively as possible whether CEA is, in fact, specific for digestive system tumors (particularly colonic cancers). In the remainder of the article we should like to consider the contradictory evidence currently available which bears on this question and to discuss the consequences of some of these findings in terms of the medical value of CEA detection.

The results obtained by Gold's group[37] indicated that circulating CEA could be detected only at significant levels (≥ 2.5 ng./ml.) in the sera of patients with cancer of the large bowel, while sera from patients with malignancies of other areas of the gastrointestinal tract and its appendages or nonmalignant diseases of these organs were negative. The negative results involving tumors of the upper digestive tract were presumed to reflect the lower CEA concentration previously reported in these tissues.[2] These results, in conjunction with their earlier studies,[1, 2] were viewed as confirmation of the specific association of CEA with colon and rectal adenocarcinoma. In fact, it was subsequently suggested that the presence of CEA be considered virtually diagnostic of these types of cancers.[38] Unfortunately, the results of other groups have raised serious doubts as to the complete specificity of this association.

Martin and Martin,[39] studying perchloric acid extracts of tumor tissue obtained in a manner somewhat different from that used by Gold and co-workers, detected two antigens associated with human colonic cancer, one of which they considered to be identical to Gold's CEA. Their antigens were analyzed by a precipitin-inhibition reaction utilizing heterologous immune rabbit sera. In this manner it was demonstrated that the CEA-like antigen could be found in perchloric acid extracts of normal colon or nonmalignant diseased colonic tissue, although at a concentration well below that of malignant colonic tissue. They concluded that CEA represents a quantitative rather than a specifically qualitative difference between cancerous and noncancerous digestive system tissues. It must be stressed that the absolute identity of the Martins' antigen with CEA has not yet been established. In addition, experiments such as these which are dependent upon heterologous immunizations are subject to the danger of incomplete absorption of anti-normal activity from anti-tumor sera. Furthermore, more recent studies in which perchloric acid tissue extracts were also utilized support the conclusions of Gold. These investigations[40] also reported the presence of two antigenic determinants, one of which was shown by immunodiffusion to be identical to Gold's CEA. Most importantly, both these antigens were detected only in extracts of colonic adenocarcinomas and were not present in the corresponding normal tissues.

Other workers have also utilized heterologous sera raised in rabbits against perchloric acid extracts of digestive system tumor tissue and reported the presence of tumor-specific antigens which cross reacted with antigens from normal fetal intestinal tissue.[41] Although an association with entodermally derived tissue was not examined, the authors concluded that the antigen involved was identical to CEA. Subsequent studies of this determinant in tissue sections by the indirect immunofluorescence technique demonstrated its localization to the luminal region of the intestinal mucosa.[42] However, this conclusion must be viewed with great caution since the tissue sections examined were frozen and fixed, techniques which can alter membrane structure. To definitively demonstrate the surface localization of their antigen these studies should be repeated with unfixed colonic tumor cells in suspension. Nevertheless, utilizing fixed tissue sections, this antigen has been reported to be present in hemorrhoidal and ulcerative colitis mucosa, as well as in the mucosa of benign polyps of the colon, with its content directly related to the degree of polyp differentiation.[43] Similar results were obtained with anti-CEA serum provided by Gold. Of great significance, however, was the inability of Gold to confirm these results with the same specific antiserum, but using unfixed target cells. The implication that the tissue must be fixed before the antigen can be detected[42, 43] raises serious doubts as to its identity with CEA, since it has already been shown that CEA can be demonstrated on the surface of unfixed cells by immunofluorescence.[28, 30]

Still other antigens have been reported to be present in, and associated with, human colonic cancer.[44-46] However, the nature of these antigens and their relationship to CEA remain undefined at this time. As important as the previously described studies of colon cancer-associated antigens may be in facilitating our understanding of the nature of the CEA and the mechanism of its appearance in tumor cells, their relevance to the question of whether CEA can be utilized in a clinically significant way is minimal. Even assuming the identity of some of these antigens[39, 41] with CEA, the fact remains that the diagnostic and/or prognostic value of CEA rests with the ability to detect it in the serum of cancer patients, and not in the tumor tissue itself. In addition, since the circulating CEA is presumably derived from the tumor tissue, the levels of CEA found in nonmalignant tissue, in general, or nonentodermally derived malignant tissues are so small[39] that its presence in these tissues has little real impact on the potential medical application of circulating CEA. Thus, it is clear that our consideration of the clinical usefulness of CEA concerns those studies which deal with the detection of CEA in the serum or plasma of patients with various malignant and nonmalignant disorders.

A series of investigations along these lines have been carried out by Zamcheck and his colleagues. Using the radioimmunoassay technique for circulating CEA developed by Gold's group,[37] they were able to confirm the presence of CEA in the sera of patients with colonic cancer and, in addition, found it in all cases examined of adenocarcinoma of the pancreas.[47] However, positive results were also obtained with sera from patients with tumors outside the digestive system (lung) as well as from patients with non-neoplastic disorders of the gastrointestinal tract and other organs (particularly renal disease and alcoholic liver disease). Although Gold was unable to detect CEA in extracts of lung carcinomas or fetal lung and bronchial tissue,[2] it is possible that the presence of circulating CEA in sera from patients with lung cancers reflects the entodermal origin of this tissue. These initial results[47] also supported the earlier conclusion[37] that postoperative monitoring of serum CEA levels could give an early indication either of tumor regrowth due to incomplete resection or of the presence of tumor metastases.

The association of circulating CEA with colon carcinoma and other diseases has also been reported by other workers. Thus, utilizing a somewhat different radioimmunoassay[48] for circulating CEA from that of Gold's groups (an important point which is considered in detail later), the great majority (~85 per cent) of patients with gastrointestinal and pancreatic tumors were found to contain elevated levels of CEA in the blood.[49, 50] Furthermore, in the latter studies the strict gastrointestinal tract tumor specificity previously reported for CEA could not be confirmed. LoGerfo et al.[49] not only detected CEA in sera from some patients with non-neoplastic diseases (11 of 299, including 10 of 31 patients examined with ulcerative colitis), but also reported its presence in sera from over half the patients with carcinoma of nondigestive system tissues (76 of 131, including lung, breast, prostate, and ovarian cancers). Likewise, Reynoso et al.[50] found abnormal serum CEA levels to be associated with a wide variety of malignancies originating in nonentodermally derived tissues (90 of 281), including a particularly high incidence (six of seven) in children with neuroblastoma.

Subsequent investigations by Zamcheck and co-workers,[51] again utilizing Gold's radioimmunoassay, have revealed a lower percentage of positive CEA values (72 per cent) in patients with colon cancer than reported in their previous study (91 per cent).[47] These more recent results are similar to those obtained by other investigators employing the same technique (74 per cent);[52] in addition, abnormal CEA levels were again found to be associated with non-malignant disorders of the gastrointestinal tract and cancers of other tissues. Recent studies[53] employing the modified radioimmunoassay procedure[48, 49] have reaffirmed a clear association between circulating CEA and chronic inflammatory diseases of the intestine. Whether this is related to a predisposition of these tissues to become malignant, and can thus be considered to represent an early indicator of neoplastic change,[54] may be revealed by future studies. Alternatively, its association with these conditions may merely reflect its appearance in inflamed bowel tissue.

Thus, it is apparent that the previously reported[1, 3, 37] association of CEA with tumors of entodermally derived tissues, as well as its purported specificity only for neoplastic adult cells, has been seriously challenged. However, before we discard the concept of a specific relationship between CEA and gastrointestinal cancers, several relevant points must be very carefully considered. Of prime importance is the question of what precise antigenic specificity the various assay procedures are detecting. The zirconyl phosphate gel radioimmunoassay technique[48] utilized in several of the studies mentioned previously,[49, 50, 53] is known to detect ion-sensitive sites. The discrepancy between results obtained with this assay and those of Gold's group[37] may thus reflect reactions with different antigenic specificities, possibly present on the same molecule or representing different forms of the same antigen. It may be that the antigenic site detected by the zirconyl phosphate gel technique is partially cross reactive with the primary CEA site and similar to a specificity found in the sera of a broader range of patients. Recognizing the possibility that their assay procedure is detecting a determinant not identical to that measured by Gold's CEA technique, LoGerfo et al.[55] have wisely chosen to refer to their antigen as "tumor-associated antigen" (TAA). It would be advantageous if other workers would follow suit in employing similar terminology for related antigens under study and restrict the name CEA only to antigens identical to that described by Gold. The studies of TAA have confirmed its relationship to colon carcinoma,[55] but do not support a strict specificity with either entodermally derived tissue or the neoplastic state. In particular, it has been found in the circulation of patients with various lung tumors[56] and its presence in low concentrations in normal colon and lung tissues and in the plasma of healthy adults has recently been reported.[57, 58] It would be of interest to determine whether TAA is present in fetal tissues, since it was initially found to be absent in the sera of pregnant females.[49] That the radioimmunoassays of Gold and Lo Gerfo may be detecting the same antigenic site, however, is suggested by the parallel results obtained with these two procedures in preliminary studies.[51]

The critical role of the assay procedure used is well illustrated by the recent results of Egan and co-workers.[59, 60] Employing still another modified radioimmunoassay for CEA, in this case based on the double antibody technique,[59] two different forms of CEA, distinguished by size (6.8S and 10.1S), were found to be present in perchloric acid extracts of digestive system tumors.[60] The smaller material was found more often and was shown to be identical to Gold's CEA. Neither form could be detected in extracts of normal liver or colon tissue. Thus, this modified radioimmunoassay is capable of distinguishing between two forms of CEA not previously detected by other procedures. The presence of such different forms could account for the varying distribution pattern of CEA and TAA (and other related determinants). Alternatively, the serum and plasma processing procedures used in other studies may themselves result in the conversion of the CEA molecule to altered configurations revealing related, but distinguishable, antigenic sites.[49, 61]

That CEA represents a complex molecule with multiple antigenic sites is indicated by the immunologic activity of several amino acid-free heterosaccharide groups obtained from purified CEA,[62] as well as the reported relationship of CEA with blood group A antigen.[63] In addition, a normal antigen present on the surface of colonic cells has been detected by immunofluorescence which co-purifies with CEA up to the final purification step and which may represent another antigenic site on the CEA molecule.[30] These studies emphasize the caution which must be displayed in interpreting results which relate to the tissue distribution of CEA, but which are obtained with differing assay procedures, whether radioimmunoassays or other.[64]

The second major factor to be considered in resolving the discrepancies reported with respect to the specificity of CEA concerns the selection of the patient sample. This may be particularly relevant in accounting for the contrasting results obtained by Zamcheck's and Gold's groups,[37, 47, 51, 65] since the former workers utilized Gold's radioimmunoassay technique and, in many cases, antigen and antisera supplied by him. The importance of the patient sample studied is demonstrated by the finding that while elevated serum CEA levels were present in all patients with metastatic disease, only 19 per cent of those with localized tumors were positive.[51] Such a relationship between the level of circulating antigen and the extent of the neoplastic disease has also been reported for TAA.[55] Although Reynoso et al.[50] reported no direct correlation between the size of the gastrointestinal tract tumor, or the extent of metastatic spread, and the level of circulating CEA, they did claim that the more advanced cases tended to have higher values. The above studies emphasize the need to carefully define the patient sample investigated in future analyses of the distribution of serum CEA and its relationship to various disease conditions, and further suggest that at least some of the conflicting results of earlier studies may reflect differences in the patients examined. In addition, such studies have indicated that CEA's major clinical significance may be as a prognostic, rather than diagnostic, tool in the detection and treatment of colon carcinoma.

As mentioned, Gold and co-workers,[37] based on preliminary results, were the first to suggest that postoperative monitoring of serum CEA levels could give an early indication either of tumor regrowth at the primary site (due to incomplete resection) or of previously undetected metastases. Subsequent studies carried out in other laboratories[50, 51, 55] have supported and extended this postulate. The correlations found between the CEA level detected and the extent of tumor growth[51, 55] led to the suggestion that both the preoperative and postoperative serum CEA levels could be used as important predictive indicators. Thus, absence of CEA reactivity preoperatively implied localization of the tumor, while a strongly positive result suggested metastases. Likewise, successful tumor resection was indicated by continuing negative postoperative serum CEA assays, regardless of whether the patient had been negative or positive preoperatively. Conversely, a continuing positive serum CEA level after surgery, or the increase of CEA concentration in a patient whose level had initially decreased postoperatively, was taken to indicate residual tumor. Thus, the preoperative serum CEA content can provide an indication of the extent of tumor spread and of the likelihood that the cancer is amenable to curative resection, while the postoperative levels indicate whether such surgery has been successful. These guidelines are not absolute, however, since tumor recurrence has been reported in some patients with negative postoperative CEA levels.[51]

Thus, to return to the original questions, what is the value of CEA as a diagnostic or prognostic tool, or both, and how do the conflicting results concerning its specificity affect its usefulness? It is clear that the radioimmunoassays for circulating CEA have a high degree of reliability in patients with primary carcinoma, particularly those with more extensive disease. Nevertheless, the current confusion concerning the specific association of circulating CEA with large bowel cancer demands that the use of large-scale serum-screening programs for CEA as a diagnostic test for such tumors be held in abeyance. Hopefully, additional studies of large numbers of patients with a variety of disorders, both malignant and nonmalignant, may help to reconcile the divergent results presently being reported. Also, standardization of the assay technique used and more data on the structure and composition of the CEA molecule would be extremely helpful toward this end. Serious thought must also be given to the question of what constitutes a reasonable cutoff value for CEA positivity. As has been pointed out,[65] the generally accepted value currently used, 2.5 ng./ml., represents a relatively low threshold of positivity which, while detecting a higher proportion of tumors, leads to the inclusion of more "false positives." It is worthwhile to consider whether a somewhat higher cutoff value would be more desirable. Thus, more reliable positive diagnoses would be achieved, although some cancers would not be detected by this procedure. It is also possible that, as the sensitivity of CEA detection procedures improves, an equally low, if not lower, threshold value can be employed which will allow the discrimination of the appropriate neoplastic conditions from other disorders with which CEA has been associated.

The uncertainty as to the specificity of CEA notwithstanding, it is clear that the assay of circulating CEA can provide a valuable prognostic tool. Initially it can give an indication as to the approximate extent of tumor growth and the chances of successful tumor resection. Continuous postoperative monitoring of humoral CEA can provide a clue as to the effectiveness of the surgical procedure or can indicate the presence of previously undetected metastases. Whether such information can be obtained early enough to actually improve patient survival will be determined only by long-term follow-up studies of large numbers of patients.

Thus, the results of CEA studies available at the present time suggest that serum CEA assays are not yet sufficiently specific to allow the presence of elevated

CEA levels to be considered diagnostic of colonic carcinoma. At the same time, there is no doubt that by selection of the appropriate assay technique (e.g., Gold's radioimmunoassay), the desired antigenic site (or forms) of the CEA can be tested for and, in combination with appropriate clinical and histologic observations, can be of value prognostically both pre- and postoperatively with certain cancers. Should future investigations strengthen the specific association of CEA with gastrointestinal cancer there is every reason to believe that a test diagnostic for large bowel tumors involving the assay of circulating CEA can be utilized. Presently the results of Gold and co-workers[37, 38] are the strongest support for such a possibility. It is hoped that the exchange of coded patient samples between the various laboratories involved in the measurement of circulating CEA may help to resolve the questions concerning the specificity of CEA and the differences in the results obtained by the various assays. Until this is achieved, the diagnostic value of CEA is definitely limited, although its prognostic value is considerable when used in conjunction with standard clinical tests.

References

1. Gold, P., and Freedman, S. O.: Demonstration of tumor-specific antigens in human colonic carcinomata by immunological tolerance and absorption techniques. J. Exp. Med. 121:439–462, 1965.
2. Gold, P., and Freedman, S. O.: Specific carcinoembryonic antigens of the human digestive system. J. Exp. Med. 122:467–481, 1965.
3. Abelev, G. I., Assecritova, I. V., Kraevsky, N. A., et al.: Embryonal serum α-globulin in cancer patients: Diagnostic value. Int. J. Cancer 2:551–558, 1967.
4. Alpert, M. E., Uriel, J., and de Nechund, B.: Alpha₁ fetoglobulin in the diagnosis of human hepatoma. New Eng. J. Med. 278:984–986, 1968.
5. Mawas, C., Kohen, M., Lemerle, J., et al.: Serum α₁ foeto-protein (fetuin) in children with malignant ovarian or testicular teratomas: Preliminary results. Int. J. Cancer 4:76–79, 1969.
6. Masopust, J., Kithier, K., and Rádl, J.: Occurrence of fetoprotein in patients with neoplasms and non-neoplastic diseases. Int. J. Cancer 3:364–373, 1968.
7. Edynak, E. M., Old, L. J., Vrana, M., et al.: A fetal antigen associated with human neoplasia. New Eng. J. Med. 286:1178–1183, 1972.
8. Häkkinen, I., and Viikari, S.: Occurrence of fetal sulphoglycoprotein antigen in the gastric juice of patients with gastric diseases. Ann. Surg. 169:277–281, 1969.
9. Stolbach, L. L., Krant, M. J., and Fishman, W. H.: Ectopic production of an alkaline phosphatase isoenzyme in patients with cancer. New Eng. J. Med. 281:757–762, 1969.
10. Nathanson, L., and Fishman, W. H.: New observations on the Regan isoenzyme of alkaline phosphatase in cancer patients. Cancer 27:1388–1397, 1971.
11. Tal, C., and Halperin, M.: Presence of serologically distinct protein in serum of cancer patients and pregnant women: An attempt to develop a diagnostic cancer test. Israel J. Med. Sci. 6:708–716, 1970.
12. Pearson, G., and Freeman, G.: Evidence suggesting a relationship between polyoma virus-induced transplantation antigen and normal embryonic antigen. Cancer Res. 28:1665–1673, 1968.
13. Duff, R., and Rapp, F.: Reaction of serum from pregnant hamsters with surface of cells transformed by SV40. J. Immunol. 105:521–523, 1970.
14. Coggin, J. H., Ambrose, K. R., and Anderson, N. G.: Fetal antigen capable of inducing transplantation immunity against SV40 hamster tumor cells. J. Immunol. 105:524–526, 1970.
15. Ambrose, K. R., Anderson, N. G., and Coggin, J. H.: Interruption of SV40 oncogenesis with human fetal antigen. Nature (London) 233:194–195, 1971.

16. Hanna, M. G., Tennant, R. W., and Coggin, J. H.: Suppressive effect of immunization with mouse fetal antigens on growth of cells infected with Rauscher leukemia virus and on plasma-cell tumors. Proc. Nat. Acad. Sci. USA 68:1748–1752, 1971.
17. Baranska, W., Koldovsky, P., and Koprowski, H.: Antigenic study of unfertilized mouse eggs: Cross-reactivity with SV40-induced antigens. Proc. Nat. Acad. Sci. USA 67: 193–199, 1970.
18. Koprowski, H., Sawicki, W., and Koldovsky, P.: Immunologic cross-reactivity between antigen of unfertilized mouse eggs and mouse cells transformed by simian virus 40. J. Nat. Cancer Inst. 46:1317–1323, 1971.
19. Berman, L. D.: The SV40 S antigen: A carcinoembryonic antigen of the hamster? Int. J. Cancer 10:326–330, 1972.
20. Brawn, R. J.: Possible association of embryonal antigens(s) with several primary 3-methylcholanthrene-induced murine sarcomas. Int. J. Cancer 6:245–249, 1970.
21. Alexander, P.: A cross-reacting fetal antigen in primary chemically induced sarcomas of rats and its relation to immunotherapy. In Anderson, N. G., and Coggin, J. H. (eds.): Proceedings of the 1st Conference on Embryonal and Fetal Antigens. Oak Ridge, Tenn., U.S. Atomic Energy Commission, 1971, pp. 217–222.
22. Baldwin, R. W., Glaves, D., Harris, J. R., et al.: Tumor-specific antigens associated with aminoazo dye-induced rat hepatomas. Transplant. Proc. 3:1189–1191, 1971.
23. Black, P. H., Collins, J. J., and Culp, L. A.: Altered surface properties of neoplastic cells. In Clark, R. L., Cumley, R. W., McCay, J. E., and Copeland, M. M. (eds.): Oncology 1970, Proceedings of the 10th International Cancer Congress, Vol. I. Chicago, Year Book Medical Publishers, Inc., 1971, pp. 210–225.
24. Häyry, P., and Defendi, V.: Surface antigen(s) of SV40-transformed tumor cells. Virology 41:22–29, 1970.
25. Burger, M. M.: A difference in the architecture of the surface membrane of normal and virally transformed cells. Proc. Nat. Acad. Sci. USA 62:994–1001, 1969.
26. Nicolson, G. L.: Difference in topology of normal and tumour cell membranes shown by different surface distributions of ferritin-conjugated Concanavalin A. Nature New Biol. 233:244–246, 1971.
27. Krupey, J., Gold, P., and Freedman, S. O.: Physicochemical studies of the carcinoembryonic antigens of the human digestive system. J. Exp. Med. 128:387–398, 1968.
28. Gold, P., Gold, M., and Freedman, S. O.: Cellular location of carcinoembryonic antigens of the human digestive system. Cancer Res. 28:1331–1334, 1968.
29. Gold, P., Krupey, J., and Ansari, H.: Position of the carcinoembryonic antigen of the human digestive system in ultrastructure of tumor cell surface. J. Nat. Cancer Inst. 45:219–225, 1970.
30. Collins, J. J., Gold, P., Black, P. H.: In preparation.
31. Gold, P.: Circulating antibodies against carcinoembryonic antigens of the human digestion system. Cancer 20:1663–1667, 1967.
32. Collatz, E., von Kleist, S., and Burtin, P.: Further investigations of circulating antibodies in colon cancer patients: On the autoantigenicity of the carcinoembryonic antigen. Int. J. Cancer 8:298–303, 1971.
33. LoGerfo, P., Herter, F. P., and Bennett, S. J.: Absence of circulating antibodies to carcinoembryonic antigen in patients with gastrointestinal malignancies. Int. J. Cancer 9:344–348, 1972.
34. Hellström, I., Hellström, K. E., and Sheppard, T. H.: Cell-mediated immunity against antigens common to human colonic carcinomas and fetal gut epithelium. Int. J. Cancer 6:346–351, 1970.
35. Hollinshead, A., Glew, D., Bunnag, B., et al.: Skin-reactive soluble antigen from intestinal cancer-cell-membranes and relationship to carcinoembryonic antigens. Lancet 1:1191–1195, 1970.
36. Lejtenyi, M. C., Freedman, S. O., and Gold, P.: Response of lymphocytes from patients with gastrointestinal cancer to the carcinoembryonic antigen of the human digestive system. Cancer 28:115–120, 1971.
37. Thomson, D. M. P., Krupey, J., Freedman, S. O., et al.: The radioimmunoassay of circulating carcinoembryonic antigens of the human digestive system. Proc. Nat. Acad. Sci. USA 64:161–167, 1969.
38. Gold, P.: The role of immunology in human cancer research. Canad. Med. Ass. J. 103: 1043–1051, 1970.
39. Martin, F., and Martin, M. S.: Demonstration of antigens related to colonic cancer in the human digestive system. Int. J. Cancer 6:352–360, 1970.

40. Kleinman, M. S., Harwell, L., and Turner, M. D.: Studies of colonic carcinoma antigens. Gut 12:1–10, 1971.
41. von Kleist, S., and Burtin, P.: Isolation of fetal antigen from human colonic tumors. Cancer Res. 29:1961–1964, 1969.
42. von Kleist, S., and Burtin, P.: Cellular localization of an embryonic antigen in human colonic tumors. Int. J. Cancer 4:874–879, 1969.
43. Burtin, P., Martin, E., Sabine, M. C., et al.: Immunological study of polyps of the colon. J. Nat. Cancer Inst. 48:25–32, 1972.
44. Norland, C. C., Maass, E. G., and Kirsner, J. B.: Identification of colon carcinoma by immunofluorescent staining. Cancer 23:730–739, 1969.
45. McNeil, C., Ladle, J. N., Helmick, W. M., et al.: An antiserum to ovarian mucinous cyst fluid with colon cancer specificity. Cancer Res. 29:1535–1540, 1969.
46. Nairn, R. C., Nind, A. P. P., Guli, E. P. G., et al.: Immunological reactivity in patients with carcinoma of colon. Brit. Med. J. 4:706–709, 1971.
47. Moore, T. L., Kupchik, H. Z., Marcon, N., et al.: Carcinoembryonic antigen assay in cancer of the colon and pancreas and other digestive tract disorders. Amer. J. Dig. Dis. 16:1–7, 1971.
48. Hansen, H. J., Lance, K. P., and Krupey, J.: Demonstration on an ion sensitive antigenic site on carcinoembryonic antigen: Assay using zirconyl phosphate. Clin. Res. 19:143, 1971.
49. LoGerfo, P., Krupey, J., and Hansen, H. J.: Demonstration of a common neoplastic antigen: Assay using zirconyl phosphate gel. New Eng. J. Med. 285:138–141, 1971.
50. Reynoso, G., Chu, T. M., Holyoke, D., et al.: Carcinoembryonic antigen in patients with different cancers. J. A. M. A. 220:361–365, 1972.
51. Dhar, P., Moore, T., Zamcheck, N., et al.: Carcinoembryonic antigen (CEA) in colonic cancer. J. A. M. A. 221:31–35, 1972.
52. Nugent, F. W., and Hansen, E. R.: Radio-immunoassay of carcinoembryonic antigen as a diagnostic test for cancer of the colon: A preliminary report. Lahey Clin. Found. Bull. 20:85–88, 1971.
53. Rule, A. H., Straus, E., Vandevoorde, J., et al.: Tumor-associated (CEA-reacting) antigen in patients with inflammatory bowel disease. New Eng. J. Med. 287:24–26, 1972.
54. Zamcheck, N., and Moore, T. L.: Ulcerative colitis/colon cancer: Immunologically linked disorders? New Eng. J. Med. 287:43, 1972.
55. LoGerfo, P., LoGerfo, F., Herter, F., et al.: Tumor-associated antigen in patients with carcinoma of the colon. Amer. J. Surg. 123:127–131, 1972.
56. LoGerfo, P., Herter, F. P., Braun, J., et al.: Tumor associated antigen with pulmonary neoplasms. Ann. Surg. 175:495–500, 1972.
57. LoGerfo, P., Herter, F., and Hansen, H. J.: Tumor associated antigen in normal lung and colon. J. Surg. Oncol. 4:1–7, 1972.
58. Chu, T. M., Reynoso, G., and Hansen, H. J.: Demonstration of carcinoembryonic antigens in normal human plasma. Nature (London) 238:152–153, 1972.
59. Egan, M. L., Lautenschleger, J. T., Coligan, J. E., et al.: Radioimmune assay of carcinoembryonic antigen. Immunochemistry 9:289–299, 1972.
60. Coligan, J. E., Lautenschleger, J. T., Egan, M. L., et al.: Isolation and characterization of carcinoembryonic antigen. Immunochemistry 9:377–386, 1972.
61. Collins, J. J., and Black, P. H.: Specificity of the carcinoembryonic antigen. New Eng. J. Med. 285:175–177, 1971.
62. Gold, P.: Personal communication.
63. Gold, J. M., Freedman, S. O., and Gold, P.: Human anti-CEA antibodies detected by radioimmunoelectrophoresis. Nature New Biol. 239:60–62, 1972.
64. Lange, R. D., Chernoff, A. I., Jordan, T. A., et al.: Experience with a hemagglutination inhibition test for carcinoembryonic antigen: preliminary report In Anderson, N. G., and Coggin, J. H. (eds.): Proceedings of the 1st Conference on Embryonal and Fetal Antigens. Oak Ridge, Tenn., U.S. Atomic Energy Commission, 1971, pp. 379–388.
65. Zamcheck, N., Moore, T. L., Dhar, P., et al.: Immunologic diagnosis and prognosis of human digestive-tract cancer: Carcinoembryonic antigens. New Eng. J. Med. 286:83–86, 1972.

Comment

Evaluation of Carcinoembryonic Antigen in Diagnosis of Cancer of the Colon

Our intention was to have this topic discussed in the usual format of presentation of alternative points of view by two essayists; but one who accepted our invitation to participate failed to honor his agreement. Because of this circumstance, we sent the comprehensive and scholarly paper submitted by Drs. Collins and Black to Drs. Phil Gold and Samuel O. Freedman and asked them to express their agreement or disagreement. They were kind enough to submit, on very brief notice, the following comments.

—EDITORS

Doctors Collins and Black have done a most admirable job in reviewing the literature concerning the carcinoembryonic antigen (CEA) of the human digestive system. The paper describes the present applications and future potentials, rather than the limitations, of CEA detection as a diagnostic and prognostic tool.

In examining the question of whether or not the CEA is qualitatively tumor-specific, the point made by Collins and Black concerning the molecular heterogeneity of CEA is well taken and is worthy of re-emphasis. Although at least one region of the protein component of the molecule appears to be constant,[1] CEA contains a number of different immunogenic groupings other than the tumor-specific determinant. These include a blood group A-like site,[2] a zone which apparently cross reacts with the fetal sulfoglycoprotein antigen (FSA) of human gastric cancers,[3] and one or more areas which appear to cross react with materials detectable in normal human tissues.[4-6] The antigenic determinants for these normal tissue sites are quite distinct from the tumor-specific area on the CEA molecule and will be considered briefly later.

In addition to this intramolecular variation, it has also been found that different batches of CEA, and even one preparation of this material, may demonstrate intermolecular heterogeneity when examined by certain biologic and physicochemical criteria.[7, 8] Remaining cognizant of the fact that the CEA and other CEA-like molecules have always been defined by the use of heterologous sera prepared against CEA preparations of variable purity, which have subsequently been absorbed to different degrees, it is hardly surprising that the question of the tumor-specificity of the CEA molecule has arisen from studies in some laboratories. However, a number of recent experimental findings have served to reaffirm the initial impression that the CEA is specific for entodermally derived digestive system tumors in the adult.[5, 6, 9, 10] Moreover, the demonstration of components in normal human tissues, such as the normal glycoprotein (NGP) of Mach et al.,[4] the nonspecific crossreacting antigen (NCA) of von Kleist et al.,[5] and the $\beta\hat{E}$ of Ørjasaeter et al.,[6] which cross react with an area, or areas, of the CEA molecule distinct from the tumor-specific site, may explain the apparent demonstration of CEA-like materials in tissues other than gastrointestinal cancers. The ultimate resolution of this aspect of the problem will likely require extensive physicochemical, immunochemical, and structural analyses of the CEA, as well as of those other molecules which may bear antigenic similarities to the CEA.

Virtually identical, theoretical arguments may be put forward in consideration of the so-called false positive results obtained by radioimmunoassay for CEA when the individual in question is truly free of any form of gastrointestinal cancer, even in its earliest stages. It would, of course, be difficult to make a substantial argument for the existence of circulating CEA in conditions other than digestive system tumors unless it can be clearly shown that this molecule is, indeed, being produced by the diseased tissue under consideration. Hence, the relationships between circulating CEA, CEA-like serum constituents, and the group of moieties which have been termed tumor-associated antigens (TAA) remain to be determined. Here again, the physicochemical characterization of the molecular entities under consideration will be required for the resolution of the problem. The possibility that there may be a family of circulating CEA-like molecules, each of which is pathognomonic of a specific disease entity, is, however, most attractive.

A few other points in the manuscript by Collins and Black warrant comment. In the matter of the natural immunogenicity of the CEA, a specific humoral immune response, exclusively of the IgM class of antibody molecule, has been demonstrated by at least two techniques.[2, 11] It has, further, been observed that the methodology employed for antibody detection is of major importance in determining the data ultimately obtained. Hence, BDB-hemagglutination produced positive results with the sera of patients bearing digestive system cancers only if the tumor had not undergone metastatic spread.[11] On the other hand, the technique of radioimmunoelectrophoresis was able to detect anti-CEA antibodies in the sera of patients with disseminated cancers.[2] The use of a modified Farr technique, even with acid-dissociation for the detection of antibody bound to antigen, was unable to detect anti-CEA antibodies under any circumstances.

Upon turning to the area of cell-mediated immune responsiveness to the CEA, no substantial evidence for such a phenomenon has ever been put forward. Although cell-mediated immunity against antigens common to human colonic carcinomas and fetal gut epithelium has been demonstrated by the use of the colony inhibition technique,[12] it was simply suggested that the CEA might be the common factor involved. No direct evidence for this was ever presented, or even sought. Using another in vitro model of cell-mediated immunity, Lejtenyi et al.[13] were unable to demonstrate any significant degree of transformation when lymphocytes of patients with digestive system tumors were exposed to CEA. By skin testing patients bearing digestive system cancers with extracts of their own tumors, it was found that CEA was present in fractions of the material which were capable of eliciting a delayed hypersensitivity reaction.[14] It was, however, subsequently found that the CEA and the skin reactive material could be separated by polyacrylamide gel electrophoresis.[15]

The recent studies of Denk et al.[9] serve to answer the question, raised by Doctors Collins and Black, concerning the use of immunofluorescence with and without tissue fixation for the detection and localization of CEA in tissue sections. In contradiction to the findings of Burtin et al.,[16,17] these investigators were unable to find CEA in alcohol-fixed sections of any tissues other than gastrointestinal tumors. These results are in agreement with the findings made in our laboratory, where unfixed tissues and explanted cells have been studied.

Finally, brief and pragmatic consideration may be given to the present status of the various radioimmunoassays for the CEA in the sera of patients. The literature review presented by Collins and Black coupled with the preceding paragraphs leave very little to be said. It seems obvious that standardization of reagents and technology will prove most helpful in interpreting the various sets of data which will be forthcoming. It has become increasingly evident that the specificity of the assay is dependent upon the purity of the CEA employed as a standard for both immunization and testing, and the extent to which the final preparation of anti-CEA antiserum is absorbed. Moreover, the technique utilized in the radioimmunoassay may be another parameter in determining the conditions which will give rise to positive results—be they due to CEA or CEA-like materials in the circulation.

At the moment it would appear that the radioimmunoassays for CEA are of greatest value when utilized in conjunction with other diagnostic procedures in the search for cancer. Moreover, a major and immediate role for the detection of circulating CEA is in the prognosis of cancer in a patient who has had either surgery or chemotherapy for the treatment of a tumor. It has been repeatedly demonstrated, as Collins and Black point out, that the presence of metastases will produce high circulating levels of CEA, while persistent levels of circulating CEA following surgical resection of the primary lesion strongly suggest the presence of residual tumor. The value of serial determinations for CEA during cancer chemotherapy is presently under evaluation in a number of centers, and early results are rather encouraging.

On the basis of the foregoing observations, therefore, it is difficult to understand why Doctors Collins and Black conclude that it is "clear that the radioimmunoassays for circulating CEA have a high degree of reliability in patients with primary carcinoma, particularly those with more extensive disease"—unless "extensive" disease is meant to indicate metastases.

There seems little doubt that a good deal of further study will be required to elucidate the theoretical and practical implications of the structure and biologic function of the CEA and the use of this and related materials in the diagnosis of human disease. Nevertheless, a start has been made, and rapid progress will, we hope, be forthcoming.

PHIL GOLD and SAMUEL O. FREEDMAN

References

1. Terry, W. D., Henkart, P. A., Coligan, J. E., et al.: Structural studies of major glycoprotein in preparations with carcinoembryonic antigen activity J. Exp. Med. 136:200–241, 1972.
2. Gold, J. M., Freedman, S. O., and Gold, P.: Human anti-CEA antibodies detected by radioimmunoelectrophoresis. Nature, New Biology 239:60–62, 1972.
3. Hakkinen, I. P. T.: Immunological relationship of the carcinoembryonic antigen and the fetal sulfoglycoprotein antigen. Immunochemistry 9:1115–1119, 1972.
4. Mach, J.-P., and Pusztaszeri, G.: Carcinoembryonic antigen (CEA): Demonstration of a partial identity between CEA and a normal glycoprotein. Immunochemistry 9:1031–1034, 1972.
5. von Kleist, S., Chavanel, G., and Burtin, P.: Identification of an antigen from normal human tissue that crossreacts with the carcinoembryonic antigen. Proc. Nat. Acad. Sci. USA 69:2492–2494, 1972.
6. Ørjasaeter, H., Fredriksen, G., and Liavag, I.: Studies on carcinoembryonic and related antigens in malignant tumors of colon-rectum. Acta Path. Microbiol. Scand. (Section B) 80:599–608, 1972.
7. Shuster, J., Silverman, M., and Gold, P.: Metabolism of carcinoembryonic antigen in xenogeneic animals. Cancer Res. 33:65–68, 1973.
8. Banjo, C.: Unpublished data.
9. Denk, H., Tappeiner, G., Eckerstorfer, R., et al.: Carcinoembryonic antigen in gastrointestinal tumors and extra gastrointestinal tumors and its relationship to tumor cell differentiation. Int. J. Cancer 10:262–272, 1972.
10. Coligan, J. E., Lautenschlager, J. T., Egan, M. L., et al.: Isolation and characterization of carcinoembryonic antigen. Immunochemistry 9:377–386, 1972.
11. Gold, P.: Circulating antibodies against carcinoembryonic antigen of the human digestive system. Cancer 20:1663–1667, 1967.
12. Hellström, I., Hellström, K. E., and Sheppard, T. H.: Cell mediated immunity against antigens common to human colonic carcinomas and fetal gut epithelium. Int. J. Cancer 6:346–351, 1970.
13. Lejtenyi, M. C., Freedman, S. O., and Gold, P.: Response of lymphocytes from patients with gastrointestinal cancer to the carcinoembryonic antigen of the human digestive system. Cancer 28:115–120, 1971.
14. Hollinshead, A. C., Glew, D., Bunnag, B., et al: Skin-reactive soluble antigen from intestinal cancer-cell membranes and relationship to carcinoembryonic antigens. Lancet 1:1191–1194, 1970.
15. Hollinshead, A. C., McWright, C. G., Alford, T. C., et al.: Separation of skin reactive intestinal cancer antigen from the carcinoembryonic antigen of Gold. Science 177:887–889, 1972.
16. von Kleist, S., and Burtin, P.: Cellular localization of an embryonic antigen in human colonic tumors. Int. J. Cancer 4:874–879, 1969.
17. Burtin, P., Martin, E., Sabine, M. C., et al.: Immunological study of polyps of the colon. J. Nat. Cancer Inst. 48:25–32, 1972.

29

The Treatment of Hodgkin's Disease

The Treatment of Hodgkin's Disease—A Conservative View
    by John Horton

The Case for an Aggressive Chemotherapeutic Approach for Patients with Advanced Hodgkin's Disease
    by Joseph R. Bertino

Comment
    by Jerome B. Block and Thomas C. Chalmers

The Treatment of Hodgkin's Disease—A Conservative View

JOHN HORTON

Albany Medical College of Union University, Albany New York

All I mean by truth is what I can't help thinking.

O. Wendell Holmes, Jr.

Although the recent increase in interest in the disease named after him would surely gladden the heart of Sir Thomas Hodgkin, he might be dismayed to realize that its cause is still unknown, its biology poorly understood and its treatment largely empirical. It is then perhaps somewhat surprising that the medical profession seems to accept with little question the current dogma that all patients should receive an absolute maximum of this empirical treatment. It will be my argument that currently available data support equally well the judgment that overall mortality and morbidity can be minimized by systematically and specifically adjusting more conservative treatment regimens to the needs of each patient and his disease.

Patients who are labeled with the diagnosis of Hodgkin's disease may have any one of several diseases, each of which may well have a different etiology, as well as a different biology and prognosis.[1] It is no longer possible to follow the course of untreated Hodgkin's disease, but studies such as those of Jackson and Parker[2] demonstrate that a proportion of patients given little or no therapy lived for long periods of time. The clinical course of some patients who have symptoms of fever or episodic lymphadenopathy for several years before a specific diagnosis of Hodgkin's disease can be made suggests that an appreciable period of survival without treatment is still a very real phenomenon. The resemblance of the pathology and clinical behavior of some patients to that of an unusual systemic reaction to an infectious or toxic stimulus cannot be ignored. Agreed, the course of most untreated patients with Hodgkin's disease suggests the behavior of a malignant

731

process, but the malignant cells may be difficult to define. The pleomorphic reactive inflammatory cells which make up the majority of the physical bulk of Hodgkin's tissue are benign, and the Reed Sternberg cell, the hallmark of the disease, is probably a nonproliferating cell.[3] It seems likely, however, that it represents the end stage of an abnormal mononuclear reticulum cell having malignant properties. Perhaps we should consider what may occur in an area of Hodgkin's disease when it shrinks after treatment with radiation or chemotherapy. Both these modalities have cytotoxic and immunosuppressive properties. The shrinkage might be due to either death or change of the malignant cells, thereby resulting in loss of the surrounding benign reactive cells, or merely due to an inhibition of these reactive cells without destruction of the malignant ones. Achievement of just the latter effect could certainly result in what we now term a "complete remission" as well as amelioration of symptomatology, although it would not, of course, achieve cure.

Let us examine some of the steps we might consider in the investigation and management of a patient who presents with Hodgkin's disease.

Staging

The prognosis and treatment of our patient certainly depends in large part on the extent of disease when he or she first presents. Investigation will include a history, physical examination, and hematologic, chemical, and radiologic studies. The real questions are whether lower limb lymphography and surgical abdominal exploration will be performed.

The usual rationale stated for performing lower limb lymphography is to delineate areas of nodal involvement below the diaphragm. This is obviously superfluous when Stage III or IV disease is already apparent. Since demonstration of nodes above the level of L2 by this technique is unusual, it is of little help in evaluating disease in this region. The interpretation of lymphograms is difficult, even for experienced radiographers, and the degree of correlation between the observed changes and pathological interpretation is often poor. In our own institution, for example, there was concurrence on only 50 per cent of patients studied. Many physicians place a great deal of reliance on this radiographic examination, but recognition of its inaccuracy was a major factor in prompting the movement toward celiotomy as an adjunct in the definition of disease below the diaphragm.[4] This latter procedure, performed in centers that have the facilities for complete evaluation of findings, has unquestionably produced valuable information. Celiotomy, I believe, is still primarily an investigational tool, and unless it is being performed as part of a specific program by experienced and interested personnel who can make and report the appropriate correlations, it should not be done in an indiscriminate fashion.

Abdominal exploration with splenectomy and liver and multiple node biopsies cannot be considered to be a "minor" operation and will be associated with appreciable morbidity and a definite risk of mortality, especially since the usual close temporal relationship of lower limb lymphography has, in our hands, seemed to increase the risk of postoperative thromboembolic complications. Johnson[5] has questioned the value of celiotomy, and even such a pioneer as Rosenberg[6] now feels that its value is limited essentially to evaluation of the spleen. It seems likely that, in the future, recognition of disease patterns requiring synthesis of knowledge of the peripheral characteristics of the lymphadenopathy, the histologic pattern, and the overall clinical picture, will give a good indication of the extent of disease and will probably obviate the necessity for celiotomy. It can already be stated, for example, with a good deal of confidence that a young girl having a slow onset in her neck of a few large nodes showing a nodular sclerosing pattern, a widened upper mediastinum, but no systemic symptoms or splenomegaly, is most unlikely to have lower abdominal node or liver involvement. In contrast, as another example, a young male with small, shotty axillary and cervical nodes of a mixed cellularity pattern without mediastinal widening will virtually always have disease in the retroperitoneal nodes.

The ultimate place of "surgical staging" measured in terms of patient survival will not be established until several years hence. There is one prospective and randomized study[7] now being performed at the Roswell Park Memorial Institute that should answer this question. This will compare the survival of groups of patients whose treatment will be based on a staging process either including or excluding surgical exploration.

Treatment

The choice of treatment for the patient depends on many factors, including the patient-related ones of extent of disease, histologic pattern, and host condition. In general, patients with the classic Stages I, II, or III will be treated primarily with radiation, and those with Stage IV primarily with chemotherapy. Factors not related directly to the patient, such as the experience and expertise of medical personnel, availability and adequacy of treatment equipment, facilities for management of complications, and adequacy of follow-up, tend less often to be considered but are equally as important as the patient characteristics when the extent of therapy to be offered is determined.

SPLENECTOMY

The routine performance of splenectomy as an adjunct in the staging process has been advocated as a therapeutic modality to reduce the extent of hematologic toxicity induced by treatment. This is probably not justified for several reasons. Most importantly, the majority of patients can receive adequate therapy without excessive damage to the bone marrow. Data supporting the effectiveness of removing a normal spleen for this purpose is sparse, and Tartaglia et al.[8] have been unable to demonstrate that splenectomy in dogs ameliorates the extent of hematologic toxicity induced by the administration of nitrogen mustard. The higher measured levels of white cell, platelet, and lymphocyte counts that are noted after splenectomy may well induce a false sense of security. It is more likely that these changes in values represent a shift of blood cells into the circulating pool rather than an enhancement of bone marrow reserve. In fact, in a recently reported study,[9] asplenic patients treated with chemotherapy sustained more marrow suppression than their counterparts with intact spleens as reflected by a proportionately greater fall in their blood counts during therapy.

Removal of the spleen following trauma in a normal person probably leaves few sequelae.[10] The role of the spleen in protection against severe infections is not well understood, but a recent case report[11] highlights the possibility that splenectomy may increase further the risk of severe infection by common pathogens in the immunologically impaired patient with Hodgkin's disease. Nevertheless, the presence of an enlarged spleen, especially if it is producing the hematologic effects of hypersplenism, may be an indication for its removal.

RADIATION THERAPY

Gilbert[12] and Hynes and Frelick[13] lit the fires of radiotherapeutic aggression in Hodgkin's disease several years ago. These fires are being fanned by such radiotherapists as Kaplan[15] and Johnson et al.,[16] who now recommend that very high doses of radiation therapy be given to all lymph node-bearing areas in all patients except, perhaps, some poor risk patients in Stage IV. Is this approach justified? The real criterion for success would be demonstration of prolongation of survival of a population with Hodgkin's disease that has received such treatment. It is impossible to be sure that such goals have been achieved. Interpretation of data is also complicated by variability in other therapy given. Reported survival statistics are almost always hospital or institution based and therefore subject to all the vagaries of referral patterns. The End Results Section of the National Cancer Institute has data (Table 1) that show an improvement of survival, but the input into this registry, too, is more from medical centers than from geographic areas.[17] Two states, New York and Connecticut, that have mandatory cancer reporting have not been able to provide me with figures that will answer this question. The degree of improvement in survival noted by the End Results Section is similar to that for localized lung cancer, and it seems reasonable to suggest that these changes might just as easily be due to increased gravitation to a reporting treatment center of motivated younger patients, who have a more favorable prognosis, as to any change in therapy. This could explain the observation that the number of patients being reported from centers to the End Results

Table 1. *Survival Rate in Four Time Periods of Patients with Hodgkin's Disease Reported from Three Centralized and Six Medical Center Registries**

TIME PERIOD	1940–49	1950–59	1960–64	1965–69
Number of Patients	1013	2008	1324	1990
Survival Rate (%)				
3 years	35	44	53	61
5 years	25	34	42	—
10 years	14	22	—	—

*Courtesy S. Cutler, Sc.D, End Results in Cancer, Report No. 4, January, 1972.

Section continues to increase (Table 1) even though the overall incidence of Hodgkin's disease in this country is probably stable. Further evidence to support this suggestion is that incidence of the relatively benign nodular sclerosis histologic pattern is considerably higher in the patient population receiving treatment at Stanford Medical Center[18] than would be expected in a general population.

The next question is: Should this high-dose, extensive radiotherapy be given to all patients with Hodgkin's disease? I believe the answer is no. The authors supporting high-dose intensive radiotherapy can undoubtedly themselves give the treatment they recommend with relative impunity. They are well trained, skillful, and have the best equipment. Outside these centers the situation is entirely different. The majority of patients will receive treatment in community hospitals from part-time radiotherapists who have had limited training and experience. In addition, mere availability of supervoltage equipment by no means implies that large port therapy can be given. For example, a recent survey of radiation facilities serving a population of 2,000,000 people located in an area of the Northeast United States demonstrated that only one facility could administer extensive radiation through double large ports as advocated by Kaplan. Six other institutions in this area have to use multiple small ports in the administration of high-dose therapy. The result has been an inordinately high incidence of such severe and sometimes fatal complications as transverse myelitis, esophageal perforation, and mediastinitis. The logic for development of radiotherapy centers in this country seems clear, but this is not the current situation. Undoubtedly many hospitals are upgrading their equipment, but the change is slow and trained radiotherapists are still scarce. The dictum that physicians should do more good than harm is still sound.

The next question is: Even if the facilities and personnel are available, should everyone receive "total nodal" radiation? Opinions vary, but the results of Peters[19] certainly indicate that less than "total nodal" irradiation gives excellent results in patients with limited disease and favorable histologic patterns. The increased morbidity and toxicity, the lessened tolerance for subsequent chemotherapy, and the probable increased risk of development of other cancers or leukemia[20] following total nodal radiation are factors that must be considered, although "total nodal" radiation is probably valid for patients with Stage III A disease. Of interest is that the survival data of up to 18 years follow-up of patients with clinical Stage I disease treated at the Albany Medical Center using minimally sized ports and doses, and usually without radiation of contiguous but apparently uninvolved areas, paralleled those described by Easson and Russell.[14] Kaplan[15] has popularized the attempts to maximize dosage as well as field size of radiation treatment, but many of our attempts to emulate him have been thwarted by treatment-limiting toxicity. The results of Easson and Russell, which were good enough to make them talk of cure, were achieved with conventional equipment and what would now be considered very modest doses of radiation. The determination of what is optimal radiation therapy in terms of the radiation dose and dose rate, the energy, and the shape and size of fields for any particular stage still needs study in a careful, prospective, randomized, and comparative fashion.

CHEMOTHERAPY

Chemotherapy undoubtedly plays an important role in alleviating symptomatology in those patients who present with extensive disease or who have recurrences after radiotherapy. As with radiotherapy, it is difficult to document prolongation of survival, although Aisenberg and Goldman[21] have attempted to do this based on experience with a hospital population. They concluded that patients under the age of 50 were living about two years more in the period after 1963 as compared with the period before 1961 and attributed this increased survival to the advent of agents such as vinblastine (Velban) and procarbazine (Matulane). Comparative studies such as those performed by the Eastern Cooperative Oncology Group[22] have demonstrated that a higher incidence of complete remissions can be obtained with combination rather than single agent chemotherapy, although the overall incidence of remissions (complete and partial) is similar. In many of these studies, treatment was continued for what would now be considered to be much too short a period of time, and the single drugs were usually not administered in an optimal fashion.

The current vogue is for high-dose, intensive combination therapy with "MOPP" (nitrogen mustard [Mustargen], vincristine [Oncovin], procarbazine [Matulane] and prednisone). The original study of this combination[23] was on a highly selected, well motivated group of patients and gave impressive figures in terms of complete remission, but this treatment was not compared directly with any other therapy. Certainly the incidence of complete remissions is higher with such therapy than that previously achieved with single agents, but the true significance of a complete remission is not clear, and the question of whether achievement of this will result in longer survival is not fully answered. Progressive disease that has previously responded to high-dose, intensive combination chemotherapy usually develops in areas that were clinically involved before treatment. This suggests that the major effects of the chemotherapy might have been on the reactive inflammatory component of the disease and that control of the malignant cells had not been achieved. Few studies have been performed that compare the survival of patients treated with "MOPP" with those treated with single agents. One preliminary report by Brook and Gocka[24] suggests that patients treated with "MOPP" may be living longer, but the numbers of patients followed are still very small. Even if the final results of this study confirm these preliminary suggestions, I believe that patients should not invariably be offered "MOPP" or a similar high-dose, intensive combination, especially since those who need chemotherapy and have had prior extensive radiotherapy will have prolonged bone marrow suppression.[25]

Cooperative groups studying combination chemotherapy generally exclude patients from the study protocol who, they believe, will not do well. These exclusions are often not emphasized in published reports, and an unwarranted impression of treatment usefulness is generated. Of course, bad results are rarely published. An exception is a recent report of the deleterious effects of combination therapy in some patients with advanced lymphosarcoma involving extranodal sites.[26] Similar poor risk patients with Hodgkin's disease would probably fare better with appropriate single agent chemotherapy used in an optimal fashion and given for a prolonged period of time than they would with high-dose, intensive combination therapy. Many classes of chemotherapeutic agents are known to be highly active in Hodgkin's disease, and the degree of cross resistance tends to be low. As an example, the nitrosourea compounds are very effective, even for patients previously treated with alkylating agents, procarbazine, vinca alkaloids and prednisone.[27] It would seem reasonable to tailor any chemotherapy program both on patient factors and on the availability of medical expertise and facilities. At the present time, planned combinations of radiation and chemotherapy must still be considered to be an experimental treatment.

Conclusion

There is currently a paucity of hard data to support the claim that aggressive staging procedures, intensive, extensive, and high-dose radiation therapy, and high-dose, intensive combination chemotherapy have significantly changed the survival of patients with Hodgkin's disease. Evaluation, comparison, and improvement of treatments must continue, but this can reasonably be done only in centers with specialized and sophisticated personnel and equipment. The majority of patients in this country will not be managed in such a setting, and since close adherence to the "maximal therapy" concept under less than ideal circumstances will be likely to result in an excess of treatment-induced morbidity and mortality, a more conservative approach is justified. Much more evidence is needed to prove that high dosage "total nodal" radiation and/or combination chemotherapy will "cure" Hodgkin's disease, or even prolong and improve the quality of survival of all patients with this disorder.

References

1. MacMahon, B.: Epidemiology of Hodgkin's disease. Cancer Res. 26:1189–1200, 1966.
2. Jackson, H., Jr., and Parker, F., Jr.: Hodgkin's Disease and Allied Disorders. New York, Oxford University Press, 1947.
3. Peckham, M. J., and Cooper, E. H.: Proliferation characteristics of the various classes of cells in Hodgkin's disease. Cancer 24:135–146, 1969.
4. Lowenbraun, S., Ramsey, H., Sutherland, J., and Serpick, A. A.: Diagnostic laparotomy and staging for Hodgkin's disease. Ann. Intern. Med. 72:655–663, 1970.
5. Johnson, R. E.: Is staging laparotomy routinely indicated in Hodgkin's disease? Ann. Intern. Med. 75:459–462, 1971.
6. Rosenberg, S. A.: A critique of the value of laparotomy and splenectomy in the evaluation of patients with Hodgkin's disease. Cancer Res. 31:1737–1740, 1971.
7. Stutzman, L.: Personal communication.
8. Tartaglia, A. P., Scharfman, W., and Lempert, N.: Unpublished data.
9. Panettiere, F., and Coltman, C. A.: Effect of splenectomy on chemotherapy (MOPP) for Hodgkin's disease. Proc. Amer. Soc. Clin. Oncol., Abstract No. 49, 1972.
10. Ek, J. I., and Rayner, S.: An analytical study of splenectomized cases after traumatic rupture of healthy spleens. Acta Med. Scand. 137:417–435, 1950.
11. Stiver, G., Sharrar, R., Kendrick, M., and Eickholl, T.: Bacterial risk in staging splenectomy. Ann. Intern. Med. 76:670, 1972.
12. Gilbert, R.: Radiotherapy in Hodgkin's disease. Malignant granulomatosis. Amer. J. Roentgenol. 41:198–241, 1939.

13. Hynes, J. F., and Frelick, R. W.: Roentgen therapy of malignant lymphoma with special reference to segmental radiation therapy. Amer. J. Roentgenol. 70:247–257, 1953.
14. Easson, E. C., and Russell, M. H.: The cure of Hodgkin's disease. Brit. Med. J. 5347:1704–1797, 1963.
15. Kaplan, H. S.: Role of intensive radiotherapy in the management of Hodgkin's disease. Cancer 19:356–367, 1966.
16. Johnson, R. E., Thomas, L. B., Schneiderman, M., et al.: Preliminary experience with total nodal irradiation in Hodgkin's disease. Radiology 97:425–432, 1970.
17. Preliminary Release. End Results in Cancer, Report No. 4. End Results Section, National Cancer Institute, Bethesda, Maryland, January, 1972.
18. Dorfman, R.: Relationship of histology to site in Hodgkin's disease. Cancer Res. 31:1786–1793, 1971.
19. Peters, M. V.: Prophylactic treatment of adjacent areas in Hodgkin's disease. Cancer Res. 26:1232–1243, 1966.
20. Anderson, R. E., Nishiyaina, H., Li, R., Ishada, K., and Okabe, N.: Pathogenesis of radiation-related leukemia and lymphoma. Lancet 1:1060–1062, 1972.
21. Aisenberg, A. C., and Goldman, J. M.: Prolongation of survival in Hodgkin's disease. Cancer 27:802–805, 1971.
22. Lenhard, R. E., Jr., and the Eastern Cooperative Oncology Group: Combination chemotherapy of Hodgkin's disease. Proc. Amer. Ass. Cancer Res. 11:48, 1970. (Abstract.)
23. De Vita, V., Jr., Serpick, A. A., and Carbone, P. P.: Combination Chemotherapy in the treatment of advanced Hodgkin's disease. Ann. Intern. Med. 73:881–895, 1970.
24. Brook, J., and Gocka, E. F.: Comparison of single agents with combination therapy in Hodgkin's disease. Proc. Amer. Ass. Cancer Res. 13:79, 1972. (Abstract.)
25. Curran, R. E., and Johnson, R. E.: Tolerance to chemotherapy after prior irradiation for Hodgkin's disease. Ann. Intern. Med. 72:505–510, 1970.
26. Mukherji, B., Yagoda, A., Oettgen, H. F., and Krakoff, I. H.: Cyclic chemotherapy in lymphoma. Cancer 29:886–893, 1972.
27. Selawry, O. S., and Hansen, H. H.: Superiority of CCNU (1-(2-chloroethyl)-3-cyclohexyl-1-nitrosourea; NSC 79037) over BCNU (1,3-bis (2 chloroethyl)-1-nitrosourea; NSC 409962) in treatment of advanced Hodgkin's disease. Proc. Amer. Ass. Cancer Res. 13:46, 1972. (Abstract.)

The Case for an Aggressive Chemotherapeutic Approach for Patients with Advanced Hodgkin's Disease

JOSEPH R. BERTINO

Yale University School of Medicine

Improvements in the therapy of advanced Hodgkin's disease in recent years have resulted from the introduction of new, effective, antilymphoma drugs in the clinic, the use of these drugs in combination in maximum dose and, in some programs, from the addition of radiation therapy. This improved outlook has paralleled the development of more precise histologic and clinical staging methods[1-3] (Table 1) and more sophisticated radiation therapy techniques.[4,5] The purpose of this article is to review these advances, with emphasis on intensive drug treatment of this disease.

Table 1. *Clinical Staging of Hodgkin's Disease*

Stage I. Involvement of a single lymph node region (I) or a single extralymphatic organ or site (I_E).
Stage II. Involvement of two or more node regions on the same side of the diaphragm (II) or localized involvement of extralymphatic organ or site and of one or more node regions on the same side of the diaphragm (II_E).
Stage III. Involvement of node regions on both sides of the diaphragm (III), which may also be accompanied by localized involvement of extralymphatic organ or site (III_E) or by involvement of the spleen (III_S), or both (III_{SE}).
Stage IV. Diffuse or disseminated involvement of one or more extra lymphatic organs or tissues with or without associated lymph node enlargement.

Drugs Capable of Causing Tumor Regression in Patients with Hodgkin's Disease

The drugs available to the clinician and investigator for the treatment of Hodgkin's disease are listed in Table 2. In no other neoplastic disease, except possibly for acute lymphocytic leukemia, does the clinician have at his disposal so many effective antitumor drugs. Three of these drugs, nitrogen mustard, vinblastine, and a nitrosourea (CCNU), are each capable of producing long-term (ca. six months) remissions in approximately 60 per cent of treated patients with advanced Hodgkin's disease; in 10-20 per cent of patients the remissions are complete,[6,7] as defined by the absence of all objective findings of disease by physical examination, laboratory tests, and appropriate x-rays. The other agents listed (prednisone, procarbazine, vincristine, adriamycin, bleomycin) are also capable of producing a high percentage of remissions (50 to 70 per cent), but these are usually of short duration (two or three months).

COMBINATION CHEMOTHERAPY

The modern use of combination chemotherapy in Hodgkin's disease was guided by two important theoretical principles:[8,9] (1) drugs with independent mechanisms of action and differing from each other in dose-limiting side effects may have additive or even synergistic effects based upon kinetic or biochemical considerations, and (2) the use of drug combinations may prevent emergence of drug-resistant mutant cells, a common problem encountered in the clinic, especially with single-agent therapy of Hodgkin's disease.

Based upon the recognized limitations of single agent therapy as was prac-

Table 2. *Drugs Useful in the Treatment of Hodgkin's Disease*

DRUG	YEAR INTRODUCED	% RESPONDING	% COMPLETE REMISSION
I. *Alkylating Agents*			
Nitrogen mustard	1943	50–60	20–30
Cyclophosphamide	1961	40–50	10–20
II. *Vinca Alkaloids*			
Vinblastine	1961	60–70	10–20
Vincristine	1963	60–70	10–20
III. *Nitrosoureas*			
Carmustine (bischloroethyl nitrosourea, BCNU)*	1961	50	10–20
Lomustine (cyclohexyl chloroethyl nitrosourea, CCNU)*	1970	60–70	20–30
IV. *Miscellaneous*			
Prednisone	1952	60–70	10–20
Procarbazine	1963	60–70	10–20
Adriamycin*	1969	50–60	10–20
Bleomycin*	1969	50–60	< 10

*Investigational drugs.

Table 3. *The MOPP Program*

DAY OF CYCLE	1	8	14	28
Vincristine (I.V.)	1.4	1.4	Rest Interval	
Nitrogen mustard (I.V.)	6	6		
Procarbazine (oral)	100	→		
Prednisone (oral)	40	→		

All drug doses listed are in mg/sq.m. The cycle indicated above is repeated six times. Prednisone is administered only at cycles one and four.

ticed in the clinic in the early 1960's, several early studies served to provide encouragement for this approach. Lacher and Durant,[10] in 1963, utilizing a combination of chlorambucil and vinblastine, reported a complete remission rate of 40 per cent of the patients with advanced Hodgkin's disease. A four-drug combination study, called MOMP (cyclophosphamide, vincristine, methotrexate and prednisone), was initiated at the NCI in 1963 and produced an 81 per cent complete remission rate.[11] These programs led to the first MOPP (the newly introduced procarbazine was substituted for methotrexate and nitrogen mustard was substituted for cyclophosphamide) trial (Table 3), and 80 per cent of the 43 patients entered into this program from 1964 to 1967 achieved a complete remission.[12,13]

In a sense, it is unfortunate that drug combinations were not evolved using sequential studies, with each new combination adding a single drug, so that results achieved with single sequential use of the other drugs employed in the combination could be compared. However, with the large number of drugs available, and the infinite number of dosage schedules and sequences possible, together with the limited number of patients available (properly stratified as to histologic and clinical staging), it is perhaps not surprising that "enlightened empiricism" prevailed, leading to the "MOPP" regimen. Other programs utilizing drug combinations have also resulted in an increased number of complete remissions as compared to single agent therapy (Table 4), and other groups have confirmed the high complete response rate of patients with Hodgkin's to

Table 4. *Drug Combination Program in Hodgkin's Disease*

DRUG COMBINATION	DURATION OF TREATMENT (MOS.)	COMPLETE REMISSION (%)	REFERENCES
Vinblastine, chlorambucil	Continuous	40	10
MOMP (vincristine, cyclophosphamide methotrexate, prednisone)	2.5	80	11
MOPP (vincristine, nitrogen mustard, procarbazine, prednisone)	6	81	12, 13, 16
MVPP (vinblastine, nitrogen mustard, procarbazine, prednisone)	6	71	17
Yale Program (nitrogen mustard, prednisone, vincristine, procarbazine, vinblastine)	12*	81	20, 23

*With radiation therapy. (See Table 4.)

MOPP.[14-17] In general, combination therapy has been utilized for the more advanced stages of Hodgkin's disease (III B, IV B); however, in the earlier NCI MOPP study, it should be noted that of the patients with stage III A and IV A disease treated, all achieved a complete remission, and only one of these patients has relapsed thus far.[13] Thus, when studies are compared, it seems clear that the larger the number of asymptomatic patients in a given trial (III A, IV A), the better the response rate. Age also appears to be of importance in the response rate expected; children less than 16 years of age had a response rate of only 50 per cent in the NCI program.[13]

The critics of combination chemotherapy programs may well argue that appropriate control single agent therapy has not been employed. A randomized study performed by Acute Leukemia Group B compared MOPP to a five-drug program (vincristine, vinblastine, procarbazine, chlorambucil, and prednisone) and to each of these drugs used singly in sequence.[14] Both combinations produced equivalent complete responses, and each was superior to the use of the same drugs in sequence. The use of a single agent (vinblastine) was compared to a combination of three drugs (prednisone, vinblastine, and cyclophosphamide) by the Eastern Cooperative Oncology Group.[18] A complete remission (CR) rate of 10 per cent was produced by the vinblastine alone, as compared to a 41 per cent CR rate with the three-drug combination. Nevertheless, an intensive sequential use of drugs in full dose, but at short intervals (e.g., three or four weeks), has not been compared to combination chemotherapy, an approach that could produce similar results in terms of overall complete remissions calculated after the fourth or fifth drug was administered. However, it should be noted that a cyclic drug approach of this type was of only limited benefit in the treatment of acute lymphocytic leukemia.[19] Other combinations of these approaches, i.e., both combination and sequential use of drugs (as in the Yale program) may prove to be equally efficacious in inducing complete remission, perhaps with less toxicity.[20-23]

Remission Duration and Survival

Although it seems reasonable that an increased complete remission rate would correlate well with an increased expectancy for survival, the long-term follow-up data from the initial MOPP trial has now established this premise. The median duration of remission from the end of six cycles of MOPP in this series is 36 months. Of the patients who achieved a complete remission, 70 per cent are alive at six years, and the survival of the entire group is in excess of 60 per cent at six years.[13] Thus, a direct correlation exists between achieving a complete remission and subsequent survival. While no data comparing survival achieved with single agents to that with drug combinations are available, the earlier experience with single agent therapy in patients with advanced Hodgkin's yielded median survivals of only one to two years.[6, 24, 25] Perhaps of even more value is the fact that most of the patients treated with MOPP therapy have been off all therapy following the initial treatment for six months. Thus, combination therapy appears to produce not only long disease-free intervals, but long treatment-free intervals as well. It is also highly encouraging that no relapses have been noted in patients who have had a disease-free remission of 42 months or longer.[13] Since the follow-up time in this group is five to seven years, it is not yet possible to use the word "cure" in conjunction with this program, but it appears likely, based on analogy with the radiation therapy data, that a minimum of 33 per cent of the patients initially treated with MOPP are potential "cures."

TREATMENT OF RADIATION THERAPY RELAPSES

Most centers undertake to treat all Hodgkin's disease except III B, IV A, and IV B with extended field x-ray therapy without accompanying or preceding chemotherapy. Five-year disease-free survivals ranging from 80 to 90 per cent in Stage I A and II A to 60 per cent for stage III A Hodgkin's have been reported, with poorer results if patients have systemic symptoms.[24] Thus, it is important to consider chemotherapy for these radiation therapy failures. A high rate of complete remissions (70 to 80 per cent) using combination chemotherapy has also been reported for radiation failures by the NCI group,[13] the English group,[17] the Southeastern Cooperative group, and in our series of patients.[23] In our experience, tolerance to chemotherapy was somewhat impaired, especially if patients had total nodal irradiation, but as a rule, most of the chemotherapeutic program could be administered safely.

COMBINATION CHEMOTHERAPY AND RADIATION THERAPY

Several years ago we noted that failure of combination chemotherapy in patients with advanced Hodgkin's was associated with recurrence of tumor at previously involved areas. This led to the development of a treatment program utilizing combination chemotherapy, followed by low-dose irradiation to areas of known involvement with tumor, followed by two additional cycles of chemotherapy.[20-23] Details of this combination chemotherapy-radiation therapy program are given in Table 5. Similar considerations have also led to a combination chemotherapy–x-ray program initiated recently by the Southwest group.[9]

Table 5. *The Yale Combination Chemotherapy plus Low Dose Radiation Therapy for Hodgkin's Disease*

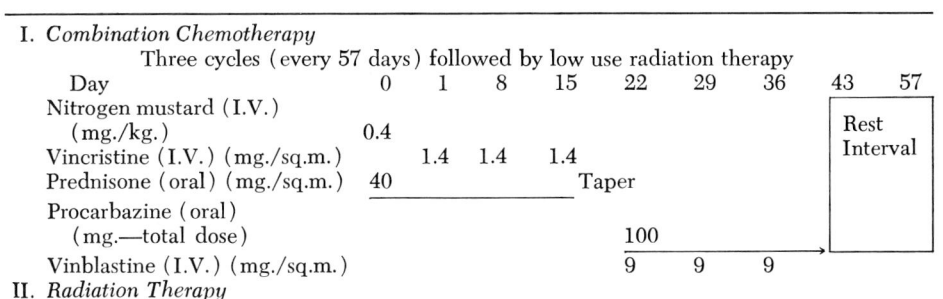

I. *Combination Chemotherapy*
Three cycles (every 57 days) followed by low use radiation therapy

Day	0	1	8	15	22	29	36	43	57
Nitrogen mustard (I.V.) (mg./kg.)	0.4							Rest Interval	
Vincristine (I.V.) (mg./sq.m.)		1.4	1.4	1.4					
Prednisone (oral) (mg./sq.m.)	40				Taper				
Procarbazine (oral) (mg.—total dose)					100				
Vinblastine (I.V.) (mg./sq.m.)					9	9	9		

II. *Radiation Therapy*
1500 to 2000 rads in three or four weeks to all previously involved sites except bone marrow.

III. *Combination Chemotherapy*
After one-month interval, two more cycles of chemotherapy as above, separated by a three-month interval.

Of 17 previously untreated patients entered into the Yale combination x-ray program, 15 have achieved a complete remission; no patient (11 at risk) who has achieved a complete remission and completed radiation therapy and two additional chemotherapy cycles has relapsed thus far (one to four-year follow-up).

It is also reasonable in previously untreated patients with advanced disease to utilize the combination of chemotherapy with more extensive radiation therapy, and a program comparing total nodal radiation therapy with total nodal radiotherapy followed by MOPP chemotherapy has been initiated by the Stanford group.[16, 26] This study, which includes patients with intermediate stages of Hodgkin's disease (II B, III A, and III B), indicates thus far that the addition of chemotherapy to radiation therapy in this group of patients may improve the percentage of patients free of disease at two to three years after treatment and, thus, the cure rate. However, as is pointed out by these authors, further follow-up is necessary before this conclusion can be established. The administration of MOPP chemotherapy to the total nodal radiotherapy patient group was somewhat more difficult, since a longer period of time was necessary (27 vs. 22 weeks) and doses of some of the agents (nitrogen mustard, vincristine, procarbazine) were reduced as compared to the doses achieved in the NCI study.[16, 26] An advantage of the Yale program is that the addition of low-dose radiation therapy allows primary radiation therapy failures the opportunity for further combination x-ray, since most of these patients will tolerate this additional low-dose radiation therapy treatment. Results to date indicate that patients previously irradiated who have relapsed do just as well as untreated patients.[22, 23]

Toxicity

The acute toxic effects of drug therapy with potential risk of infection and bleeding, the risks accompanying splenectomy, and radiation therapy side effects are well known and have been described,[6, 24, 25] and will not be discussed further. Possible long-range toxicities of combination chemotherapy programs are now receiving more attention as the numbers of long-term survivors accumulate. The possible side effects to be considered are bone marrow damage, immunologic damage, damage to gonads, and carcinogenic potential.

In patients treated with MOPP and in the patients treated at Yale with combination chemotherapy and x-ray, despite significant and sometimes prolonged marrow depression following chemotherapy, patients examined six months or more after completion of therapy have essentially normal leukocyte and platelet counts and hematocrits.[13, 23] Furthermore, in our small series, as in the original MOPP group, no unusual susceptibility to infection has occurred, once therapy has been stopped and blood counts have returned to normal.

Damage to the immunologic system of patients treated with MOPP therapy, or with total nodal irradiation therapy, has not been documented; in fact, the NCI studies have shown that established delayed hypersensitivity commonly returns to normal in anergic patients who respond to treatment.[13, 27]

Male patients treated with prolonged use of alkylating agents and also with MOPP have had evidence of damage to spermatogenesis. The majority of these patients studied showed either complete azoospermia or very low sperm counts, and thus are presumably infertile.[13, 28] Absence of ovarian function in a substantial number of lymphoma patients treated with combination chemotherapy programs has also been documented.[28, 29]

In the NCI series three of 21 patients who relapsed after extensive irradiation and subsequently were treated with MOPP developed second malignancies.[30] The three malignancies occurred among seven patients who had received both chemotherapy and irradiation within a 12-month period. Fortunately we have not noted any secondary malignancies as yet in our small series of patients treated with chemotherapy and irradiation, nor has the Stanford group noted secondary malignancies in their series of patients treated with both modalities sequentially.

Conclusions

Combination chemotherapy programs and combinations of drugs with x-ray therapy in patients with intermediate and advanced stages of Hodgkin's disease have remarkably altered the expected natural history of this disease in recent years. A patient with Hodgkin's lymphoma, presenting at any stage, if treated at a major center with expertise in handling this disease, now has an excellent chance of obtaining a complete remission. Chance for potential cure decreases with the severity of disease as judged by clinical and perhaps histologic staging, but may be higher than 33 per cent, even in patients with stage IV B Hodgkin's. Clearly there is still room for improvement, and combinations of drugs and x-ray, and programs utilizing additional new drugs with longer duration of treatment, have been initiated in an attempt to further improve these results.

Since more patients are surviving longer, it is only appropriate that the risks of staging, including exploratory laparotomy and splenectomy, irradiation, and chemotherapy be carefully documented and identified. Sterility in this young adult population appears to be a common problem; long-term marrow depression and immunologic deficiency do not seem to be important considerations at this writing. Fatal complications due to radiation therapy programs and to chemotherapy have occurred even in the best centers, but appear to be in the order of 5 per cent or less. Finally, the possibility of secondary malignancies recurring, especially in patients treated with both x-ray and chemotherapy, has been raised in one small series of patients followed at the NCI.

However disconcerting the side effects noted above, the encouraging results obtained thus far with the treatments outlined appear to far outweigh the possible risks. Further refinements in techniques of radiation therapy and possibly of selection of drugs for combination chemotherapy programs may decrease these risks even further.

References

1. Carbone, P. P., Kaplan, H. S., Musshoff, K., Smithers, D. W., and Tubiana, M.: Report of the Committee on Hodgkin's Disease Staging Classification. Cancer Res. 31:1860, 1971.
2. Lukes, R. J.: Criteria for involvement of lymph node, bone marrow, spleen and liver in Hodgkin's disease. Cancer Res. 31:1755, 1971.
3. Rosenberg, S. A.: A critique of the value of laparotomy and splenectomy in the evaluation of patients with Hodgkin's disease. Cancer Res. 31:1737, 1971.
4. Kaplan, H. S.: The radical radiotherapy of regionally localized Hodgkin's disease. Radiology 78:553, 1962.
5. Johnson, R. F.: Modern approaches to the radiotherapy of lymphoma. Seminars Hemat. 6:357, 1969.
6. Ultmann, J. C.: Current status. The management of lymphoma. Seminars Hemat. 7:441, 1970.
7. Selawry, O. S., and Hansen, H. H.: Superiority of CCNU (1-(2-chloroethyl)-3-cyclohexyl-1-nitrosourea; NSC 79037) over BCNU (1,3-bis (2-chloroethyl)-1-nitrosourea; NSC 409962) in treatment of advanced Hodgkin's disease. Proc. Amer. Ass. Cancer Res. 13:46, 1972.
8. Hryniuk, W., and Bertino, J. R.: Rationale for the selection of chemotherapeutic agents. Advances Intern. Med. 15:267–297, 1969.
9. Frei, E., III: Combination cancer therapy. (Presidential Address.) Cancer Res. 32:2593, 1972.
10. Lacher, M. T., and Durant, J. R.: Combined vinblastine and chlorambucil therapy of Hodgkin's disease. Ann. Intern. Med. 62:468, 1965.
11. DeVita, V. T., Moxley, J. H., III, Brace, K., and Frei, E., III: Intensive combination chemotherapy and X-irradiation in the treatment of Hodgkin's disease. Proc. Amer. Ass. Cancer Res. 6:15, 1965.
12. DeVita, V. T., Serpick, A. A., and Carbone, P. P.: Combination chemotherapy in the treatment of advanced Hodgkin's disease. Ann. Intern. Med. 73:881, 1970.
13. DeVita, V. T., Canellos, G. P., and Moxley, J. H., III: A decade of combination chemotherapy of advanced Hodgkin's disease. Cancer 30:1495, 1972.
14. Carter, S. R.: Clinical trials and combination chemotherapy. Cancer Chemother. Rep. 2:81, 1971.
15. Moores, R. R.: Comparison of combination therapy vs. nitrogen mustard in Hodgkin's disease. Proc. Amer. Ass. Cancer Res. 11:58, 1970.
16. Rosenberg, S. A., Moore, M. R., Bull, J. M., Jones, S. E., and Kaplan, H. S.: Combination chemotherapy and radiotherapy for Hodgkin's disease. Cancer 30:1505, 1972.
17. Nicholson, W. M., Beard, M. E. J., Crowther, D., Stansfeld, A. G., Vartan, C. P., Malpas, J. S., Fairley, G. H., and Scott, R. B.: Combination chemotherapy in generalized Hodgkin's disease. Brit. Med. J. 3:7, 1970.
18. Lenhard, R.: Personal communication.
19. Zuelzer, W. W.: Implications of long-term survival in acute stem cell leukemia of childhood treated with composite cyclic therapy. Blood 24:477, 1964.
20. Levitt, M., DeConti, R. C., Pearson, H. A., Marsh, J. C., Zanes, R. P., Mitchell, M. S., Kaetz, H. W., and Bertino, J. R.: The Yale combination chemotherapy program for advanced Hodgkin's disease: A preliminary report. Connecticut Med. 34:862, 1970.
21. Farber, L. F., Levitt, M., DeConti, R. C., Mitchell, M. S., Marsh, J. C., Skeel, R. T., Pearson, H. A., Zanes, R. P., and Bertino, J. R.: Combination-sequential chemotherapy in Hodgkin's disease. Proc. Amer. Ass. Cancer Res. 12:87, 1971.
22. DeConti, R. C., Farber, L. R., Hubbard, S. P., Prosnitz, L., and Bertino, J. R.: Combination-sequential chemotherapy followed by low dose radiotherapy in advanced Hodgkin's disease. American Society of Hematology, 15th Annual Meeting, December, 1972, p. 132.
23. Prosnitz, L., Farber, L. R., Fischer, J. J., and Bertino, J. R.: Low dose radiation therapy and combination chemotherapy in the treatment of advanced Hodgkin's disease. Radiology. 107:187, 1973.
24. Kaplan, H. S.: On the natural history, treatment, and prognosis of Hodgkin's disease. Harvey Lect. 64:215–259, 1970.
25. Karnofsky, D. A.: Chemotherapy of Hodgkin's disease. Cancer 19:371, 1966.

26. Moore, M. R., Bull, J. M., Jones, S. E., Rosenberg, S. A., and Kaplan, H. S.: Sequential radiotherapy and chemotherapy in the treatment of Hodgkin's disease: A progress report. Ann. Intern. Med. 77:1, 1972.
27. Young, R. C. Corder, M. P., Haynes, H. A., and DeVita, V. T.: Delayed hypersensitivity in Hodgkin's disease. Amer. J. Med. 52:63, 1972.
28. Kumar, R., Biggart, J. D., McEvoy, J., and McGeown, M. G.: Cyclophosphamide and reproductive function. Lancet 1:1212, 1972.
29. Sobrinho, L. G., Levine, R. A., and DeConti, R. C. Amenorrhea in patients with Hodgkin's disease treated with antineoplastic agents. Amer. J. Obstet. Gynec. 109:135, 1971.
30. Arsenau, J. C., Sponzo, R. W., Levin, D. L., Schnipper, L. E., Bonner, H., Young, R. C., Canellos, G. P., Johnson, R. E., and DeVita, V. T.: Non-lymphomatous malignant tumors complicating Hodgkin's disease. New Eng. J. Med. 287:1119, 1972.

Comment

The Treatment of Hodgkin's Disease

   Analysis of the articles by Horton and by Bertino indicates that this controversy cannot be factually resolved at this time. There is a paucity of unassailable data which could establish superiority of aggressive therapy over conservative therapy for Hodgkin's disease or vice versa. Both authors are respected therapists and both are right (or wrong) as they marshal the pertinent uncontrolled data to support their "extreme" opinions. Indeed, some may feel that aggressive combination chemotherapy for Hodgkin's disease is of an order of effectiveness entirely similar to penicillin therapy for pneumococcal pneumonia or vitamin B_{12} for pernicious anemia, so that establishing relative efficacy with older single agent therapy is trivial and not in the best interests of care of patients with the disease. None of the very few attempted comparative efficacy trials for combination chemotherapy have yet been published in full.[1-3] Have these data remained in abstract form because the uncontrolled trials of combination therapy have suggested an incontrovertible degree of efficacy as compared with previous experience with single agents? The abstracts do support the role of combined drug therapy but are readily criticized by Dr. Horton, who notes their study design as inadequate to the issue. Dr. Bertino's "penicillin" is "sulfadiazine" in Dr. Horton's view until proved otherwise.
   Is the issue worth being addressed, or is it enough to know that MOPP therapy will produce complete remissions in somewhere between 60 and 85 per cent of selected patients? Treatment of Hodgkin's disease with a combination of drugs does exact an appreciable toll on normal host tissues, as noted by the authors. To a large part these appear reversible. However, the aggressive approach to cure of the disease has imperceptibly and predictably led to combining intensive drug therapy with high dose radiotherapy in accordance with that part of our American credo which says, "More is better." We agree with Dr. Horton's call for caution in these rapid developments and plead for controlled trials of the ever more aggressive combinations. Newly emerging risks make this need even more imperative. The isolated initial observations of the development of a second neoplasm in aggressively treated patients[4] have continued, so that the risk of such second cancers or acute leukemias in groups receiving both radiotherapy and chemotherapy may now approach 30 times that of normal.[5]
   Given a continuing uncertainty about the efficacy of increasingly aggressive therapy, the physician will base his decision on multiple elements such as eco-

nomic factors and the area's clinical support services. These are undeniably responsible aspects of patient management, but they pale in importance beside clearly specific, definitive therapeutic guidelines. The lack of controlled data facilitates controversy and prevents scientific impetus from forcing responsible changes in medical practice.

Dr. Bertino notes that Hodgkin's disease is now so complex with regard to staging, histologic type, symptom prognosis, and drugs available, that in a practical sense there are not enough patients to do a well designed study to see whether more and more aggressive treatments are more effective than harmful. The *reductio ad absurdum* is that we now know too much about the disease ever to learn how best to treat it. Dr. Bertino may be correct, and he thereby strengthens our view that the first trials of every new therapeutic regimen should include a valid comparison with standard therapy.

JEROME B. BLOCK and THOMAS C. CHALMERS

References

1. Moores, R. R.: Comparison of combination therapy vs. nitrogen mustard in Hodgkin's disease. Proc. Amer. Ass. Cancer Res. *11*:58, 1970.
2. Lenhard, R.: Combination chemotherapy of Hodgkin's disease. Proc. Amer. Ass. Cancer Res. *11*:48, 1970.
3. Brook, J., and Gocka, E. F.: Comparison of single agents with combination therapy in Hodgkin's disease. Proc. Amer. Ass. Cancer Res. *13*:79, 1972.
4. Arsenau, J. C., Sponzo, R. W., Levin, D. L., Schnipper, L. E., Bonner, H., Young, R. C., Canellos, G. P., Johnson, R. E., and DeVita, V. T.: Nonlymphomatous malignant tumors complicating Hodgkin's disease. New Eng. J. Med. *287*:1119, 1972.
5. Arsenau, J. C.: Cancer treatment as a cause of host disease. *In International Conference on the Paraneoplastic Syndromes*. New York, The New York Academy of Sciences, 1973.

30

The Marihuana Debate

The Marihuana Debate: Doubts About Legalization
    by Donald B. Louria

Marihuana Is Not a Public Health Menace: It Is Time to Relax Our Social Policy
    by Richard C. Pillard

The Marihuana Debate: Doubts About Legalization

DONALD B. LOURIA

*Department of Preventive Medicine
and Community Health,
New Jersey Medical School*

An unseemly and silly polemic over the alleged charms and dangers of marihuana is currently sweeping the United States. I have elected to start with the null hypothesis: marihuana needs to be controlled. In an attempt to support that hypothesis, I shall focus on three areas: the dangers of single or repetitive usage; the problem of escalation to other drugs; and the issue of the number of intoxicants our society wishes to legitimatize.

Dangers of Single or Repetitive Use

These are listed in Table 1. Since the drug is illegal, there are, of course, no incidence figures. It does seem clear that each of the adverse effects listed occurs infrequently, but each does occur, and this removes marihuana from the innocuous category.

Panic and/or depression after use of marihuana or hashish is well described. Indeed, panic was reported in the French literature of the mid 1800's by a variety

Table 1. *Most Frequent Serious Untoward Effects Following Marihuana Use*

Panic
Depression
Paranoia
Psychiatric abnormalities
Thinking difficulties
Intellectual impairment
Psychological deterioration
Loss of control of drug ("pothead")
Amotivational syndrome

of authors, including the writer Charles Baudelaire and the eminent psychiatrist Jacques-Joseph Moreau; the latter was also acutely aware of the likelihood that such adverse effects were dose-related.[1] Similar reactions were reported about the same time by the American educator Fritz Ludlow.[1] Thereafter, panic was virtually ignored in the American literature until the 1930's, when Bromberg[2] described a variety of adverse effects, including panic, in 14 patients. Five years later panic reactions were mentioned in the famed LaGuardia report, often used to buttress arguments that marihuana is innocuous; thus, one experimental subject was described who "smoked one cigarette and became restless, agitated, dizzy, fearful of his surroundings and afraid of death."[3] Perhaps the most concise description is that of the well known author, William Burroughs, written in 1956.[4] Said Burroughs: "Marihuana is a sensitizer, and the results are not always pleasant. It makes a bad situation worse. Depression becomes despair; anxiety, panic. I once gave a marihuana cigarette to a guest who was mildly anxious. After smoking half a cigarette, he suddenly leaped to his feet screaming, 'I got the fear' and rushed out of the house." More recently Grossman[5] reported severe fright lasting for 45 minutes in an apparently healthy young man after ingestion of the mild cannabis product, bhang.

Weil[6] reports that, in his experience, panic may occur in as many as 25 per cent of certain groups, but Blum and his colleagues[7] in their intensive study do not list panic among the major untoward effects reported by students themselves. These differences are probably related to a different understanding of the word "panic;" Weil appears to be comingling mild to moderate anxiety and true panic, thus augmenting his figures.

Other significant adverse psychologic effects may occur even in moderate users, albeit infrequently. Dally[8] reported a bizarre self-inflicted injury in a 24 year old cannabis user, and Talbott and Teague[9] recorded psychotic reactions in 12 men serving in the armed forces in Vietnam who used a form of cannabis more potent than that ordinarily smoked in the United States. In these patients, as in those reported by others,[10] there is rarely any adequate assessment of the patient's personality before use of marihuana. Consequently it is unclear how often marihuana in conventional dose causes major psychiatric difficulties in ostensibly normal persons, and how often the drug acts as a precipitating agent in those with already established personality aberrations. Presumably marihuana usually plays the latter role, as a precipitating agent. But this does not justify the facile statement of the marihuana proponents that any major psychologic abnormality precipitated by marihuana can be ignored on the grounds that the individual was not normal and would eventually have undergone the same psychiatric manifestations as a result of other life stresses. Surely if a pharmacologic agent can promote a psychosis in a predisposed individual, the drug should be assiduously avoided by that individual, and it cannot be considered innocuous. To consider precipitation of psychologic abnormalities as unimportant is as ridiculous as maintaining that a thermal inversion is in reality not dangerous because ordinarily the only persons who die or become seriously ill are those with underlying lung disease. In this regard, it is of interest that a few cases have been reported of alleged schizophrenia in which virtual remission occurred after the use of marihuana was discontinued.[11, 12]

Additional dangers to those who smoke repetitively include loss of motivation, difficulty in thinking, psychologic deterioration, and total loss of control (becoming a "pothead").[10-15] Farnsworth, in particular, has stressed the so-called amotivational syndrome in chronic marihuana users.[13, 14] Dr. Henry Brill has called this the "vagabond" syndrome. Whatever the name, it is clear that some marihuana users lose goal-directed orientation. In some cases they seek help, stop use of marihuana, and thereafter experience a return to pre-marihuana goal-directed activity.

It is well established that the administration of cannabis acutely impairs learning ability.[16, 17] Consequently it is hardly surprising that some young persons have mentation difficulties for a period of hours after its use. Chronic, heavy use of cannabis does cause psychologic deterioration in some persons, but it is unclear whether modest use can result in such untoward effects. Studies by Zinberg and Weil,[18] Tylden and Wild,[11] and Kolansky and Moore[10] suggest this possibility, but in these studies lack of a careful assessment of the pre-marihuana personality makes any firm conclusions unwarranted.

Certain of those who repeatedly smoke marihuana lose control of the drug completely, becoming so-called "potheads."[15] For them, the cannabis becomes the center of a progressively more solipsistic existence.

Although there are no firm data on the incidence of these untoward effects, the percentage of users experiencing all of them considered together certainly does not exceed 1 to 4 per cent. It has also been suggested that cannabis may cause hepatitis[19] and brain damage,[20] but the former observation has not been confirmed, and the latter is clouded by the possibility that the investigations were not adequately controlled.

Escalation to Other Drugs

The mainstay of the argument against legalization of marihuana lies not with the side reactions just enumerated, but rather with another potentially serious adverse effect, namely, escalation to other more dangerous mind-altering agents. For years there has been a bitter polemic over the relationship of marihuana to use of other drugs. In the late 1930's, 1940's, and 1950's, the public tended to accept the dogmatic insistence of law enforcement agencies that marihuana use ineluctably led to use of heroin. Then, in the early 1960's, opponents of that simplistic view pointed out that some 200,000,000 persons in the world used cannabis products, but only a tiny fraction of them eventually use heroin. Despite the data showing that heroin use follows marihuana smoking only rarely, the myth has persisted, supported only by selected epidemiologic data showing that the overwhelming majority of heroin users first had tried marihuana.[19, 21, 22]

The marihuana opponents have doggedly clung to the marihuana-heroin connection despite the solid antithetical arguments; conversely, the marihuana acolytes, having punctured the myth of linkage to heroin, have then assumed inappropriately that the entire concept of escalation is erroneous.

The relevant question for the United States currently is not how often marihuana users subsequently become involved with heroin, but rather how often they move on to any potentially dangerous mind-altering agent. Our studies, among others, show clearly that marihuana use ordinarily precedes use of such drugs as LSD, and that the likelihood of current marihuana users experimenting with LSD is dose-related (Fig. 1).[23-26] Thus, in our studies on suburban high school students,[23, 24] an individual who uses marihuana rarely has a 4 per cent chance of using LSD; if he smokes marihuana monthly, the likelihood of LSD experimentation increases to 9 per cent. Weekly marihuana use is associated with a 22 per cent chance of LSD use, and this percentage doubles for those smoking marihuana at least twice a week. In similar studies by Goode[25] and Popoff[26] the daily marihuana user had a 77 to 82 per cent chance of also using LSD. Clearly the relationship between LSD and marihuana in the school and college populations studied is far more impressive than between marihuana and heroin. On the basis of the various data available, it is difficult to avoid the conclusion that a substantial percentage of marihuana users will subsequently experiment with LSD, and that the likelihood of such experimentation is directly related to the frequency of marihuana use. I have recently reviewed 20 studies of marihuana-LSD use among high school and college students; these investigations suggest that among those using marihuana more than a few times, approximately one in five will also use LSD. As noted first by Eells,[27] LSD use is very unlikely in an individual who does not use marihuana.

Since the various epidemiologic studies buttress the escalation hypothesis, the obvious derivative question is why should the phenomenon occur. There appear to be at least seven possibilities, none of which is adequately documented. First, there is the common seller hypothesis; according to this concept, the same person selling marihuana also sells LSD and other more dangerous agents in the street market place. Second, the thrill of illegality may cause young persons starting with one illegal drug, marihuana, to move to other illicit agents. Separat-

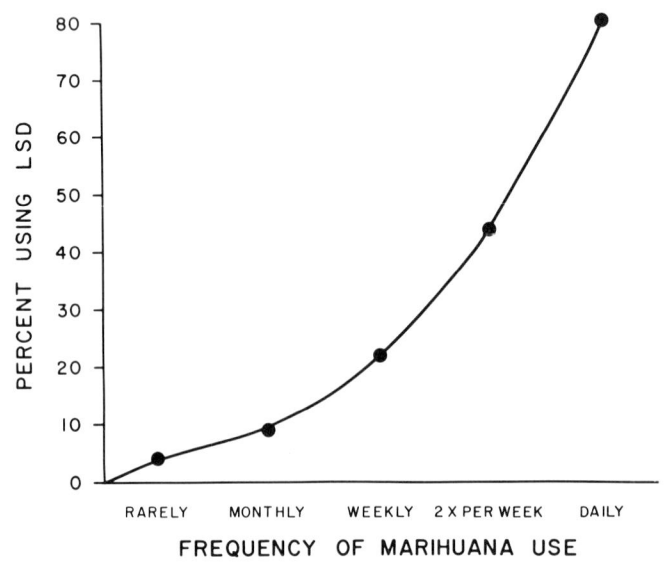

Figure 1. Relation of frequency of marihuana use to likelihood of LSD use. (Data compiled from three studies; see references 23, 24, 25, and 26.)

ing marihuana from the other drugs might reduce this tendency to use multiple illegal agents. Third, there may be differences in physiological or biochemical reactions to cannabis that relate to who will or will not escalate from marihuana to a drug such as LSD. (There are, of course, no current data that bear directly on this possibility.) Fourth, it may be that the same curiosity that plays such an important motivational role in initial use of mind-altering drugs[23, 24] continues to influence those who progress to more potent agents. This would hardly be surprising. An old saying notes that "a man should live if only to satisfy his curiosity," and epidemiologic survey data indicate that curiosity remains one of the major reasons for drug experimentation. Fifth, there is a growing consensus that peer group pressure has enormous influence in individual drug use patterns. If the marihuana user's peer group uses drugs such as LSD extensively, then the likelihood of a given member of the group following the multiple drug use behavior of the group is obviously very substantial. Sixth, in a society dominated by hedonism, the search for pleasure may in itself account for the phenomenon of escalation. Any of the drugs being used illicitly today has the capacity to either induce or augment pleasure, and pleasure, like curiosity, is a major motivational force in initial experimentation with marihuana.[23, 24] For some pleasure-oriented individuals, marihuana will not satiate their sensate drives; once the pleasurable effects of marihuana-induced mind alteration have been experienced, they seek stronger mind-altering agents such as LSD. Finally, there are informal data suggesting that marihuana users who suffer from substantial underlying personality aberrations are far more likely to become multiple drug users.

Escalation from marihuana to a drug such as LSD does not, of course, constitute an isolated event. There are multiple predisposing and converging influences. The proponents of legalized marihuana point to these, admit that marihuana may be associated with experimentation with more dangerous agents, and then dismiss the entire concept of escalation on the grounds that marihuana has not been shown to be *the* causative factor in escalation to a more dangerous drug. Obviously causation is difficult to document beyond peradventure, and it will take years to adequately investigate the seven possible reasons for escalation just listed. Important societal decisions must be made long before the issue of escalation is settled. To me, the clearly shown association is in itself important; the evidence indicates that a user of marihuana may well become involved with a drug such as LSD, whereas a nonuser of cannabis is not likely to become so involved. The reasons underlying escalation may not be adequately delineated, but anyone urging legalization of marihuana must accept this as one of the potential untoward effects the marihuana smoker may experience; legalization of marihuana and consequent increased use may result in increased prevalence of use of far more dangerous drugs.

How Many Intoxicants Shall We Legitimatize?

Perhaps the major issue surrounding the marihuana debate has been almost assiduously ignored. This is the question of the total number of intoxicants we wish in our society. It is difficult to decide what the total acceptable number should be. Some societies have had one, others at least several drug escape mechanisms. Obviously what has been done in the period prior to the technological revolution or in primitive societies cannot be uncritically applied to the United States in the late 20th century. Nevertheless, it seems clear that if each intoxicant has significant adverse effects, the medical-psychiatric-social risks from unlimited intoxicants would be an enormous burden for a society and could even threaten the very viability of that society. Even the most ardent admirers of marihuana do not usually advocate an unlimited number of intoxicants and insist that the question is merely the addition of a single new agent, a euphoriant. But it should be obvious that if marihuana were to be legalized, there will be other pressure groups urging legalization of other agents, each group advocating its favorite drug on the basis of its being no more dangerous than marihuana. In Sweden, between 1965 and 1970, the drug urged upon the society by the drug subculture was not cannabis, but rather central nervous system stimulants.[28, 29]

Even if one chooses to disregard the possibility of serious attempts to introduce additional intoxicants were marihuana to be accepted, even if we confine the debate to the parochial issue of marihuana per se, there are ample reasons for substantial reservations over expanding the list of legitimatized intoxicants. Currently, we have three such drugs—caffeine, nicotine, and ethyl alcohol. Caffeine, despite the possibility that it may promote bladder tumors,[30] and despite the fact that it is, under certain experimental conditions, a mutagen and teratogen,[31, 32] appears to be, for the most part, harmless for virtually all users consuming it in conventional amounts.[33] Nicotine in the form of tobacco is, of course, hardly innocuous. Ochsner[34] estimates that the yearly cost in lives and money from cigarette smoking is 300,000 lives and 19 billion dollars. This figure may be somewhat inflated, but the data do seem reasonably convincing that the pack-a-day smoker incurs considerable risk from heart or lung disease, even if the loss in lives and money is not so great as indicated by Ochsner. The risk from alcohol is similarly great. There are an estimated six to nine million alcoholics in the United States, approximately 20,000 lethal automobile accidents yearly ascribed to alcohol use, and marked additional costs in money and lives due to job absenteeism, marital disruption, hepatic cirrhosis, central nervous system abnormalities, and so forth.

The question is, then, do we wish to add to the problems already created by our current legal intoxicants?

Should we opt to add marihuana to our legitimatized intoxicants, the following issues must be carefully considered:

1. How can we assess the role of marihuana in automobile and other accidents unless we can accurately measure the drug and its metabolites in body fluids? Such techniques may be available soon, but currently there are no such techniques suitable for general use.

2. If marihuana is legalized, it would be very difficult to deny users access to more potent forms of cannabis such as hashish. Even if standards of strength were adopted, we should realize that if marihuana were legalized, hashish use would concomitantly increase. Since hashish is considerably more potent than American marihuana, the incidence of adverse effects would be expected to be greater. The

careful studies of Isbell, Gorodetzsky and Jasinski[35] on the effects of tetrahydrocannabinol on human volunteers support this notion; so does the report of Keeler,[36] who recorded hallucinations in six of 56 persons using marihuana, particularly after larger doses.

3. If marihuana were legalized (or "regulated," so that its use is not considered a crime), use will almost surely increase and, consequently, so will the number of acute and chronic adverse effects, including panic, depression, psychiatric abnormalities, loss of motivation, and psychologic deterioration.

4. Legalization of marihuana would result in the presence in society of a considerable number of individuals who had lost control of the drug ("potheads"). Nobody can predict the number accurately, but if marihuana began to rival alcohol in prevalence of use (and this might well occur), the number of "potheads" burdening society might then be counted in the millions.

5. If marihuana were legalized, the number of individuals escalating to other drugs would ineluctably increase. Even if the present 20 per cent escalation rate for repeated users diminished substantially, this would be countered by increased total number of users. Additionally, the acceptability of marihuana would increase chronic use (as contrasted to ephemeral experimentation). Since the likelihood of escalation is dose-related,[24-26] the number of individuals moving to more dangerous drugs out of curiosity, hedonism, peer group pressure, or personality abnormalities would likely be quite substantial. The derivative question is whether society is willing to chance a profound increase in the number of users of LSD, mescaline, parenteral stimulants, and so forth, consequent to marihuana legalization.

6. If marihuana were legalized, and lower age limits for use set at age 17 or 18, some proponents of legalization aver that those under the established age would not use the drug, because they would know that at a given age, use would be permitted. Such thinking is patently ridiculous. If those over age 17 ebulliently pronounce the glories of marihuana, their younger, underage colleagues will surely experiment with the drug in large numbers. To think otherwise would be foolhardy. Currently the illegal intoxicant used most frequently by adolescents is alcohol, which is legally proscribed for those under a statutorily defined age. Many feel that the likelihood of adverse effects from cannabis is not only dose- but also age-related; the younger the individual, the more likely a given dose will produce untoward effects. If this be true, and if marihuana use were to rise precipitously in the under-17 age group, a large number of adverse effects might be anticipated. Surely this would not be acceptable to society at large. Other proponents of legalization say the laws will prevent such underage use, regardless of the desires of the very young; they propose that selling to that segment of the population be punished severely. Our experience with alcohol does not support their glib pronouncements. If marihuana is legal for those over 17 or 18, the laws pertaining to possession by or sale to younger persons will, as with alcohol, of necessity be relatively mild and will not deter use. In this regard, it is well to remember that spread of marihuana is from user to neophyte within the peer group; stringent laws would be ineffective and could result in the same cruelties inherent in the pre-1972 marihuana laws in most states.

If society should elect to legalize marihuana, we will not collapse as a society. But if we are either to legalize or to continue to reject legalization, it must not be on the basis of insular or emotional arguments; instead, the decision should be made after a dispassionate assessment of the potential public health risks of the drug and an analysis of the complex issue of the number and nature of intoxicants we wish to have in our society during the coming decades.

References

1. Bloomquist, E. R.: *Marihuana. The Second Trip*. Beverly Hills, Calif., Glencoe Press, 1971.
2. Bromberg, W.: Marihuana: A psychiatric study. J.A.M.A. *113*:4–12, 1939.
3. Mayor's Committee on Marihuana: *The Marihuana Problem in the City of New York*. Lancaster, Penn., Jacques Cattrell Press, 1944.
4. Burroughs, W.: Letter from a master addict to dangerous drugs. Brit. J. Addict. *53*:119–131, 1956.
5. Grossman, W.: Adverse reactions associated with cannabis products in India. Ann. Intern. Med. *70*:529–533, 1969.
6. Weil, A. T.: Adverse reactions to marihuana. New Eng. J. Med. *282*:997–1000, 1970.
7. Blum, R., and associates: *Students and Drugs*. San Francisco, Jossey-Bass, Inc., 1970.
8. Dally, P.: Undesirable effects of marihuana. Brit. Med. J. *3*:367, 1967.
9. Talbott, J. A., and Teague, J. W.: Marihuana psychosis. J.A.M.A. *210*:299–302, 1969.
10. Kolansky, H., and Moore, W. T.: Effects of marihuana on adolescents and young adults. J.A.M.A. *216*:486–492, 1971.
11. Tylden, E.: A case for cannabis? Brit. Med. J. *3*:556, 1967.
12. Keeler, M. H.: What are the questions concerning marihuana? N. Carolina Med. J. *30*:41–43, 1969.
13. Farnsworth, D. L., and Weiss, S. T.: Marihuana: The conditions and consequence of use and the treatment of users. In Wittenborn, J. R., Brill, H., Smith, J. P., and Wittenborn, S. A. (eds.): *Drugs and Youth*. Springfield, Ill., Charles C Thomas, 1969, p. 168.
14. Farnsworth, D. L.: The drug problem among young people. West Virginia Med. J. *63*:433–437, 1967.
15. Goldstein, R.: *One in Seven: Drugs on Campus*. New York, Walker and Co., 1966.
16. Weil, A. T., Zinberg, N.E., and Nelsen, J. M.: Clinical and psychological effects of marihuana in man. Science *162*:1234–1242, 1968.
17. Clark, L. D., and Nakashima, E. N.: Experimental studies of marihuana. Amer. J. Psychiat. *125*:379–384, 1968.
18. Zinberg, N. E., and Weil, A. T.: A comparison of marihuana users and non-users. Nature (London) *226*:119–123, 1970.
19. Kew, M. C., Bersohn, I., and Siew, S.: Possible hepatotoxicity of cannabis. Lancet *1*:578–579, 1969.
20. Campbell, A. M. G., Evans, M., Thomson, J. L. G., and Williams, M. J.: Cerebral atrophy in young cannabis smokers. Lancet *2*:1219–1224, 1971.
21. Ball, J. C., and Chambers, C. D.: *The Epidemiology of Opiate Addiction in the United States*. Springfield, Ill., Charles C Thomas, 1970.
22. Chapple, P. A. L.: Cannabis: A toxic and dangerous substance: A study of eighty takers. Brit. J. Addict. *61*:269–282, 1966.
23. Wolfson, E. A., Lavenhar, M. A., Blum, R., Quinones, M. A., Einstein, S., and Louria, D. B.: Survey of Drug abuse in six New Jersey high schools: I. Methodology and general findings. Proceedings of the First International Conference on Student Drug Surveys. New York, Baywood Publishing Co. Inc., 1972.
24. Lavenhar, M. A., Wolfson, E. A., Sheffet, A., Einstein, S., and Louria, D. B.: Survey of drug abuse in six New Jersey high schools: II. Characteristics of drug users and non-users. Proceedings of the First International Conference on Student Drug Surveys. New York, Baywood Publishing Co. Inc., 1972.
25. Goode, E.: Multiple drug use among marihuana smokers. Soc. Prob. *17*:48–64, 1969.
26. Popoff, D.: Feedback on drugs. Psychology Today, April, 1970, p. 51.

27. Eells, A.: A survey of student practices and attitudes with respect to marihuana and LSD. J. Counseling Psych. 15:459–467, 1968.
28. Louria, D. B.: *The Drug Scene.* New York, McGraw-Hill Book Company, 1968.
29. Bejerot, N.: *Addiction and Society.* Springfield, Ill., Charles C Thomas, 1970.
30. Cole, P.: Coffee drinking and cancer of the lower urinary tract. Lancet 1:1335–1337, 1971.
31. Snigorska, B., and Bartel, H.: Studies on the teratogenic influence of caffeine on white mouse fetuses. Folia Morph. 29:316–325, 1970.
32. Kuhlmann, W., Fromme, H., Heege, E., and Ostertag, W.: The mutagenic action of caffeine in higher organisms. Cancer Res. 28:2375–2389, 1968.
33. Bateman, A. J.: A storm in a coffee cup. Mutat. Res. 7:475–478, 1969.
34. Ochsner, A.: *Smoking: Your Choice Between Life and Death.* New York, Simon and Schuster, 1970.
35. Isbell, H., Gorodetzsky, C. W., Jasinski, D., et al.: Effects of (−) Δ 9-Transtetrahydrocannabinol in man. Psychopharmacologia 11:184–188, 1967.
36. Keeler, M. H.: Marihuana induced hallucinations. Dis. Nerv. System 29:314–315, 1968.

Marihuana Is Not a Public Health Menace: It Is Time To Relax Our Social Policy*

RICHARD C. PILLARD

Boston University School of Medicine

The use and abuse of marihuana is controversial enough, but in a rather different way from the issues debated in the previous volume in this series. Marihuana has no established therapeutic value, and very few smokers indeed come to attention for the treatment of adverse effects. It is a recreational drug; its use is a personal decision, and regulation is a matter of public social policy to be decided finally in the voting booth, not in the clinic. Of course, the opinion of physicians will exert great influence. Our clinical experience and pharmacologic researches will provide the data base upon which wise judgments can be made. Two documents have recently appeared which should serve just this purpose. *Marihuana and Health*[1] is the second report from the Secretary of Health, Education, and Welfare summarizing the large body of research in progress (more than 150 of the references are to articles published in 1971 or in 1972). *Marihuana: A Signal of Misunderstanding*[2] is a report of the National Commission on Marihuana and Drug Abuse. It is both a summary of current knowledge and a recommendation for social policy.

The evidence presented in these reports suggests that marihuana is not harmless, but neither is it a major threat to public health. The Commission recommends that criminal penalties for private use be removed and that "a social control policy seeking to discourage marihuana use . . . concentrating primarily on the prevention of heavy and very heavy use" be undertaken. These recommendations are the more impressive because they were unanimously endorsed by all 13 commissioners chosen from various political and professional backgrounds

---

* Preparation of this chapter was supported in part by grant #MH-20484 and by Research Scientist Development Award MH-32,896 from the National Institute of Mental Health.

(four are physicians) and because they are in accord with the findings of other commissions in this country,[3] Canada,[4] and England.[5]

We hope that the Commission's report will become the basis for a new sense of agreement on what our national marihuana policy should be. Rather than review it in detail, I shall use the opportunity provided by this chapter to offer some additional comments and several supporting recommendations.

Reasons for Casual Use

Many surveys have examined the frequency of marihuana use and they all show that it is increasing. A Gallup poll[6] in early 1972 revealed that 51 per cent of college students have smoked at least once; this was up from 5 per cent in 1967. "Curiosity" is by far the commonest reason for first use and "peer social pressure" in some form is second. Of those who have ever smoked, over 40 per cent say that they have stopped. Adverse reactions, though fairly common, are rarely given as the reason for quitting. More frequent is a comment such as, "My curiosity was satisfied."

The willingness of adolescents and young adults to behave contrary to the customs of adult society is neither new nor pathological; youth has always done so. The young in primate colonies are compulsively curious and often exceed the restraints which adults try to impose on them. There is a powerful tendency to acquire new experiences at the time of life when information is most easily assimilated and behavior patterns most easily changed. This does not, of course, imply that drug taking must be judged as a wise or useful experiment. It does imply that those who do it need not be seen as trying to escape lives of desperation; they may simply be expressing a normal aspect of development. For the unlucky individual, curiosity for its own sake can be a disaster; for the species, it is probably a trait with high survival value.

There remains a substantial group—about 30 per cent of young adults—who plan to continue smoking. For them marihuana is not a fad but a form of enjoyment which they see as a normal part of life. Occasional users cannot easily be summarized, for they represent every personality type and life style.[7] They endorse such values as education, money, marriage, and job security as much as do nonusers. Political liberalism and rejection of religious values have been associated with drug use, but these factors become less discriminating as the prevalence of use increases.

Tart[8] surveyed marihuana effects in a sample of 150 persons. His informants repeatedly spoke of the enhancement of sensory perceptions and of using the drug chiefly to enjoy the pleasure of this effect. An increase in visual imagery is prominent. It is more evident to the subject when he is relaxing with eyes closed than when attending to a task. Accompanying this is a feeling of novelty, of perceiving subtle aspects of visual, tactile, and auditory stimuli. For this reason, smoking is usually a leisuretime activity in an environment where music, pictures, or simply one's own thoughts can be enjoyed.

These reports of sensory enhancement are heard so regularly that they probably refer to a true drug effect, although no pharmacologic basis for it is known. The possibility that perceptual thresholds are lowered and that stimuli are truly more discriminable has been tested and is so far without support. Another possible explanation is that the process of adaptation or habituation to stimuli is being slowed. Adaptation is a simple but powerful concept and has recently become an important area of study.[9] As examples, we will tend to become indifferent to a fearful experience like skydiving or the pleasure of a favorite dessert if we are repeatedly exposed to them. Adaptation can be demonstrated to all sorts of affective and sensory stimuli. It is generally studied as an organismic response but has also been demonstrated at the synaptic level.[10]

Marihuana may have as one of its actions the slowing or temporary stoppage of the adaptation process. Thus, attention is continually directed to sensory experience. Familiar objects regain their novelty: the experience of pleasant sensations is intensified, and perhaps of unpleasant sensations as well, since smokers will try to avoid stressful or esthetically unpleasing settings. This speculation can be tested. Adaptation to a stimulus can be studied physiologically by observing changes in palmar skin conductance and in the Contingent Negative Variation, an aspect of evoked electrocortical activity.

The novelty-enhancing effect is most often a matter of enjoyment, but some individuals find it a source of creative insight. Grinspoon[11] provides a fascinating example. He reports a biographic fragment by "Mr. X," a leading scientist, who is an occasional user of marihuana. Mr. X describes insights obtained while high and his strategy for integrating them into normal consciousness: "There is a myth about such highs: the user has an illusion of great insight but it does not survive scrutiny in the morning. I am convinced that this is an error, and that the . . . insights achieved when high are real. . . . The main problem is putting [them] in a form acceptable to the quite different self we are when we're down the next day. Some of the hardest work I've ever done has been to put such insights down on tape or in writing. . . . I find that reasonably good insights can be remembered the next day, but only if some effort has been made to set them down another way. If I write the insight down or tell it so someone, then I can remember it with no assistance the following morning; but if I merely say to myself that I must make an effort to remember, I never do. . . .

"I have made a conscious effort to think of a few particularly difficult current problems in my field when high. It works, at least to a degree. I find I can bring to bear . . . a range of relevant experimental facts which appear to be mutually inconsistent. . . . Then in trying to conceive of a way of reconciling the disparate facts, I was able to come up with a very bizarre possibility, one that I'm sure I would never have thought of down" (pp. 113–116).

Does getting high really increase creativity? Probably not. Mr. X was already a successfully creative man. He already had a highly developed imagination and the discipline to use it for work. He stressed the effort required to focus attention on a task and the need to transcribe the resulting ideas so that they would be available for examination in the normally conscious state. The contribution of marihuana was, he felt, to enhance imagery and facilitate novel associations. Many observers have had similar impressions and have suggested that marihuana be used to enhance self-understanding, as a psychotherapy adjunct, or, for the artist, to provide a new repertoire of images.

Until more evidence is collected on this issue, we take a skeptical view. The hypnosis literature provides a parallel: a well-hypnotized subject can, for instance, be "age regressed." He will play in a sandbox and write an awkward scrawl in a convincingly child-like manner. Is this "real" regression? No, because an unhypnotized control subject can, if he is properly motivated, put on as good an act. Also, both the hypnotized subject and the control behave in ways crucially different from true child behavior. There is no difference in performance between hypnotized subject and control; the former, like the marihuana smoker, has a feeling of powerfully intensified subjective experience, whereas the latter does not.[12]

The feeling that one's human capabilities have been enhanced is convincing to the subject and seductive for the experimenter. Just for this reason we should be especially cautious about claims which gratify optimistic wishes. The chances are very strong that by spending equal time a motivated subject could produce as many novel associations sober as high—the process would just not seem so interesting.

Other Uses

Work adjunct. Cannabis products of low potency are widely used in India[13] and in other countries by persons required to put in long hours of monotonous labor. Workers apparently smoke neither for oblivion nor to enjoy sensory enhancement. They claim that a small amount of marihuana is a physical stimulant which delays fatigue, and they use it as we use coffee.

Reduction of hostility. There is now good evidence that the psychoactive ingredient, tetrahydrocannabinol, reduces attack and fighting behavior in animals, including the mouse, rat,[14] and the Siamese fighting fish.[15] This seems to be a true antihostility effect; i.e., it occurs at doses which do not cause sedation or incoordination. Carlini and Masur[16] have made a particularly interesting observation: well fed rats treated with marihuana extract are less inclined to fight, but animals which are chronically starved and chronically drugged are significantly *more* inclined to do so. It has also been observed in humans that undernourished cannabis users are irritable and sometimes violent. The antihostility effect is not well sustained; it wears off after several days of treatment. However, these observations may form the basis for a study of psychopharmacologic ways to control hostile behavior.

Drug withdrawal. Marihuana has been tried as an agent to reduce the symptoms of opiate withdrawal but its use in this manner has never really been effective. A recent report[17] describes cross-tolerance between marihuana and alcohol, suggesting the possibility of using it in the treatment of alcoholic withdrawal syndrome.

We have recently investigated the possibility that marihuana intoxication increases susceptibility to hypnotic induction; however, we found no increase as measured by the Stanford Hypnotic Susceptibility Scale.[18]

Other therapeutic possibilities include reduction of intraocular pressure,[19] nonaddicting analgesia,[20] and use as a fast-acting antidepressant.

Adverse Reactions

About half the users of marihuana report occasional unpleasant effects,[21] and for 20 per cent these are severe.[8] They usually occur the first time the subject is severely intoxicated. Disorientation, paranoid thoughts, and anxiety or panic are the common symptoms. If the drug is taken by smoking, these uncomfortable reactions subside within an hour or so, but occasionally there are residual effects for several days. Medical treatment is hardly ever needed; reassurance and rest are usually enough.

As to chronic effects, this serious issue has not been resolved. A three-week free-access study in Boston[1] and a 14-week study in Canada have recently been completed. These have not been published in detail, but preliminary reports show that users: (1) did not tend to increase their dose of marihuana throughout the study period, (2) were able to maintain a stable and adequate level of simple task performance, (3) did not show deterioration in their personal relations or in their appearance, and (4) did not have withdrawal reactions.

Heavy Users

Studies of very heavy users, i.e., those who smoke every day or so (5 per cent of the male college student population[6]) are reported from the United States, Greece, and Jamaica.[1] In the United States these are almost invariably multiple drug users. Two generalizations from these studies are offered: (1) On psychomotor performance tests (reaction time, attention, decoding, or tracking tasks) the constant users do better than occasional users.[22] This might be expected since they have so much more practice performing while high. (2) The daily users are able to work and maintain an adequate overall life style, but their college grades are lower,[23] they often work at jobs below their intellectual level, the incidence of psychopathology is high, sexual deviation is more common, and self reports of psychologic dependence on marihuana are frequent.[24] Marihuana may not be the cause of these shortcomings; however, all the evidence suggests that if there are long-term adverse effects, they will be found in the daily user group.

Recommendations

1. The recommendations of the National Commission on Marihuana and Drug Abuse should be actively supported. These include: removal of penalties for personal possession, removal of penalties for casual distribution without profit;

a small fine for public use; retention of penalties for crimes committed while intoxicated or for sale of cannabis for profit.

The report of the Commission is a particularly thoughtful and informative document which deserves the attention of everyone interested in the field.* Proponents of complete legalization should be pleased to see an important part of their case acknowledged as reasonable. Proponents of the status quo should reflect: the growing number of voting age users will soon give them the power to have things as they wish. The frustration and the sense of injustice being felt by many on this issue may result in a legalization policy motivated more by rebelliousness than by wisdom. The National Commission has prepared policy guidelines which are both scientifically and politically reasonable. They deserve support from the medical profession.

2. If the recommendations of the National Commission are effected it will mean that demand is legalized but supply is not. This would seem to create a situation favorable for an underworld of unregulated smuggling. Feasibility studies should be undertaken to determine how supply can best be regulated. Perhaps a government-manufactured, -sold, and -taxed marihuana of known potency would be appropriate. Users might be required to register, and their tax money could be applied to drug abuse treatment and research. Studies need also to be done on the context of drug use so that social factors which might contribute to excess use can be identified and changed.

3. The procedure to obtain marihuana for research needs to be greatly simplified. Present regulations require the researcher to obtain approvals from his institution and from one State and three Federal agencies. This complexity and the time required to get a project going tends to discourage all but experienced and well connected researchers. Even they are starting to complain. Earlier this year 101 members of the American College of Neuropsychopharmacology, including three Nobel Laureates, sent a telegram to the President protesting "rules, regulations, statutes, procedures and legalisms" which create "barriers to research and threaten the continued existence of research itself."[25] Marihuana should be no different from any other drug in its availability as a research tool.

4. Education about drugs should be part of high school and college curricula. Fair and objective educational materials should make available to the student a variety of opinions about drug use. Too often drug education relies on slogans—"stay away from drugs"—which imply that all drug use is uniformly bad. Cannabis is not heroin, and youthful users know it. It is more useful to teach discrimination between drugs and use habits which are more dangerous or less so than to teach the generalization that all drugs are bad. Excellent teaching aids are now available and are being increasingly used in junior and senior high schools.

In conclusion, this is a good place to recommend to the reader that marihuana use is more than a question of identifying certain pharmacologic effects of a drug and judging them as good or bad. That approach considers but one element in a system. The effect of an individual's drug use must be appraised as it affects him physically, psychologically, and socially, since it may increase or decrease his use

---

* Available from U.S. Government Printing Office and at Regional Government Centers for $1.00

of other drugs, and it may affect his family and associates. A simple verdict on drug use is never possible. At best we can hope that our increasing knowledge and collective social wisdom can help us to extract more benefit than harm from the experience of drug use.

References

1. Secretary of Health, Education, and Welfare: *Marihuana and Health.* Second Annual Report to Congress 1972. Washington, D.C., Supt. of Documents, Government Printing Office.
2. National Commission on Marihuana and Drug Abuse: *Marihuana: A Signal of Misunderstanding.* Washington, D.C., Supt. of Documents, Government Printing Office.
3. President's Commission on Law Enforcement and Administration of Justice, Task Force Report: *Narcotics and Drug Abuse: Annotations and Consultants' Papers, 1967.* Washington, D.C., Supt. of Documents, Government Printing Office.
4. LeDain, G.: *Interim Report of the Commission of Inquiry into the Non-Medical Use of Drugs.* Ottawa, Queen's Printer, 1970.
5. Advisory Committee on Drug Dependence: *Cannabis.* London, Her Majesty's Stationery Office, 1968.
6. Gallup finds rise in marijuana use. New York Times, February 6, 1972.
7. Coles, R., Brenner, J. H., and Meagher, D.: *Drugs and Youth.* New York, Avon Printing, 1971.
8. Tart, C. T.: Marijuana intoxication: Common experiences. Nature (London) 226(5247): 701, 1970.
9. Appley, M. H. (ed.): *Adaptation-Level Theory.* New York, Academic Press, Inc., 1971.
10. Kupermann, I., Castellucci, V., Pinsker, H., and Kandel, E.: Neuronal correlates of habituation and dishabituation of the gill-withdrawal reflex in aplysia. Science 167:1743, 1970.
11. Grinspoon, L.: *Marihuana Reconsidered.* Cambridge, Harvard University Press, 1971.
12. O'Connell, D. N., Shor, R. E., and Orne, M. T.: Hypnotic age regression: An empirical and methodological analysis. J. Abnorm. Psychol. 76(3):1, 1970.
13. Chopra, I. C., and Chopra, R. N.: The use of cannabis drugs in India. U.N. Bull. Narcotics 9(1):13, 1957.
14. Garattini, S.: Effects of a cannabis extract on gross behavior. In Wolstenholme, G. E. W., and Knight, J. (eds.): *Hashish: Its Chemistry and Pharmacology.* (Ciba Foundation Study Group No. 21.) Boston, Little, Brown and Company, 1965, pp. 70–82.
15. Gonzalez, S. C., Matsudo, V. K. R., and Carlini, E. A.: Effects of marihuana compounds on the fighting behavior of Siamese fighting fish. Pharmacology 6:186, 1971.
16. Carlini, E. A., and Masur, J.: Development of aggressive behavior in rats by chronic administration of cannabis patira (marihuana). Life Sci. 8:607, 1969.
17. Newman, L. M., Lutz, M. P., Gould, M. H., and Domino, E. F.: Δ^9-Tetrahydrocannabinol and ethyl alcohol: Evidence for cross-tolerance in the rat. Science 175:1022, 1972.
18. Fisher, S., Pillard, R. C., and Botto, R. W.: Hypnotic susceptibility during cannabis intoxication. In press.
19. Hepler, R. S., and Frank, I. R.: Marihuana smoking and intraocular pressure. J.A.M.A. 217(10):1392, 1971.
20. Hollister, L. E.: Marihuana in man: Three years later. Science 172:21, 1971.
21. Halikas, J. A., Goodwin, D. W., and Guze, S. B.: Marihuana effects. J.A.M.A. 217(5):692, 1971.
22. Meyer, R. E., Pillard, R. C., Shapiro, L. M., and Mirin, S. M.: Administration of marijuana to heavy and casual marijuana users. Amer. J. Psychiat. 128(2):198, 1971.
23. Goode, E.: Drug use and grades in college. Nature (London) 234:225, 1971.
24. Mirin, S. M., Shapiro, L. M., Meyer, R. E., and Pillard, R. C.: Casual versus heavy use of marijuana: A redefinition of the marijuana problem. Amer. J. Psychiat. 127(9):1134,
25. Chayet, N. L.: Legislative harassment of physicians and researchers. New Eng. J. Med. 285:1399, 1971.

31

Management of Cerebral Ischemia

MEDICAL MANAGEMENT IN CEREBRAL ISCHEMIA
  by John S. Meyer and Ninan T. Matthew

THE ADVANTAGES OF ANTICOAGULANT MANAGEMENT OF OCCLUSIVE CEREBROVASCULAR DISEASE (STROKE)
  by Clark H. Millikan

THE ROLE OF SURGERY IN CONTROLLING CEREBRAL ISCHEMIA
  by Jesse E. Thompson

Medical Management in Cerebral Ischemia*

JOHN STIRLING MEYER and NINAN T. MATHEW

Department of Neurology, Baylor College of Medicine

Medical treatment of cerebral infarction or ischemia is one of the most controversial topics in clinical medicine today.[1] Despite the controversy, or because of it, a remarkable renaissance of interest and consequent gain in knowledge of the epidemiology, natural history, pathogenesis, and treatment (both medical and surgical) of cerebral ischemia has resulted in the past two decades. Our discussion will be confined to nonhemorrhagic ischemic cerebrovascular disease, although spasm and ischemia are a common accompaniment of intracranial bleeding.

First, let us attempt to list reasons for this controversy:

1. There is considerable variation in the natural history of cerebral ischemia and infarction from one patient to another, making evaluation of treatment difficult.[1]

2. There are often differences in the type, degree, and stage of cerebral ischemia at a given point in time when the effectiveness of treatment is being assessed.[1]

3. The cerebral metabolic changes induced by ischemia which affect neuronal function are complex and variable.[2]

4. The cerebral hemodynamic changes following cerebral ischemia are complex and variable.[3]

5. In the past there has been a perhaps unjustifiable tendency to apply conclusions drawn from a few observations made of experimental cerebral ischemia in animals to patients with cerebral arteriosclerosis.

In spite of the above-mentioned problems, we believe that suitable selection of comparable groups of patients with cerebral ischemia for control purposes is possible when evaluating new forms of treatment. Furthermore, methods of

---

* This work was supported by Grant NS 09287 01 from the National Institute of Neurological Disease and Stroke.

measuring cerebral blood flow and metabolism are now available which make it possible to measure changes in cerebral hemodynamics and metabolism resulting from cerebral ischemia and to detect any modification that may result from various methods of treatment.

Treatment of patients at risk from stroke or who have suffered from cerebral ischemia may be classified according to the stage of the disease into prophylactic, primary, and secondary treatment: *Prophylactic treatment* is directed at identifying those at risk from stroke and attempting to prevent the ictus by treating risk factors such as hypertension.[4] *Primary treatment* of the acute stroke, once it has occurred, is directed toward preventing progression of cerebral infarction and further episodes of ischemia, minimizing edema and necrosis of brain tissue, and improving or restoring disordered cerebral energy metabolism so that normal neuronal function may be maintained. *Secondary treatment* of the acute ischemic stroke includes supportive and rehabilitative measures. Supportive management includes treatment of complicating infections, improving respiratory exchange in paralyzed and/or comatose patients, correcting dehydration and abnormalities of the blood chemistry and electrolytes, and providing adequate nursing care with frequent turning. Rehabilitation depends on measures such as active and passive exercises and on retraining speech and other disabilities so that an optimum return to society may be achieved.

The value of prophylactic and secondary treatment has become rapidly and universally accepted. It is the relatively new and dynamic field of primary treatment which is highly controversial at the present time and requires carefully controlled therapeutic trials in comparable groups of patients to determine the efficacy of various forms of treatment.

Prophylactic Treatment

A subcommittee was appointed by the Stroke Council of the American Heart Association[5] to make a statement concerned with risk factors which may predispose an individual to cerebral infarction. Their conclusions may be summarized as follows:

Seven risk factors have been identified which are accompanied by more than a doubling of the risk of cerebral infarction, and when they occur in combination, the risk is further compounded. The seven risk factors are:

1. Hypertension of 160/95 mm. Hg or greater.
2. Serum cholesterol values exceeding 250 mg. per cent or a pre-beta band on electrophoresis (in persons under age 50 only).
3. Cardiac enlargement by x-ray.
4. Left ventricular hypertrophy as shown by electrocardiography.
5. Clinical evidence of coronary artery disease.
6. Congestive heart failure and/or dysrhythmia.
7. Impaired glucose tolerance or a two-hour postprandial blood sugar more than 160 mg. per cent or a fasting or casual blood sugar more than 120 mg. per cent.

While it seems prudent to treat all these risk factors in order to prevent stroke, so far the only method that has been shown by a controlled clinical trial to prevent stroke effectively is antihypertensive management.[4] The Subcommittee warned that dogmatic statements concerning the risk factors are premature, and field trials to demonstrate the efficacy of preventive measures which appear to be rational are urgently needed. In order to identify patients at risk, the report also suggested that the physical examination should include evaluation of the vascular system for bruits about the head and neck and differences in pressure and pulse of the upper extremities and neck.

Prophylaxis of cerebral infarction therefore entails periodic determinations of blood pressure, blood lipids, glucose tolerance, hemoglobin, electrocardiogram, chest x-ray, as well as careful clinical evaluation. Because of the higher frequency of cerebral infarction among blacks and those with a strong family history of hypertension, diabetes, lipid disorders, and strokes, periodic asssessments should be carried out more frequently in such individuals. The American Heart Association's statement concluded that, in the long run, prophylaxis is the only hope for achieving a substantial reduction in the incidence of ischemic stroke. Primary treatments, such as surgery, may lessen the likelihood of a stroke in those with transient ischemic attacks and extracranial vascular disease—an important benefit —but they will not necessarily lengthen life.

Primary Treatment of Transient Ischemic Attacks (TIA) and Reversible Ischemic Neurologic Deficits

Approximately one third of the patients suffering from TIAs will have irreversible cerebral infarction, another one third will continue to have TIAs, and about one third will spontaneously cease having attacks in a follow-up interval of approximately five years.[6,7] It is difficult to predict into which of the three categories an individual patient with TIAs will fall, particularly if the causative mechanism is not diagnosed. Consequently it seems advisable to consider all patients with TIAs to be at risk from cerebral infarction and to identify, treat, or remove whenever possible the pathogenetic mechanisms involved in each particular patient.

Remediable mechanisms responsible for TIAs include cerebral embolization by platelet and red emboli, cardiac dysrhythmia, transient hypotension, severe hypertension with spasm of cerebral vessels, hypoglycemia, polycythemia, transient regional diversions of cerebral blood flow (e.g., the subclavian steal), as well as kinking and external compression of vessels and severe anemia.[8]

The widespread use of aortocranial arteriography has shown the frequent presence of stenotic and ulcerated plaques of the proximal carotid and vertebral arteries. This has led to debate over the relative merit of surgical removal of the offending plaque versus medical treatment. Advocated medical treatment includes vasodilator and anticoagulant drugs or medications such as dipyridamole and acetylsalicylic acid to inhibit aggregation of platelets and thus prevent repeated embolization from such a plaque.

Some of the controversy concerned with the management of TIAs and the unconvincing results of therapeutic trials in the past probably arise from the facts that the critical hemodynamic factor responsible for the transient ischemic attacks was not properly identified, and the control and treated groups of patients were not similar. Although recurrent fibrinoplatelet emboli arising particularly from ulcerated plaques in the arteries of the neck is a mechanism well supported by clinical and experimental evidence, there is no doubt that a large percentage of TIAs are due to a hemodynamic crisis of some sort other than embolism. For example, Cooper and West[9] argue cogently that the majority of episodes of cerebrovascular ischemia in patients with cardiac dysfunction are a result of hemodynamic alterations, such as a reduction of cardiac output with reduced cerebral blood flow resulting in poor cerebral perfusion, and are not due to embolism. We are convinced that the majority of transient cerebral symptoms due to ischemia within the vertebrobasilar system are postural in nature due to cerebral dysautoregulation and respond well to cerebral vasodilator drugs such as papaverine and beta-histine HCl.[10] Observations such as this explain why treatment directed toward preventing embolism are ineffective in some patients with TIAs and effective in others.

Anticoagulant Therapy

At the Fourth Princeton Conference Millikan[11] reviewed the status of anti-coagulants in relation to cerebral ischemia and re-emphasized his belief that anticoagulants are beneficial in patients with TIAs and stroke in evolution. In a national cooperative study concerned with a controlled clinical trial of anticoagulant therapy published in 1966,[12] the incidence of further ischemic episodes was reduced by anticoagulants in patients with TIAs, though the mortality of thrombotic cerebrovascular disease in the carotid territory was not improved and actually may have been worsened, since the incidence of fatal and nonfatal hemorrhagic episodes was high. It should be borne in mind that few or none of these patients had cerebral arteriograms, so that the treated and control groups may not have been the same, or even suffering from cerebral embolism at all. The conclusion of this national cooperative study was that patients suffering from TIAs are the only group in whom anticoagulants are worthwhile, and even in this group, anticoagulant treatment was contraindicated after four to six months.

The inherent dangers of hemorrhagic complications of long-term anticoagulant therapy, as well as the lack of evidence of long-term beneficial effects, must be appreciated. In general, the use of anticoagulants should be limited to selected cases of recurrent cerebral thromboembolism from a known cardiac source, and to patients with TIAs due to extracranial occlusive disease in whom surgical treatment is contraindicated and in whom platelet inhibitors are ineffective, and in rare instances to patients with progressive thrombosis within the basilar artery.

Platelet Inhibitors

When such reasons for limitations of anticoagulant therapy are considered, it should be noted that an arterial thrombus begins as a deposition of platelets releases ADP, which leads to further aggregation of platelets and deposition of fibrin with incorporation of all the blood elements and formation of a red thrombus. Decreased fibrinolysis and increased platelet adhesiveness has been found in patients with occlusive cerebrovascular disease.[13] Thus, platelet inhibitors may play an important role in the treatment of cerebral thromboembolism.

Increased consumption of platelets, as well as platelet adhesiveness, has been shown to accompany cerebral thromboembolism in patients with prosthetic cardiac valves.[14, 15] Sullivan and associates,[16] in an important trial, reported a decrease in the number of embolic episodes in patients with prosthetic heart valves who were treated with dipyridamole (Persantin) plus warfarin when compared to a control group of comparable patients treated with warfarin alone. In our hospital the use of dipyridamole alone (without anticoagulants) in doses of 100 mg. 4 times daily in patients with cerebral emboli from prosthetic heart valves resulted in cessation or reduction of further episodes of cerebral embolization.[17] It is important clinically to differentiate platelet embolism from embolism due to fragments of red thrombus, since the former responds to platelet inhibitors while the latter may require anticoagulants. Platelet emboli produce relatively minor neurologic signs of brief duration, whereas red emboli produce more severe and persistent focal neurologic signs.

Acetylsalicylic acid (aspirin)[18] and sulfinpyrazone[13] are two other drugs which prevent platelet adhesiveness and have been shown to be clinically useful. A supplementary dose of 15 gm. of aspirin at night permits reduction of effective dipyridamole dosages to 100 mg. daily from 400 mg. daily.[19] In other words, aspirin potentiates the action of dipyridamole.

Based on our experience in treating cases of cerebral embolism, especially after cardiac valve replacements and from inoperable extracranial arterial ulcerated atherosclerotic plaques, we would recommend the following:[17] Whenever recurrent fibrinoplatelet embolism with recurrent focal neurologic signs and symptoms is suspected, treatment with dipyridamole and acetylsalicylic acid is instituted. The length of time such therapy should be continued will have to be decided by the physician, based on the individual patient response. We have patients who have been treated with dipyridamole for over two years, with virtual absence of cerebral ischemic symptoms and without any untoward side effects.

Surgical Treatment

Despite reports of controlled clinical trials, the indications for extracranial arterial surgery in the treatment of cerebral ischemia are still debated. The Joint Study of Extracranial Arterial Occlusion[20] reported the incidence of TIAs and new episodes of cerebral infarction were reduced by carotid endarterectomy in patients with unilateral carotid stenosis, bilateral carotid stenosis, and unilateral stenosis with occlusion of the opposite carotid artery. In patients with bilateral carotid stenosis, a marked difference in the survival was noted in favor of surgical treatment. On the other hand, patients with severe hypertension and evidence of heart disease had a significantly greater survival rate if they were managed medically.

It is our own view that if aortocranial arteriography shows a carotid plaque with irregularities suggesting ulceration, surgical treatment is indicated, particularly if the symptoms can be related to ischemia within the territory of brain supplied by the diseased artery. Our practice is to defer surgery and utilize medical treatment (to be cited later) for at least three weeks after a cerebral ischemic episode to avoid rendering an ischemic cerebral infarction hemorrhagic. There is one possible exception to this program: In a few patients with progressive ischemia, if a "rat tail" filling defect, suggesting a recent thrombus imposed on a plaque, is noted in the extracranial portion of the internal carotid artery during arteriography, then emergency thrombectomy may be considered to prevent total occlusion of the artery by the thrombus. Recurrent retinal embolization constitutes another indication for immediate endarterectomy.[1] About 60 per cent of the patients will not prove to fulfill such indications for surgery and will remain candidates for medical treatment.

Primary Medical Treatment of Patients with Acute Cerebral Infarction

Several workers in the field of cerebrovascular disease take a nihilistic view and do not recommend any form of treatment for acute progressive cerebral infarction other than physical medicine. However, others advocate a number of methods for treating patients with acute cerebral ischemia designed to prevent extension of the infarction, reduce the neurologic disability, hasten recovery, and minimize mortality. Each of these will be discussed separately for convenience, although we advocate that they be used together as appears indicated after appraisal of each individual patient.

INHALATION THERAPY IN THE MANAGEMENT OF PATIENTS WITH ACUTE CEREBRAL INFARCTION

40 per cent oxygen inhalation. Work in experimental animals indicates that the rapid onset of the neurologic deficit, resulting from cerebral ischemia, is caused primarily by regional cerebral anoxia.[21-24] However, regional metabolic acidosis due to the accumulation of acid metabolites such as lactate, cerebral edema, and other metabolic disorders later become contributing factors. Inhalation of oxygen is generally conceded to be beneficial since it enhances the delivery of oxygen to ischemic zones of the brain. Observations in our laboratory showed that inhalation of a mixture of 95 per cent oxygen and 5 per cent carbon dioxide produces a mean increase of 14.8 mm. Hg in cerebral venous pO_2[21] and a statistically significant increase in cerebral oxygen consumption of 0.5 ml./100 gm. brain/minute in patients with subacute and chronic cerebral ischemia.

Recent reports recommend the use of 40 per cent oxygen inhalation rather than mixtures of 95 or 100 per cent oxygen in order to avoid the toxic effects of prolonged use of high concentrations. It is now our practice to administer 40 per cent oxygen, since the prolonged use of pure oxygen results in the accumulation of interstitial and alveolar fluid in the lungs, diminished replication of endothelial cells, the deposition of a hyaline membrane, and interference with alveolar surfactant activity, as well as an increase in intrapulmonary shunting and the ratio of dead space to total volume. All these factors eventually lead to a decrease in oxygen uptake by the alveolar capillaries.[26-31]

Hyperbaric oxygenation. Heyman et al.[32] found that hyperbaric oxygen could restore neurologic function and maintain neuronal viability in a small number of acute stroke patients. Hass et al.,[33] Ben-Yishay and associates,[34, 35] and Jacobs et al.[36] reported improvement in mental performances of patients with cerebral ischemia while on treatment with hyperbaric oxygen. In none of these reports has sustained improvement been documented after discontinuation of therapy. On the contrary, rapid return of the neurologic deficit has been the rule.

Recent reports suggest the advisability of combining decarboxylase or carbonic anhydrase inhibitors with hyperbaric oxygen to prevent excessive cerebral and retinal vasoconstriction.[37-39] However, a more recent report of Sarno et al.[40] is disappointing in that no sustained beneficial effect in stroke patients was found after treatment with hyperbaric oxygen. At this stage, hyperbaric oxygenation is not recommended since it is impractical, expensive, and not without danger.

Intermittent 5 per cent CO_2 inhalation. Whether intermittent 5 per cent CO_2, one of the most potent cerebral vasodilators known, should be added to the inhaled oxygen mixture for 15 minutes out of each hour during the treatment of acute stroke has been a subject of intensive study and controversy during the past five years. The controversy stemmed from the fact that paradoxical vasomotor responses to CO_2, whereby blod was deviated from the ischemic zone to normal brain ("intracerebral steal"), was reported in a few extensive and acute cerebral infarcts in experimental animals and in patients.[41, 42] Agreement has now been reached that the phenomenon of paradoxical response to CO_2 occurs only rarely in humans and is limited to the acute phase of cerebral infarction. It is virtually never seen in patients with mild or moderate infarction, subacute infarction, diffuse cerebrovascular disease, or TIAs.[43-45] Fieschi et al.[46] and Fazekas and Alman[47] reported that in patients with cerebral circulatory disturbance, the vasodilator capacitance to CO_2 was reduced or impaired in only 25 per cent of patients. Measurement of regional cerebral blood flow (rCBF), using intracarotid injection of xenon-133 and recording the clearance with the gamma camera, revealed paradoxical responses to 5 per cent CO_2 inhalation only in patients with mass lesions such as intracerebral hematoma or brain tumor.[48] rCBF was increased in all regions in all six patients with recent hemispheric infarction in whom this method was used, although the increase in infarcted zones was less than in the normal ones.

The first impression on reviewing reports of the effects of CO_2 inhalation on regional blood flow in experimentally infarcted areas of the brain is that a confusing disagreement exists, some laboratories reporting increased blood flow to ischemic hemispheres and others a reduction or steal.[49, 50] Close inspection of these reports shows differences in the concentration of CO_2 used, the species of animals, and the severity of infarction. In general, low concentrations of CO_2, such as 5 per cent mixture with oxygen, do not cause a paradoxical response unless the infarction is massive and acute. In such patients, 5 per cent CO_2 may increase intracranial pressure and cerebral edema in the infarcted zone, resulting in a "squeeze" of blood into the more normal brain.

The phenomenon of diaschisis (reduction of blood flow to the entire brain as a result of localized acute cerebral infarction) makes the therapeutic dilemma more complex.[51] Since CO_2 inhalation increases total CBF, even if the increase occurs only in the depressed but noninfarcted hemisphere, the effect may be beneficial clinically.

Our present state of knowledge suggests the following guidelines regarding the use of CO_2 inhalation in the treatment of cerebral ischemia.[10] Concentrations of CO_2 greater than 5 per cent should not be used. Intermittent 5 per cent CO_2 inhalation may be beneficial in patients with TIAs and with mild and moderate cerebral infarctions as evidenced by the clinical state of the patient and diagnostic and laboratory test findings (lumbar puncture, arteriography, brain scan). This form of treatment is contraindicated, however, in the acute stage of intracerebral hemorrhage and in massive cerebral infarction. Since the "intracerebral steal" has been reported only during the early stages of brain infarction, it is now our practice to defer 5 per cent CO_2 inhalation for the first 48 hours after severe cerebral infarction and to limit inhalation therapy to 40 per cent oxygen during this interval.

Hyperventilation. Based on clinical and experimental data concerned with what was termed the "luxury perfusion syndrome" and the possibility of an "inverse steal," Lassen[52] and Rossanda[53] at one point recommended the use of prolonged hyperventilation in the treatment of focal cerebrovascular disease. This type of therapy was recommended despite the reported adverse effects of hyperventilation, which include decreased CBF, brain pO_2, and oxygen availability due in part to the Bohr effect, increased brain and CSF lactate, increased brain tissue NADH, and cerebral anaerobiosis with impairment of oxidative metabolism, slowing of the EEG, and the production of epileptic seizures in those predisposed to convulsive disorders.[54-59]

Since the combined effects of hyperventilation increase rather than decrease cerebral acidosis by increasing cerebral ischemia, and produce the above mentioned undesirable effects, the theoretical basis for hyperventilation therapy in stroke is certainly open to question. A controlled therapeutic trial was carried out in Copenhagen in which prolonged active hypocapnic hyperventilation in patients with severe infarction was compared with a similar series of patients who underwent normocapnic active ventilation, and no statistical differences were observed between the two groups; however, survival in both groups appeared to be prolonged, possibly emphasizing the importance of maintaining an open airway and adequate pulmonary exchange.[60]

Brock et al.[61] at the Seventh Princeton Conference were the first to suggest the importance of increased regional intracranial and tissue pressures in regional cerebral hemodynamics. They suggested that any beneficial effects derived from hyperventilation in patients with disorders associated with increased intracranial pressure such as stroke, trauma, or brain tumor were due to the slight reduction of intracranial pressure resulting from decreased blood volume within the skull. These investigations pointed out that there are other means of reducing intracranial pressure without decreasing CBF which might offer a more logical approach to therapy.

Lassen argued that the systemic respiratory alkalosis induced by hyperventilation would benefit the patient with acute cerebral infarction. Studies carried out in our laboratory showed that metabolic alkalosis induced by infusion of THAM (tris-[hydroxymethyl] aminomethane) did not influence blood flow to the infarcted hemisphere.[44] However, reduction of intracranial pressure and edema by injection of mannitol and glycerol did increase the hemispheric blood flow (HBF) in patients with acute cerebral infarction.[62]

Therapeutic Measures Designed to Reduce Cerebral Edema and Improve Metabolism in Cerebral Infarction

Cerebral edema becomes maximal three or four days after infarction, has long been known to be a constant complication of cerebral infarction, and is the major cause of death during the acute stages.[63, 64] Reduction of intracranial pressure and cerebral edema in patients with stroke by the intravenous injection of mannitol or glycerol was shown to increase CBF[62]

Glycerol therapy. The beneficial effects of treatment of cerebral edema by glycerol was recently stressed by Meyer et al.[51, 62, 65] Although there are a number of agents which reduce cerebral edema by their hyperosmolar effect, glycerol administered orally or intravenously appears to be the treatment of choice, as it was shown that it not only reduces cerebral edema, increases cerebral blood flow, but also improves cerebral metabolism possibly by recoupling of uncoupled oxidative phosphorylation. This is evidenced by reduction of cerebral oxygen consumption and respiratory quotient (RQ) in the presence of normal or slightly increased glucose consumption and restoration of the inorganic phosphate and free fatty acids which are released by infarcted brain.[66] These changes were associated with EEG and clinical improvement.

Glycerol is administered orally in a dose of 1.5 gm./kg. of body weight every 24 hours. We have administered it in divided doses mixed with fruit juices to mask the unappealing taste.[65] When the intravenous route is used, we infuse 500 ml. of 10 per cent glycerol in a solution of 5 per cent glucose or normal saline over a period of three to four hours daily for the first four or six days of acute cerebral infarction. In the case of massive infarction, the daily infusion may be continued for two weeks or longer. In a prospective therapeutic trial involving 36 patients with acute cerebral infarction, the mortality was shown to be reduced. In another study carried out in this center, the results of a double-blind therapeutic trial of glycerol given intravenously for five days showed statistically significant results in favor of glycerol when the neurologic status was compared between the glycerol and the placebo group ($p<.01$).[67]

Glycerol appears to have other benefits in the treatment of patients with cerebral edema due to acute cerebral infarction since many of them also have associated diabetes mellitus and renal insufficiency. When glycerol is given in the recommended dosage we have not observed any toxic effects. Glycerol is a diuretic and has been used effectively in several patients with grossly impaired renal function, resulting in diuresis with decreased creatinine and blood urea nitrogen (BUN) following its administration. There is no evidence of hemolysis caused by infusion of 10 per cent solution at a rate of 3 ml. per minute. When given at a maximum rate in patients with impending cerebral herniation on an emergency basis at 12 ml. per minute, hemolysis is slight and no ill effects have resulted. There is no rebound phenomenon (a further increase of intracranial pressure when therapy is discontinued) such as occurs when mannitol and urea are given.

Glycerol provides an important source of carbohydrate that can be rapidly converted to glucose by the liver in the absence of insulin;[68] hence, it has the effect of sparing fatty acids and protein utilization in diabetic patients by providing a source of glucose without insulin. Glycerol also slowly but effectively passes the blood-brain barrier and thus provides a readily available source of energy at the neuronal membrane, resulting in recoupling of oxidative phosphorylation.

Steroid therapy. Corticosteroids, especially dexamethasone, are well established agents in reducing cerebral edema, particularly when caused by tumors. Their use in acute cerebral infarction was debated until Patten et al.[69] reported a double-blind study in which evidence was shown that dexamethasone is beneficial. Dexamethasone is given in daily divided doses of 16 to 20 mg. for the first 10 days, followed by gradual withdrawal. Our experience would confirm that of Patten and his co-workers that steroids are usually effective in enhancing neurologic recovery and reducing the mortality rate in the acute stage of cerebral infarction. However, steroids cause serious side effects such as gastric ulceration and hemorrhage, exacerbation of diabetes mellitus, and Cushing's syndrome, and the effect is less rapid than that of glycerol, which we recommend as the preferred treatment.

Low molecular weight dextran. Gilroy, Meyer, and Barnhart[70] reported better neurologic recovery in the treated group in a controlled study of the use of intravenous low molecular weight dextran in the treatment of a large series of cases of acute cerebral infarction.[70] This preparation reduces platelet adhesiveness and is a hyperosmolar agent. The first "loading dose" of 500 ml. was administered intravenously over a period of one hour, and thereafter 500 ml. was infused over each 12-hour period for three days. Platelet aggregation was shown to be decreased in the treated group. Other reports indicate that low molecular weight dextran infusion may stop TIAs that are refractory to anticoagulant therapy.[71, 72] Low molecular weight dextran has been reported to improve the microcirculation in areas of ischemia and to reduce the extent of experimental infarction.[73, 74]

Low molecular weight dextran therapy is contraindicated in patients with impaired renal function, since there is the danger of precipitating acute renal failure. There is also some danger of precipitating heart failure in patients with borderline cardiac reserve. Glycerol does not have these disadvantages. Low molecular weight dextran should not be used, therefore, in patients with hypertensive or diabetic nephropathy or cardiac failure associated with stroke. Daily urine output and fluid intake charts should be maintained, and periodic estimation of BUN and creatinine are essential.

Other hyperosmolar agents. The use of mannitol is not recommended since it has a transient effect in reducing brain edema, causes a rebound increase in intracranial pressure, and is metabolically inert. Likewise, urea therapy is not recommended. Furthermore, a certain number of patients with acute stroke have an associated renal insufficiency and high blood urea nitrogen.

Cerebral Vasodilator Drugs

Papaverine. Studies carried out in our stroke center in experimental animals and in patients with cerebral infarction have demonstrated that papaverine hydrochloride, given intravenously or orally, increases CBF and cerebral oxygen delivery. When given orally, the drug provides a more sustained action than when given intravenously.[75, 76] Clinical improvement also was noted in a controlled study. Our observations were confirmed by McHenry et al.,[77] who observed increased rCBF in the ischemic area in patients with cerebral infarction. Objections have been raised by some workers regarding the medical possibility. of causing an intracerebral steal with the use of cerebral vasodilator drugs in the acute stage of cerebral infarction. However, Olesen and Paulson[78] could demonstrate intracerebral steal after intracarotid injection of papaverine in only one cerebral area in 14 patients with focal cerebral ischemia, and confirmed the beneficial effects of vasodilators. Likewise, McHenry found no patients at all with intracerebral steal after intravenous papaverine therapy.

Because of this experience, we recommend the use of parenteral papaverine in the acute stage of cerebral infarction and long-term oral treatment in patients recovering from completed strokes and with TIAs in the vertebrobasilar territory, as well as in patients who are not suitable candidates for surgical excision of plaques in the cervical portion of the carotid arteries. In our experience oral papaverine has proved particularly useful in the long-term treatment of chronic cerebrovascular insufficiency.

Betahistine hydrochloride (Serc). This drug (not yet approved by the Food and Drug Administration) increases cerebral blood flow in patients with cerebral ischemia. Unpublished studies show the drug to be as effective as papaverine or hexobendine. It is particularly useful in patients with vertebrobasilar insufficiency.

Hexobendine. This drug also has not been released for general use in the United States by the Food and Drug Administration, although it has been widely used in Austria and Germany. Measurements in both animals and man have shown that hexobendine given intravenously, intramuscularly, or orally increases CBF by about 15 per cent and is associated with an increase in $CMRO_2$.[79, 80] McHenry and colleagues,[81] in an independent study, showed an increase in rCBF in areas of ischemia in patients with cerebral infarction who were given hexobendine intramuscularly. Based on these findings, a double-blind study of hexobendine in the treatment of acute and chronic cerebral ischemia was carried out in our laboratory. In patients consenting to this procedure, serial measurements of rCBF were made by the intracarotid injection of xenon-133 and measurement of the clearance with the gamma camera. When the study was completed, and the code broken, the patients who had received hexobendine showed a statistically significant increase in hemispheric blood flow and rCBF when compared to the control group who had received a similar appearing placebo.[51] There was also measurable clinical improvement in these patients.[82]

Other cerebral vasodilator drugs. Cyclandelate and isoxsuprine are presently being evaluated clinically in the treatment of cerebral ischemia and arteriosclerotic dementia in our stroke center. Other investigators have reported that these drugs are beneficial in the treatment of cerebrovascular disease and arteriosclerotic dementia.[83, 84] Our patients with arteriosclerotic dementia have shown significant improvement in psychologic tests when given cyclandelate versus placebo in double-blind manner.

THROMBOLYTIC AGENTS

Although abnormalities of the fibrinolytic system have been demonstrated in patients with stroke,[13] a randomized evaluation of intravenous streptokinase proved it to be contraindicated in cerebral infarction caused by thrombosis because of the danger of the infarct becoming hemorrhagic and of inducing a systemic hemorrhagic complication.[85] Thrombolytic agents seem more promising in treating cerebral venous thrombosis. It is possible that urokinase may prove to be more efficient than streptokinase, since unlike streptokinase, antibodies against it are not present and effective therapy is easier to maintain.[85]

Summary

Cerebral diagnostic evaluation in all patients with cerebral ischemia and infarction is essential since the cause may be entirely different from one patient to another. This includes a careful history, physical and neurologic examinations including auscultation of the neck, serial measurements of the blood pressure, and auxiliary tests such as skull and cervical spine x-rays, EEG, brain scans, and arteriograms.

If ulcerated plaques of the carotid artery are found, carotid endarterectomy is justified if embolism from this source can account for the symptoms. The majority of patients will not be surgical candidates, and medical treatment is indicated. If embolism of the heart is suspected and the neurologic signs are mild and transient, particularly if prosthetic heart valves are present, platelet embolism is a likely cause and dipyramindole and acetylsalicylic therapy should be considered. If the emboli cause larger and more persistent neurologic deficits, red embolism should be considered and anticoagulant therapy instituted.

If hypertension, hypotension, or cardiac dysrhythmia exist, these should be treated.

In patients with transient ischemic attacks within the vertebrobasilar territory, vasodilators such as papaverine, hexobendine and betahistine HCl are often effective.

In patients with acute cerebral infarction, surgical treatment is contraindicated and intravenous glycerol therapy is recommended for six days, together with inhalation of 40 per cent oxygen. Later, vasodilation therapy and rehabilitative measures should be added.

References

1. Millikan, C. H.: Summary of the Eighth Princeton Conference on Cerebral Vascular Disease, January 5–7, 1972, Princeton, New Jersey. Stroke 3:105, 1972.
2. Meyer, J. S., and Welch, K. M. A.: Relationship of cerebral blood and metabolism to neurological symptoms. In Meyer, J. S., and Schadé, J. P. (eds.): *Cerebral Blood Flow.* Vol. 35 of *Progress in Brain Research.* Amsterdam, Elsevier/North Holland, 1972, pp. 284–347.
3. Meyer, J. S., Fukuuchi, Y., Shimazu, K., Ohuchi, T., and Ericsson, A.D.: Abnormal hemispheric blood flow and metabolism in cerebrovascular disease. Disordered patterns of hemispheric metabolism. Stroke 3:141, 1972.
4. Veterans Administration Cooperative Study Group on Antihypertensive Agents: II. Results in patients with diastolic blood pressure averaging 90 through 114 mm Hg. J.A.M.A. 213:1143, 1970.
5. Kannel, W. B., Blaisdell, F. W., Clifford, R., Hass, W., McDowell, F., Meyer, J. S., and Seltzer, R.: Risk factors in stroke due to cerebral infarction. Stroke 2:423, 1971.
6. Marshall, J.: Natural history of transient ischemic cerebrovascular attacks. Quart. J. Med. 33:309, 1964.
7. Robinson, R. W., Demirel, M., and Lebeau, R. J.: Natural history of cerebral thrombosis 9–19 year follow-up. J. Chronic Dis. 21:221, 1968.
8. Bauer, R. B., Wechsler, N., and Meyer, J. S.: Carotid compression and rotation of the head in occlusive vertebral artery disease. Ann. Intern. Med. 55:283, 1961.
9. Cooper, E. S., and West, J. W.: Cardiac arrhythmias, cerebral function and stroke. Curr. Conc. Cerebrovas. Dis. (Stroke) 5:53, 1970.
10. Meyer, J. S., Mathew, N. T., and Shimazu, K.: Clinical management of cerebral ischemia. In Toole, J. F., Moossy, J., and Janeway, R. (eds.): *Cerebral Vascular Diseases, Proceedings of the Eighth Princeton Conference.* New York, Grune & Stratton, 1972.
11. Millikan, C. H.: Anticoagulant therapy in cerebrovascular disease. In Millikan, C. H., Siekert, R. G., and Whisnant, J. P. (eds.): *Cerebral Vascular Diseases, Proceedings of the Fourth Princeton Conference.* New York, Grune and Stratton, 1965, pp. 181–184.
12. Baker, R. N., Broward, J. A., Fang, H. C., Fisher, C. M., Groch, S. N., Heyman, A., Karp, H. R., McDevitt, E., Scheinberg, P., Schwartz, W., and Toole, J. F.: Anticoagulant therapy of cerebral infarction: Report of a national cooperative study. In Millikan, C. H. (ed.): *Cerebrovascular Disease.* Baltimore, The Williams & Wilkins Company, 1966, pp. 287–302.
13. Sweeny, V. P., and Naiman, S. C.: Abnormalities in fibrinolysis and platelet function associated with occlusive cerebrovascular disease. Neurology 21:402, 1971.
14. Weily, H. S., and Genton, E.: Altered platelet function in patients with prosthetic mitral valves. Circulation 42:967, 1970.
15. Lander, H., Kinlough, R. L., and Robson, H. N.: Reduced platelet survival in patients with Starr-Edwards prostheses. Brit. Med. J. 1:688, 1965.
16. Sullivan, J. M., Harker, D. W., and Gorlin, R.: Effect of dipyridamole on the incidence of arterial emboli after cardiac valve replacement. Circulation 39(Suppl. I):1, 1969.
17. Meyer, J. S., Charney, J. Z., Rivera, V. M., and Mathew, N. T.: Cerebral embolization: Prospective clinical analysis of 42 cases. Stroke 2:541, 1971.
18. Harker, L. A.: Platelet kinetics and artificial heart valves. Clin. Res. 18:176, 1970.
19. Harker, L. A., and Slichter, S. J.: Studies of platelet and fibrinogen kinetics in patients with prosthetic heart valves. New Eng. J. Med. 283:1302, 1970.
20. Fields, W. S., Maslenikov, V., Meyer, J. S., Hass, W. K., Remington, R. D., and MacDonald, M.: Joint study of extracranial arterial occlusion. J.A.M.A. 211:1993, 1970.
21. Meyer, J. S., Sawada, T., Kitamura, A., and Toyoda, M.: Cerebral oxygen, glucose, lactate, and pyruvate metabolism in stroke. Therapeutic considerations. Circulation 37:1036, 1968.
22. Meyer, J. S., Sawada, T., Tododa, M., and Kitamura, A.: Anaerobic cerebral metabolism induced by ischemia. Relation to hyperventilation and cerebrovascular disease in man. In Toole, J. F., Siekert, R. G., and Whisnant, J. P. (eds.): *Cerebral Vascular Diseases, Proceedings of the Sixth Princeton Conference.* New York, Grune & Stratton, 1968, pp. 111–122.
23. Meyer, J. S., Ryu, T., Tododa, M., Shinohara, Y., Wiederholt, I., and Guiraud, B.: Evi-

dence for a Pasteur effect regulating cerebral oxygen and carbohydrate metabolism in man. Neurology 19:954, 1969.
24. Meyer, J. S., Gotoh, F., and Takagi, Y.: Inhalation of oxygen and carbon dioxide. Effect on composition of cerebral venous blood. Arch. Intern. Med. 119:4, 1967.
25. Salford, L. G., Brierley, J. B., Plum, F., and Siesjö, B. K.: Histology and high energy substrates in rat brain after graded hypoxia. Panminerva Med. 13:185, 1971.
26. Haugaard, N.: Cellular mechanisms of oxygen toxicity. Physiol. Rev. 48:311, 1968.
27. Faridy, E. D., Permutt, S., and Riley, R. L.: Effect of ventilation on surface forces in excised dogs' lungs. J. Appl. Physiol. 21:1453, 1966.
28. Tierney, D. F.: Pulmonary surfactant in health and disease. Dis. Chest 47:247, 1965.
29. Clements, J. A., and Fisher, H. K.: The oxygen dilemma. New Eng. J. Med. 282:976, 1970.
30. Barber, R. E., Lee, J., and Hamilton, W. K., Oxygen toxicity in man. A prospective study in patients with irreversible brain damage. New Eng. J. Med. 283:1478, 1970.
31. Hedley-Whyte, J.: Causes of pulmonary oxygen toxicity. New Eng. J. Med. 283:1518, 1970.
32. Heyman, A., Saltzman, H. A., and Whalen, R. E.: The use of hyperbaric oxygenation in the treatment of cerebral ischemia and infarction. Circulation (Suppl. II):20, 1966.
33. Haas, A., Ben-Yishay, Y., and Diller, L.: The effects of enriched oxygen on respiratory pathophysiology and some concomitants in the left hemiplegia. Paper read at A.M.A. Conference on Experimental Medicine, Atlantic City, June, 1967.
34. Ben-Yishay, Y.: The effects of enriched oxygenation on sensory-motor perceptual performance of adult left hemiplegics. NYU doctoral dissertation, 1967.
35. Ben-Yishay, Y., Diller, L., and Haas, A.: The effects of oxygen inhalation on motor impersistence in brain-damaged individuals. A double blind study. Neurology 17:1003, 1967.
36. Jacobs, E. A., Winter, P. M., Alvis, H. J., and Small, S. M.: Hyperoxygenation effect on cognitive functioning in the aged. New Eng. J. Med. 281:753, 1969.
37. Kong, Y., Lunzer, S., Heyman, A., Thompson, H. K., Jr., and Saltzman, H. A.: Effects of acetazolamide on cerebral blood flow of dogs during hyperbaric oxygenation. Amer. Heart J. 78:229, 1969.
38. Kong, Y., Lunzer, S., Heyman, A., and Saltzman, H. A.: Protective effects of acetazolamide and hyperbaric oxygenation on experimentally induced syncope. Stroke 1:69, 1970.
39. Hart, G. B., and Thompson, R. E.: The treatment of cerebral ischemia with hyperbaric oxygen (OHB). Stroke 2:247, 1971.
40. Sarno, J. E., Rusk, H. A., Diller, L., and Sarno, M. T.: The effect of hyperbaric oxygen on the mental and verbal ability of stroke patients. Stroke 3:10, 1972.
41. Høedt-Rasmussen, K., Skinhøj, E., Paulson, O., Ewald, J., Bjerrum, J. K., Fahrenkrug, A. and Lassen, N. A.: Regional cerebral blood flow in acute apoplexy; the "luxury perfusion syndrome" of brain tissue. Arch. Neurol. 17:271, 1967.
42. Fieschi, C.: Regulation of cerebral vessels to CO_2 in acute brain disease and its importance to therapy. In Toole, J. F., Moossy, J., and Janeway, R. (eds.): Cerebral Vascular Diseases, Proceedings of the Seventh Princeton Conference. New York, Grune & Stratton, 1971, pp. 130–139.
43. McHenry, L., Jr., Formal discussion of paper by C. Fieschi (Regulation of cerebral vassels to CO_2 in acute brain disease and its importance to therapy.) In Toole, J. F., Moossy, J., and Janeway, R. (eds.): Cerebral Vascular Diseases, Proceedings of the Seventh Princeton Conference. New York, Grune & Stratton, 1971, pp. 139–141.
44. Meyer, J. S., Fukuuchi, Y., Shimazu, K., Ohuchi, T., and Ericsson, A. D.: Abnormal hemispheric blood flow and metabolism in cerebrovascular disease. II. Therapeutic trials with 5% CO_2 inhalation, hyperventilation, and intravenous infusion of THAM and mannitol. Stroke 3:157, 1972.
45. Thompson, S.: Reactivity of cerebral blood flow to CO_2 in patients with transient cerebral ischemic attacks. Stroke 2:273, 1971.
46. Fieschi, C., Agnoli, A., and Galbo, E.: Effects of carbon dioxide on cerebral hemodynamics in normal subjects and in cerebrovascular disease studied by carotid injection of radioalbumin. Circ. Res. 13:436, 1963.
47. Fazekas, J. F., and Alman, R. W.: Maximal dilation of cerebral vessels. Arch. Neurol. 11: 303, 1964.
48. Mathew, N. T., Meyer, J. S., Bell, R. L., and Ericsson, A. D.: New method for measuring regional cerebral blood flow and blood volume in man using the gamma camera. Trans. Amer. Neurol. Ass. 96:273, 1971.
49. Waltz, A. G.: Regional cerebral blood flow: Responses to changes in arterial blood pres-

sure and CO_2 tension. *In* Toole, J. F., Siekert, R. G., and Whisnant, J. P. (eds.): *Cerebral Vascular Disease, Proceedings of the Sixth Princeton Conference.* New York, Grune & Stratton, 1968, pp. 66–76.
50. Kogure, K., Fujishima, M., Scheinberg, P., and Reinmuth, O. M.: Effects of changes in carbon dioxide pressure and arterial pressure on blood flow in ischemic regions of the brain in dogs. Circ. Res. 24:557, 1969.
51. Meyer, J. S., Shinohara, Y., Kanda, T., Fukuuchi, Y., Ericcson, A. D., and Kok, N. K.: Diaschisis resulting from acute unilateral cerebral infarction: Quantitative evidence in man. Arch. Neurol. 23:241, 1970.
52. Lassen, N. A.: The luxury perfusion syndrome and its possible relation to acute metabolic acidosis localized within the brain. Lancet 2:1113, 1966.
53. Rossanda, M.: Prolonged hyperventilation in treatment of unconscious patients with severe brain injuries. Scand. J. Lab. Clin. Invest. (Suppl. 102):XIII E, 1968.
54. Meyer, J. S., and Gotoh, F.: Hyperventilation and the electroencephalogram. Recording brain oxygen and carbon tensions, pH, EEG and blood flow during hyperventilation. Trans. Amer. Neurol. Ass., 1960, pp. 155–160.
55. Meyer, J. S., and Gotoh, F.: Metabolic and electroencephalographic effects of hyperventilation. Experimental studies of brain oxygen and carbon dioxide tension, pH, EEG, and blood flow during hyperventilation. Arch. Neurol. 3:539, 1960.
56. Gotoh, F., Meyer, J. S., and Takagi, Y.: Cerebral effects of hyperventilation in man. Arch. Neurol. 11:410, 1965.
57. Plum, F., and Posner, J. B.: Blood and cerebrospinal fluid lactate during hyperventilation. Amer. J. Physiol. 212:864, 1967.
58. Granholm, L., Lukjanova, L., and Siesjö, B. K.: Evidence of cerebral hypoxia in pronounced hyperventilation. Scand. J. Clin. Lab. Invest. (Suppl. 102):IV C, 1968.
59. Betz, E., Pickerodt, V., and Weidner, A.: Respiratory alkalosis: Effect on CBF, pO_2, and acid-base relations in cerebral cortex with a note on water content. Scand. J. Clin. Lab. Invest. 22(Suppl. 102):4 D, 1968.
60. Christensen, M. S., and Paulson, O. B.: Prolonged artificial hyperventilation in severe cerebral apoplexy. Clinical results and CSF findings in a controlled study. Panminerva Med. 13:201, 1971.
61. Brock, M., Hadjidimos, A. A., Deruaz, J. P., Fischer, F., Dietz, H., Kohlmeyer, K., Poll, W., and Schurmann, K.: Effects of hyperventilation on regional cerebral blood flow on the role of changes in intracranial pressure and tissue perfusion pressure for shifts in rCBF distribution. *In* Toole, J. F., Moossy, J., and Janeway, R. (eds.): *Cerebral Vascular Diseases, Proceedings of the Seventh Princeton Conference,* New York, Grune & Stratton, 1971, pp. 114–123.
62. Meyer, J. S., Fukuuchi, Y., Shimazu, K., Ohuchi, T., and Ericsson, D.: Effect of intravenous infusion of glycerol on hemispheric blood flow and metabolism in patients with acute cerebral infarction. Stroke 3:168, 1972.
63. Ng, L. K. Y., and Nimminnitya, J.: Massive cerebral infarction with severe brain swelling. Stroke 1:158, 1970.
64. Shaw, C., Alvord, E. C., and Berry, R. G.: Swelling of brain following ischemic infarction with arterial occlusion. Arch. Neurol. 1:161, 1959.
65. Meyer, J. S., Charney, J. Z., Rivera, V. M., and Mathew, N. T.: Treatment of cerebral edema due to acute cerebral infarction. Lancet 2:993, 1971.
66. Meyer, J. S., Stoica, E., Giri, N. Y., and Shimazu, K.: Cerebral metabolic changes accompanying ischemia of the brain. *In* Lazorthes, G., Bés, A., Guiraud, B., and Géraud, J. (eds.): *Proceedings of the Journées Internationales de Circulation Cérébrale de Toulouse,* 1972.
67. Mathew, N., Meyer, J. S., Rivera, V. M., Charney, J. L., and Hartmann, A.: Double-blind evaluation of glycerol therapy in acute cerebral infarction. Lancet 2:1227–1229, 1972.
68. Freund, G.: The metabolic effects of glycerol administration to diabetic patients. Arch. Intern. Med. 111:123, 1968.
69. Patten, B. M., Mendell, J., Bruun, B., Curtin, W., and Carter, S.: Double-blind study of the effects of dexamethasone on acute stroke. Neurology 22:377, 1972.
70. Gilroy, J., Barnhart, M. I., and Meyer, J. S.: Treatment of acute stroke with dextran 40. J.A.M.A. 210:293, 1969.
71. Leak, D., and Price, R. K.: Low molecular weight dextran in cerebral ischemic episodes. Lancet 1:772, 1964.
72. Browne, T. R., III, and Poskanzer, D. C.: Treatment of strokes. New Eng. J. Med. 218:594, 1964.

73. Meiselman, H. J., Merrill, E. W., and Salzman, E. W.: Effect of dextran on rheology of human blood: Low shear viscometry. J. Appl. Physiol. 22:480, 1967.
74. Cantu, R. C., and Ames, A., III: Experimental prevention of cerebral vasculature obstruction produced by ischemia. J. Neurosurg. 30:50, 1969.
75. Meyer, J. S., Gotoh, F., Gilroy, J., and Nara, M.: Improvement in brain oxygenation and clinical improvement in patients with strokes treated with papaverine hydrochloride. J.A.M.A. 194:957, 1965.
76. Meyer, J. S., Teraura, T., Sakamoto, K., and Hashi, K.: The effect of Pavabid (oral papaverine) on cerebral blood flow and metabolism in the monkey. Cardiov. Res. Cent. Bull. 9:105, 1971.
77. McHenry, L. C., Jr., Jaffe, M. E., Kawamura, J., and Goldberg, H. I.: Effect of papaverine in regional cerebral blood flow in focal vascular disease of the brain. New Eng. J. Med. 282:1167, 1970.
78. Olesen, J., and Paulson, O. B.: The effect of intra-arterial papaverine on regional cerebral blood flow in patients with stroke or intracranial tumor. Stroke 2:148, 1971.
79. Meyer, J. S., Kondo, A., Szewczykowski, J., Nomura, F., and Teraura, T.: The effect of a new drug (hexobendine) on cerebral hemodynamics and oxygen consumption. J. Neurol. Sci. 11:137, 1970.
80. Meyer, J. S., Kanda, T., Shinohara, Y., Fukuuchi, Y., Shimazu, K., Ericsson, A. D., and Gordon, W. H., Jr.: Effect of hexobendine on cerebral hemispheric blood flow and metabolism: Preliminary clinical observations concerning its use in ischemic cerebrovascular disease. Neurology 21:691, 1971.
81. McHenry, L. C., Jr., Jaffe, M. E., Kawamura, J., and Goldberg, H. I.: The effect of hexobendine on regional cerebral blood flow in stroke patients. Neurology 20:375, 1970.
82. Baer, P. E., Faibish, G., Meyer, J. S., and Gay, J. R.: Psychological assessment of vasodilator effects in older cerebrovascular patients. Presented at Gerontological Society annual meeting, December, 1972.
83. Dhrymiotis, A. D., and Whittier, J. R.: Effect of a vasodilator, isoxsuprine, on cerebral ischemic episodes. Curr. Ther. Res. 4:124, 1962.
84. Kuhn, R. A.: Effect of cyclandelate upon cerebral blood flow in patients with "stroke." Angiography 17:422, 1966.
85. Meyer, J. S., Gilroy, J., Barnhart, M. I., and Hohnson, J. F.: Therapeutic thrombolysis in cerebral thrombo-embolism. Randomized evaluation of intravenous streptokinase. In Millikan, C. H., Siekert, R. G., and Whisnant, J. P. (eds.): *Cerebral Vascular Diseases, Proceedings of the Fourth Princeton Conference*. New York, Grune & Stratton, 1965, pp. 200–213.
86. Fletcher, A. P., Alkjaersig, N., O'Brien, J., and Tulevski, V. G.: Blood hypercoagulability and thrombosis. Trans. Ass. Amer. Physicians 83:159, 1970.

Anticoagulant or Surgical Treatment of Cerebral Ischemia*

CLARK H. MILLIKAN

Mayo School of Medicine, Mayo Cerebrovascular Clinical Research Center

Physicians are aware that neurologists constitute a group, some of whom are most reluctant to accept a new idea, particularly if that new idea is a method of treatment. The treatment of a series of serious disorders such as the various categories of cerebrovascular disease is a subject which stimulates almost endless argument, particularly about the most common general subdivision, occlusive cerebrovascular disease, in which the primary pathophysiological event is focal brain ischemia. Some neurologists are not only reluctant to take to the idea of using the stethoscope and ophthalmoscope for the detection of carotid bruits, retinal emboli, ischemic change, and so forth, but are unwilling to even journey to a medical library and inspect the evidence concerning the use of anticoagulants, carotid thromboendarterectomy, vasodilators, steroids, or agents which change the function of blood platelets.

The need to learn a new classification of cerebrovascular disease, pay additional heed to eliciting a complete and accurate history, and add a neurovascular examination to the standard general physical and neurologic examinations before undertaking new methods of treatment may be too much for some to accomplish. However, precise definitions of subcategories of occlusive cerebrovascular disease are mandatory to selection of patients for comparing various methods of treatment; i.e., anticoagulants, thromboendarterectomy, or vasodilators. A classic example of inattention to accuracy is represented by Browne and Poskanzer,[1] who write that there are "no data available affecting the decision . . . of whether to give anticoagulation or perform operation." If the clinical investigator makes

---

* This investigation was supported in part by Research Grant NDS 06663–07 from the National Institutes of Health, Public Health Service.

no distinction between patients with carotid system transient ischemic attacks with ipsilateral amaurosis in some episodes and ipsilateral retinal emboli, patients with global aphasia and right hemiplegia of 36 hours' duration, or patients with a lateral medullary syndrome of 72 hours' duration, he will indeed become more and more confused about "the treatment of choice."

What is the evidence concerning anticoagulant treatment and surgical therapy? First one must define categories. The term "clinical stage" refers to that portion of the temporal profile in which the patient is at a given point in time. The three commonly used categories of clinical stage are: transient ischemic attacks (incipient stroke or impending stroke), progressing stroke (stroke-in-evolution), and completed stroke.

Transient ischemic attacks. TIA are episodes of temporary and focal cerebral dysfunction of vascular origin which are variable in duration, commonly lasting two to 15 minutes but occasionally lasting as long as a day (24 hours). They leave no focal neurologic deficit.

It is important to distinguish between attacks in the carotid arterial system and in the vertebrobasilar system. (Fields et al.[19] confuse the two systems, so that it is impossible to determine the clinical picture of their patients having carotid thromboendarterectomy or no surgery.) Transient ischemic attacks in the carotid system are characterized by weakness or numbness limited to one side of the body or a part of one side of the body, dysphasia if the dominant hemisphere is involved, and impaired vision (amaurosis fugax) limited to the eye on the side of temporarily defective blood flow. In some patients there may be physical signs of appropriate arterial occlusive disease, including diminished pulsation in the carotid artery, a bruit over the carotid artery or eye, emboli in the retinal vessels, ischemic retinopathy, and/or relative hypotension in the retinal arteries measured with the ophthalmodynamometer. These are only signs of arterial disease and may be present in the absence of a history of transient ischemic attacks or may be absent in the presence of a history of transient ischemic attacks!

Transient ischemic attacks in the vertebrobasilar arterial system are also characterized by swift onset, average duration of five to 20 minutes, and rapid disappearance, leaving the patient normal. The variety of manifestations produced by focal ischemia in this arterial distribution is considerably more variable and complex than in the carotid system. The matter of the relative significance of a symptom or a pattern of symptoms is important. For instance, if one asks the question, "Have you ever had any dizziness?" almost all adults will answer, "Yes." This question is almost completely nonselective (nondiagnostic), and if answered affirmatively must be followed by a series of direct and branching questions to establish the meaning and impact (significance) of the symptom (dizziness) on the patient. While vertigo is the most common of all vertebrobasilar TIA symptoms, a diagnosis of a vertebrobasilar TIA should *not* be made with a history of a few minutes of vertigo as the only symptom. When vertigo is accompanied by one or more symptoms such as monoplegia, diploplia, bilateral defects in the visual fields, dysarthria, or dysphagia the diagnosis is probably correct. Limb weakness or defect in sensation is commonly bilateral and may shift from place to place in different attacks. Convulsive events are uncommon, and loss of consciousness is rare. While there may be bruits suggesting compromise of flow in the innominate artery, in either subclavian artery, or at the origin of either vertebral artery, the absence or presence of such sounds does not weigh heavily in the diagnosis. The diagnosis is dependent upon the history of the attacks.

Progressing strokes. A stroke-in-evolution is that temporal category in which there has been progression (increased severity of the neurologic signs) within recent minutes; this value judgment may be made from analysis of the history or by repeated examination of the patient. It may be difficult to be certain from minute to minute or even from hour to hour whether progression will occur. However, if there has been definite worsening of the neurologic deficit during the few minutes immediately prior to making a judgment about a particular patient's status, the situation should be classified as a progressing cerebral infarction (stroke-in-evolution). If the site of focal ischemia is in the carotid system, 18 to 24 hours without progression is ordinarily sufficient time to mean that further progression is unlikely and that the status of the temporal profile should no longer be categorized as "progressing stroke." If the lesion is in brain supplied by the vertebrobasilar system, a longer period of time (up to 72 hours) should probably elapse before the patient is removed from the progressing stroke category and is designated as a "completed stroke," since there is a tendency for periods of progression to be separated by many hours. In some instances, at a given point in time, it may be impossible to be certain whether a patient is having a TIA of unusually long duration or is having the initial component of a progressing stroke. There are also situations, difficult to classify in a precise fashion, when there are frequent TIA's close together in time in which mild residual neurologic deficit accumulates and is detected on neurologic examination; the physician suspects that a small cerebral infarct is present, even though the patient denies any symptoms between the episodes.

Completed stroke. This refers to a category in which the focal neurologic deficit is stable; the number of hours suggested for making this decision has just been discussed under progressing stroke. The word "completed" does not imply that a particular neurologic sign has become maximal in quantity, i.e., hemiplegia as distinguished from hemiparesis, but refers only to the temporal aspect of the event. A cerebral infarct may be judged to be completed when the neurologic deficit is minor, but also when the neurologic deficit is severe.

Evidence Concerning Anticoagulant Treatment of Transient Ischemic Attacks

A number of studies of the natural history of transient ischemic attacks have been published. The results of these studies are summarized in Table 1. Three studies report that less than 20 per cent of patients with transient ischemic attacks developed cerebral infarction (completed stroke). Ziegler's[2] patients did not include individuals with severe heart disease or hypertension, and 62 per cent of those having angiography had less than 10 per cent stenosis of any cervical-

Table 1. *Natural History of Untreated Transient Ischemic Attacks*

STUDY	NUMBER OF PATIENTS	FOLLOW-UP (MONTHS)	NORMAL	CEREBRAL INFARCT (TOTAL)	CEREBRAL INFARCT (LETHAL)	CEREBRAL HEMORRHAGE
Mayo Clinic[6]	160	60	83 (52%)	51 (32%)	18 (11%)	7 (4%)
Cooperative Study[7]	20	20	?	5 (25%)	1 (5%)	0
Fisher[8]	23	?	?	8 (34%)	0	0
Pearce et al.[3]	20	10.6	11 (55%)	2 (10%)	?	?
Baker et al.[9]	30	40.6	?	7 (23%)	?	?
Baker et al.[10]	79	41	?	17 (22%)		
Friedman et al.[11]	23	27.4	?	8 (35%)	0	1 (2%) SAH
Marshall[4]	61	45 ?	54 (89%)	1 (2%)	1 (2%)	
Ziegler and Hassanein*[2]	135	36	?	22 (16%)	5 (3.7%)	?

*62 per cent of 93 patients having angiography had less than 10 per cent stenosis of any cervical-cerebral artery.

cerebral artery. Pearce and associates[3] followed the patients for less than a year. Their results suggest that had their patients been observed for 50 or 60 months the percentage of those developing cerebral infarction would have been the highest recorded. The experience noted by Marshall[4] is the only one that is entirely different from any other reported in the literature. This observation is particularly strange, as Marshall[5] reported earlier that same year that 68 (43 per cent) of 158 patients with TIA's developed cerebral infarction during a follow-up of nearly five years! One can, therefore, only conclude that the series reported by Marshall (in Table 1) is not only entirely different from those of other authors, but is even different from his own experience and does not represent the natural history of transient ischemic attacks. Based on the available data, 25 to 40 per cent of patients with transient ischemic attacks (presuming that each patient has had more than one attack) will eventually have cerebral infarction if followed as long as five years.

Six studies have been done in which a direct attempt was made to compare the results of anticoagulant therapy of transient ischemic attacks with no treatment. The results are summarized in Table 2. Variations in patient response to a particular dose of anticoagulant occur, as with attempted control of diabetes or hypertension; however, the treatment was supervised by expert personnel and the control of anticoagulant was as well maintained as is practical. In Table 2 the number of months of follow-up are listed; in the study of Pearce and associates[3] the time was less than a year. This means that there is little or no difference in their results compared to those of the other investigators. Although five of the reports contain too few patients to permit traditional statistical evaluation of the results, it is of special interest that the percentage of individuals developing cerebral infarction was so similar (a spread of from 3 to 7 per cent) in all the treated groups. Cerebral hemorrhage occurred in 7 per cent of the patients receiving anticoagulants in the series reported from the Mayo Clinic.[6] However, during five years' observation of similar untreated patients, the Mayo investigators reported that 4 per cent had intracerebral hemorrhage. Apparently this type of patient (with cerebrovascular disease) is at high risk for cerebral hemorrhage, and some

Table 2. *Anticoagulant Therapy and Transient Ischemic Attacks*

STUDY	NUMBER OF PATIENTS	FOLLOW-UP (MONTHS)	NORMAL	CEREBRAL INFARCT (TOTAL)	CEREBRAL INFARCT (LETHAL)	CEREBRAL HEMORRHAGE
Mayo Clinic[6]						
Control	160	60	83 (52%)	51 (32%)	18 (11%)	7 (4%)
Treated	175	60	131 (75%)	7 (4%)	3 (2%)	13 (7%)
Cooperative Study[7]						
Control	20	20	?	5 (25%)	1 (5%)	0
Treated	24	18	?	1 (4%)	0	2 (8%)
Fisher[8]						
Control	23	?	?	8 (34%)	0	0
Treated	29	30	?	1 (3%)	0	0
Pearce et al.[3]						
Control	20	10.6	11 (55%)	2 (10%)	?	?
Treated	17	11.1	7 (41%)	2 (5%)	?	?
Baker et al.[9]						
Control	30	40.6	?	7 (23%)*	?	2
Treated	30	37.9	?	2 (7%)	?	0†
Friedman et al.[11]						
Control	23	27.4		8 (35%)‡	0	1 (4%) SAH
Treated	21	27.4		0	0	0

*Three patients randomized as treated had CVA after A/C stopped.
†One cerebral hemorrhage in treated group, but while *off* anticoagulant.
‡One patient had been on A/C, but A/C was discontinued before the cerebral infarction.

of the instances of intracerebral hemorrhage in the patients receiving anticoagulant might have occurred had the individual not been taking such a drug. In Table 2 the number of TIA's reported (by either treated or untreated patients) is not recorded since all authors mention that for all practical purposes TIA's stop while the patient is receiving an anticoagulant; in many instances the untreated patients continue to have attacks.

From the observations of cessation of transient ischemic attacks in patients receiving anticoagulants and, particularly, of the lowered incidence of cerebral infarction during therapy, it is concluded that anticoagulant therapy significantly decreases the risk of cerebral infarction in patients with transient ischemic attacks. In a carefully selected group of such patients, anticoagulant therapy is very worthwhile, provided the anticoagulant program is so managed as to keep the number of complications at a minimum.

Evidence Concerning Results of Surgical Treatment of Transient Ischemic Attacks

It is shocking to realize that although the first operation on a carotid artery for TIA was reported by Eastcott, Pickering, and Rob[12] in 1954, there are no valid data available in the literature concerning the effect of surgery in preventing subsequent cerebral infarction. Table 3 lists data from some of the reports. Reports

Table 3. Surgical Therapy and Transient Ischemic Attacks

SERIES	NUMBER OF PATIENTS	OPERATIVE DEATHS	OPERATIVE MORBIDITY	FOLLOW-UP (MONTHS)	NORMAL	TOTAL CEREBRAL INFARCT	TOTAL DEATHS
Thompson[14]	151	2	0	24–30	114 (75%)	10 ? (7%)	22 (15%)
Wylie and Ehrenfeld[13]	129	0	0	48	?	?	36 (28%)
Joint Study[19]	169	6 (3%)	13 (8%)	42	70 (41%)	25 (15%)	20 (12%)
DeWeese et al.[22]	187	4 (2%)	18 (10%)	24 ?	109 ? (58%)	37 ? (20%)	50 (27%)
Kuster and Wallace[23]	66	1	?	?	50 (75%)	7 ?	7 (11%)
Siekert, Whisnant, and Millikan[21]	32	1	5 (15.6%)	30	24 (75%)	9 (28%)	5 (15.6%)

from individual institutions leave many questions unanswered, or leave the reader incredulous. For example, Wylie and Ehrenfeld[13] write of 129 operated patients without any operative mortality and *not a single* complication; but while the reader learns that after 48 months' follow-up 28 per cent of the patients are dead, the crucial information (number of patients having cerebral infarcts) is not mentioned. Thompson[14] reported two operative deaths in 151 patients and *not a single* complication. Definite information concerning the duration of follow-up and the incidence of cerebral infarction is not available.

Over seven million dollars has been spent on the "Joint Study of Extracranial Arterial Occlusion."[15-19] It was hoped that valuable information concerning the results of surgical treatment would come from this tremendous expenditure. Unfortunately there are so many defects in the project that the practicing physician cannot find the answers he seeks—answers necessary for the successful treatment of individual patients. Defects in the study include:

1. No information concerning the frequency or severity of the attacks.

2. More patients with unilateral carotid stenosis as the only arterial abnormality had vertebrobasilar TIA's than had carotid TIA's. This has produced a group of patients which members of the study agree do not actually exist;[20] indicating a fundamental defect in the design of the investigation.

3. The content of the attacks is not available; i.e., how many carotid patients had amaurosis as part of the attacks.

4. No information is available about bruits.

5. Patients were not fully examined; there are no data about retinal artery pressures and no mention is made of retinal emboli.

6. There is no correlation of the type of lesion in the arteriogram (degree of stenosis, ulceration, and so forth) with the physical signs or symptoms.

7. Variations in the type of surgical operation (hypercarbia, anticoagulant, shunt, patch-graft, anesthesia) eliminate the possibility of even knowing which operation has the lowest morbidity and mortality.

8. There is no way to assess the quality of any of the data: how many patients were contributed by a particular institution; even more important, who saw the patients and filled out the forms—secretaries, clerks, medical students, interns.

9. No data are available about the natural history of TIA's; there is no way to know which patients received anticoagulants, antihypertensive drugs, digitalis, weight reduction, insulin, clofibrate, and so forth.

Each of these defects is significant enough to put the conclusions of the Joint Study to serious question; the total impact of so many defects makes the conclusions worthless.

Years ago Siekert et al.[21] reported initial observations of a small group of surgically treated carotid TIA patients. After 30 months of follow-up, 12 per cent of the patients had a cerebral infarct, compared to 20 per cent of similar untreated patients. However, inclusion of operative morbidity and mortality changed the figure to 28 per cent. When one recalls that TIA patients are neurologically normal at the time of surgery, a mortality-morbidity rate of 28 per cent, or even the 11 per cent reported by the Joint Study, is unacceptable.

Although millions of dollars have been made by surgeons operating on the carotid arteries, we don't know that strokes have been prevented or improved!

There is, however, a special group of carotid TIA patients who are at high risk of *immediate* cerebral infarction. These are individuals who have evidence of a carotid lesion which is actively producing pathophysiological events at that moment. The evidence includes a history of recent carotid system TIA (generally with amaurosis fugax as a part of the pattern) and one or more of the following: (1) a long >2/6 (on a basis of 6) carotid bruit, sometimes changing; (2) retinal emboli; (3) significant unilateral ↓ retinal artery pressure; or (4) ischemic retinopathy. Experience at Mayo Clinic with patients having this clinical constellation of symptoms and signs indicates that immediate intravenous administration of heparin (unless some unique contraindication is present) followed promptly by arteriography to display the cervical and intracranial cerebral circulation (again presuming no contraindications) is the proper method of management. Appropriate arterial surgery is performed immediately after the arteriogram.

Evidence Concerning Anticoagulant Treatment of Progressing Stroke

Unfortunately there is considerable variation in the type of patient accepted into this category. The patient should be placed in the "progressing stroke" group when there is a prehospital history of progressing symptoms and signs during the very immediate few minutes (up to two or three hours) before admission or when there has been an increase in severity or distribution of the neurologic deficit after admission to the hospital. If patients are included whose neurologic deficit reached its maximum degree 24 hours prior to admission or certainly as long as 48 or 72 hours before admission, one will find that the "progressing stroke" category includes many individuals in whom the dynamic pathophysiological process has stopped its progression. Inclusion of such patients can only accrue to the relative advantage of any scheme of treatment, since in such patients there is no progression to treat! That is, the absence of progression indicates that the pathophysiological process has reached its maximum degree, and from that point in time on, the natural history of such patients is usually one of improvement, sometimes at a fairly rapid rate. An example of this incorrect categorization is in a study by Gilroy, Barnhart, and Meyer[24] concerning the use of low molecular weight dextran in the treatment of "progressing stroke." Patients were included in the treated group in whom progression had not occurred for 72 hours; observations by Jones and Millikan[25] show that 96 per cent of such patients would have no further progression!

Another variation in the type of patient accepted into this category was pointed out by Whisnant.[26] He mentioned that little distinction is made in some instances between progressing stroke in the territory of the vertebrobasilar system as contrasted to the carotid system. Whisnant reported a mortality of 8.5 per cent with anticoagulant treatment of patients having progressing stroke in the vertebrobasilar system, whereas 58.9 per cent of a similar untreated group died. He went on to say: "The confusion has arisen in the literature regarding the mortality of vertebral-basilar thrombosis from the inclusion in this category of limited brain stem infarcts—that is, well localized infarcts in the distribution of a single arterial branch. Since these limited lesions in the stem have a fairly good prognosis, the inclusion of these obviously lowers the mortality rate." Thus, Whisnant found that of 140 patients treated with anticoagulant, where there had been progression with fluctuation or stepwise accumulation of the neurologic deficit related to the territory of more than a single arterial branch of the vertebral artery or vertebrobasilar system, 12 patients died; whereas of 39 not receiving anticoagulant, 23 died.

There are few reports in the literature in which the term "progressing stroke" is used in relatively uniform fashion and in which a comparison is made between a group of patients treated with anticoagulant medication and a group not receiving such treatment. Because of the acute, often emergent, nature of the disorder, the intravenous administration of heparin is generally the way that anticoagulant treatment is initiated, and it is common practice to then continue with an oral anticoagulant, at least during the period of hospitalization. The extraordinary variability in the natural history of acute progressing stroke makes it mandatory that comparison be made by the individual investigator or group of investigators of treated and untreated patients of similar type. An example of this variability was demonstrated objectively at Mayo Clinic[27] about two decades ago when the natural history of 204 consecutive patients with acute onset of progressing stroke in the carotid system was observed. At 14 days after the onset, 12 per cent of the patients were normal, 5 per cent (using motor phenomena as a basis for comparison) had varying degrees of monoparesis, 69 per cent had varying degrees of hemiparesis, and 14 per cent were dead. It should be obvious that the quality of the observations made at the bedside of such patients must be of high order or valid inferences cannot be drawn from either group or from a comparison.

Table 4 summarizes those studies reported in the literature which, in general, fulfill the above qualifications. In each investigation a primary determination was

Table 4. *Anticoagulant Treatment for Progressing Stroke*

STUDY	NUMBER OF PATIENTS	FOLLOW-UP (MONTHS)	CEREBRAL INFARCT (LETHAL)	CEREBRAL HEMORRHAGE (LETHAL)	PROGRESSIVE INFARCT	TOTAL PROGRESSIVE
Mayo Clinic[28]						
Control	60	12	25 (42%)	0	8 (13%)	55%
Treated	181	12	12 (7%)	0	25 (14%)	20%
Carter[29]						
Control	38	6	7 (17%)	0	12 (33%)	50%
Treated	38	6	3 (7%)	0	9 (24%)	32%
Cooperative Study[7]						
Control	67	15	10 (15%)	0	21 (31%)	46%
Treated	61	12	5 (8%)	1 (2%)	8 (13%)	23%
Fisher[8]						
Control	14	?	0	0	9	64%
Treated	14	?	0	0	3	21%
Fisher (National Study)[30]						
Control	49	7.4	7		14 (29%)	20 (40%)
Treated	51	5.7	4	1	7 (14%)	7 (14%)

made of the state of the patient at the time of the patient's admission to the study —progression of the neurologic deficit had taken place in the preceding few minutes. There was frequent re-evaluation of the neurologic deficit, and subsequently comparison was made between the maximal defect developed and the defect present at the point of entry into the study. The percentage of patients showing progression of neurologic deficit (after primary assessment) in the control and treated groups of each report is in the right hand column of the table. In each instance the treated group fared considerably better than those not receiving anticoagulant; that is, in the Mayo study[28] 20 per cent of those treated showed evidence of neurologic progression after entry into the study, whereas 52 per cent of patients not receiving anticoagulant showed progression after initial evaluation. The figures concerning the Fisher (National) Study[30] are difficult to interpret but are included, since the patients were said to be randomized. Fisher said, "In regard to progression of the infarction, the number of patients is 14 in the control and 7 in the treated group. Now, if we analyze the number of episodes of progression and classify them as early (within two weeks of randomization) and late (after two weeks) there were in the control group 11 early and 9 late and in the treated group 6 early and 1 late. If one adds these together, one gets 20 episodes in the control group and 7 episodes in the treated group; this suggests that anticoagulants were having a beneficial effect on the process of thrombosis and infarction."

In Fisher's[8] own personally observed patients it is apparent that the total number of subjects is too small to provide a statistically significant result. However, the trend was very definite, with only 21 per cent of the treated patients showing progression, as contrasted to 64 per cent of those not receiving anticoagulant. The observations of the cooperative group,[7] in 1962, confirmed this trend, with twice as many nontreated patients having progression after entry into the study compared with those individuals receiving anticoagulant. Thus, it is evident that in a few carefully performed investigations of the use of anticoagulant for acute progressing stroke, the evidence in each study points to a lack of progression in patients receiving anticoagulant as contrasted to those individuals not getting such drugs.

Evidence Concerning the Surgical Treatment of Progressing Stroke

Blaisdell[31] writes, "At the present time (arteriographic) evaluation is not considered indicated in the following three groups of patients, either because of the high risk of surgery or because of the small possibility of a favorable result: (1) patients with an acute neurologic deficit, (2) those with severe disability from a previous stroke, and (3) those with heart disease." The first of these contraindications was probably a result of experience in the Joint Study,[18] in which the mortality was 42 per cent in 50 patients operated upon within two weeks following an acute stroke and was 20 per cent for patients not having surgery. Bruetman et al.[32] and Wylie and his associates[33] have reported intracerebral hemorrhage as a complication of carotid surgery. In these reports all one can learn about the patients is that they were in coma, semicoma, or stupor and had arteriography and surgery. No information is available about the nature and quantity of the focal neurologic lesion, carotid bruits, retinal artery pressures, retinal emboli, and so forth. It is most unfortunate that the Joint Study[15-19] did not include neurovascular examination of the patients and some effort to record accurately the neurologic status of the patients during the first few hours of entry into the study. If attention had been directed to these matters, an important group of progressing stroke patients would have appeared, a group in which emergency anticoagulant treatment and surgery are indicated. At Mayo Clinic over 20 patients, similar to the one reported at Princeton[34] in January, 1972, have been examined and treated. From our current experience the indications for this emergency treatment are:

I. Clinical events

    A. Cluster of frequent severe carotid TIA's (a persisting mild neurologic deficit accumulates as evidence of mild progressing stroke), or

    B. Recent mild cerebral infarction (carotid system), followed by a cluster of TIA's or

    C. Onset of a focal neurologic deficit during or soon after arteriography or

    D. Immediate postoperative thrombosis (following carotid thromboendarterectomy)

AND

II. Physical signs (which, added to the clinical events, suggest that the basic pathologic process is currently active):

    A. Retinal emboli (most commonly cholesterol), or

    B. Long systolic or systolic-diastolic bruit of grade 2 or 3 or more (on the basis of 6) over the carotid bifurcation, or

    C. Ipsilateral decrease in retinal artery pressure

A changing carotid bruit[34] suggests a change in the morphology of the carotid lesion; further experience may show that this phenomenon should be added to the above list of physical signs.

Blaisdell's[31] second contraindication (those with severe disability from a recent or old cerebral infarct) has been used at Mayo Clinic since 1955. Emergency or elective angiography and endarterectomy are not indicated in patients with acute or old completed cerebral infarction when the neurologic deficit is severe, for example, when there is aphasia and/or hemiplegia.

The third contraindication listed by Blaisdell[31] (patients with heart disease), if followed precisely, would eliminate most patients. It seems likely that Blaisdell is actually referring to patients with recent myocardial infarction, heart failure, severe angina, and so forth, rather than including all patients with any evidence of heart disease.

As has been implied in the above discussion, it is mandatory that the physician take a careful history and do a careful general, neurologic, and neurovascular examination in order to make correct decisions about the use of surgery in progressing stroke. Each patient must be correctly categorized and the indications for emergency surgery must be followed as listed above.

Evidence Concerning the Anticoagulant Treatment of Completed Stroke

The objective of anticoagulant treatment in this category is to prevent recurrent thrombosis or embolism in all parts of the body, including the brain. There has never been any theoretical or practical reason to believe that anticoagulation would promote healing of damaged brain tissues or return of injured neurons to normal function other than by the protection of the existing blood supply and the prevention of further occlusive events, either embolic, thrombotic, or thromboembolic. The subject is made additionally complex, since often no distinction is made between (1) patients with massive neurologic damage as the residua of cerebral infarction (patients for whom only custodial care remains as a way of life) and individuals who have so little damage that return to their usual occupation is feasible, and (2) cerebral infarcts caused by emboli from a cardiac source (myocardial infarction with mural thrombus, abnormalities of cardiac rhythm, and so forth) and emboli from an intramural source (ulcerated carotid plaque, thrombus, or atherosclerosis). Arranging the components of (1) and (2) produces patient problems with important differences. For instance, the relatively young person with atrial fibrillation who has mild neurologic impairment from a cardiac embolus might philosophically be a fine candidate for long-term anticoagulant therapy (if the patient were at high risk and anticoagulant would significantly lower the risk), while a person of 70 years, aphasic and hemiplegic from an embolus from a myocardial infarct, would be a very inappropriate candidate for such treatment. Likewise, anticoagulant therapy and surgical reconstruction of a carotid artery may also be viewed with varying enthusiasm, related to the degree of permanent brain damage after the completed stroke and the morphology of the carotid lesion at the time for decision about treatment.

Unfortunately the literature concerning anticoagulant therapy in completed stroke does not make these distinctions; this may account for the difference of opinion about the value of the treatment. Table 5 is a summary of those reports in which the authors used a standard definition of "completed stroke" and compared groups of treated and untreated patients. Three of the five investigations report fewer cerebral infarcts in the treated than in the control patients; in one instance there is a dramatic difference in favor of treatment (McDowell et al.[37]). Severe hemorrhage was related almost exclusively to treated patients and in two series was 10 or more per cent. Variable periods of follow-up make evaluation of the data difficult. In the study by Howell et al.,[39] as listed in Table 5, the treated patients were followed for only 16 months, while the control patients had a follow-up of 36 months and, therefore, over twice as long a time period during which to have repeated cerebral infarcts. The authors counted the number of strokes in the first 16 months in both series; in the control there were 12 and in the treated group there was one; there continued to be a suggestion of beneficial prevention by the medication. The Cooperative Group[7] found a recurrence of cerebral infarct in 42 per cent of treated patients followed only 10 months, while only 27 per cent of the control group followed 16 months had one or more recurrent infarcts. The treated patients had a 10 per cent incidence of severe

Table 5. *Anticoagulant Therapy for Completed Stroke*

STUDY	NUMBER OF PATIENTS	FOLLOW-UP (MONTHS)	CEREBRAL INFARCTS (TOTAL)	CEREBRAL INFARCTS (LETHAL)	SEVERE HEMORRHAGE
Cooperative Group[7]					
Control	60	16	16 (27%)	5 (8%)	0
Treated	72	10	30 (42%)	6 (8%)	7 (10%)
Hill et al.[36]					
Control	65	31	19 (29%)	1 (2%)	0
Treated	66	28	22 (33%)	5 (8%)	7 (11%)
McDowell et al.[37]					
Control	99	33.5	22 (22%)	7 (7%)	2 (2%)
Treated	92	42.2	1 (1%)	1	7 (7.6%)
Enger and Boyesen[38]					
Control	49	39.2	8 (16%)	3 (6%)	0
Treated	51	22.8	4 (8%)	1 (2%)	3 (6%)*
Howell et al.[39]					
Control	92	36	28 (30%)	?	0
Treated	103	16	7 (7%)	?	4 (4%)

*Patients hypertensive—not treated.

hemorrhage. This combination of events, on the basis of this one study, shows that anticoagulant therapy is contraindicated for completed stroke.

In another type of study Marshall and Shaw[40] tried "to assess the influence of anticoagulant treatment on the immediate mortality—i.e., within six weeks of the cerebrovascular accident." The criterion for admission into the study, either into the group treated with anticoagulant or into a group not so treated, was that within *72 hours* before admission the patient had sustained a severe focal neurologic deficit thought to be due to cerebral infarction. By using the paired patient technique, the authors observed that the treatment could not possibly be effective, so the study was stopped at a point at which the results were inconclusive in that there was no statistical evidence that the treatment was dangerous.

Therefore, there continues to be a definite difference of opinion about the results of the use of anticoagulants in this broad category (completed stroke) of cerebrovascular disease. Anticoagulants, administered on a long-term basis, must be considered dangerous, and every effort should be made to control precisely the level of the anticoagulant action. Hypertension must be effectively controlled; certain relative contraindications to the use of the medicine are impaired hepatic, renal, or gastroenterologic function.

Prevention of Recurrent Thromboembolic Events (Cardiac Source) with Long-Term Anticoagulant Therapy

Currently it is very important to distinguish a cerebral embolic event of cardiac source (rheumatic heart disease, atrial fibrillation, myocardial infarction with mural thrombus, and so forth) from a cerebral embolic event of intra-arterial source (ulcerated carotid plaque, carotid or other arterial friable thrombus with

Table 6. *Anticoagulant Therapy and Recurrent Thromboembolic Events from a Cardiac Source*

	OFF ANTICOAGULANT				ON ANTICOAGULANT		
	Number of Patients	Patient Months	Total No. Thromboembolic Events	Cerebral Emboli	Patient Months	Total No Thromboembolic Events	Cerebral Emboli
Askey and Cherry[41]	20	?	?	?	260	Says decreased	
Cosgriff[42]	18	?	?	?	200	2	?
Wright and McDevitt[43]	57	795	205	81	1162	23	6
McDevitt[44]	47	1437	132	33	1315	27	5

embolus, and so forth). The former makes up almost all the traditional literature about cerebral embolism and the latter, the most common phenomena, appeared about two decades ago in discussion of the pathogenesis of transient ischemic attacks. This section concerns long-term prevention of cerebral emboli from a cardiac source.

Although it is common practice to administer anticoagulant orally (long-term) to prevent recurrent thromboembolic events from a cardiac source, there has been little actual comparison of treated and untreated patients. The triad of rheumatic heart disease, mitral stenosis, and atrial fibrillation has long been associated with emboli to various organs, often the brain. Table 6 lists some of the meager data in the literature. Mainly on the basis of the observations by Wright and McDevitt,[43] internists and neurologists administer oral anticoagulant, often starting treatment after the first embolic event. Carter[45] states that recurrence rate after embolism (from a cardiac source) is about 50 per cent in the first year and writes, "I have found that this incidence could be significantly reduced in the first six months by continuing anticoagulant therapy as a prophylactic measure." He cautions that if rheumatic atrial fibrillation is the source of cerebral embolism, the anticoagulant therapy must be continued indefinitely unless sinus rhythm is restored.

Cardiac sources of emboli include prosthetic heart valves. The usual treatment for prevention (long-term oral anticoagulant) is being reinvestigated. Sullivan et al.[46] reported that only one patient of 42 (553 months' follow-up) had two embolic events while receiving dipyridamole and anticoagulant, whereas nine patients of 50 (695 months' follow-up) had 17 embolic events while receiving anticoagulant and a placebo.

Summary

The clinical stages of cerebrovascular disease must be defined in order to accurately assess the value of a method of treatment. The three commonly used clinical stages are: (1) transient ischemic attacks (incipient or impending stroke); (2) progressing stroke (stroke-in-evolution); and (3) completed stroke.

The evidence in the medical literature is that:

1. Treatment with anticoagulant generally stops transient ischemic attacks and lowers the incidence of cerebral infarction (the treatment has danger and must be carefully managed).

2. Carotid thromboendarterectomy is often performed for transient ischemic attacks. The morbidity-mortality of surgery varies widely; in the series of patients reported by the Joint Study there were so many defects in the design of the investigation that evaluation of the treatment is worthless, and the value of surgery is not really known.

3. Anticoagulant treatment of certain carefully selected patients with progressing cerebral infarction in the carotid or vertebrobasilar arterial distributions significantly decreases the amount of progression, compared to similar untreated patients.

4. There continues to be a definite difference of opinion about long-term anticoagulant therapy for completed stroke. The treatment must be considered dangerous and every effort made to control the level of anticoagulant action. Arterial hypertension must be effectively controlled.

5. It is common practice to administer anticoagulant orally (long-term) to prevent recurrent thromboembolic events from a cardiac source.

Finally, evidence from the Mayo Clinic is that emergent (intravenous heparin) anticoagulant therapy followed immediately by carotid thromboendarterectomy is indicated when the clinical events and physical signs listed on page 797 are present.

References

1. Browne, T. R., III, and Poskanzer, D. C.: Treatment of strokes (first of two parts). New Eng. J. Med. 281:594–602, 1969.
2. Ziegler, D. K., and Hassanein, R.: Prognosis in patients with transient ischemic attacks. Stroke. 4:(July) 1973.
3. Pearce, J. M. S., Gubbay, S. S., and Walton, J. N.: Long-term anticoagulant therapy in transient cerebral ischemic attacks. Lancet 1:6–9, 1965.
4. Marshall, J.: The natural history of transient ischemic cerebrovascular attacks. Quart. J. Med. 33:309–324, 1964.
5. Marshall, J.: *In* Millikan, C. H., Siekert, R. G., and Whisnant, J. P.: *Cerebral Vascular Diseases. Transactions of the Fourth Princeton Conference.* New York, Grune & Stratton, 1965, p. 194.
6. Siekert, R. G., Whisnant, J. P., and Millikan, C. H.: Surgical and anticoagulant therapy of occlusive cerebrovascular disease. Ann. Intern. Med. 58:637–641, 1963.
7. Baker, R. N., Broward, J. A., Fang, H. C., Fisher, C. M., Groch, S. N., Heyman, A., Karp, H. R., McDevitt, E., Scheinberg, P., Schwartz, W., and Toole, J. F.: Anticoagulant therapy in cerebral infarction. Neurology 12:823–835, 1962.
8. Fisher, C. M.: The use of anticoagulants in cerebral thrombosis. Neurology 8:311–332, 1958.
9. Baker, R. N., Schwartz, W. S., and Rose, A. S.: Transient ischemic attacks—a report of a study of anticoagulant treatment. Neurology 16:841–847, 1966.
10. Baker, R. N., Ramseyer, J. C., and Schwartz, W. S.: Prognosis in patients with transient cerebral ischemic attacks. Neurology 18:11–57, 1968.
11. Friedman, G. D., Wilson, S., Mosier, J. M., Colandrea, M. A., and Nichaman, M. Z.: Transient ischemic attacks in a community. J.A.M.A. 210:1428–1432, 1969.

12. Eastcott, H. H. G., Pickering, G. W., and Rob, C. G.: Reconstruction of internal carotid artery in patient with intermittent attacks of hemiplegia. Lancet 2:994, 1954.
13. Wylie, E. J., and Ehrenfeld, W. K.: *Extracranial Occlusive Cerebrovascular Disease: Diagnosis and Management*. Philadelphia, W. B. Saunders Company, 1970, pp. 220–221.
14. Thompson, J. E.: *Surgery for Cerebrovascular Insufficiency (Stroke)*. Springfield, Ill., Charles C Thomas, 1968, pp. 42–43.
15. Fields, W. S., North, R. R., Hass, W. K., Galbraith, J. G., Wylie, E. J., Ratinov, G., Burns, M. H., Macdonald, M. C., and Meyer, J. S.: Joint study of extracranial arterial occlusion as a cause of stroke. I. Organization of study and survey of patient population. J.A.M.A. 203:955–960, 1968.
16. Hass, W. K., Fields, W. S., North, R. R., Kricheff, I. I., Chase, N. E., and Bauer, R. B.: Joint study of extracranial arterial occlusion. II. Arteriography, techniques, sites, and complications. J.A.M.A. 203:961–968, 1968.
17. Bauer, R. B., Meyer, J. S, Fields, W. S., Remington, R., Macdonald, M. C., and Callen, P.: Joint study of extracranial arterial occlusion. III. Progress report of controlled study of long-term survival in patients with and without operation. J.A.M.A. 208:509–518, 1969.
18. Blaisdell, W. F., Clauss, R. H., Galbraith, J. G., Imparato, A. M., and Wylie, E. J.: Joint study of extracranial arterial occlusion. IV. A review of surgical considerations. J.A.M.A. 209:1889–1895, 1969.
19. Fields, W. S., Maslenikov, V., Meyer, J. S., Hass, W. K., Remington, R. D., and Macdonald, M.: Joint study of extracranial arterial occlusion. V. Progress report of prognosis following surgery or nonsurgical treatment for transient cerebral ischemic attacks and cervical carotid artery lesions. J.A.M.A. 211:1993–2003, 1970.
20. Hass, W.: In McDowell, F. H., and Brennan, R. W.: *Cerebral Vascular Diseases. Transactions of the Eighth Princeton Conference*. New York, Grune & Stratton, 1972, p. 31.
21. Siekert, R. G., Whisnant, J. P., and Millikan, C. H.: Surgical and anticoagulant therapy of occlusive cerebrovascular disease. Ann. Intern. Med. 58:637–641, 1963.
22. DeWeese, J. A., Rob, C. G., Satran, R., Marsh, D. O., Joynt, R. J., Lipchik, E. O., and Zehl, D. N.: Endarterectomy for atherosclerotic lesions of the carotid artery. J. Cardiov. Surg. 12:299–308, 1971.
23. Kuster, G. G. R., and Wallace, R. B.: Surgical treatment of obstructive disease of the brachiocephalic vessels. Mayo Clin. Proc. 47:572–576, 1972.
24. Gilroy, J., Barnhart, M. I., and Meyer, J. S.: Treatment of acute stroke with dextran 40. J.A.M.A. 210:293–298, 1969.
25. Jones, H. R., Jr., and Millikan, C. H.: The temporal profile of acute cerebral infarction in the distribution of the internal carotid artery. Stroke. In press.
26. Whisnant, J. P.: *In* Millikan, C. H., Siekert, R. G., and Whisnant, J. P.: *Cerebral Vascular Diseases. Transactions of the Third Princeton Conference*. New York, Grune & Stratton, 1961, pp. 156–157.
27. Millikan, C. H.: Evaluation of carbon dioxide inhalation for acute focal cerebral infarction. Arch. Neurol. 73:324–328, 1955.
28. Millikan, C. H.: Anticoagulant therapy in cerebrovascular disease. *In* Siekert, R. G., and Whisnant, J. P.: *Cerebral Vascular Diseases. Transactions of the Fourth Princeton Conference*. New York, Grune & Stratton, 1965, p. 181.
29. Carter, A. B.: Anticoagulant treatment in progressing stroke. Brit. Med. J. 2:70–73, 1961.
30. Fisher, C. M.: Anticoagulant therapy in cerebral thrombosis and cerebral embolism. A national cooperative study, interim report. Neurology 11:119–131, 1961.
31. Blaisdell, F. W.: *In* McDowell, F. H., and Brennan, R. W.: *Cerebral Vascular Diseases. Transactions of the Eighth Princeton Conference*. New York, Grune & Stratton, 1972, p. 13.
32. Bruetman, M. E., Fields, W. S., Crawford, W. S., and DeBakey, M. E.: Cerebral hemorrhage in carotid artery surgery. Arch. Neurol. 9:458–467, 1963.
33. Wylie, E. J., Hein, M. F., and Adams, J. F.: Intracranial hemorrhage following surgical revascularization for treatment of acute strokes. J. Neurosurg. 21:212–215, 1964.
34. Millikan, C. H.: *In* McDowell, F. H., and Brennan, R. W.: *Cerebral Vascular Diseases. Transactions of the Eighth Princeton Conference*. New York, Grune & Stratton, 1972, pp. 23–24.
35. Siekert, R. G., and Millikan, C. H.: Changing carotid bruit in transient cerebral ischemic attacks. Arch. Neurol. 14:302–304, 1966.
36. Hill, A. B., Marshall, J., and Shaw, D. A.: Cerebrovascular disease: Trial of long-term anticoagulant therapy. Brit. Med. J. 2:1003–1006, 1962.

37. McDowell, F., and McDevitt, E.: Treatment of the completed stroke with long-term anticoagulant: six and one-half years' experience. In Siekert, R.G., and Whisnant, J. P.: *Cerebral Vascular Diseases. Transactions of the Fourth Princeton Conference.* New York, Grune & Stratton, 1965, pp. 185–199.
38. Enger, E., and Boyesen, S.: Long-term anticoagulant therapy in patients with cerebral infarction. A controlled clinical study. Acta Med. Scand. *178*(Suppl. 438):1–61, 1965.
39. Howell, D. A., Tatlow, S. F. T., and Feldman, S.: Observations on anticoagulant therapy in thromboembolic disease of the brain. Canad. Med. J. *90*:611–614, 1964.
40. Marshall, J., and Shaw, D. A.: Anticoagulant therapy in acute cerebrovascular accidents. Lancet *1*:995–998, 1960.
41. Askey, J. M., and Cherry, C. B.: Thromboembolism associated with auricular fibrillation. J.A.M.A. *144*:97–100, 1950.
42. Cosgriff, S.: Prophylaxis of recurrent embolism of intracardiac origin. J.A.M.A. *143*:870–872, 1950.
43. Wright, I. S., and McDevitt, E.: Cerebral vascular diseases: Their significance, diagnosis and present treatment, including the selective use of anticoagulant substances. Ann. Intern. Med. *41*:682–698, 1954.
44. McDevitt, E.: Treatment of cerebral embolism. Mod. Treatm. *2*:52–63, 1965.
45. Carter, A. B.: Strokes. Natural history and progression. Proc. Royal Soc. Med. *56*:483–486, 1963.
46. Sullivan, J. M., Harken, D. E., and Gorlin, R.: Effect of dipyridamole on the incidence of arterial emboli after cardiac valve replacement. Circulation *39*(Suppl. 1):I, 149–153, 1969.

The Role of Surgery in Controlling Cerebral Ischemia

JESSE E. THOMPSON

University of Texas Southwestern Medical School

As early as 1856 Savory,[1] on the basis of clinical and postmortem observations, had noted that occlusive lesions in the extracranial segments of the main arteries supplying the brain could be associated with symptoms of cerebral ischemia. A half century later in 1914, Hunt[2] pointed out that extracranial obstructions had been largely overlooked and emphasized the importance of examining the cervical carotid system in patients with strokes. Nevertheless, until recently the prevailing notion held by most physicians was that strokes were caused by intracranial vascular disease. Management of the stroke patient consisted largely of perfunctory rehabilitation measures, since no other therapy was available.

During the past two decades, however, changing concepts of the etiology, diagnosis, and treatment of cerebrovascular insufficiency have been responsible for a widespread renewal of interest in this disease.[3] Increasing awareness of the extracranial location and segmental nature of atherosclerotic occlusive lesions in a large proportion of patients with cerebral ischemia resulted from more widespread use of cerebral arteriography as a clinical diagnostic tool. This was followed by the rapid development and employment of appropriate vascular surgical techniques for removing the obstructing plaques and restoring cerebral blood flow. It is now estimated that 75 per cent of patients with ischemic stroke syndromes have at least one obstructive lesion at a surgically accessible site and that upwards of 50 per cent have the principal occlusions confined to the extracranial vasculature. Another important factor has been the appreciation of the significance of transient ischemic attacks as forerunners of actual strokes.

While improved techniques of rehabilitation have given the patient with a completed stroke a more hopeful outlook, primary emphasis has shifted from rehabilitation to prevention of strokes. The stroke-prone patient has been identified, and measures such as cessation of smoking, reduction in weight, modification of diet, and treatment of diabetes, hypertension, and heart disease have been prescribed. There are few actual data, however, to prove that these measures have resulted in any significant reduction in the incidence of strokes. The only methods of treatment that have been shown to lower the occurrence of strokes in susceptible individuals are: (1) carotid endarterectomy, and (2) long-term anticoagulants.

Surgical measures have assumed an increasingly important role in the definitive management of properly chosen patients with cerebrovascular insufficiency syndromes. It is the author's thesis that surgical correction of accessible extracranial occlusive lesions is the preferred method of treatment if optimal results are to be obtained and strokes are to be prevented.[4]

As experience increases, the indications for surgical therapy are being clarified. However, operation is still not uniformly accepted or employed. There has been no general agreement on indications in most of the clinical categories because of the lack of adequate control data with which to compare the results reported in several large surgical series.

In 1961, therefore, a nationwide Joint Study of Extracranial Arterial Occlusion was begun "to determine the efficacy of arterial reconstructive surgery in the treatment of cerebrovascular disease."[5] Several reports of this randomized study have been published[5-9] and contain a great deal of interesting and important data. Some of the results and conclusions derived from this collaborative effort have been confusing and controversial; in many instances they are at variance with the personal results of a number of surgeons with wide experience in this field. Millikan,[10] an acknowledged authority in cerebrovascular disease, has recently raised questions regarding the value of collaborative studies in general and has leveled severe criticism at the Joint Study of Extracranial Arterial Occlusion in particular. He states "that the answers to key clinical questions have not and will not be forthcoming from the material put together by the Joint Study."

It is the purpose of this article to present my personal experience with the surgical management of cerebrovascular insufficiency, to relate this to the considerable data, both surgical and nonsurgical, available in the literature, and from this analysis to make recommendations as to the proper role of surgery in the treatment of cerebral ischemia. There is no intention of introducing a detailed critique of the Joint Study data.

Classification

The clinical syndromes of cerebrovascular insufficiency vary from a few minor symptoms to the catastrophic stroke. It is important to classify patients into specific clinical categories based on the neurologic status when the patient is first seen. Only in this way can proper therapy be selected and the results of different methods of treatment within the same category be compared. Three groups of patients will be considered here: (1) frank strokes, those patients with neurologic deficits, including acute profound strokes, progressing strokes, recent and old completed strokes, fluctuating deficits, and mild neurologic deficits of more than 24 hours' duration; (2) transient cerebral ischemia, those patients with focal attacks of neurologic dysfuction and transient symptoms of generalized cerebral ischemia lasting minutes or hours, but without residual neurologic deficit at 24 hours; (3) asymptomatic bruits, those patients without neurologic symptoms but with cervical bruits arising from occlusive carotid plaques demonstrated by arteriography.

In addition to a clinical classification, anatomic classification of occlusions by arteriography is necessary. It has been clearly demonstrated that on clinical grounds alone one cannot with any degree of accuracy localize the lesions to the extracranial or intracranial vasculature, or for that matter even to the carotid or vertebrobasilar systems in many instances. Accurate arteriography is obligatory for precise definition of the problem and proper planning of therapy.

The goals of therapy should be clearly defined in every patient with cerebrovascular insufficiency considered for operation. The basic goals of surgical removal of occlusive plaques are to increase cerebral blood flow and to eliminate sources of cerebral emboli. By so doing one hopes to relieve symptoms, improve neurologic deficits, prevent strokes and, if possible, prolong life. The goals differ in the various clinical categories, as will be discussed subsequently. With cerebrovascular insufficiency one is concerned as much with morbidity as with mortality. The disability in a patient with stroke who cannot talk, write, walk, or care for himself is catastrophic, even though he is still alive. The *quality* of survival is thus an important consideration in this field.

Indications and Contraindications

The indications and contraindications for carotid endarterectomy are listed in Table 1. It is generally agreed that patients with acute profound strokes and progressing strokes should not be considered for arteriography or surgery. Mortality rates from 20 to 60 per cent have been reported following operation in the early stages of the disease.[8, 11-13] Morbidity among survivors has been correspondingly high. Operation is contraindicated for cervical occlusions in the presence of severe intracranial disease, but mild intracranial disease is an indication rather than a contraindication. Age in itself is not necessarily a contraindication when the patient's general condition otherwise does not pose any undue hazards.

The indications for operation are based on long-term follow-up studies and will be presented in detail.

Table 1. *Indications for Carotid Endarterectomy in Cerebrovascular Insufficiency*

A. *Contraindications*
 1. Acute profound strokes
 2. Progressing strokes
 3. Severe intracranial disease
 4. Other severe generalized disorders (e.g., cancer)
B. *Indications*
 1. Frank strokes—selected
 2. Transient cerebral ischemia
 3. Asymptomatic bruits—selected

Results of Carotid Endarterectomy

During a 15-year period the author and his associates[14] have performed 879 carotid endarterectomies on 700 patients with cerebrovascular insufficiency. The operative mortality is shown in Table 2, with a breakdown into early and more recent results. In the recent period general anesthesia has been employed, together with the routine use of a temporary inlying bypass shunt for cerebral protection during carotid clamping, and operation has not been performed on patients with acute and progressing strokes. Mortality in the frank stroke group has thus been reduced to half its previous level, while that in the transient ischemia group has been reduced two thirds, to 0.6 per cent. There have been no operative deaths among patients with asymptomatic bruits.

Frank Stroke

A completed stroke is a serious disorder. A recent study[15] gives the mortality within one month of onset of an initial stroke as 33 per cent, with death from subsequent stroke adding an additional 11.5 per cent. Mortality varied with the age of the patient, from 20 per cent in patients 55 years and under to 51 per cent in patients 85 years and over.

While the goals of therapy in this group of patients are to improve neurologic status and to prevent further strokes, a more fundamental consideration is whether these strokes could have been averted in the first place, and if so, how.

The functional results of any method of treatment for frank strokes are difficult to assess since the severity of neurologic deficits at onset varies so widely and the natural history of improvement is so well known. A patient who survives an initial stroke usually improves, at least for a time and to some degree. Thus, postoperative improvement in some patients is consistent with the expected course of the disease and is not necessarily to be attributed to surgical therapy. There is no accurate method at the present time whereby one can determine whether a

Table 2. *Operative Mortality following Carotid Endarterectomy for Cerebrovascular Insufficiency*

CLINICAL CATEGORY	ENTIRE PERIOD 15 YEARS 879 OPERATIONS (PER CENT)	EARLY PERIOD 1957–1963 INCL. 260 OPERATIONS (PER CENT)	RECENT PERIOD 1964–1971 INCL. 619 OPERATIONS (PER CENT)
Frank stroke (288 operations)	6.25	8.7	4.3
Transient cerebral ischemia (478 operations)	0.8	1.7	0.6
Asymptomatic carotid bruit (113 operations)	0	0	0
Totals	2.4	5.0	1.5

neurologic deficit results from cerebral infarction or cerebral ischemia. Reversibility of deficits is unpredictable and may occur when least expected.

The long-term functional results after carotid endarterectomy in 126 surviving patients followed up to 13 years show 30.2 per cent normal, 58.7 per cent improved, 4.7 per cent unchanged, and 6.4 per cent worse. Among 75 deaths during this period, 15 were due to cerebral causes. Thus only 6.9 per cent of the entire series of frank stroke patients died of subsequent strokes.[14]

It is difficult to compare medical and surgical therapy in this group of stroke patients for reasons stated above. Table 3, however, attempts to compare one series of medically treated patients taken from the literature[16] with a similar group of patients in our recent surgical series.

It would appear that in selected patients with frank strokes, endarterectomy has lowered the incidence of recurrent strokes, has decreased the mortality from subsequent stroke, and probably has been responsible for some improvement in neurologic status beyond that to be expected from the natural course of the disease.

On the basis of results observed, the following indications for surgery in the frank stroke group are suggested: The patient with a fixed neurologic deficit from an old stable stroke is not a candidate for operation. As previously mentioned, patients with acute profound and progressing strokes should not be operated upon because of the prohibitive mortality and morbidity. For the patient with a mild, improving neurologic deficit, increase in cerebral blood flow may hasten the improvement, in some instances even to a normal status. If a patient with a previous stable stroke develops new symptoms of ischemia, arteriograms should be performed. Recurrent strokes in such patients usually result from new or different arterial lesions and not from thrombotic extension of the lesion responsible for the original stroke. If a significant carotid lesion is found, operation may well prevent a further stroke.

TRANSIENT CEREBRAL ISCHEMIA

The transient ischemic stage of cerebrovascular insufficiency should be the ideal time for definitive therapy. No neurologic deficit is present, and if the causative lesion can be removed, strokes should be prevented in the majority of patients so treated. Several series of untreated patients with transient cerebral ischemic

Table 3. *Functional Results in Medically and Surgically Treated Patients with Frank Strokes*

AUTHOR	METHOD OF THERAPY	LENGTH OF FOLLOW-UP	NUMBER OF PATIENTS	NORMAL OR IMPROVED (PER CENT)	UNCHANGED (PER CENT)	WORSE (PER CENT)	DEATHS, ALL CAUSES (PER CENT)
Bauer et al[16]	Medical	Up to 42 mos.	73	37	28.8	9.6	24.6
Thompson et al[14]	Surgical	Up to 53 mos.	82	68.2	4.9	4.9	22*

*Of 18 deaths, three were operative and 15 during follow-up. Seven deaths, 8.5 per cent, were due to strokes.

attacks have now been reported in the literature.[17,18] On the average, 35 per cent of these patients developed actual strokes if followed up to five years. In one study from England, Acheson and Hutchinson[19] report the occurrence of strokes in 151 patients with TIA's to be as high as 62 per cent. In my experience, 60 per cent of patients presenting with strokes gave a history of previous transient ischemic episodes.[4]

The goals of surgical therapy in this group are twofold: to relieve the disabling symptoms of transient ischemia, and to prevent strokes. Four parameters will be considered: operative mortality, neurologic complications of operation, long-term functional results, and long-term survival rates.

As shown in Table 2, operative mortality is quite low, being 0.6 per cent when general anesthesia and a temporary shunt are routinely employed. This is an acceptable figure for this elderly (average age 63) group of atherosclerotic patients.

The most serious complication of carotid endarterectomy is the occurrence of neurologic deficits. If one is to advocate surgery for patients with transient cerebral ischemia, it is imperative that every effort be made to avoid such complications. General anesthesia, maintenance of normal blood pressure, gentleness during dissection, routine use of a shunt, and the avoidance of postoperative hypotension and hypertension combine to give the lowest complication rates. In my series the incidence of transient deficits related to operation has been 0.76 per cent, while that of permanent deficits, both mild and severe, has been 1.5 per cent.[20] These figures are acceptable for this group of patients.

Long-term functional results following carotid endarterectomy have been quite satisfactory. Of 210 survivors followed up to 13 years, 81 per cent have had no further attacks, while an additional 15.7 per cent have had fewer attacks of less severity.[14] Table 4 shows a comparison of one group of our surgical patients with a group of untreated patients and a group of patients treated with anticoagulants, taken from the literature,[21] all having transient cerebral ischemic attacks. The occurrence of strokes, fatal and nonfatal, in the surgical group is less than one tenth that in the untreated controls. Endarterectomy is thus effective in relieving symptoms and in lowering the incidence of subsequent strokes. A number of reports with large series of surgical patients followed for long periods of time show results comparable to those reported herein and testify further to the salutary effects of carotid endarterectomy in patients with transient cerebral ischemia.[11, 22-24]

Apart from surgery the only other type of treatment beneficial for transient

Table 4. *Results of Treatment of Transient Cerebral Ischemia*

	MAYO CLINIC SERIES[21]		ENDARTERECTOMY (THOMPSON ET AL.)[14]
	UNTREATED	ANTICOAGULANTS	
Patients (no.)	160	175	142
Follow-up (mos.)	60	60	53
Normal	83 (52%)	131 (75%)	113 (80%)
Cerebral infarct (total)	51 (32%)	7 (4%)	4 (2.8%)
Lethal cerebral infarct	18 (11%)	3 (1.7%)	1 (0.7%)
Cerebral hemorrhage	7 (4.4%)	13 (7.4%)	0

ischemia appears to be long-term anticoagulant therapy.[18] Table 4 shows the results in a group of patients so treated. Endarterectomy is superior in every category and does not carry the hazard of cerebral hemorrhage, which is a serious complication seen in most series of transient ischemia patients treated with anticoagulants. Mortality and morbidity imposed by surgery are far less hazardous than cerebral hemorrhage associated with anticoagulant therapy. If anticoagulant drugs are discontinued, the rate of recurrent ischemic attacks is very high.[25]

While the series in Table 4 shows only five-year results, comparison of our surgical series at 13 years[14] with an untreated series followed 15 years[17] shows the same relative results in favor of surgical therapy. No studies with anticoagulants over a similarly long period of time are available.

Endarterectomy is a very durable operation. Our studies and those of others have demonstrated that arteries reconstructed by endarterectomy remain patent for many years, with an extremely low incidence of recurrent stenotic disease.[26, 27] On the other hand, it is well known that anticoagulants do not halt the progression of atherosclerotic lesions, and total occlusions may occur in any area of the peripheral vasculature of patients receiving these drugs. The high degree of association of acute hemiplegic strokes with acute total internal carotid occlusion has been well documented.[28]

While the long-term incidence of fatal and nonfatal strokes in transient ischemia is markedly reduced following endarterectomy, no increase in the long-term survival rates of surgically treated patients when compared with controls can be demonstrated at the present time. As yet there are inadequate data and too many variable factors for accurate statistical comparisons. Patients with cerebrovascular insufficiency usually have generalized atherosclerotic disease. Hypertension and coronary artery disease, especially when associated with previous myocardial infarction, are the limiting factors in prognosis. Follow-up studies after carotid endarterectomy have shown that over half the long-term deaths are due to heart disease, while the death rate from stroke is markedly reduced.[14] The remarks made earlier relative to "quality" of survival are appropriate to this discussion.

In summary, patients with transient cerebral ischemia are ideal candidates for surgical therapy since removal of the offending lesions eliminates sources of cerebral emboli and increases cerebral blood flow. Follow-up studies demonstrate a marked reduction in the occurrence of transient ischemic attacks and a significant lowering in the expected incidence of subsequent strokes, both fatal and nonfatal. At the same time, operative mortality and morbidity are low and are acceptable for this group of elderly atherosclerotic patients.

ASYMPTOMATIC BRUIT

The most controversial area in this field concerns the advisability of performing arteriography and surgery on patients with asymptomatic carotid bruits. Asymptomatic subclavian bruits, even with a demonstrated subclavian-steal syndrome, do not require operative intervention. The midcarotid bruit, however, reflecting the presence of atherosclerosis at the common carotid bifurcation, is another matter. Ninety per cent of such bruits arise from internal carotid plaques, the rest coming from external carotid plaques or other uncommon lesions.[4]

Several studies have been done on patients with overt cerebrovascular insufficiency, correlating stenotic lesions demonstrated on arteriograms with carotid bruits heard in the neck.[29-31] The degree of correlation is very high when bruits are audible, ranging from 75 to 85 per cent. Overall correlation between demonstrable carotid disease and bruits is about 60 per cent, since lesions may be present on the arteriogram, yet no bruit be audible. These include stenoses of less than 50 per cent, severe stenoses with a lumen diameter of 1 mm. or less, and total occlusions of the internal carotid artery. A carotid bruit, when present, thus constitutes a significant finding in patients with cerebrovascular insufficiency. The controversy arises as to the significance of the bruit in the absence of cerebral symptoms.

It does not appear unreasonable to consider the asymptomatic carotid bruit as part of the total picture of cerebrovascular insufficiency rather than an isolated finding on physical examination. The natural history of ischemic thrombotic stroke due to extracranial lesions must begin somewhere. It may begin as a plaque at the common carotid bifurcation and its first physical manifestation be an asymptomatic bruit. With time the asymptomatic lesion becomes symptomatic from ulceration and embolization or from impairment of cerebral blood flow. Hopefully, the first symptom is a TIA, when therapy can be initiated. At times, however, the first symptom is hemiplegia, especially if a stenotic carotid undergoes acute total occlusion. This sequence of events is seen repeatedly in retrospective studies of patients with completed strokes. Many other factors enter in to complicate this simplistic scheme; namely, multiple lesions both extracranial and intracranial, anatomic configurations of cerebral collateral pathways, rate of progression of atherosclerosis in the individual patient, hypertension, diabetes, etc., to mention some of the more important ones. The length of time during which these bruits are present is also important.

Javid et al.[32] have studied the natural history of carotid atheromas on serial arteriograms over a period of one to nine years. They noted no change in size of the atheromas in 38 per cent of the lesions studied, but found a significant increase in 62 per cent of the atheromas. The increase was greater than 25 per cent per year in 34 per cent of lesions, was less than 25 per cent per year in 20 per cent while recurrent stenosis or thrombosis occurred in 7.4 per cent.

We have followed, up to eight years, 59 patients with asymptomatic carotid bruits who were not operated upon when the bruit was first detected. During this time 30 (51 per cent) of the patients have remained asymptomatic. In 15 (25 per cent) transient cerebral ischemia has developed. Four of these had disappearance of the bruit with total occlusion of the internal carotid artery demonstrated by arteriography. Fourteen patients (24 per cent) had frank strokes, usually without transient ischemic attacks from two days to four years following detection of the bruit. Eleven of these patients developed total carotid occlusions, with disappearance of the bruit associated with onset of stroke. Thus, in 29, or 49 per cent, of the 59 patients transient ischemia or frank strokes developed during the follow-up period.

For a comparative surgical series we have performed 76 elective operations on 49 patients with asymptomatic bruits. General anesthesia was used together with a temporary shunt for cerebral protection. There was no operative mortality. Two patients had operation-related deficits. One had a right hemiparesis and dysphasia which cleared completely. The other has a permanent visual field defect in the ipsilateral eye, probably owing to embolism from the necrotic plaque. During long-term follow-up no patient has died of stroke, one patient had a mild stroke with full recovery, and a second had a severe stroke one year after operation and has a residual deficit.

In the experience reported, asymptomatic carotid bruits have proved not to be innocent lesions but have represented potential stroke hazards in certain individuals. The clinical hazard depends directly upon the lesion giving rise to the bruit and the status of all vessels supplying the brain, both primary and collateral. Thus, little hazard is posed by bruits arising from stenosis of the external carotid or from loops or kinks. On the other hand, bruits coming from atherosclerotic plaques involving the internal carotid probably become symptomatic in most instances if followed long enough.

In the final analysis arteriography is the definitive diagnostic maneuver necessary to establish the etiology of a carotid bruit and to determine its significance as a stroke hazard. As cerebral arteriography has become increasingly safer, it should be recommended more often for studying patients with asymptomatic carotid bruits of grade II intensity or greater, especially if these occur bilaterally. The overall general status of each patient should be considered very carefully, however, before recommending this procedure. It should not be done if some contraindication to endarterectomy already exists or if multiple risk factors are present, such as generalized atherosclerosis or severe hypertension associated with heart disease. Careful clinical judgment must be exercised.

If the arteriograms show a significant atherosclerotic stenosis in the internal carotid artery, endarterectomy may be cautiously considered. Specific indications include: (1) bilateral stenoses, (2) unilateral stenosis with contralateral occlusion, (3) stenosis in the artery to the dominant hemisphere, (4) known progressive atherosclerotic lesions elsewhere in the peripheral vasculature, especially in younger patients, and (5) contemplated major surgery of another sort when a hypotensive episode might well result in a stroke.[14]

Since no unnecessary risks should be taken, appropriate measures for cerebral protection must be employed during carotid endarterectomy to avoid producing neurologic deficits. Operative mortality should be below 1 per cent and complications no more than 2 per cent.

In summary, asymptomatic carotid bruits may originate in the internal carotid artery from atherosclerotic plaques which predispose to strokes in certain individuals over the age of 40. Arteriography is necessary to determine the significance of these bruits. If hazardous lesions are demonstrated, carotid endarterectomy may be recommended for selected patients without multiple risk factors to prevent the occurrence of ischemic cerebral episodes. Further long-term studies of the natural history of asymptomatic carotid bruits and follow-up studies of patients already operated upon are needed.

References

1. Savory, W. S.: Case of a young woman in whom the main arteries of both upper extremities and of the left side of the neck were throughout completely obliterated. Med.-Chir. Tr. (Lond.) 39:205, 1856.
2. Hunt, J. R.: The role of the carotid arteries in the causation of vascular lesions of the brain, with remarks on certain special features of the symptomatology. Amer. J. Med. Sci. 147:704, 1914.
3. Millikan, C. H : The pathogenesis of transient focal cerebral ischemia. Circulation 32:438, 1965.
4. Thompson, J. E.: *Surgery for Cerebrovascular Insufficiency (Stroke)*. Springfield, Ill., Charles C Thomas, 1968.
5. Fields, W. S., North, R. R., Hass, W. K., Galbraith, J. G., Wylie, E. J, Ratinor, G., Burns, M. H., Macdonald, M. C., and Meyer, J. S.: Joint study of extracranial arterial occlusion as a cause of stroke: I. Organization of study and survey of patient population. J.A.M.A. 203:955, 1968.
6. Hass, W. K., Fields, W. S., North, R. R., Kricheff, I. I., Chase, N. E., and Bauer, R. B.: Joint study of extracranial arterial occlusion: II. Arteriography, techniques, sites, and complications. J.A.M.A. 203:961, 1968.
7. Bauer, R. B., Meyer, J. S., Fields, W. S., Remington, R., Macdonald, M. C., and Callen, P.: Joint study of extracranial arterial occlusion: III. Progress report of controlled study of long-term survival in patients with and without operation. J.A.M.A. 208:509, 1969.
8. Blaisdell, F. W., Clauss, R. H., Galbraith, J. G., Imparato, A. M., and Wylie, E. J.: Joint study of extracranial arterial occlusion. IV. A review of surgical considerations. J.A.M.A. 209:1889, 1969.
9. Fields, W. S., Maslenikov, V., Meyer, J. S., Hass, W. K., Remington, R. D., and Macdonald, M.: Joint study of extracranial arterial occlusion: V. Progress report of prognosis following surgery or nonsurgical treatment for transient cerebral ischemic attacks and cervical carotid artery lesions. J.A.M.A. 211:1993, 1970.
10. Millikan, C. H.: Summary of the Eighth Princeton Conference on Cerebral Vascular Diseases, January 5–7, 1972, Princeton, New Jersey. Stroke 3:105, 1972.
11. DeWeese, J. A., Rob, C. G., Satran, R., Norris, F. H., Lipchik, E. O., Zehl, D. N., and Long, J. M.: Surgical treatment for occlusive disease of the carotid artery. Ann. Surg. 168:85, 1968.
12. Thompson, J. E., Kartchner, M. M., Austin, D. J., Wheeler, C. G., and Patman, R. D.: Carotid endarterectomy for cerebrovascular insufficiency (stroke): Follow-up of 359 cases. Ann. Surg. 163:751, 1966.
13. Wylie, E. J., Hein, M. F., and Adams, J. E.: Intracranial hemorrhage following surgical revascularization for treatment of acute strokes. J. Neurosurg. 21:212, 1964.
14. Thompson, J. E., Austin, D. J., and Patman, R. D.: Carotid endarterectomy for cerebrovascular insufficiency: Long-term results in 592 patients followed up to thirteen years. Ann. Surg. 172:663, 1970.
15. Whisnant, J. P., Fitzgibbons, J. P., Kurland, L. T., and Sayre, G. P.: Natural history of stroke in Rochester, Minnesota, 1945 through 1954. Stroke 2:11, 1971.
16. Bauer, R. B., Meyer, J. S., Gotham, J. E., and Gilroy, J.: A controlled study of surgical treatment of cerebrovascular disease—42 months experience with 183 cases. In Millikan, C. H., Siekert, R. G., and Whisnant, J. P. (eds.): *Cerebral Vascular Diseases*. New York, Grune & Stratton, 1966, p. 254.
17. Goldner, J. C., Whisnant, J. P., and Taylor, W. F.: Long-term prognosis of transient cerebral ischemic attacks. Stroke 2:160, 1971.
18. Millikan, C. H.: Reassessment of anticoagulant therapy in various types of occlusive cerebrovascular disease. Stroke 2:201, 1971.
19. Acheson, J., and Hutchinson, E. C.: The natural history of focal cerebral vascular disease. Quart. J. Med. 40:15, 1971.
20. Thompson, J. E.: Prevention of complications of cerebral arteriography and surgery. In Dale, W. A. (ed.): *Management of Arterial Occlusive Disease*. Chicago, Year Book Medical Publishers, Inc., 1971, p. 353.
21. Siekert, R. G., Whisnant, J. P., and Millikan, C. H.: Surgical and anticoagulant therapy of occlusive cerebrovascular disease. Ann. Intern. Med. 58:637, 1963.

22. DeBakey, M. E., Crawford, E. S., Cooley, D. A., Morris, G. C., Jr., Garrett, H. E., and Fields, W. S.: Cerebral arterial insufficiency: one to 11-year results following arterial reconstructive operation. Ann. Surg. *161*:921, 1965.
23. Wylie, E. J., and Ehrenfeld, W. K.: *Extracranial Occlusive Cerebrovascular Disease: Diagnosis and Management.* Philadelphia, W. B. Saunders Company, 1970.
24. Young, J. R., Humphries, A. W., Beven, E. G., and de Wolfe, V. G.: Carotid endarterectomy without a shunt. Arch. Surg. *99*:293, 1969.
25. Marshall, J., and Reynolds, E. H.: Withdrawal of anticoagulants from patients with transient ischemic cerebrovascular attacks. Lancet *1*:5, 1965.
26. Blaisdell, F. W., Lim, R., and Hall, A. D.: Technical result of carotid endarterectomy. Amer. J. Surg. *114*:239, 1967.
27. Edwards, W. S., Wilson, T. A. S., and Bennett, A.: The long-term effectiveness of carotid endarterectomy in prevention of strokes. Ann. Surg. *168*:765, 1968.
28. Thompson, J. E., Austin, D. J., and Patman, R. D.: Endarterectomy of the totally occluded carotid artery for stroke: Results in 100 operations. Arch. Surg. *95*:791, 1967.
29. Gilroy, J., and Meyer, J. S.: Auscultation of the neck in occlusive cerebrovascular disease. Circulation *25*:300, 1962.
30. McDowell, F., Rennie, L., and Ejrup, B.: Arterial bruit in cerebrovascular disease. *In* Millikan, C. H., Siekert, R. G., and Whisnant, J. P. (eds.): *Cerebral Vascular Diseases.* New York, Grune & Stratton, 1966, p. 124.
31. Thompson, J. E., and Patman, R. D.: Endarterectomy for asymptomatic carotid bruits. Heart Bull. *19*:116, 1970.
32. Javid, H., Ostermiller, W. E., Hengesh, J. W.: Dye, W. S., Hunter, J. A., Najafi, H., and Julian, O. C.: Natural history of carotid bifurcation atheroma. Surgery *67*:80, 1970.

Index

Abruptio placentae, disseminated
    intravascular coagulation in, 625
  heparin in, 630
Acetohexamide in diabetes, 404
Acetylsalicyclic acid. See *Aspirin*.
Achlorhydria, aspirin and, 503
Acid clearing test in gastroesophageal
    reflux, 515
Acid perfusion test in gastroesophageal
    reflux, 515
Acidity, gastric, control of, 13
Acidosis, lactic, 399
  arterial, 285
    phenformin and, 400
    shock and, 285
  respiratory, artificial ventilation and, 282
Acne, glucocorticoid therapy in, 442
Acute granulocytic leukemia, chemotherapy
    in, aplastic crisis in, 613. See also
    Acute myelocytic leukemia.
  induction of, 615
  cytosine arabinoside in, 612
  differential diagnosis of, 616
  in aged, treatment of, 614
  management of, aggressive, 601-609
    tempered, 610-619
  6-mercaptopurine in, 611
  remissions in, 611
    criteria of, 615
  staging of, 617
  survival in, quality of, 614
  treatment of, failures in, 616
Acute myelocytic leukemia, 601. See also
    Acute granulocytic leukemia.
  age and, 602
  antibiotics in, 604
  chemotherapy of, 605
    intermittent, 606
    maintenance, 606
  immunotherapy in, 607
  marrow examination in, 606
  6-mercaptopurine in, 605
  obesity and, 604
  remission in, 602
    induction of, 605
  transfusions in, 604
  treatment in, 604

Acute myelocytic leukemia (*Continued*)
  treatment in, supportive, 604
Adenocarcinoma(s), disseminated
    intravascular coagulation in, 625
  5-fluorouracil in, 30
  of pancreas, carcinoembryonic
    antigen in, 718
Adenopathy, transient, Kveim reaction
    in, 342
Adrenal insufficiency, corticosteroid
    therapy and, 441
Adrenocortical steroids, in Crohn's
    disease, 455-459
  in rheumatoid arthritis, 28
Adrenogenital syndrome, corticosteroid
    therapy in, 446
Adriamycin in Hodgkin's disease, 740
Aerosols, IPPB and, 264
Age, acute myelocytic leukemia and, 602
  tolerance of aspirin and, 501
Aged, acute granulocytic leukemia in,
    treatment of, 614
Airway, resistance in, IPPB and, 258
Alcohol, aspirin and, in gastrointestinal
    bleeding, 497
  hyperlipidemia and, 212
  peptic ulcer and, 504
Alimentation, parenteral, central venous
    pressure and, 181
Alkalis, gastroesophageal reflux and, 527
Alkalosis, respiratory, IPPB and, 260
Allergy, therapy of, 256
  glucocorticoid, 442
Amotivational syndrome, marihuana and, 755
Amyloidosis, steroids and, 651
Anastomosis(es), coronary, patency of, 127
Anemia, dialysis and, 671
  iron deficiency, aspirin and, 504
  microangiopathic hemolytic, disseminated
    intravascular coagulation and, 637
  pernicious, 26
Anesthesia for cardiopulmonary bypass, 299
Anesthetists, halothane hepatitis and, 580
Angina pectoris, coronary bypass
    grafts in, 137-141
  history of, 126
  ileal bypass and, 235

815

Angina pectoris (*Continued*)
　surgery in, placebo effect of, 140
Angiography, pulmonary, in embolization, 295, 304
Antacids, gastroesophageal reflux and, 519
Antibiotic(s), in acute myelocytic leukemia, 604
　preoperative, in surgery of bowel, 31
Antibody, formation of, etiology of, 26
Anticoagulant therapy, in cerebral ischemia, 774
　in completed stroke, 798
　in myocardial infarction, 10
　in progressing stroke, 794
　in transient cerebral ischemia, 789
　long-term, recurrent thromboembolism in, prevention of, 799
Anti-GBM disease, 705
　etiology of, 705
　pathogenic mechanisms in, 705
Antigen, Australia, liver disease and, 17
　fecal, Crohn's disease and, 462
　tumor-associated, 719
Antiglomerular basement membrane, 686
Anxiety, drugs and, 33
Appendectomy, acute ileitis and, 471
Arbor viruses, disseminated intravascular coagulation and, 638
Arteriography, aortocranial, in cerebral ischemia, 773
　in classification of cerebrovascular insufficiency syndrome, 806
Artery(ies), carotid, asymptomatic bruit in, endarterectomy in, 810
　mammary, use in bypass grafts, 138
　pulmonary, catheterization of, central venous pressure and, 181
　　pressure in, balloon flotation catheters for, 191
　　　end-diastolic, in, 182
　　　wedge, 182
　　　hypovolemia and, 182
Arthritis, preventive maintenance services in, 87
　rheumatoid, treatment of, 28
Aspirin, acute gastrointestinal bleeding and, 493-499
　blood coagulation and, 505
　buffered, 506
　　action of, 503
　dyspepsia from, 501
　enteric-coated, 506
　gastric ulcer and, 506
　in cerebral ischemia, 775
　in rheumatoid arthritis, 28
　injury to gastric mucosa by, 502
　intravenous, 507
　sodium bicarbonate and, 506
　tolerance of, age and, 501
　vitamin C deficiency and, 506
Atelectasis, lobar, oxygenation in, 275
Atherogenesis, hyperlipidemia and, 214

Atherogenesis (*Continued*)
　hypertension and, 210
Atheroma(s), beta lipoproteins and, 212
　carotid, arteriography in, 811
　diet and, 210
　plasma lipids and, 209
　pulmonary, 210
Atherosclerosis, cholesterol and, 218
　coronary, history of, 126
　diabetics and, 213
　factors in, 208
　heart disease and, 217
　hypercholesterolemia and, 221
　myocardial infarction and, 217
　prevention of, by dietary control of hyperlipidemia, 208-216
　　dietary changes for, 224
Atherosclerotic vascular disease, dialysis and, 679
Atrium, right, and left, pressures in, relation of, 188
　pressure in, central venous pressure and, 186
Atropine, esophageal sphincter and, 517
Australia antigen, liver disease and, 17
Auto-antibodies, 26
Autograft(s), saphenous vein, patency of, 126
Autoimmune disease, 26
Azathioprine, carcinogenicity of, 465
　in Crohn's disease, 460-469, 473
　superinfection from, 466
　withdrawal of, 465

Bacillus Calmette Guérin, British and U.S.A. tests of, comparison of, 324
　in tuberculosis, advantage of, 322-331
Back, problems with, preventive maintenance services in, 87
Bacterial infections, glomerular disease and, 700
Bacteriuria, asymptomatic, 19
Betahistine hydrochloride in cerebral ischemia, 781
Betamethasone, 440
Biguanides in adult-onset diabetes, 395, 398
Bile, composition of, bile salt secretion rate and, 550
Bile acid, feedback of, oversensitive, 552
Bile salt, loss of, excessive, 552
　secretion rate of, bile composition and, 550
　synthesis of, phenobartibal and, 556
Biliary tract disease, coronary heart disease and, 539
　surgical treatment of, 534
Biopsy, renal, in nephrotic syndrome, 653, 655, 658
Bleeding, gastrointestinal, acute, aspirin and, 493-499. See also *Hemorrhage(s)*.

INDEX

Bleeding (*Continued*)
   gastrointestinal, acute, aspirin, and other factors in, 496
     major, aspirin and, 504
     minor, aspirin and, 504
   uterine, functional, glucocorticoid therapy in, 442
Bleomycin in Hodgkin's disease, 740
Blood, coagulation of, aspirin and, 505
   for transfusion, mismatched, disseminated intravascular coagulation and, 637
   Hageman factor of, disseminated intravascular coagulation and, 636
   sampling of, central venous pressure and, 180
   volume of, central venous pressure and, 178
Blood gas, analysis of, 276
Blood vessels, microsurgical techniques for, 127
Bone disease, renal, dialysis and, 671
Bone marrow, examination of, in acute myelocytic leukemia, 606
Bowel, surgery of, antibiotic preparation for, 31
Bronchitis, 254
   emphysema and, 254
Bronchodilator, nebulized, administration of, 257
Bronchospasm, IPPB and, 259
Bronchus(i), irritation of, 255
   spasm of, 255
Buformin in diabetes, 404

Carbohydrate(s), plasma cholesterol and, 212
Carbon dioxide, inhalation of, intermittent, in cerebral ischemia, 777
Carbon dioxide narcosis, 259
Carbutamide in diabetes, 404
Cancer, BCG in, 322
   Crohn's disease and, 461
   disseminated intravascular coagulation in, 635
   of colon, diagnosis of, carcinoembryonic antigen in, 715-724
   of lung, carcinoembryonic antigen in, 718
   of thyroid, diagnosis of, 429
     prevalence of, 429
Carcinoembryonic antigen, depressive-dedifferentiation and, 716
   detection of, value of, 716
   immunogenicity of, 716
   in adenocarcinoma of pancreas, 718
   in diagnosis of cancer, of colon, 715-724
     of lung, 718
   in neuroblastoma, 719
   postoperative monitoring of, 721
   preoperative, 721
   tumor-associated antigen and, 720

Carcinoma, chronic disseminated intravascular coagulation and, 638
   heparin in, 629
   of gallbladder, 538
     cholelithiasis and, 534
Cardia, esophageal, prevention of gastroesophageal reflux and, 513-523
Cardiac output, decreased, IPPB and, 259
Cardiac surgery, IPPV in, 279
Cardiopulmonary bypass in embolectomy, 298
Carotid artery, asymptomatic bruit in, endarterectomy in, 810
Cataracts, oral hypoglycemic agents and, 408
Catheter(s), balloon, flotation, for central venous pressure, 191
Catheterization, arterial, complications of, 183
   central venous. See *Central venous catheterization.*
   pulmonary artery, central venous pressure and, 181
   urethral, 21
   venous, complications of, 183
Celiac disease, Kveim test and, 341
Celiotomy in Hodgkin's disease, 732
Central venous pressure, acute left ventricular failure and, 190
   atrial electrogram and, 180
   balloon flotation catheters for, 191
   blood sampling and, 180
   blood volume and, 178
   clinical application of, 189
   interpretation of, errors in, 179
   measurement of, errors in, 179
   monitoring of, limited value of, 185-193
   parenteral alimentation and, 181
   phlebotomy and, 180
   physiology of, 186
   pulmonary artery catheterization and, 181
   right ventricular pressure and, 187
   significance of, 177
   value of, 185
   venous infusions and, 178
   venous pressure and, 186
Central venous catheterization, routine, in critically ill, 177-184
Cerebral edema, glycerol therapy in, 779
Cerebral ischemia, acetylsalicylic acid in, 775
   acute, inhalation therapy in, 776
     treatment of, medical, 776
   anticoagulant therapy in, 774
   antihypertensive, 773
   aortocranial arteriography in, 773
   betahistine hydrochloride in, 781
   control of, surgery in, 804-814
   cyclandelate in, 782
   dipyridamole in, 775
   edema in, reduction of, 779
   hexobendine in, 781

Cerebral ischemia (*Continued*)
   hyperbaric oxygenation in, 777
   hyperventilation in, 778
   intermittent CO_2 inhalation therapy
      in, 777
   isoxsuprine in, 782
   oxygen inhalation in, 776
   papaverine in, 781
   platelet inhibitors and, 774
   progressive, 789
   streptokinase in, 782
   sulfinpyrazone in, 775
   therapy of, choice of, 787-803
      medical, 771-786
      prophylactic, 772
      surgical, 775
   transient. See *Transient cerebral ischemia*.
   urokinase in, 782
   warfarin in, 775
Cerebrovascular insufficiency syndrome,
      classification of, arteriography in, 806
   surgery in, 805
      classification of, 805
Chenodeoxycholic acid in gallstone
      disease, 542, 556
Child(ren), nephrotic syndrome in, focal
      sclerosis and, 660
   remission in, cyclophosphamide and,
      654
      steroids and, 652, 658
   poststreptococcal glomerulonephritis in, 20
   smallpox vaccination in, hazards of
      discontinuation of, 379
Chlorambucil in Hodgkin's disease, 741
Chlorpropamide, hypoglycemia and, 398
   in diabetes, 404
Cholangiography, 538
Cholecystectomy, 534, 549
   prophylactic, 536
Cholecystitis, acute, 534, 537
Cholecystography, 534
Cholecystokinin, in diagnosis of gallstone
      disease, 546
Choledocholithiasis, 538
   gallstones and, 534
Cholelithiasis, carcinoma of gallbladder
      and, 534
Cholesterol, atherosclerosis and, 218
   heart disease and, 199
   in xanthomas, 210
   metabolism, partial ileal bypass and, 229
   plasma, alcohol and, 212
      carbohydrates and, 212
      dietary cholesterol and, 212
      polyunsaturated fats and, 212
      saturated fats and, 212
   secretion of, excessive, 552
   serum, coronary disease and, 7
      levels of, death rates and, 223
         heart disease and, 223
         jejuno-ileal bypass and, 228

Cholesterol (*Continued*)
   serum, levels of, normal, 222
Chrysotherapy in rheumatoid arthritis, 28
Chylomicrons, xanthomatous, 209
Chylomicronemia, diet and, 211
Cimino arteriovenous fistula, dialysis
      and, 670
Cirrhosis, alcoholic, disseminated
      intravascular coagulation in, 635
   hepatic, 17
Colectomy, total, in Crohn's colitis, 475
Colitis, azathioprine in, 463, 465
   Crohn's, 475
   granulomatous, 470
   right-sided, 474
   ulcerative, 470
      Kveim test and, 341
      segmental, 474
      vs. Crohn's disease, 474
Colloid osmotic pressure, changes in, 182
Colon, cancer of, diagnosis of,
      carcinoembryonic antigen in, 715-724
Colonoscope, polypectomy by, 16
Coma, hepatic, halothane and, 570
Community medicine, internal medicine
      and, 44
Consumption-coagulopathy, 623
   heparin in, 629
Cor pulmonale, right heart failure and, 256
Coronary artery disease, dietary prophylaxis
      of, 7
   randomization of patients with, 131
      bias in, 132
Coronary bypass graft(s), effect of, on
      history of disease, 138
      myocardial ischemia, 138
   future of, 132
   history of, 125
   in angina pectoris, 136-141
   in mycardial ischemia, 125-136
   occlusive lesions following, 139
Coronary problems, preventive maintenance
      services in, 87
Corticosteroid therapy, dosage in, 448.
      See also *Glucocorticoid therapy*.
   in Crohn's disease, 473
   in osteoarthritis, 447
   prolonged, hazards of, 446-449
      termination of, 449
   sucrose and, 206
   systemic, 448
   topical, 448
   withdrawal syndrome of, 449
Cortisone, 441, 443
   in rheumatoid arthritis, 439
Crohn's disease, adrenocortical steroids in,
      benefits of, 455
      complications of, 457
      contraindications to, 457
      dosage of, 456
      indications for, 445-459
      surgery and, 458

Crohn's disease (*Continued*)
  azathioprine in, 460-469
  cancer and, 461
  chronic, 471
  colonic, 470, 474
  diet in, 485
  epidemiology of, 483
  etiology of, 482
  fecal antigen and, 462
  granuloma in, 461
  incidence of, 483
  milk and, 485
  natural history of, 483
  personality of patients with, 484
  recurrence of, 471
    incidence of, 460
  rest in, 484
  salicylazosulfapyridine in, 486
  surgery in, 458, 470-481, 486
    fecal fistula following, 471
  treatment for, 484
    antibacterial, 486
    conservative, 482-488
    corticosteroid, 487
    immunosuppressive, 461
  vs. ulcerative colitis, 474
Cryoglobulinemia, nephritis and, 698, 703
Cyclandelate in cerebral ischemia, 782
Cyclophosphamide, in Hodgkin's disease, 741
  nephrotic syndrome and, 661
Cytotoxic drugs, in rheumatoid arthritis, 29
  nephrotic syndrome and, 661

Death, alternatives in, 113-121
  as you wish it, 110-112
  cholesterol-lowering diet and, 241
  definition of, 114
  dignity and, 107
  fear of, 117
  life after, 104
  patient knowledge of, 116
  patient planning for, 111
Defibrination syndrome, 623
Dexamethasone, 440
Dextran in cerebral edema, 780
Diabetes mellitus, adult-onset, biguanides in, 395-398
  capillary basement membrane thickness and, 392
  control of, value of, 390
  insulin in, 396
  oral antidiabetic agents in, limitations of, 389-403
  atherosclerosis and, 213
  chylomicronemia and, 211
  complications of, 25
  glucocorticoid therapy and, 441
  preventive maintenance services in, 87
  sucrose and, 205
  weight control in, importance of, 393

Diagnosis(es), clinical, internal medicine and, 46
  screening programs in, reliability of, 95
Dialysis, anemia and, 671
  atherosclerotic vascular disease and, 679
  Cimino arteriovenous fistula in, 670
  costs of, 679
  complications of, avoidance of, 671
  during sleep, 670
  frequency of, 669
  gonadal function and, 672
  growth and, 671
  heart failure and, 672
  hepatitis and, 672
  home, 668
  hyperlipidemia and, 679
  hypertension and, 672
  in uremia, 667-674
    cost effectiveness of, 668
  psychiatric problems in, 667
  Quinton-Scribner shunt in, 670
  renal bone disease and, 671
  shortcomings of, 677
  vs. renal transplantation, 676
Diaphragm, esophageal hiatus of, 518
Diet, change in, in prevention of atherosclerosis, 224
  cholesterol-lowering, death and, 241
  control of hyperlipidemia by, atherosclerosis prevention and, 208-216
  fat composition of, change in, 224
  fat controlled, for all, 217-227
  in Crohn's disease, 485
  plasma lipids and, 240
  ulcer, 13
  vascular disease and, 240
Diet program, national, skeptical view of, 239-244
Dipyridamole in cerebral ischemia, 775
Disease, early detection of, benefits of, 90
Disseminated intravascular coagulation, causes of, 625
  chronic, 627
    carcinoma and, 638
  clinically significant, heparin in, 633-648
  diagnosis of, 625, 626
    differential, 628
  etiology of, 623
  fulminant meningococcemia and, 637
  Hageman factor and, 636
  hemorrhage and, 640
  heparin in, 640
  injured red cells and, 637
  interrupting, 627
  intrauterine fetal death and, 639
  leukemia and, 626
  lupus erythematosus and, 639
  management of, heparin in, cautions, 623-632
    contraindications to, 626
    indications for, 627
    rationale for, 625

Disseminated intravascular
    coagulation (*Continued*)
  shock and, 626, 630
  thrombin and, 634
  thromboplastin and, 636
  viral infections and, 638
Drugs, anxiety and, 33
  efficacy of, regulation of information of, 71
  hallucinogenic, 756
  new, development of, FDA and, 79
  package circular on, 72
  prescription, sources of information on, 69
  quality of, prevention of variations in, 70
  regulation of, benefits of, 75
    losses from, 76
  safety of, control of, 71
  withdrawal from, marihuana and, 765
Dying, prolongation of, vs. prolongation of life, 106. see also *Patient, dying.*
Dyspepsia, aspirin, 501
  chronic, sucrose and, 205
Dyspnea, IPPB and, 259

Eczema vaccinatum, 364
Edema, cerebral, dextran in, 780
  glycerol therapy in, 779
  in cerebral ischemia, reduction of, 779
  steroids in, 780
  pulmonary, indications of, 182
    IPPB in, 250
Electrogram, atrial, central venous pressure and, 180
Embolectomy, pulmonary, 298
  advantages of, 303-309
  evaluation of, 307
  history of, 303
  in pulmonary embolism, 293
  indications for, 300
Embolism, pulmonary. See *Pulmonary embolism.*
Emphysema, 254
  bronchitis and, 254
  management of, 23
Encephalitis, postvaccinial, 364, 374
Endarterectomy, carotid, contraindications to, 806
  in cerebral ischemia, 775
  indications for, 806
  results of, 807
Endocarditis, glomerulonephritis and, 700
Endoplasmic reticulum, halothane and, 567
Enteritis, acute, 470
  chronic, 471
  regional, 474. See also *Crohn's disease.*
Epsilon aminocaproic acid, fibrinolysis and, 638, 644
Erythema nodosum, Kveim reaction in, 342
Erythroleukemia, 617
Esophagitis, gastroesophageal reflux and, 515

Esophagoscopy in esophagitis, 515
Esophagus, muscles of, 516
  sphincters of, 516
    atropine and, 517
    gastrin and, 517
Euthanasia, vs. suicide, 104
Exanthematous diseases, disseminated intravascular coagulation and, 638
Exercise, capacity for, defined, 147
  physical training and, 152
  following myocardial infarction. See *Myocardial infarction* and also *Physical training.*
  tolerance of, following vascular surgery, 130
Exercise performance, defined, 147

Family medicine, internal medicine and, 44
Fat(s), dietary, change in, 224
  heart disease and, 203
  polyunsaturated, effect of, 221
  saturated, effect of, 221
  plasma cholesterol and, 212
Federal Trade Commission, drugs and, 67
Fetus, intrauterine death of, disseminated intravascular coagulation and, 639
Fibrin, formation of, factors in, 623
Fibrinolysis, epsilon aminocaproic acid and, 638, 644
Fibrinolytic therapy, in myocardial infarction, 11
Fistula, fecal, following surgery in Crohn's disease, 471
5-Fluorouracil in adenocarcinoma, 30
Fluroxene, 565
  metabolism of, 567
Food and Drug Administration, deficiencies of, 74
  differing standards within, 77
  regulations of, appeals against, 78
    new drug development and, 79
  role of, 67
Fungal infections, heparin in, 630

Gallbladder, carcinoma of, 538
  cholelithiasis and, 534
Gallstone(s), asymptomatic, follow-up of, 535
  incidence of, 535
  bile pigment, 545
  cholesterol, and bile acid, 545
    classification of, 550
    stages of disease, 545
  dissolution of, 549
  growth of, active, 548
    stable, 548
  prevention of, 548
  silent, 533

Gallstone(s) (*Continued*)
  silent, chemotherapy for, 542
    individualized therapy for, advantages of, 545-559
  surgery for, advantages of, 533-544
Gallstone disease, extrahepatic, primary, 552
Gangrene, postinfectious, heparin in, 629
Gastric mucosa, aspirin injury to, 502
Gastrin, esophageal sphincter and, 517
  peptic ulcer and, 13
Gastritis, atrophic, aspirin and, 503
Gastroesophageal junction, competence of, hormones affecting, 526
  mechanisms of, 525
  extraluminal pressure in, intra-abdominal pressure and, 526
  intraluminal pressure at, measurement of, 524
  sphincter at, importance of, 524-528
Gastroesophageal reflux, alkalis and, 527
  antacids and, 519
  diagnosis of, 514
  esophageal peristalsis and, 519
  esophagitis in, 515
  prevention of, cardia and, 513-523
    mechanisms in, 526
  signs and symptoms of, 514
  surgery in, 520
    effects of, 521
  vs. hiatal hernia, 513
Gastrointestinal disease, preventive maintenance services in, 87
Gastrointestinal lesion, hemorrhage from, aspirin and, 495
Glomerular basement membrane, antigens in, glomerulonephritis and, 685
Glomerular disease, bacterial infections and, 700
  immunologic, experimental, 694
    mechanisms in, evaluation of, 694-709
    importance of, 685-693
Glomerulonephritis, anti-GBM, 694, 705. See also *Nephritis*.
  Australian antigen positive hepatitis and, 690
  causes of, 685
  hydrocephalus and, 690
  hypocomplementemic membranoproliferative, 687
  immune complex, 694, 698
    etiology of, 696
  malaria and, 701
  membranous, 659, 704
  poststreptococcic, 20, 690, 698
  proliferative, 659
  rapidly progressive, 705
  thyroiditis and, 690
Glomerulosclerosis, diabetic, 691
Glucocorticoid therapy, 439-445. See also *Corticosteroid therapy*.
  dangers of, 440
  in adrenal insufficiency, 441

Glucocorticoid therapy (*Continued*)
  in infertility, 442
  low dosage, investigation of, 444
Glybenzcyclamide in diabetes, 404
Glycerol therapy in cerebral edema, 779
Goiter belt, 428
Gonadal function, dialysis and, 672
Goodpasture's syndrome, 688, 705
Gout, sucrose and, 205
Graft(s), coronary bypass. See *Coronary bypass graft(s)*.
  saphenous vein, aorto-coronary, 127
Granulocytopenia, septicemia and, 607
Graves' disease, nodes in, 425
Growth, dialysis and, 671
Guillain-Barré syndrome, ventilation in, 277

Halothane, advantages of, 565
  as hepatotoxin, 567
  disadvantages of, 566
  endoplasmic reticulum and, 567
  hepatic coma and, 570
  hypersensitivity to, 565
    clinical stigmata of, 587
  impurities in, 568
  liver disease and, 572
  metabolism of, 566, 588
  methylcholanthrene and, 567
  mitochondria and, 568
  phenobarbitol and, 567
  repeated administration of, 585, 586
Halothane hepatitis, 565-579
  anesthetists and, 580
  clinical features of, 569
  differential diagnosis of, 572
  jaundice in, 569
  pathology of, 570
  prevalence and epidemiology of, 568
  vs. jaundice, 573
  vs. viral hepatitis, 573, 590
Hashimoto's thyroiditis, nodes in, 424
Health, maintenance of, multiphasic testing in, 86
  preventive, 86, 87
Health care, 87
  benefits of, measurement of, 60
  community, modernization of, 60
  evaluation of, 52
  paramedical personnel and, 86, 88
  primary, nurse specialists and, 58, 59, 60
    physicians' assistants and, 59
    teamwork in, 56, 59
    units for, 58
  regional, modernization of, 60
  therapeutic and rehabilitative, 86
  vs. sick care, 86
Health examinations, periodic, 85
Heart, output of, depressed, IPPB and, 259
Heart disease, atherosclerosis and, 217
  cholesterol and, 199
  coronary, biliary tract disease and, 539

Heart disease (*Continued*)
  epidemiology of, limitations of, 202
  fats and, 203
  manifestations of, multiple, 205
  physical activity and, 146
  rehabilitation in, guidelines for, 157
    with physical training, 155
      benefits of, 145-161
      risks of, 158
  serum cholesterol levels and, 223
  sugar and, 199-207
Heart failure, dialysis and, 672
  right, cor pulmonale and, 256
Heartburn in gastroesophageal reflux, 514
Hemangioma, giant, disseminated intravascular coagulation in, 625
Hematemesis, aspirin and, 493
Hemochromatosis, phebotomy in, 18
Hemolytic uremic syndrome, heparin in, 630
Hemorrhage(s), acute, aspirin as cause, 495. See also *Bleeding*.
  disseminated intravascular coagulation and, 640
  heparin and, 640
Hemorrhagic fevers, disseminated intravascular coagulation and, 638
Hemorrhagic pulmonary disease, anti-GBM, nephritis and, 688
Heparin, hemorrhage and, 640
  in disseminated intravascular coagulation and, 640
  in fungal infections, 630
  thrombin and, 634
Hepatitis, Australian antigen positive glomerulonephritis and, 690
  dialysis and, 672
  drug-induced, 565
  halothane. See *Halothane hepatitis*.
  isoniazid and, 317
  methoxyflurane, 572
  viral, vs. halothane hepatitis, 573, 590
Hepatitis associated antigen, 591
Herd immunity, vaccination and, 364
Heredity, thyroid cancer and, 425
Hernia, hiatal. See *Hiatal hernia*.
Heroin, marihuana and, 755
Hexobendine, in cerebral ischemia, 781
Hiatal hernia, diagnosis of, 514
  gastroesophageal competence in, 525
  Müller maneuver in, 525
  sliding, 513
  Valsalva maneuver in, 525
  vs. gastroesophageal reflux, 513
Hirsutism, glucocorticoid therapy and, 442
Hodgkin's disease, advanced, therapy of, aggressive, 739-747
  celiotomy in, 732
  chemotherapy in, 736
    combination, 740
    spermatogenesis and, 744
    toxicity of, 744
  lymphography in, 732

Hodgkin's disease (*Continued*)
  nitrosourea in, 737, 740
  radiation therapy in, 734
    chemotherapy and, 743
    complications of, 735
    relapses from, 743
  remission in, complete, 732
    duration of, 742
  splenectomy in, 732, 733
  staging of, 732, 739
    surgical, 733
  survival in, 742
  treatment of, 733
    conservative, 731-738
Homograft, rejection of, heparin in, 630
Hormone(s), effect on gastroesophageal competence, 526
Hostility, reduction of, by marihuana, 765
Hydrocephalus, glomerulonephritis and, 690
Hydrocortisone, 441, 443
  in Crohn's disease, 456
Hypercapnia, impending respiratory failure in, 277
Hypercarbia, intubation in, 275
  therapy of, 256
Hypercholesterolemia, atherosclerosis and, 221
Hyperglycemia, weight control and, 393
Hyperlipidemia, alcohol and, 212
  atherogenesis and, 214
  carbohydrate-induced, 213
  chemotherapy for, 214
  control of, dietary, atherosclerosis prevention and, 208-216
    surgical, 228-238
  dialysis and, 679
  Type III, xanthomas in, 210
Hyperlipoproteinemia, chylomicronemia and, 211
Hypertension, atherogenesis and, 210
  benign, treatment of, 9
  dialysis and, 672
  glucocorticoid therapy and, 441
  malignant, antihypertensive drugs in, 9
  preventive maintenance services in, 87
  renovascular, 22
Hyperthyroidism, radioiodine therapy in, 432
  surgery in, 432
Hypertriglyceridemia, management of, 243
Hyperuricemia, fructose and, 205
Hyperventilation in cerebral ischemia, 778
Hypoglycemia, glucocorticoid therapy and, 441
  sulfonylureas and, 398
Hypoglycemic agents, oral, benefits of, 404-415
  cataracts and, 408
  effectiveness of, 395
  infection and, 407
  macroangiopathy and, 409
  microangiopathy and, 409
  neuropathy and, 408

INDEX

Hypokalemia, IPPB and, 260
Hypovolemia, pulmonary artery wedge, pressure and, 182
Hypoxemia, lactic acidosis and, 285
Hypoxia, artificial ventilation in, 286
    therapy of, 256

Ileal bypass, angina pectoris and, 235
    complications of, 234
    partial, cholesterol metabolism and, 229
        lipid levels and, 231
        technique for, 229
Ileal disease, azathioprine in, 463, 465
Ileitis, acute, 470
    appendectomy and, 471
    postcolectomy, 478
    prestomal, 478
    regional, Kveim test and, 341
Ileocolitis, 470, 474
Ileostomy, in Crohn's colitis, 475
Illness, terminal, guidelines for management of, 118
Immunosuppressive therapy, in Crohn's disease, 461
    in rheumatoid arthritis, 28
    nephrotic syndrome and, 661
    superinfection from, 466
Indigestion, incidence of, 514
Infarction, cerebral. See *Cerebral ischemia.*
    myocardial. See *Myocardial infarction.*
Infection, oral hypoglycemic agents and, 407
Infertility, gluococorticoid therapy in, 442
Infusions, venous, central venous pressure and, 178
Inspiration, pressure of, measurement of, 252
Institutions, modification of, for dying patients, 120
Insulin, sucrose and, 206
Intermittent positive pressure breathing, aerosols and, 264
    airway resistance and, 258
    bronchospasm and, 259
    chronic obstructive lung disease and, 249-262
    circulatory effects of, 251
    dangers and limitations of, 263-271
    defined, 249
    development of, 264
    dyspnea and, 259
    effect on patient, 252
    gas used for, 252
    humidification in, 252
    in chronic obstructive pulmonary disease, 256
    indications for, 260
    intubation and, 268
    misconceptions about, 269
    response to, 252
        adverse, 259
    sympathomimetic effects of, 259

Intermittent positive pressure breathing (*Continued*)
    therapy with, complications of, 267
        postoperative, 268
        results of, 261
    uses of, 249
    ventilatory failure and, 266
    ventilation and, 257
Intermittent positive pressure ventilation, advantages of, 278
    disadvantages of, 278
    supervision of, 278
Internal medicine, certification in, 5
    clinical diagnosis and, 46
    community medicine and, 44
    family medicine and, 44
    functions of, 48
    future of, 45, 64
    identity crises in, 34-50
    Osler definition of, 42
    secondary patient care and, 47
    subspecialties in, growth of, 43
Internist(s), as consultant, 54. See also *Physician(s).*
    broadly based, importance of, 51-63
    general, education of, 55
    function of, 53
Intoxicants, legal, number desirable, 757
Intubation, advantages of, 278
    disadvantages of, 278
    in hypercarbia, 275
    IPPB and, 268
    supervision of, 278
IPPB. See *Intermittent positive pressure breathing.*
IPPV. See *Intermittent positive pressure ventilation.*
Ischemia, cerebral. See *Cerebral ischemia.*
    myocardial, coronary bypass grafts in, 125-136, 138
Islet cell function, sulfonylureas and, 406
Isoniazid, chemoprophylaxis with, 313
    effectiveness of, 315
    hepatitis and, 317
    hypersensitivity to, 317
    jaundice and, 317
    side effects of, 316
Isoxsuprine in cerebral ischemia, 782

Jaundice, halothane and, 569
    isoniazid and, 317
    postoperative, 591
    vs. halothane hepatitis, 573
Jejuno-ileal bypass, serum cholesterol and, 228
Joint Study of Extracranial Arterial Occlusion, defects of, 793

Ketonemia, therapy of, 396
Kidney infections, preventive maintenance services in, 87

Kveim reaction, mechanism of, 342
  study of, importance of, 346
Kveim test, diagnostic value of, 345
  errors in, sources of, 350
  in sarcoidosis, nonspecificity of, 339-348
    reliability of, 349-358
  international trials of, specificity of, 352
  interpretations of, conflicting, 344
    histologic, 345
  materials used in, 343
  regional ileitis and, 341
  specificity of, 340
  suspensions for, CSL, comparison of, 354
    satisfactory, criteria for, 356
    unsatisfactory, 350, 352

Leukemia, acute granulocytic. See *Acute granulocytic leukemia* and also *Acute myelocytic leukemia*.
  BCG in, 322
  chronic lymphatic, Kveim test and, 341
  disseminated intravascular coagulation and, 626, 630
  myelomonocytic, 617
  promyelocytic, heparin in, 629
Life, after death, 104
  cost of preservation, 108
  definition of, 108
  prolongation of, physician and, 103-109
    vs. prolongation of dying, 106
  quality of, definition of, 116
  respect for, 117
  uniqueness of, 108
Lipid(s), plasma, atheromas and, 209
  diet and, 240
Lipogenesis, sucrose and, 205
Lipoproteins, coronary disease and, 7
Liver, disease of, Australia antigen and, 17
    halothane and, 572
  dysfunction of, postoperative, factors in, 582
  failure of, acute, heparin in, 630
LSD, marihuana and, 756
Lung, cancer of, carcinoembryonic antigen in, 718
  disease of, chronic obstructive, IPPB in, 249-262
  shock, IPPB in, 250
  ventilation of, pressure required for, 251
Lupus erythematosus, disseminated, intravascular coagulation and, 639
  Kveim test and, 341
Lupus nephritis, 690, 698, 701
  steroids and, 651
Luxury perfusion syndrome, 778
Lymphography in Hodgkin's disease, 732
Lymphoma, chemotherapy in, ovarian function and, 745
  disseminated intravascular coagulation in, 635
Lymphosarcoma, chemotherapy in, 736

Macroangiopathy, oral hypoglycemic agents and, 409
Malaria, disseminated intravascular coagulation and, 637, 638
  glomerulonephritis and, 701
Marihuana, amotivational syndrome and, 755
  as stimulant, 765
  drug withdrawal and, 765
  escalation to other drugs from, 755
  heroin and, 755
  hostility reduction by, 765
  legalization of, adverse effects of, 753-761
    advocacy of, 762-768
  LSD and, 756
  mentation and, 755
  panic following, 754
  reactions to, adverse, 766
  schizophrenia and, 754
  use of, heavy, 766
    reasons for, 763
    repetitive, dangers of, 753
    single, dangers of, 753
Marrow, bone, examination of, in acute myelocytic leukemia, 606
Mastitis, chronic cystic, glucocorticoid therapy in, 442
Masugi nephritis, 696
Medical care, multiphasic testing in, 85-91. See also *Health care*.
Medicines, patent, abuses of, 68
Melena, aspirin and, 493
Meningococcemia, fulminant, disseminated intravascular coagulation and, 637
6-Mercaptopurine, in acute myelocytic leukemia, 605
Metabolism, aerobic, maximal oxygen intake and, 148
Metformin in diabetes, 404
Methotrexate in Hodgkin's disease, 741
Methoxyflurane, 565
  metabolism of, 567
  renal toxicity and, 568
Methoxyflurane hepatitis, 572
Methycholanthrene, halothane and, 567
Methyl prednisolone, 440
Methyl prednisone in Crohn's disease, 456
Microangiopathy, oral hypoglycemic agents and, 409
Milk, Crohn's disease and, 485
Mitochondria, halothane and, 568
Müller maneuver in hiatal hernia, 525
Multiphasic testing, as triage to medical care, 85-91. See also *Screening programs*.
  benefits of, 88
  guidelines for, 88
Muscle(s), respiratory, fatigue of, 256
Myasthenia gravis, IPPV in, 279
  ventilation in, 277
Myocardial infarction, anticoagulants in, 10
  atherosclerosis and, 217

INDEX 825

Myocardial infarction (*Continued*)
  exercise therapy following, disadvantages of, 162-172
    eligibility for, 165
    in hospital, 165
    studies of, 163
      problems in, 166
Myocardial ischemia, coronary bypass grafts in, 125-136
Myocardium, delivery of oxygen to, augmented, 128

Narcosis, carbon dioxide, 259
Neck, radical dissection of, in thyroid cancer, 432
Nephritis, anaphylactoid, in purpura, 702. See also *Glomerulonephritis*.
  anti-glomerular basement membrane, 686, 687
    hemorrhagic pulmonary disease and, 688
  chronic, etiology of, 20
  cryoglobulinemia and, 703
  immune complex, 689
  in anaphylactoid purpura, 702
  in cryoglobulinemia, 698
  in periarteritis nodosa, 702
  lupus, 690, 698, 701
    steroids and, 651
  malarial, 698
  Masugi, 696
  nephrotoxic serum, 696
  phases of, 687
  Steblay, 696
Nephropathy, diabetic, steroids and, 651
Nephrosclerosis, 691
Nephrosis, lipoid, 706
  malarial, 690
Nephrotic syndrome, cyclophosphamide in, 661
  cytotoxic drugs in, 661
  immunosuppressive therapy, 661
  in children, focal sclerosis and, 660
    remission in, cyclophosphamide in, 654
    steroids and, 652, 658
  renal biopsy in, 653, 655, 658
  steroids in, advantages of, 658, 662
    limited role of, 651-657
    relapses in, 661
  syphilis and, 700
Neuroblastoma, carcinoembryonic antigen in, 719
Neuropathy, diabetic, in adult-onset diabetics, 392
  oral hypoglycemic agents and, 408
Nitrogen mustard in Hodgkin's disease, 740, 741
Nitrosourea in Hodgkin's disease, 737, 740
Nurse specialists, primary health care and, 58, 59, 60

Obesity, acute myelocytic leukemia and, 604
  control of, 24
  preventive maintenance services in, 87
  sucrose and, 205
Oligospermia, glucocorticoid therapy in, 442
Osteoarthritis, corticosteroid therapy in, 447
Oxygen, delivery of, to myocardium, augmented, 128
  inhalation of, in cerebral ischemia, 776
  intake of, maximal, 148
    physical training and, 152
    symptom-limited, 148
  therapy with, 283
Oxygen toxicity, artificial ventilation and, 286
  IPPB and, 260
Oxygenation, hyperbaric, in cerebral ischemia, 777
  impaired, 275

Pain, relief of, 104
Pancreas, adenocarcinoma of, carcinoembryonic antigen in, 718
Papaverine in cerebral ischemia, 781
Paramedical personnel, preventive maintenance services and, 88
Patient(s), ambulant, care of, 56
  critically ill, central venous catheterization in, routine, 177-184
  death and, 110
  document for, defining therapy wanted, 111
    time of use, 112
  dying, at home, 120
    modification of institutions for, 120
    physician and, 115
    treatment of, legal aspects of, 119
  effect of IPPB on, 252
  knowledge of imminent death, 116
  physician's contract with, 107
  primary care of, 46
  response to IPPB, mental, 253
    physical, 252
  secondary care of, 47
  tertiary care of, 47
Periarteritis nodosa, nephritis in, 702
Peristalsis, esophageal, gastroesophageal reflux and, 519
Peritonitis, IPPV in, 279
pH reflux test in gastrointestinal reflux, 515
Pharmacotherapy, disadvantages of, 74-80
  federal regulation of, importance of, 67-73
Phenformin, complications of use, 411
  in adult-onset diabetes, 399, 404
  lactic acidosis and, 400
Phenobarbital, bile salt synthesis and, 556
  halothane and, 567
Phlebotomy, central venous pressure and, 180
  in hemochromatosis, 18

Physical activity, heart disease and, 146
Physical training. See also *Myocardial infarction, exercise therapy following.*
  effects of, 145
    physiological, 148
    psychological, 154
  exercise capacity and, 152
  in heart disease, benefits of, 145-161
    rehabilitative, 155
    studies of, experimental, 146
  maximal oxygen intake and, 152
Physician, assistants to, primary health care and, 59. See also *Internist(s).*
  contract with patient, 107
  dying patient and, 115
  generalist, primary patient care and, 46
  omniscience of, 105
  personal, numbers needed, 57
  role of, 51
Pituitary gland, prednisolone and, 440
Plasma, coagulation of, injuries activating, 636
  cholesterol in. See *Cholesterol, plasma.*
  lipids in, atheromas and, 209
    diet and, 240
  triglyceride levels of, lowering of, 243
Platelets, inhibitors of, cerebral ischemia and, 774
Pleural effusion, oxygenation in, 275
Pneumonia, IPPB in, 250
  nosocomial, 259
Pneumothorax, IPPB and, 259
Polycythemia, therapy of, 256
Polyneuritis, ascending, IPPV in, 279
Polyp(s), colonic, management of, 16
Polypectomy by colonoscope, 16
Prednisolone, 439, 443
  peptic ulcer and, 440
  pituitary gland and, 440
Prednisone, 439-443
  in Crohn's disease, 456
  in Hodgkin's disease, 740, 741
Pregnancy, smallpox vaccination in, 375
Procarbazine in Hodgkin's disease, 736, 740, 741
Proteinuria, remissions in, steroids and, 652
Protozoan infections, disseminated intravascular coagulation and, 638
Psychosocial problems, preventive maintenance services in, 87
Pulmonary disease, chronic obstructive, IPPB in, 256
  indications for, 260
  pathophysiological abnormalities in, 253
  therapy of, 255
  increase in, with IPPB, 260
Pulmonary embolism, diagnosis of, 295
  drug therapy for, disadvantages of, 308
  embolectomy in, 293
    advantages of, 303-309
  etiology of, 294
  heparin in, 296

Pulmonary embolism (*Continued*)
  massive, diagnosis of, 304
    shock and, 306
  shock in, 297
  thrombolytic therapy in, 293-302
  urokinase in, 296
    bleeding complications of, 297
    contraindications to, 298
Pulmonary insufficiency, acute, advantages of aggressive therapy for, 275-279
Purpura, anaphylactoid nephritis in, 702
  thrombotic thrombocytopenic, heparin in, 630
Purpura fulminans, disseminated intravascular coagulation in, 625, 638
  heparin in, 629
Pyelonephritis, 691

Quinton-Scribner shunt in dialysis, 670

Radiation therapy in Hodgkin's disease, 734
  complications of, 735
Radiography in gastroesophageal reflux, 514
Red blood cells, disseminated intravascular coagulation and, 637, 638
Reed Sternberg cell in Hodgkin's disease, 732
Regurgitation in gastroesophageal reflux, 514
Rehabilitation, cardiac, physical training in, 155
Renal bone disease, dialysis and, 671
Renal disease, disseminated intravascular coagulation in, 635
  nonimmunologic, 691
Renal toxicity, methoxyflurane and, 568
Renal transplantation, costs of, 678
  in transfused patients, 679
  in uremia, 675-680
  psychiatric problems following, 677
  survival rates of, 677
  vs. dialysis, 676
Respiratory distress syndrome, disseminated intravascular coagulation in, 625
  heparin in, 630
Respiratory failure, acute, advantages of aggressive therapy for, 275-279
  causes of, 276
  postoperative, ventilation in, 277
  impending, symptoms of, 276
  tracheostomy in, 278
Respiratory fatigue, 258
Rheumatoid arthritis, corticosteroid therapy in, dangers of, 447
  cortisone in, 439, 442
  disseminated intravascular coagulation in, 635
Rickettsial disease, disseminated intravascular coagulation and, 638
  heparin in, 630

Salicylazosulfapyridine in Crohn's
     disease, 473, 486
Sarcoidosis, defined, 339
     Kveim test in, nonspecificity of, 339-348
          reliability of, 349-358
Scanning, isotope, of thyroid nodules, 423
Schizophrenia, marihuana and, 754
Sclerosis, focal, in nephrotic syndrome
     in children, 660
Screening program(s), costs and benefits
     of, 97. See also *Multiphasic testing.*
     diagnosis by, reliability of, 95
     ethics of, 99
     evaluation of, 94
     operational problems of, 97
     risks of, assessment of, 96
     treatment services and, 96
     unvalidated procedures in, 92-98
Scrub typhus, disseminated intravascular
     coagulation and, 638
Septicemia, disseminated intravascular
     coagulation and, 625-637
     granulocytopenia and, 607
Serum, cholesterol in. See
     Cholesterol, serum.
     lipid levels of, partial ileal bypass
          and, 231
Shock, disseminated intravascular
     coagulation and, 626, 630
     pulmonary embolism and, 306
     lactic acidosis and, 285
Shock lung, IPPB in, 250
Shunt, Quinton-Scribner, in dialysis, 670
Sick care vs. health care, 86
Smallpox, Global Eradication Program for,
     365
     importation of, 367
          probability of, 376
          spread following, 376
     incidence of, 365, 368
     outbreaks of, character of, 366
     risk of, 365
     vaccination for, abolition of, 363-370
          complications following, risk of, 373
          cost of, 378
               human, 364
          in children, hazards, discontinuation
               of, 379
          indications for, 371-381
          pregnancy and, 375
Sodium taurocholate in gallstone
     therapy, 549
Sphincter, gastroesophageal, importance
     of, 524-528
Splenectomy in Hodgkin's disease, 732,
     733
Statistics, medical, usefulness of, 35
Steblay nephritis, 696
Steroids, in cerebral edema, 780
     in nephrotic syndrome, limited role
          of, 651-657
          relapses in, 661

Stomach, cardia of, defined, 516
     erosion of, aspirin and, 502
Streptokinase in cerebral ischemia, 782
Stroke, completed, 789. See also
     Cerebral ischemia.
     carotid, endarterectomy in, 807
     treatment of, anticoagulant, 798
     progressing, 789
     treatment of, anticoagulant, 794
          surgical, 796
Sucrose, corticosteroids and, 206
     diabetes mellitus and, 205
     experiments with, 204
     heart disease and, 200
     increased consumption of, 201
     insulin and, 206
     lipogenesis and, 205
     plasma triglycerides and, 204
Sugar, coronary disease and, 199-207
Suicide vs. euthanasia, 104
Sulfinpyrazone in cerebral ischemia, 775
Sulfonylureas, hypoglycemia and, 398
     in adult-onset diabetes, 395
     islet cell function and, 406
     therapy with, hazards of, 397
Surgery, metabolic, 228
     placebo effect of, in angina pectoris, 140
     vascular, exercise tolerance following, 130
          operative mortality from, 131
Syphilis, nephrotic syndrome and, 700
Systemic lupus erythematosus, disseminated
     intravascular coagulation in, 635

Terminal illness, guidelines for
     management of, 118
Therapy, interruption of, consequences
     of, 106
     patient document defining, 111
          time of use, 112
     omission of, 104
Thermography, thyroid, 424
Thrombectomy in cerebral ischemia, 776
Thrombin, action of, 633
     disseminated intravascular coagulation
          and, 634
     heparin and, 634
Thromboembolism, recurrent, in
     anticoagulant therapy, prevention of, 799
Thrombolytic therapy in pulmonary
     embolism, 293-302
Thromboplastin, disseminated intravascular
     coagulation and, 636
Thrombosis, mural, venous, 211
Thymectomy, IPPV following, 279
Thyroid, cancer of, death from, 429
     diagnosis of, 429
     prevalence of, 429
     enlargement of, 433
     scan of, 431

Thyroid nodule(s), cancerous, factors
    in, 423
  heredity and, 425
  incidence of, 422
 cold, 431
 hot, 431
 in Graves' disease, 425
 isotope scanning of, 423
 lobectomy for, 425
 pathogenesis of, 430
 prevalence of, 428
 solitary, removal of, 421-427
 thermography of, 424
 thyroid hormone therapy in, 432
 thyroidectomy for, 425
 thyrotoxicosis and, 425
 treatment of, 431
 warm, 431
Thyroidectomy, total, indication for, 432
Thyroiditis, glomerulonephritis and, 690
 Hashimoto's, nodes in, 424
Thyrotoxicosis, thyroid nodules and, 425
Tolazamide, in diabetes, 404
Tolbutamide, complications of use, 411
 in diabetes, 404
  adult-onset, 395
Toxicity, oxygen, artificial ventilation
    and, 286
 IPPB and, 260
Tracheostomy, in peritonitis, 279
 in respiratory failure, 278
Transfusions, blood, in acute myelocytic
   leukemia, 604
Transient cerebral ischemia, carotid
   arterial system, 788
 carotid endarterectomy in, 808
 defined, 788
 treatment of, anticoagulant, 789
  primary, 773
  surgical, 791
 vertebrobasilar system, 788
Transplantation, renal. See *Renal
   transplantation.*
Triamcinolone, 440
Triglyceride(s), coronary disease and, 7
 plasma, sucrose and, 204
 xanthomatous, 209
Tuberculin conversion, 314
Tuberculin test, value of, 328
Tuberculosis, BCG for, advantage of,
   322-331
 chemoprophylaxis for, preventive,
    rationale for, 318
 chemotherapy of, continuation of, 313-321
  multiple-drug, 320
  preventive, cost of, 316
 foci of, latent, 313
  factors in, 314
 glandular, Kveim test and, 341
 ileocecal, 462
 incidence of, 325
 new cases of, source of, 326

Tuberculosis (*Continued*)
  risk of, 314
Tumor-associated antigen, 719
 carcinoembryonic antigen and, 720

Ulcer(s), duodenal, aspirin and, 500
  intractability of, 501
  sucrose and, 205
 gastric, aspirin and, 500, 506
  management of, 15
 peptic, alcohol and, 504
  aspirin and, danger of, 500-508
  management of, 13
  prednisolone and, 440
University Group Diabetes Program, 390
 interpretation of, 411
Uremia, blood transfusions in, renal
    transplantation and, 679
 dialysis in, 667-674
  cost effectiveness of, 668
  home, 668
 renal transplantation in, 675-680
Urokinase, in cerebral ischemia, 782
 in pulmonary embolism, bleeding
    complications of, 297
  contraindications to, 298
Urokinase Pulmonary Embolism Trial, 295
Urokinase-Streptokinase Pulmonary
   Embolism Trial, 296
Uterine bleeding, functional, glucocorticoid
   therapy in, 442

Vaccination, smallpox. See *Smallpox
   vaccination.*
Vaccinia, generalized, 364, 375
Vaccinia necrosum, 364, 374
Valsalva maneuver in hiatal hernia, 525
Vascular disease, diet and, 240
Vascular surgery, exercise tolerance
    following, 130
 operative mortality from, 131
Vasoconstrictor, nebulized, administration
   of, 257
Venous pressure, central venous pressure
    and, 186
Ventilation, artificial, hazards of, 281
  hypercapnia and, 282
  in hypoxia, 286
  indications for, limitations of, 280-287
  respiratory acidosis and, 282
  vs. oxygen toxicity, 286
 failure of, IPPB and, 266
 IPPB and, 257
 of lung, pressure required for, 251
 perfusion, abnormalities of, 256
Ventilators, pressure-cycled, 251
 volume-cycled, 251

Ventricle, left, acute failure of, central venous pressure and, 190
  augmentation of performance, 128
  right, hypertrophy of, 187
    pressure in, central venous pressure and, 187
Ventriculoatrial shunt, infected, glomerulonephritis and, 700
Vinblastine in Hodgkin's disease, 736, 740, 741
Vincristine in Hodgkin's disease, 740, 741

Vitamin C, deficiency of, aspirin and, 506
  in gastrointestinal bleeding, 497

Warfarin, in cerebral ischemia, 775
"Worried well," preventive maintenance services for, 88

Xanthelasma(s), beta lipoproteins and, 212
Xanthoma(s), cholesterol in, 210
  diabetic, biopsies of, 209